Raptors, Pigeons and Waterfowl

General Editor

Peter H Beynon
BVSc MRCVS

Scientific Editors

Neil A Forbes
BVetMed MRCVS

and

Nigel H Harcourt-Brown
BVSc FRCVS

Published by
British Small Animal Veterinary Association Limited
Kingsley House, Church Lane
Shurdington, Cheltenham
Gloucestershire GL51 5TQ

A Company Limited by Guarantee in England
Registered Company Number 2837793
Registered as a Charity

Typeset, Repro and Printed by J Looker Printers, Poole, Dorset BH16 5SL

First Published 1996

ISBN 0 905214 29 3

Contents

Part Two - Raptors

Part Three - Pigeons

Part Four - Waterfowl

Contributors

Richard Best BVSc MRCVS
The Veterinary Centre
32 West Hill Portishead
Bristol BS20 9LN

Ian P Boydell BVetMed CertVOphthal MRCVS
Animal Medical Centre Referral Services
511 Wilbraham Road Chorlton-cum-Hardy
Manchester M21 1UF

Martin J Brown
Wildfowl and Wetlands Trust
Slimbridge
Gloucestershire GL2 7B

Graham Butterworth
Hillbank Gillotts
Chadderton Oldham
Lancashire OL1 2SU

John E Cooper BVSc CertLAS DTVM FRCPath CBiol FIBiol FRCVS
Durrell Institute of Conservation and Ecology
University of Kent
Canterbury Kent CT2 7PD

Ruth L Cromie BSc PhD
Durrell Institute of Conservation and Ecology
University of Kent
Canterbury Kent CT2 7PD

Gerry M Dorrestein DVM PhD
Department of Veterinary Pathology
Faculty of Veterinary Medicine University of Utrecht
3584 CL Utrecht The Netherlands

Neil A Forbes BVetMed MRCVS
Clockhouse Veterinary Hospital
Wallbridge Stroud
Gloucestershire GL5 3JD

David A R Hannam BVSc DBR MRCVS
Bramblings Well Lane
Sproxton York YO6 5EY

Nigel H Harcourt-Brown BVSc FRCVS
30 Crab Lane
Bilton Harrogate
North Yorkshire HG1 3BE

Frank D W Harper BVSc MRCVS
97 Vivian Road
Sketty Swansea
West Glamorgan SA2 0UN

Patrick N Humphreys MSc MRCVS
Lower Coed Morgan
Abergavenny
Monmouthshire

Ivan B Jennings AIBS
Grange Laboratories
Sandbeck Way Wetherby
West Yorkshire LS22 4DN

Martin P C Lawton BVetMed CertVOphthal CertLAS CBiol MIBiol FRCVS
12 Fitzilian Avenue
Harold Wood Romford
Essex RM3 0QS

J (Sjeng) T Lumeij DVM PhD
Department of Clinical Sciences of Companion Animals
Faculty of Veterinary Medicine University of Utrecht
3508 TD Utrecht The Netherlands

A Dermod Malley BA MVB MRCVS
South Beech Veterinary Surgery
40 Southend Road Wickford
Essex SS11 8DU

Jemima Parry-Jones
National Birds of Prey Centre
Newent
Gloucestershire GL18 1JJ

David G Parsons BVetMed MSc CertPMP MRCVS
77 The Downs
Trowbridge
Wiltshire BA14 7NG

Tom W Pennycott BVM&S CertPMP MRCVS
Scottish Agriculture Colleges Veterinary Investigation Centre
Auchincruive Ayr
Ayrshire KA6 5AE

Patrick T Redig DVM
The Raptor Center
University of Minnesota College of Veterinary Medicine
1920 Fitch Avenue St Paul
Minnesota 55108 United States of America

Tony Richardson
Wildfowl and Wetlands Trust
Slimbridge
Gloucestershire GL2 7BT

Ian Robinson BVSc CertSHP MRCVS
RSPCA Norfolk Wildlife Hospital Station Road
East Winch Kings Lynn
Norfolk PE32 1NR

Greg N Simpson BVSc (Pret) MRCVS
Clockhouse Veterinary Hospital
Wallbridge Stroud
Gloucestershire GL5 3JD

Alan S Wallis BVSc MRCVS
117 Mains Lane
Little Singleton Poulton le Fylde
Lancashire FY6 7LD

Jason C Waine BVetMed MRCVS
97 Mount Pleasant
Redditch
Worcestershire B97 4JD

Trevor J Whitbread BVSc BSc MRCVS
Abbey Veterinary Services
14 Oak Place Newton Abbot
Devon TQ12 2HW

Foreword

At some stage in their working life, most veterinary surgeons in practice will be asked to treat raptors, pigeons or waterfowl. Many practitioners have felt the need for a concise text such as this, the *Manual of Raptors, Pigeons and Waterfowl*, which is the latest addition to the internationally acclaimed BSAVA Manual Series. This new title will enable veterinary surgeons presented with raptors, pigeons or waterfowl to provide the first class treatment that their clients have rightly come to expect. Many of these birds are presented as wildlife casualties, so the ability to respond in an appropriate manner will further enhance the public's opinion of the veterinary profession.

The *Manual of Raptors, Pigeons and Waterfowl* will give practitioners and students, and others involved in keeping the three groups of birds described, a fundamental understanding of the problems they are likely to encounter, and it may provide a platform upon which a developing special interest can be built.

The publication is laid out in four parts. The first section deals with the clinical examination and follow-up procedures and investigations which are the basis of good veterinary practice. The following three sections are dedicated to describing the diseases and clinical and surgical problems, and their treatment, for each of the three groups of birds. The format of the manual should allow rapid access to essential information as required. Much of the information in this manual cannot be found in any other single veterinary text. The detail encompassed is evidenced by the comprehensive list of twenty six authors, including experts in their field from continental Europe and the USA as well as from the UK, who, with the scientific editors, Neil Forbes and Nigel Harcourt-Brown, and the general editor, Peter Beynon, are to be congratulated for bringing this title to fruition. The *Manual of Raptors, Pigeons and Waterfowl* will certainly establish itself as an essential component of the library of every veterinary practice and centre where such birds are treated.

The BSAVA thanks all the authors and editors for their contribution to this manual. The continued high regard in which the BSAVA Manual Series is held the world over is a tribute to the hard work of the many authors and editors and to the dedication and guidance of the Association's Publications Committee, which is currently chaired by Simon Petersen-Jones.

John Robert Dalton BVMS MRCVS
President BSAVA 1995-96

CHAPTER ONE

Introduction

John E. Cooper

This manual is concerned with three groups of birds that are kept in captivity and which are regularly presented for veterinary attention.

The term 'raptor' is an ancient one. It is Latin for a bird with a hooked beak and sharp claws and is perpetuated in the French and Italian words 'rapace'. In theory it could embrace a range of different species of birds but in practice it is normally used for birds of prey of the Orders Falconiformes (hawks, falcons, eagles, vultures) and Strigiformes (owls) (Cooper, 1985). Recently, Sibley and Ahlquist (1990) suggested a different classification for raptors based on DNA studies, but this does not significantly alter the situation. There is some disagreement as to the use of the term 'raptor' as it is taken from an Order that was abandoned in the Victorian era as a classification of owls, hawks, falcons and vultures; however, the term 'raptor' is used regularly, even in scientific circles, eg. The Raptor Research Foundation in the USA.

The word 'pigeon' is taken to include 'dove': the distinction between the two is perpetuated in many English names but is artificial. These birds all belong to the Order Columbiformes (Lockwood, 1984).

'Waterfowl' needs explanation. There are many species of birds that frequent water but not all of these are properly termed 'waterfowl'. In this manual only members of the Order Anseriformes (ducks, geese and swans) are covered specifically, but there is mention of other aquatic birds where this is relevant to veterinary work.

The main characteristics of raptors, pigeons and waterfowl are given in Table 1.1.

Table 1.1. Characteristics of the different groups of birds.

Feature	Raptors		Columbiformes	Anseriformes
	Falconiformes	**Strigiformes**		
Lifestyle	Generally diurnal. Spend much of time on land, perching or in flight.	Mainly nocturnal. Spend much of time on land, perching or in flight.	Diurnal. Spend much of time on land, perching or in flight.	Generally diurnal. Spend much of time on water, sometimes on land, or in flight.
Diet	Carnivorous - whole animals, including invertebrates and carrion.	Carnivorous.	Herbivorous - seeds, leaves, fruit.	Some species predominantly carnivorous, some herbivorous, some omnivorous.
Moult	Usually annual, after breeding season. In sequence, gradual.	Usually annual, after breeding season. In sequence, gradual.	Usually annual, after breeding season.	Usually annual, after breeding season. Anserines, ie. geese and swans, moult once a year; Anatinae, ie. ducks, moult twice a year. Some species go into 'eclipse plumage' when flight may be impaired due to loss of primary and secondary feathers.

Table 1.1. Continued.

Feature	Raptors		Columbiformes	Anseriformes
	Falconiformes	**Strigiformes**		
Reproduction	Sexual dimorphism sometimes marked, often slight. Young are altricial.	Sexual dimorphism generally slight. Young are altricial.	Sexual monomorphism. Young are altricial.	Sexual dimorphism often marked. Young are precocial.
Anatomy	Hooked beak and claws (talons) for holding and eating whole animals.	Hooked beak and claws for holding and eating whole animals.	Relatively slender beak for holding vegetable matter; short claws.	Highly modified and sensitive beak for seeking and processing different types of food; webbed feet.
	Crop present.	Crop absent.	Crop present.	Crop variable.
	Generally no grit in small gizzard (thin walled).	Generally no grit in small gizzard (thin walled).	Grit in large gizzard (thick walled).	Grit in large gizzard (thick walled).
	Caeca small.	Caeca large.	Caeca small or absent.	Caeca large.
	No distinct penis (phallus).	No distinct penis (phallus).	No distinct penis (phallus).	Distinct penis (phallus) in most species.
	Trachea and syrinx unremarkable.	Trachea and syrinx unremarkable.	Trachea and syrinx unremarkable.	Trachea and syrinx often highly modified, in males especially.
	Anisodactyl - perch with three digits forward, one back. **NB**. The Osprey is semi-zygodactyl.	Owls perch with two digits forward and two back, but they are semi-zygodactyl - can be two toes cranial and two caudal or three cranial and one caudal (digit IV rotates).	Anisodactyl - perch with three digits forward, one back.	Anisodactyl, palmate - perch with three digits (webbed) forward, one (often vestigial) back. (Anhimidae are semi-palmate.)

It will be seen that, although they have much in common as members of the Class Aves, the three groups also show significant differences that are of relevance to their husbandry, examination and treatment.

One feature that the three groups do share is that members of each have long been associated with humans. In the case of pigeons and waterfowl, some species have been truly 'domesticated', in the sense that their breeding and maintenance have been continuously controlled by man (Wood-Gush, 1985). Raptors have only relatively recently been regularly bred in captivity, but are clearly on their way to domestication.

Table 1.2 provides some background information on the maintenance and use by humans of raptors,

pigeons and waterfowl. An understanding of this history can help practitioners when discussing breeds, management and biology with owners.

Although this manual covers the three groups, it must not be forgotten that only a relatively small number of species from each Order are regularly kept in captivity. Those that are likely to come to the attention of the practising veterinary surgeon, including species specifically referred to elsewhere in the manual, are listed in Table 1.3. The list is taken mainly from *A Complete Checklist of the Birds of the World* (Howard and Moore, 1994). Commonly used alternatives to the listed common names are given in brackets.

Table 1.2. Maintenance and use of raptors, pigeons and waterfowl.

Order	Background
Falconiformes	Certain species (mainly falcons, hawks and eagles) have been kept and trained for falconry for over 2,000 years. Much published literature in different languages. Since 1970 considerable success in breeding several species in captivity. Hybrids have been produced. Falconiform birds are now widely available for falconry, exhibition and research.
Strigiformes	Not traditionally used for falconry. Revered in certain cultures, eg. Ancient Greece. Associated with fear and superstition in some parts of the world. For several decades certain species have been bred in captivity: these are now widely available for aviculture, exhibition and research.
Columbiformes	*Columba livia* domesticated in Middle East over 3,000 years ago. From there it spread all over the world. Feral pigeons are descended from the same species. Domestic pigeons are still used for racing, ornamental purposes, food and research.
Anseriformes	Some species, eg. goose, domesticated for over 2,000 years - notably by the Romans. Muscovy Duck kept by South Americans, taken to Europe in 16th Century and now common in many parts of the world. Mute Swan has long tradition of association with humans and in Britain, since 1592, swans 'swimming in open and common river' have been the property of the Crown. Many varieties of domestic ducks and geese are kept for food and ornamental purposes. Other species of ducks, geese and swans are maintained in waterfowl collections.

Table 1.3. Common and scientific names.

Order Falconiformes	
Family Cathartidae (New World Vultures)	
Andean Condor	*Vultur gryphus*
Family Pandionidae (Osprey)	
Osprey	*Pandion haliaetus*
Family Accipitridae (Hawks, Eagles)	
American Bald Eagle	*Haliaeetus leucocephalus*
Old World Vultures	*Gyps* spp.
Harriers	*Circus* spp.
Northern Sparrow Hawk	*Accipiter nisus*
Great (Black) Sparrow Hawk	*Accipiter melanoleucus*
Northern Goshawk	*Accipiter gentilis*
Harris' Hawk	*Parabuteo unicinctus*
Red-tailed Hawk	*Buteo jamaicensis*
Eurasian Buzzard	*Buteo buteo*
Rough-legged Buzzard	*Buteo lagopus*
Feruginous Hawk	*Buteo regalis*
Tawny Eagle	*Aquila rapax*
Golden Eagle	*Aquila chrysaetos*
Family Sagittariidae	
Secretary Bird	*Sagittarius serpentarius*

Table 1.3. Continued.

Family Falconidae (Falcons, Caracaras)	
African Pygmy Falcon	*Polihierax semitorquatus*
American Kestrel	*Falco sparverius*
Common Kestrel	*Falco tinnunculus*
Mauritius Kestrel	*Falco punctatus*
Merlin	*Falco columbarius*
Lanner Falcon	*Falco biarmicus*
Lagger (Lugger) Falcon	*Falco jugger*
Saker Falcon	*Falco cherrug*
Gyr Falcon	*Falco rusticolus*
Peregrine Falcon	*Falco peregrinus*
Order Strigiformes	
Family Tytonidae (Barn Owls)	
Barn Owl	*Tyto alba*
Family Strigidae (Owls)	
Spectacled Owl	*Pulsatrix perspicillata*
Great Horned Owl	*Bubo virginianus*
Northern Eagle Owl	*Bubo bubo*
Indian Eagle Owl	*Bubo bengalensis*
Snowy Owl	*Nyctea scandiaca*
Eurasian Tawny Owl	*Strix aluco*
Ural Owl	*Strix uralensis*
Little Owl	*Athene noctua*
Order Columbiformes	
Family Columbidae (Doves, Pigeons)	
Feral (Native) Rock Pigeon (Dove)	*Columba livia*
(Garden) Fantail Pigeon (Dove)	*Columba livia* (*domestica*)
Collared Dove	*Streptopelia decaocto*
African Collared Dove	*Streptopelia roseogrisea*
Barbary and Java Doves	*Streptopelia roseogrisea* (*domestica*)
Order Anseriformes	
Family Anhimidae (Screamers)	
Family Anatidae (Swans, Geese, Ducks)	
Mute Swan	*Cygnus olor*
Black-necked Swan	*Cygnus atratus*
Trumpeter Swan	*Cygnus buccinator*
Tundra Swan	*Cygnus columbianus*
Whistling Swan	*Cygnus c. columbianus*
Bewick's Swan	*Cygnus c. bewickii*
Coscoroba Swan	*Coscoroba coscoroba*
Magpie Goose	*Anseranas semipalmata*

Table 1.3. Continued.

Pink-footed Goose	*Anser brachyrhynchus*
Bar-headed Goose	*Anser indicus*
Grey Lag (Domestic) Goose	*Anser anser*
Lesser Snow Goose	*Anser c. caerulescens*
Hawaiian Goose	*Branta sandvicensis*
Canada Goose	*Branta canadensis*
(Cackling) Canada Goose	*Branta canadensis minima*
Barnacle Goose	*Branta leucopsis*
Red-breasted Goose	*Branta ruficollis*
Cereopsis (Cape Barren) Goose	*Cereopsis novaehollandiae*
Freckled Duck	*Stictonetta naevosa*
Andean Goose	*Chloephaga melanoptera*
Egyptian Goose	*Alopochen aegyptiacus*
Spur-winged Goose	*Plectropterus gambensis*
Muscovy Duck	*Cairina moschata*
White-winged Wood Duck	*Cairina scutulata*
Comb Duck	*Sarkidiornis melanotos*
Hartlaub's Duck	*Pteronetta hartlaubii*
Wood Duck	*Aix sponsa*
Mandarin Duck	*Aix galericulata*
Torrent Duck	*Merganetta armata*
European Wigeon	*Anas penelope*
Green-winged Teal	*Anas crecca*
New Zealand Teal	*Anas aucklandica*
Mallard	*Anas platyrhynchos*
Bronze-winged Duck	*Anas specularis*
Crested Duck	*Anas specularioides*
Northern Pintail	*Anas acuta*
Northern Shoveller	*Anas clypeata*
Pink-eared Duck	*Malacorhynchus membranaceus*
Tufted Duck	*Aythya fuligula*
Common Eider	*Somateria mollisima*
Long-tailed Duck	*Clangula hyemalis*
Scoters	*Melanitta* spp.
Common Goldeneye	*Bucephala clangula*
Sawbills	*Mergus* spp.
Hooded Merganser	*Mergus cuculatus*
Ruddy Duck	*Oxyura jamaicensis*
Musk Duck	*Biziura lobata*
White-backed Duck	*Thalassornis leuconotis*
Other Birds Mentioned	
Chilean Flamingo	*Phoenicopterus chilensis*
Gentoo Penguin	*Pygoscelis papua*
Cormorants	*Phalacrocorax* spp.
Herring Gull	*Larus argentatus*
Lesser Black-backed Gull	*Larus fuscus*
Northern Fulmar	*Fulmaris glacialus*
Black-billed Magpie	*Pica pica*
Crows	Corvidae
Jackdaws	*Corvus monedula*
Rook	*Corvus frugilegus*
Carrion Crow	*Corvus corone*

There are certain general points that must be borne in mind when dealing with all these birds. The first is that for most species there are import and export controls, and the veterinary surgeon should be aware of these and where detailed information may be sought. Some controls are related to animal health and are implemented by the Ministry of Agriculture, Fisheries and Food (England), the Department of Agriculture and Fisheries for Scotland (Scotland) and the Agricultural Department (Welsh Office) (Wales), or its equivalent in other countries. Other controls are concerned with conservation, particularly the protection of endangered species, and are generally under the jurisdiction of the Department of the Environment in Britain, or its equivalent in other countries. The controls are summarised in Table 1.5.

The second general point concerns quarantine. Although the health provisions already referred to usually include a statutory quarantine period, this is generally aimed primarily at excluding conditions such as Newcastle disease that can present a threat to the national (poultry) flock. Other diseases and pathogens may still get through the net and present a threat to established birds. The veterinary surgeon should, therefore, encourage his/her clients to have an 'in-house' quarantine/isolation period of at least 14 days before any new bird is introduced to the collection. Before, during and after quarantine it is also important to introduce health precautions and these are outlined in Table 1.4.

Table 1.4. Health precautions before, during and after quarantine.

Before being brought into collection.	Request health certificates and other relevant data. Possibly visit the vendor's premises. Consider a) faecal, blood and other tests, and b) preventive measures, including vaccination.
During quarantine/ isolation.	Maintain strict hygiene. Observe the bird carefully and investigate any signs of ill-health. Undertake comprehensive *post-mortem* examination of any birds that die. Perform faecal, blood and other tests. Instigate preventive measures, including vaccination.
After introducing into collection.	Continue hygiene and observation and introduce any changes in management necessary to reduce stress. Investigate ill-health. Undertake thorough cleaning and disinfection of the quarantine/ isolation premises. Keep full detailed histories so that disease introduction can be followed retrospectively if necessary.

The third general point relates to welfare and ethics. Although in most countries there is legislation that protects birds and makes it an offence to cause them unnecessary suffering, sections of the public are sometimes critical of the keeping of such species in captivity and of some of the methods - for example, pinioning of waterfowl, tethering of raptors and separation of pairs of pigeons - that are used to facilitate management. As a result there is wisdom in drawing up and adhering to codes of practice which, whilst not enforceable by law, help to maintain standards and will discourage criticism or vindictive actions. One such code has been produced for birds of prey (British Field Sports Society/Hawk Board, undated) and this can usefully be adapted to individual collections and premises. The veterinary surgeon should assist his/her clients by drawing attention to the value of such self-regulation and offer help in compilation of appropriate guidelines.

For advice relating to UK animal health requirement contact:

>Ministry of Agriculture, Fisheries and Food
>Hook Rise South, Tolworth
>Surbiton Surrey KT6 7NF
>Tel: 0181.330.4411

For advice relating to UK conservation requirements contact:

>Department of the Environment
>Trade in Endangered Species Branch
>Room 810, Tollgate House
>Houlton Street
>Bristol BS2 9OL
>Tel: 0117.987.8148

Further information about the above and other legislation is available in:

Cooper JE and Cooper ME (1991) Legal cases involving birds: the role of the veterinary surgeon. *Veterinary Record* **129**, 505.

Cooper ME (1987) *An Introduction to Animal Law*. Academic Press, London.

Royal College of Veterinary Surgeons (1994) *Legislation Affecting the Veterinary Profession in the United Kingdom*. RCVS, London.

Table 1.5. Some British legislation relating to raptors, pigeons and waterfowl.

Area of law	Comments
Import and export of live birds and eggs (Animal Health)	All three groups are covered by the Animal Health Act 1981 and various Orders and Directives (European Union [EU]). Imported birds need to be covered by a licence and quarantined on arrival in the UK. Eggs require permits subject to conditions.
Import and export of live birds and eggs (Conservation)	Certain species in each group are covered by the Convention on International Trade in Endangered Species of Wild Fauna and Flora (CITES) (the Washington Convention) and by relevant EU Regulations. Permits are needed for importation and exportation of such species, whether live or dead, and their derivatives, eg. feathers, tissues, blood.
Maintenance in captivity (Conservation)	Certain indigenous raptors (Golden Eagle, Northern Goshawk, Peregrine Falcon, Merlin, or hybrids including any of these species as a parent) are covered by the Wildlife and Countryside Act 1981 (Variation of Schedule 4) Order 1994 and must be ringed and registered if kept in captivity. Some other globally threatened species also still require ringing. If in doubt contact the Department of the Environment. There are exemptions for sick and injured birds for a six week period if under the care of a veterinary surgeon. No specific legislation relates to those species of pigeons or waterfowl that are commonly kept in captivity.
Maintenance in captivity (Welfare)	All captive birds are subject to the provisions of the Protection of Animals Act 1911.
Veterinary treatment	Waterfowl kept on agricultural land may not be surgically pinioned (The Welfare of Livestock (Prohibited Operations) Regulations 1982). All birds are covered by the Veterinary Surgeons Act 1966; any diagnosis or treatment, other than first aid or emergencies, must be carried out by a registered veterinarian.
Welfare in transport.	The Transit of Animals (General) Order 1973 (as amended) covers all three groups of birds and provides general protection for them while in transit.

Assistance over specific problems or involving a point of law should be sought from a solicitor in private practice.

This manual has been produced in order to help the practitioner. It is not intended to be the authoritative text. Nevertheless, the contributors are all experienced and knowledgeable and, as a result, the chapters contain useful material, much of it not easy to locate elsewhere and not previously brought together in one volume.

The reader is encouraged to keep the manual in the practice and to use it on a regular basis. Sometimes it will prove helpful - and can promote good client relations - to go through the book with the owner, especially when trying to unravel a problem.

The manual is essentially divided into three parts, covering raptors, pigeons and waterfowl respectively. However, the editors have wisely decided to preface the manual with eleven chapters covering topics - for example, basic investigation, therapy, haematology and anaesthesia - that are relevant to all three groups of birds. Reference should be made to this part first, before moving on to the specific chapter heading that deals with different diseases and syndromes. This is facilitated by the use of cross referencing in the text.

The Appendix at the end of the manual provides separate Formularies for the three groups of birds. These three Formularies bring together the information contained within the text with regard to trade names, manufacturers, dosages, routes of administration and main indications for the various generic drugs mentioned. The dosages and routes of administration are generally the standard ones for treatment of the relevant condition(s) and group of birds, but in some instances different doses etc. are required for certain conditions and readers must make reference to the specific chapter. Veterinary surgeons must use their own clinical judgement when assessing the duration of treatment with some therapeutic agents, especially antibodies.

The Index should also be used. It has been carefully compiled and can help the practitioner to find the appropriate information during a busy consultation or when dealing with an emergency. The editors are aware that the Index cannot be totally comprehensive and would welcome feedback and comments from colleagues so that additions and changes can be made to future editions.

Finally, the reader should not assume that all his/her problems are likely to be found in this manual.

Avian medicine is now a speciality in its own right on both sides of the Atlantic, and there are colleagues to whom difficult or sensitive cases can be referred. A proper referral, however, means that the first veterinary surgeon takes a history and carries out a clinical examination: he/she then decides to seek the advice of a more knowledgeable colleague, who is sent a letter and relevant background information as well as the client and the bird. A good history is often of great value to the specialist and will save him/her valuable time. Sometimes, preliminary treatment by the referring veterinarian - for example, administration of fluids to counter dehydration - will also be necessary in order to maintain the patient until expert advice is obtained. This manual will, if properly used, assist the clinician in these tasks as well as, in other cases, providing the information that will permit a definitive diagnosis and specific therapy.

REFERENCES

British Field Sports Society/Hawk Board (undated). *Code of Welfare and Husbandry of Birds of Prey and Owls*. BFSS, London.

Cooper JE (1985) *Veterinary Aspects of Captive Birds of Prey*. Standfast Press, Gloucester.

Cooper ME (1987) *An Introduction to Animal Law*. Academic Press, London.

Cooper ME (1989) Legal considerations in the movement and submission of avian specimens. In: *Disease and Threatened Birds*. Ed JE Cooper. International Council for Bird Preservation, Cambridge.

Howard R and Moore A (1994) *A Complete Checklist of the Birds of the World*. 2nd Edn. Academic Press, London.

Lockwood WB (1984) *The Oxford Book of British Bird Names*. Oxford University Press, Oxford.

Sibley CE and Ahlquist JE (1990) *Phylogeny and Classification of Birds: a Study in Molecular Evolution*. Yale University Press, New Haven.

Wood-Gush D (1985) Domestication. In: *A Dictionary of Birds*. Eds B Campbell and E Lack. T & AD Poyser, Calton.

CHAPTER TWO

Examination, Basic Investigation and Handling

Neil A Forbes

INTRODUCTION

Birds that are presented for clinical examination may be divided arbitrarily into four groups:
- Healthy birds.
- Healthy birds with subclinical infections.
- Ill birds demonstrating no or insignificant signs of disease.
- Ill birds showing signs of disease.

Many birds that are unwell, especially in the early stages of disease, will appear healthy when examined at the surgery or in strange surroundings. The excitement caused by unfamiliar surroundings, the clinician and other animals makes the sick bird appear more healthy and alert than it really is. Birds that are found to be unwell often seem to be more ill than would be expected from the believed duration of the illness. This is because all species of birds have adapted over the generations to be highly adept at hiding the signs of ill health, as any sign of illness renders a bird a likely target for a predator. Subclinical infections may or may not have the potential to become pathogenic. For example, apparently healthy birds suffering from avian tuberculosis or *Capillaria* spp. infection will appear healthy, but render a great risk of contamination of their environment and infection of their neighbours. Such birds and their infections must be identified, diagnosed and treated.

The key factors which affect the classification of a bird may be divided into 'host factors' and 'environmental factors'.

Host Factors
- The immune status of the individual.
- Inherent genetic resistance to a particular disease varies between species and individuals.
- The age of the individual.
- The sex of the individual.

Environmental Factors
- Composition of diet.
- Feeding regime.
- Accommodation.
- Hygiene.
- Interference from other animals or birds, whether captive or wild, including predators such as cats.
- Interference by humans - keeper, trainer or others.
- Climatic conditions.

Figure 2.1 illustrates the differing health states. If the mechanism for the disturbance of this balance can be understood, the host and environmental factors can be controlled in order to reduce the chance of clinical disease. Due attention to this balance by the owner, trainer and clinician will assist in the identification of the 'healthy but subclinically infected bird', as well as early detection of symptomatic and asymptomatic 'ill birds'.

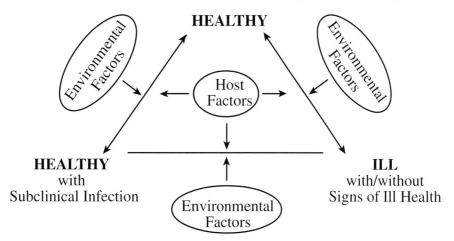

Figure 2.1: The health pyramid.

QUARANTINE AND EXAMINATION OF APPARENTLY HEALTHY BIRDS

Infectious diseases are rarely spread between raptors; examples of infectious diseases include *Salmonella* spp., falcon herpesvirus, Newcastle disease virus and avipoxviruses (via insect vectors). More commonly, disease is spread between birds by contamination of the environment, particularly the recovery or rehabilitation accommodation, eg. *Mycobacterium avium, Syngamus trachea, Capillaria* spp. (see Chapter 23). However, in view of the rapid rate of pathogenesis of many avian diseases, together with the possibility of subclinical infection, latent infection and carrier status, the avian clinician should encourage bird keepers to have all new birds examined at the start of their quarantine period. It should be stressed to the owner that, even following a very thorough examination, some diseases (especially virus infections) will not be found, hence standard quarantine procedures are still essential. Quarantine should last for at least 35 days, and the following basic principles should be adhered to:
● New birds should be isolated in a separate area or air space.
● They should be handled by a different keeper; if this is impossible, they should be fed and handled last.
● Protective clothing, which can be changed and cleaned, should be worn.
● The quarantine area should be easily cleaned and disinfected.
● Perches and any other impervious structures should be disposable.
● Daily inspection by the keeper of the bird, its food and water intake, and its weight, faeces and urates. Full notes should be kept.
● Sentinel birds, preferably from the same genus, may be used during quarantine, depending on the source of the birds, the health status of the collection and the value of the birds involved.

A routine health examination should be carried out prior to quarantine. At this consultation any signs of illness, malnutrition or poor conformation may be discussed. A full physical examination, haematology and biochemistry profiles and a faecal examination should be performed. If the bird is under Ministry of Agriculture Fisheries and Food (MAFF) quarantine regulations, no samples may be removed from the quarantine area, unless by prior agreement of the Divisional Veterinary Officer (DVO). Whilst carrying out this initial health examination, the species, age, sex, physical conformation, presence of imprinting, etc. should be assessed in relation to the purpose for which the bird has been purchased.

All birds in a collection should be fully examined by an experienced clinician at least annually. The aim is to detect infection or disease early in the pathogenesis. As with all health checks, a range of tests should be made available to the owner, so that he can select what is suitable and affordable for his bird.

RECOGNITION OF ILL HEALTH

Avian veterinary surgeons should assist and educate their clients in the recognition of ill health. Owners should carry out daily inspections of their birds. They should be fully conversant with the signs of good health in each of their species; only then will minor deviations from the normal be recognised. At the first sign of ill health, some action should be taken; delay may lead to rapid deterioration and death. Equally, the clinician should be aware that a healthy looking bird which is described by its owner as being 'not quite right', does in fact require investigation and treatment.

TRANSPORT

The transport requirements of birds varies greatly between the three groups covered by this manual as well as within each group. However, the same basic principles apply. Birds should be transported in a secure, darkened and well-ventilated container. Pigeons and smaller waterfowl can be carried in small disposable cardboard boxes. Boxes should have ventilation holes low on their sides (to minimise light at eye level) and have a new piece of carpet or similar material on the floor to allow the bird adequate grip. The size of the box should not permit wing flapping, but must allow the bird room to stand up in a natural position and turn around. Swans and large geese may be restrained in purpose made restraints (see Figures 2.2.1, 2.2.2). Long-legged birds such as flamingos must not only be able to stand up in transit, but also have their bodies supported ventrally, eg. by a hesian sling, in order to prevent collapse. Wild raptors should be transported in a small, strong cardboard box. Wooden boxes can allow the bird to damage itself as it flaps about. A small box will reassure and restrain the bird; a large box gives it room to panic. Storage of a box in a damp site or repetitive use of the same box will allow the build-up of pathogens, in particular *Aspergillus* spp. Many falconers bring their birds to the surgery on their fists. This is acceptable but can cause problems in the waiting room. Birds should be kept outside (beware overheated cars) until they are ready to be seen.

AVIAN CONSULTATIONS

Birds arriving for consultation may be divided into different categories. The ailments and treatments of each group are likely to differ (see Flow Chart 2.1). Assessment and categorisation will vary between raptors (R), pigeons (P) and waterfowl (W); however, the same principles apply.

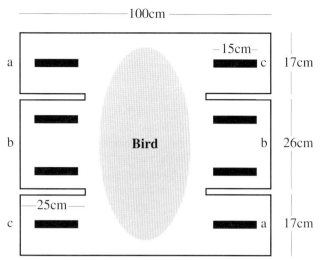

Figure 2.2.1: Swan restraint jacket. The jacket is made from water resistant, cleanable material, eg. old sail cloth. Jacket flap b is taken to meet b, then a to a and c to c. Each flap is attached to the other by way of velcro strips (marked in black). The swans legs are crossed over each other at the level of the distal metatarsi, and tied against each other using a soft bandage or similar.

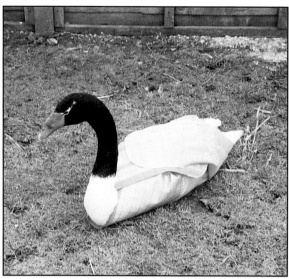

Figure 2.2.2: Black-necked Swan restrained in a swan jacket.

Flow Chart 2.1: Approach to avian consultations.

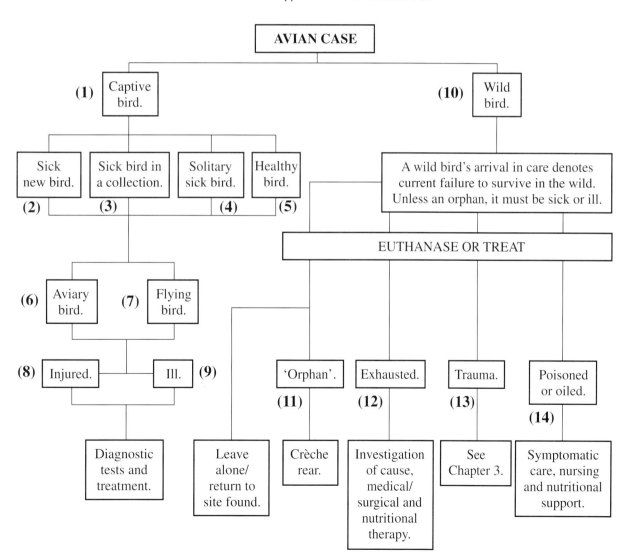

(1) Captive birds. Whether R, P or W, captive birds may be used for flying, breeding, education or conservation, or simply kept as pets; hence, full flight outcome may not be imperative. Captive birds may be subdivided into groups 2, 3, 4 and 5.

(2) Newly acquired sick birds. These birds are likely to have had contact with other birds of the same or differing species, or may have been carrying subclinical disease which has now become overt. Infectious or stress related disease must be considered.

(3) Sick birds which have been long-term resident in a collection. Husbandry standards, in particular in relation to quarantine of new arrivals, should be assessed first. How recently has a new bird been introduced? When dealing with a collection, a comprehensive diagnostic work-up should be performed. It is imperative to discover as soon as possible whether the condition is infectious. The bird and any in-contact birds should be isolated pending results. If an infection of unknown aetiology is suspected, it may be prudent to cull a sick bird, so that a more rapid complete diagnosis may be made.

(4) Sick birds kept individually. These are more likely to be suffering from a stress-related management or traumatic condition.

(5) Healthy birds. Owners should be encouraged to have all their birds examined thoroughly once or twice a year.

(6) Aviary birds. These are often not observed as closely as they should be and so may have been ill for several days prior to presentation to the clinician.

(7) Flying birds (either demonstration or hunting birds). These are handled daily and there is a close association between handler and bird. The bird may not appear ill to the clinician, but if the handler states it is 'not quite right' this should be acted upon rather than ignored.

(8) Injured captive birds. (See Chapter 3 - Flow Chart 3.3).

(9) Ill captive birds. These should always be considered as an infectious risk to others in the collection now or in the future. If an infectious agent is responsible, this should be isolated, the source detected and action taken to prevent disease in additional birds.

(10) Wild birds. The aim must always be to return the bird to the wild as soon as possible in a totally fit condition. If a wild bird is brought into captivity, it has in some way failed the test of fitness in the wild, however well it may look. These birds have an unknown history and should always be considered as a potential source of infection to other birds which are placed in close proximity. Unless extremely rare, an injured wild bird should be euthanased as soon as it becomes apparent that it is never going to be fit for return to the wild. The following injuries will prevent release of the bird to the wild:

- Psychological cripples (imprints).
- Visual impairment (even unilateral).
- Wing, leg or foot amputee.
- Loss of a hind claw.
- Loss of beak.
- Intact bird incapable of adequate flight.

On occasions, flight impaired waterfowl can be released into 'secure accommodation' where there is an island to allow protection from vermin, small numbers of birds only, and supplemental feeding as and when required. Many pigeons will survive after foot or leg amputation, but raptors over 200g should not have leg amputations performed, as this will invariably lead to bumblefoot in the remaining sound limb.

Members of the public may wish to look after injured wild birds, but their well intentioned endeavours often result in disaster. The suitability of the handler should be assessed prior to considering the care of any wild injured wild bird in captivity.

Rehabilitation techniques are described in Chapter 23. When injured wild birds are presented, an information card (see Figure 2.3) should always be completed.

When dealing with any injury to a wild bird, it should be remembered that 35-65% of wild birds carry parasitic burdens. Such infestations are generally well tolerated by fit birds in the wild, but following trauma and captivity, burdens of such parasites may become significant. All birds coming into captivity should be dosed with fenbendazole (100mg/kg p/o) or ivermectin (200mcg/kg s/c, p/o or percutaneously).

(11) 'Orphan' birds. These are usually birds which have ventured from the nest, hopped along a branch, and then fallen off. They are always found in the vicinity of the nest. The parents are generally close at hand and the orphans will usually only require feeding for a few days before they can fly themselves. Such birds should be lifted up into a high box or similar to give protection from predators, and be left where they were found. As birds have no sense of smell, the parents will not be concerned if the chick has been handled by humans. The parents will normally return to feed them. If the chick has already been removed and cannot be returned, every attempt should be made to 'crèche' rear the chick with others of the same or a similar genus. Taking in stray youngsters of uncertain health status and mixing them with others does present a considerable risk of cross-infection. However, if wild offspring are reared only with wild young of similar genera, and kept well away from resident birds, the benefit of successfully raising considerable numbers of psychologically well adjusted young for release to the wild does, in the author's opinion, outweigh the risk of cross-infection, or of imprinting birds if young are reared individually. Human contact must be prevented in order to avoid imprinting.

(12) Exhausted birds. Exhausted birds may be presented for a number of reasons: they may have been on migration and have been exhausted by inclement

Figure 2.3: Information request card for wild birds admitted.

Information to be obtained at the time of admission of a wild casualty bird.

1. Name of rescuer:

2. Address: Telephone No:

3. Exact location of recovery: Map reference:

4. Circumstances of recovery:

5. Date and time of recovery:

6. Was any traumatic incidence witnessed:

7. What was the condition of the bird at the time of recovery: Weight: grams

8. What fluid, food or treatments have already been administered:

9. Is there any knowledge or history of avian toxin exposure in the area:

10. Date: Time of admission: Signature:

---

weather, or they may be young birds which have been pushed out of their normal habitat at the dispersal phase of the breeding season. Others may be presented in states of starvation because they are unable to hunt effectively, due to a visual defect, inclement weather, destruction of prey species habitat, retarded reactions due to subclinical pesticide or other poisoning, or any physical injury or disease which prevents them from hunting effectively. Frequently, veterinary surgeons are presented with racing pigeons which have become exhausted or lost during a flight, or have sustained injury. Many racing pigeons have the name and telephone number of the fancier stamped on the dorsal aspect of one of the outer primary feathers. Failing this, the fancier can be traced via the ring number by contacting the British Pigeon Racing Association (Tel: 01452.713529 or 01443.833161).

(13) Traumatised birds. Trauma is a common cause of presentation. For a wild bird to allow itself to be caught, it either has a major injury or a minor injury which has prevented hunting, leading to weakness, emaciation and an inability to avoid capture. In pigeons, the commonest presenting traumatic injury is caused by impacts with telegraph wires; these commonly lead to extensive lacerations of the cervical skin, frequently involving the crop wall. It is essential that the crop wall is properly repaired. Swans are commonly presented following collision with electricity wires. Injuries are caused either on impact with the

wire, or on impact with the ground after the collision. These birds are often weakened and incoordinate due to low grade chronic lead poisoning. Trauma cases are discussed fully in Chapter 3.

(14) Poisoned birds (see Chapter 20); **oiled birds** (see Chapter 35).

CONSIDERATIONS PRIOR TO AVIAN EXAMINATION

Avian cases, with the exception of minor simple procedures such as 'coping' (see Chapter 15), should not be examined in the middle of a normal small animal clinic. Most birds view a dog or cat as a predator, thereby further increasing the stress of the visit. When a client requests an appointment, the receptionist should be trained to inform the client correctly. The urgency of the case must be assessed. A bird which appears sick is generally in need of urgent attention and therapy.

A full detailed history must be taken. A simple history form is often beneficial: an example is shown in Figure 2.4. This form allows the clinician not only to assess the health status and possible causes of ill health, but also informs the clinician as to the owner's level of knowledge. The time taken for 'clerking' gives the patient time to settle in the consulting room, so that a more realistic assessment of its behaviour can be made.

Figure 2.4: Specimen avian history form.

AVIAN HISTORY FORM

Owner's name and address: ....

....

Telephone number: ....

Species: .... Age: .... Sex: ....

Name: ....

Has the bird been examined by another vet?   Yes/No   Name: ....

                  Telephone Number: ....

Duration of ownership? ....

Source (if acquired in last year)? ....

Do you or have you kept other birds (list species)?   Yes/No ....

Any previous disease history with this or other birds? ....

Reason for presentation and clinical signs? ....

Duration of problem? ....

Any other birds/pets (own or friends) affected/ill? ....

Have you had any new birds in the last six months? ....

Does the bird have contact with feral birds? ....

Any change of food (type or source)? ....Duration of food storage? ....

Has the bird received any medication? ....

Is the bird confined to perch/aviary/pond? .... Size? .... Inside/Outside? ....

Has anything changed in the bird's environment in the previous three months? ....

How long ago? ....

Change of appetite? ....

What diet is fed? .... Are any other birds fed on the same diet? ....

Any change in the bird's behaviour? ....

List any supplements, additives or tonics administered: ....

Any change in water consumption? ....

What is the bird's reproductive status? ....

Has the bird's plumage changed at all in previous six months, ie. moulted or changed in appearance? ....

Has the appearance of the bird's excreta changed? ....

If yes, is it the coloured part (faeces) or the white part (urates) which has altered? ....

If flown, is there any exercise intolerance? ....

Have any nasal or ocular discharges been apparent? ....

Has there been any change in vocalisation? ....

What is the bird's body condition or weight? .... What is the bird's normal weight? ....

Has the bird required more/same/less food to maintain its weight? ....

Is the bird perching normally on one leg or two, or lying down? ....

Is there excessive heat in either foot or any leg joint? ....

If a raptor, has it been casting normally? ....

Observe from a distance, clinically assess and tick the following:

	Yes	No		Yes	No
Normal activity/reactions.			Lameness.		
Normal flight.			Ruffled appearance.		
Normal walking.			Mouth breathing or panting.		
Normal perching.			Tail bobbing.		
Alteration of voice.			Any abnormal nervous signs.		
Normal position of wings.			Weight or condition change.		
Shutting eyes.			Eye shape normal (round).		

The following key points should be noted if possible prior to physical examination:
- The bird's attitude and demeanour.
- Body conformation and contour.
- Appearance of the eye (round and bright or ovoid and slit like).
- Rate, depth and nature of breathing.
- Condition of feathers, beak, cere and feet.

Gross examination of the faeces is often useful. Table 2.1 lists some of the common findings and interpretations.

Table 2.1. Gross faecal examination.

Faecal appearance	Possible aetiologies
Reduced volume	Decreased food intake; decreased gastrointestinal tract (GIT) transit time; food deprivation; obstruction.
Small dry faeces	Water deprivation or GIT obstruction.
Dark discolouration	Upper GIT haemorrhage or blockage.
Blood	GIT (bacterial, parasitic or viral enteritis, neolplasia, foreign body, etc); coagulopathies; diseases of kidney, testicle, ovary (pre- or post-laying), cloaca.
Voluminous	Malabsorption, eg. GIT disease, bacterial enteritis or bacterial overgrowth, pancreatitis, parasitism, peritonitis; diabetes; renal neoplasia.
Bright green faeces + yellow, brown or green urates	Indicates haemolysis or hepatitis caused by toxic damage, eg. lead poisoning; bacterial or viral infections; erythrocytic parasitism or ornithosis (chlamydiosis). Bruising or surgery may cause brown discolouration of urates. B complex vitamins or proflavine dressings may cause yellowing of the urates.
Clay coloured faeces	Maldigestion or malabsorption; bacterial or *Candida* spp. overgrowth.
Undigested food (differentiate from regurgitation)	Malabsorption, maldigestion, hypermotility (due to inflammation, infection or parasitism), pancreatitis, proventriculitis.
Excess urine	Renal failure (infection, neoplasia, immune, toxic); any cause of polydipsia.

Undigested food in faeces (variable pH in different species) must be differentiated from regurgitation (if from the crop it is neutral or alkaline) and vomition (from the proventriculus it is acidic).

All birds should have microscopic examination of fresh faeces carried out:
- Direct examination for motile protozoa, fluke, etc.
- Flotation for parasite ova or oocysts.
- Diff Quik stain for bacteria, yeast, anti-inflammatory cells.

PREPARATION

Tables 2.2 and 2.3 provide check lists of standard equipment and medications which may be used during avian consultations.

Table 2.2. Equipment which may be used during the consultation.

Equipment	Used for
Secure room which may be darkened. Gloves and clean towel.	Stress free 'casting' and restraint of patient.
Pen torch.	Examination.
Stethoscope.	Auscultation.
Auriscope.	Examining orifices.
Sterile Foley catheter/air sac breathing tube.	Emergency airway.
Sterile surgical pack.	Surgical repair/insertion of air sac tube.
Weighing scales.	Daily weighing.
Hospital sheets.	Daily records.
Examination table, illumination, magnification.	Examination.
Syringes, needles, spinal needles, catheters, crop and gavage tubes.	Fluid therapy (see Chapter 3).
Microbiology swabs, blood and faeces pots, microscope slides.	Collection of diagnostic samples.
Laboratory equipment for packed cell volume, biochemistry, haematology testing on-site.	Rapid accurate diagnosis, prognosis, monitor response to therapy.
Haemostatic swabs, cautery or chemicals, eg. potassium permanganate.	Haemostasis.
Vaporiser + oxygen, mask, endotracheal tubes, anaesthetic monitoring equipment.	Anaesthesia (see Chapter 9).
2.7mm or 4.0mm rigid 0° endoscope.	Endoscopy of trachea, syrinx, cloaca, air sacs, crop (see Chapter 23).
Radiographic equipment.	Diagnostic radiographs (see Chapter 10).
Skin dressings, eg. Granuflex, Kaltostat, Preparation H, Orobase.	Stimulation of epithelialisation (see Chapter 14).
Heated pads or lamps.	Correction of hypothermia.
Refractometer (not reliable - see Chapter 8).	To assess total protein as a prognostic indicator.
Bandaging, splinting (including extension splint) materials.	Wound management and stabilisation.
Intensive care cage (to provide oxygen, increased temperature and increased humidity).	Critical care.
Nebulisation equipment.	Treatment of respiratory infections.

Table 2.3. Medications that might be useful at the time of initial examination.

Medication	Used for
Isoflurane (halothane or injectable agents if not available).	Anaesthesia (see Chapter 9).
Diazepam (0.5-1.5mg/kg i/v or i/m).	Control of fits (see Chapter 10).
Lactated Ringers (Hartmann's) solution (LRS) (10ml/kg i/v, repeat every two hours as required).	Fluid therapy (see Chapter 3).
Plasma expander (Haemaccel, Hoechst).	Blood loss.
Whole avian blood (preferably homologous).	Blood loss (only of very short-term value).
Dextrose 5% solution (1-5ml/kg by slow i/v injection, mixed 50:50 with LRS).	Hypoglycaemia.
Dexamethasone (1-2mg/kg i/v or i/m, sid or bid).	Shock, allergies, spinal injuries.
Iron dextran (10mg/kg i/m weekly).	Anaemia.
B complex vitamins (i/m to provide 10mg/kg thiamine on alternate days).	Inappetence, shock, debilitation.
Amoxycillin LA (150mg/kg i/m daily).	Broad-spectrum antibiosis.
Enrofloxacin (15mg/kg i/m or p/o on an empty crop and proventriculus).	Broad-spectrum antibiosis; can cause emesis in raptors if food is present in the crop or proventriculus.
Marbofloxacin (15mg/kg p/o bid).	As above but does not cause emesis.
Piperacillin (200mg/kg i/v or i/m, bid).	Broad-spectrum antibiosis.
Trimethroprim (12-60mg/kg i/m or p/o, bid).	Antibiosis.
Frusemide (0.5-2mg/kg i/m or s/c, bid).	Pulmonary congestion.
Metoclopramide (2mg/kg i/v, i/m or p/o).	Gut stasis or vomition.
Atropine (0.1mg/kg i/m every 3-4 hours).	Cholinesterase anti-inhibitor antidote.
Activated charcoal (2-8g/kg p/o as required).	Binding of gastrointestinal tract toxins.
Sodium Calciumedetate (25-35mg/kg i/m bid for five days).	Heavy metal poisoning (especially lead).
Povidone-iodine and chlorhexidine.	Wound cleansing.
Non-steroidal anti-inflammatories, eg. ketoprofen (2mg/kg i/m or p/o, daily).	Non-steroidal anti-inflammatory and analgesic.
Hills A/d or equivalent (20-40ml/kg every two hours by crop tube as required).	Nutritional support.
Endoparasitic and ectoparasitic preparations.	Parasite control.

ARRIVAL AT THE SURGERY

The equipment and medication listed in Tables 2.2 and 2.3 should be prepared in advance so that once the bird is handled there will be no delay. However, it is not possible to predict all possible requirements; for this reason the author advises the use of a 'panic button' within reach of the examination table, so that assistance may be summoned without releasing one's grip on the bird. Wild birds in particular are unaccustomed to human proximity; this will increase stress levels and should therefore be minimised. The use of isoflurane anaesthesia for basic examination is encouraged. It is not contraindicated even in severely debilitated birds, and its use facilitates full examination and treatment without the bird becoming stressed (see Chapter 9). If isoflurane is not available, or its cost is prohibitive for wild birds, sedation (ketamine 5mg/kg i/m), especially in larger birds such as swans and eagles, not only facilitates restraint but reduces the stress caused to the bird.

HANDLING

Raptors should be safely restrained by 'casting' in a clean towel. Wearing gloves prevents safe effective restraint and precludes proper examination of the bird, due to loss of digital sensitivity. The feet and claws are the most dangerous part of the bird. Usually, only vultures, some large owls and eagles tend to bite. If vultures have any food in their crop, this is likely to be vomited over the handler. The majority of raptor keepers are adept at handling their birds and will catch and restrain the bird for an inexperienced veterinarian. Raptors may be caught and cast in one of the following methods:
- 'Hooded' or steady bird on the fist or perch: the bird is approached from above and behind. The bird is grasped swiftly about the shoulders with a clean towel (to minimise feather damage) (see Figure 2.5). The fingers are readjusted to restrain the legs (see Figure 2.7).
- Unjessed or wild bird: will generally be presented in a cardboard box. A large clean towel is draped over

the top of the box. The top flaps of the box are folded back and the towel is dropped down over the bird. The bird's position can be seen. The bird is caught around the shoulders, from behind, with the thumbs positioned dorsally (see Figure 2.6). The fingers are then repositioned so that the legs are restrained between the penultimate fingers on either side as shown in Figure 2.7.
- Jessed, nervous or unmanned bird: the bird is held on the fist with the 'jesses' pulled down tight in the handler's gloved hand. The bird is grasped around the ankles (with a finger between the legs to prevent rubbing) (see Figure 2.8). The bird is then pushed down onto the table in dorsal recumbency, and the wings are caught and folded up before the bird is restrained.

In all the above methods the bird should be restrained on a padded (Vetbed, blanket, towel or covered cushion) examination table in order to prevent trauma as the bird struggles against a hard surface. Except whilst being examined itself, the head should be covered at all times by either a hood or lightweight towel, as this will assist in subduing the bird.

Pigeons are easily restrained and handled. They are traditionally held in the cup of one hand. The tail is held between the thumb and forefinger, and the legs held between subsequent fingers (see Figure 2.9).

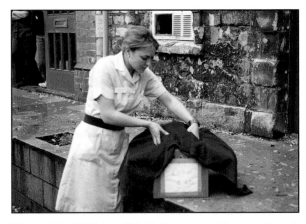

Figure 2.6: *Wild injured bird being removed from cardboard box.*

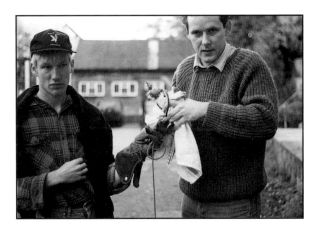

Figure 2.7: *Lanner Falcon: fingers readjusted to control the legs.*

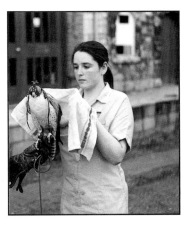

Figure 2.5: *Lanner Falcon being cast.*

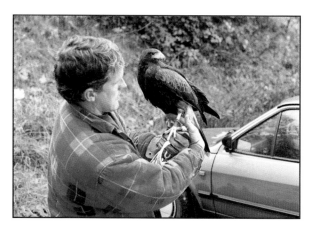

Figure 2.8: *Uncooperative Harris' Hawk being cast by grasping the feet.*

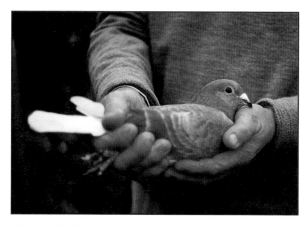

Figure 2.9: *Pigeon being restrained in the hand.*

Waterfowl are generally easily handled. Swans have an undeserved reputation for aggression. A swan should be approached confidently, the neck grasped with one hand, and then the body encircled and restrained with the other arm. Great care must be taken to prevent self-trauma when handling long-legged birds such as flamingos. As soon as the bird is restrained the legs must be grasped with one hand, with a finger between the legs to prevent them rubbing against each other. Herons, in particular, must be handled with great caution. The beak must be restrained as soon as the bird is caught; a ball of cotton wool or similar is attached to the point of the beak to prevent its use (typically aimed at the eyes) against the handler.

EXAMINATION

After the bird has been cast a routine, methodical examination protocol should be carried out. With practice, this procedure should take no longer than 3-4 minutes in routine cases. All bilaterally similar anatomical structures should be compared.

Head (for further details see Chapters 15, 25, 34)

Beak and Cere
The beak and cere should be healthy and shiny, and should meet evenly. Poor beak condition may be caused by poor diet, lack of moisture, poor management or systemic disease.

Nares
The nares should be clear, round and open, with a centrally placed shiny operculum. Discharge, occlusion or rhinolith may be present (see Chapter 18).

Oral Cavity
All parts of the mouth, in particular the tongue, under the tongue, the choana, the oral membrane and the glottis, should be visualised. Any unusual discolorations, necrotic areas or plaques should be gently scraped and smears prepared for microscopic examination.

Eyes
The eyes, sinuses and rhinarium are all anatomically interrelated. Infection of any one may lead to, or be indicative of, infection in all three. The eyelids should be opened widely to expose a round (not ellipsoid) expanse of cornea. The eyes should be clear, moist and shining, with no epiphora, and appear healthy in all respects.

Peri-Orbital Areas
The peri-orbital areas often show swellings indicative of sinusitis (see Chapter 18).

Ear
The aural canal is situated ventrocaudal to the lateral canthus. Problems in this area are uncommon. Polyps, neoplasia or infections may be present.

Respiratory System and Auscultation (see Chapter 18).
The nature and rate of the bird's respiration should be studied prior to handling and may be compared with the normal values listed in Table 2.4.

Once the bird is handled, the heart and respiratory rates will increase; rates that might be expected are shown in Table 2.4. If the bird is permitted to exercise, eg. flap its wings, its respiratory rate will increase further but should return to normal within two minutes of the end of exercise (Harrison and Ritchie, 1994).

Faecal examination for nematode ova should be carried out on all birds showing respiratory signs. Microbiological testing of the choana and trachea, and tracheal endoscopy, should also be performed.

Auscultation is relatively unrewarding in avian patients. The heart rate can be too fast to count, and may be better recorded with an electrocardiogram (ECG) (100cm/minute paper speed is required) or heart monitor. The lung field is smaller and more rigid compared with the mammalian lung and is fixed to the internal curvature of the ribs (see Chapter 18). It is often

Table 2.4. Normal respiratory and heart rates per minute.

Weight	Heart rate (resting)	Heart rate (restrained)	Respiratory rate (resting)	Respiratory rate (restrained)
25g	274	400-600	60-70	80-120
100g	206	500-600	40-52	60-80
200g	178	300-500	35-50	55-65
500g	147	160-300	20-30	30-50
1000g	127	150-350	15-20	25-40
1500g	117	120-200	20-32	25-30
2000g	110	110-175	19-28	20-30

(Harrison and Ritchie, 1994)

possible to hear a faint short inspiratory noise in a normal bird. If other noises are heard, they are likely to be associated with diseases of the nares or sinuses, restriction of air flow in the trachea, eg. syringeal aspergilloma, trichomoniasis or *Syngamus trachea*, or severe air sac disease, eg. aspergillosis, *Serratospiculum* spp., bacterial infection, chlamydiosis. Upper respiratory disease should be differentiated clinically from air sac disease. If the latter is suspected, radiography and endoscopy is indicated (see Chapters 10, 18, 23).

Neck
The oesophagus should be palpated and the mucosal thickness assessed. If there is doubt, the overlying skin should be wetted with spirit and the area transilluminated. Birds which are regurgitating should have their oesophagus and crop examined endoscopically. This can be done in a conscious bird or under anaesthesia. The crop lining is visualised better during endoscopy if the crop is insufflated with air. Oesophagus and crop smears or flushings are readily collected for screening for trichomoniasis, capillariasis, candidiasis or bacterial infections.

Plumage
The condition of the plumage (see Chapters 14, 26, 35) may be indicative of the bird's overall health.

Body Condition
The pectoral muscles will become wasted in cases of starvation or illness. The volume of pectoral muscle varies normally between species. Pigeons are always well covered while owls have much less mass in this area. The clinician should be familiar with the normal levels of musculature in different species. Body condition is best assessed by regular weighing of birds together with condition scoring of muscle covering, ie. score 1 (thin) to score 6 (fat). Loss of condition will give some indication of the chronicity of the disease. In-patients should be weighed daily. Most raptors are weighed daily during the flying season, therefore the keeper should be able to inform the clinician of the flying and fat weights of the individual bird.

Cloaca
Visual external examination and digital (or auriscope) internal examination of the cloaca should be performed (sedation or anaesthesia may be advisory). This can often reveal signs not evident on examination of the faeces. Chronic soiling of the plumage in this area may be caused by cloacitis, cloacal uroliths, diarrhoea, polydipsia, etc.

Abdominal Palpatation
Abdominal palpatation should be carried out transabdominally or *per cloacum*. The proventriculus and kidneys are palpable in most species. The abdomen sould be examined for obesity, distensions or unexpected masses, eg. hepatomegaly, eggbinding, neoplasia or abscessation.

Uropygial Gland
The uropygial gland (see Chapters 14 and 35) is situated dorsally and immediately cranial to the insertion of the central tail feathers. The gland produces the oil used during preening to help with feather condition and waterproofing. The gland should be symmetrical and smooth, and it should be possible to express a small volume of oily secretion. Birds can suffer from dysfunction, abscessation or neoplasia of the uropygial gland.

Wings
The long bones, joints and soft tissue of the wings are examined (see Chapters 17, 27, 36).

Legs and Feet
The legs and feet should be examined from the pelvis to the toes, palpating the length of each long bone and the articulation of each joint. Each leg should be compared with the opposite leg to help highlight any abnormalities. Raptors, in particular, frequently suffer from foot infections, eg. bumblefoot. A thorough examination should be made of the scaly skin, especially under the jesses if they are worn, and of the plantar aspect of the feet. (See Chapters 16, 27, 36)

COLLECTION OF DIAGNOSTIC SAMPLES

The presence of air sacs, lack of a diaphragm and accessibility of most parts of their anatomy mean that members of the Class Aves are well adapted to the collection of a wide range of diagnostic samples. Many 'sick' birds present with non-diagnostic clinical signs, but they may in fact be suffering from advanced disease. A rapid definitive diagnosis may often only be achieved following clinical pathology.

Although laboratory results may be distorted by the use of a sedative or anaesthetic, this may also be due to sampling from stressed birds. Depending on the experience of the handler and the clinician, as well as the species and origin of the patient, a mild sedative or short-acting anaesthetic (isoflurane) may aid a full, rapid and stress-free examination. Samples may be taken at the same time. Ideally, avian clinicians should be capable of extensive in-house clinical pathology, as a rapid laboratory result is essential. Blood samples are often indicated for haematology and biochemistry. Swabs and aspirates from the oesophagus, crop, choana, trachea, air sacs and cloaca can be extremely useful on occasions. The clinician should be confident with haematology (see Chapter 8), biochemistry (see Chapter 7), parasitology (see Chapter 19) and the preparation and interpretation of impression smears (see Chapter 6) and Gram stains, etc.

Swabs

Swabs for bacteriology or impression smears may be taken from many parts of the body, eg. mouth, choana, crop, trachea, cloaca, skin, feathers, etc.

Aspirates

Aspirates are often useful. They may be taken from fluid or soft tissue swellings, as well as from sinuses, joints, wounds, trachea, crop and body cavities, eg. air sacs.

Endoscopy

No avian clinician should be without a good quality endoscope (see Chapter 23). Either a 4.00mm or a 2.7mm rigid endoscope with a 0° direction of view may be used. A 30° endoscope with a piggy-back cannula (sheath) is ideal for the passage of a biopsy punch, grasping forceps, aspiration nozzle, etc. The 30° direction of view allows these instruments to be seen by the operator through the endoscope. Endoscopy is invaluable for examination of the crop, proventriculus, trachea, all the air sac cavities and the cloaca.

Radiology

Radiology is invaluable (see Chapter 10). Some practitioners will have radiographic equipment which is too powerful for most bird tissue. Fine grain, intensifying screens or rare earth screens will increase the exposure requirements and hence bring the exposures within the scope of most machines. High quality diagnostic pictures are required and can be easily attained by most practitioners. In view of the great variability of normal anatomy and, therefore, the radiological anatomy between even closely related species, it is imperative to radiograph the normal as well as the abnormal for comparison - an extra joint in a toe can easily be confused with a fracture. Two views at right angles should always be taken. Contrast studies can be useful where they are employed for visualisation of the crop, proventriculus, ventriculus, small and large intestine, cloaca and abdominal masses. Excretory urograms and arteriograms can also be of value

STABILISATION AND SHOCK THERAPY

By the time wild birds and most captive birds are examined, they will be suffering from a degree of shock, dehydration and circulatory collapse. Excessive handling and examination whilst compromised may be fatal, particularly in wild birds. Stabilisation and shock therapy is required immediately (see Chapter 3 - Appendices 3.1, 3.2).

TRAUMA CASES

The source and type of bird will affect the interpretation of the findings (see Figure 2.3). Flowchart 3.3 in Chapter 3 illustrates a schematic approach to trauma cases.

NURSING CARE (see Chapter 4)

REFERENCES AND FURTHER READING

Coles BH (1985) *Avian Medicine and Surgery*. Blackwell Scientific Publications, London

Cooper JE (1978) *Veterinary Aspects of Captive Birds of Prey*. Standfast Press, Saul.

Cooper JE and Greenwood AG (1981). Eds *Recent Advances in the Study of Raptor Diseases*. Chiron Publications. Keighley.

Harrison GJ and Ritchie BW (1994) Making distinctions in the physical examination. In: *Avian Medicine: Principles and Application*. Eds BW Ritchie, GJ Harrison and LR Harrison. Wingers, Lake Worth.

Redig PT, Cooper JE, Remple JD and Hunter DB (1993) Eds *Raptor Biomedicine*. University of Minnesota Press, Minneapolis.

Ritchie BW, Harrison GJ and Harrison LR (1994) Eds *Avian Medicine: Principles and Application*. Wingers, Lake Worth.

CHAPTER THREE

Avian Emergencies

Patrick T Redig

INTRODUCTION

This chapter provides a decision making model for the major emergencies that are most frequently encountered among raptors, pigeons and waterfowl. It is intended to serve as a quick reference to help the clinician obtain pertinent diagnostic information and implement first stage treatment plans for these problems.

Each Flow Chart and its associated text addresses a major clinical problem or presenting sign. Vertical lines are pathways to diagnoses and treatment regimens. Principal clinical signs that characterise an important aspect of any given line of development are presented in capitals and lower case letters along the line. Diagnostic information and procedures that advance one towards a diagnosis or treatment are depicted as information carried in from the side. Black boxes indicate important points of diagnosis or treatment that are especially relevant to that situation. Other diagnoses, treatments, procedures or other considerations are contained in open white boxes.

Since this section addresses typical emergency situations, it is relevant to consider preparations within the clinic that must be in a state of readiness in order to respond effectively. Lists of equipment and medications that are indispensable in providing for such a state can be found in Chapter 2 (see Tables 2.2, 2.3). Ideally, an area of the clinic should be designated for these procedures and the equipment and expendable items should be immediately available at that site. Training sessions and drills with staff on the use of equipment and on developing proficiency in execution of the techniques is recommended.

Emergency situations notwithstanding, obtaining a thorough history, even if it is done whilst the bird is undergoing examination and routine stabilisation, is important to diagnosis and treatment. Therefore, this item is at or near the top of every Flow Chart. The pertinent information that needs to be obtained when a wild bird is admitted is shown in Figure 2.3.

The priorities for examination and treatment in avian emergencies are as follows:

● Assure respiratory function by establishing a patent airway or relieving dyspnoea.

● Correct circulatory deficits, especially hypovolaemia, and otherwise stabilise the patient.
● Stop haemorrhage.
● Stabilise fractures or luxations.
● Treat wounds and soft tissue injuries.
● Establish a definitive diagnosis and management plan once survival has been assured.

The major emergencies that may be encountered in avian practice are described in more detail under specific headings in the rest of this chapter. Repetitions of the priorities listed above are spread throughout the various protocols suggested, but these elements of examination and treatment are the important initial actions.

DYSPNOEA (see Flow Chart 3.1)

(1) Factors within and without the respiratory system may be responsible for dyspnoea. Intrinsic events include inhalation of a foreign body or growth of a granuloma in the upper airway. These cause inspiratory stridor or changed vocalisation in an otherwise healthy bird. Diseases of the air sacs and lungs are typically accompanied by other signs of chronic debilitation. Expiratory stridor accompanies blockages from granulomata and exudates in the intrathoracic airways. If gas exchange itself is not compromised by inflammation or oedema, the most pronounced sign of such a condition will be a prolonged expiratory phase. Radiography may reveal overinflated abdominal air sacs. Since avian airways do not collapse under forced expiration, moist or dry rales are heard as opposed to the wheezes usually heard in mammalian lungs. Extrinsic causes of apparent respiratory distress include space occupying lesions in the thorax and abdomen, eg. swollen livers or tumours; pericardial effusion leading to pulmonary congestion; and anaemia.

(2) Note whether the dyspnoea is mild or severe; the latter is indicated by extension of the tongue and glottis on inspiration. If mild, note the degree of 'tail bob' and ventral abdominal muscle excursion. Note whether stridor accompanies inspiration or expiration. An oxygen enriched environment (100% oxygen in a holding container or critical care unit) is recommended for

Flow Chart 3.1: The dyspnoeic bird.

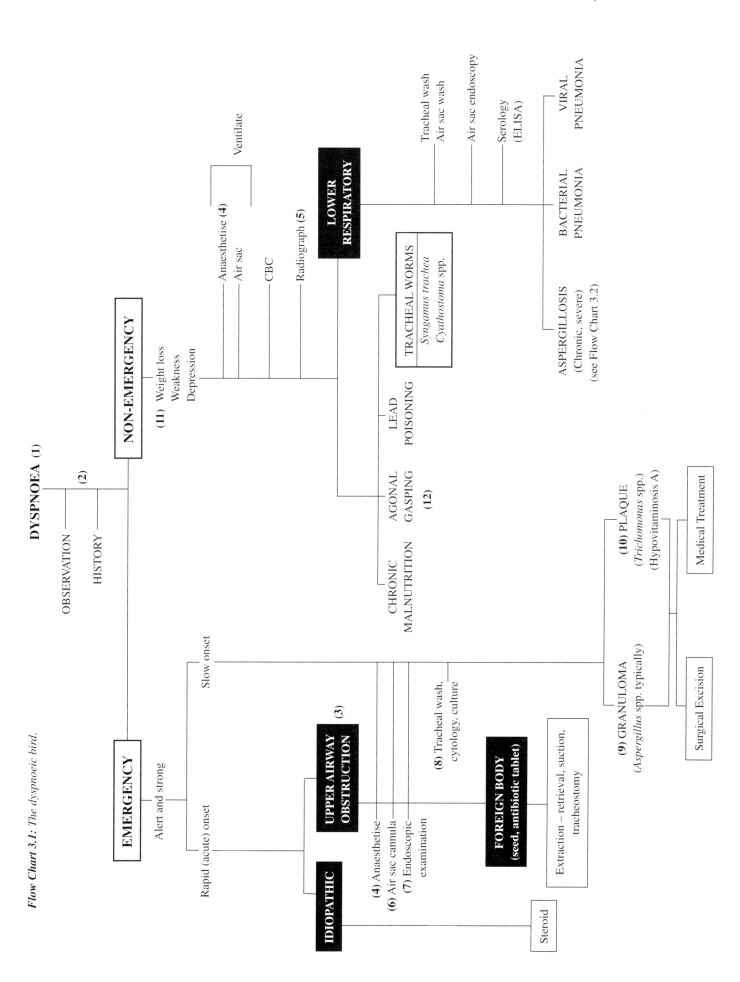

DYSPNOEA (1)

(2)

OBSERVATION

HISTORY

EMERGENCY

Rapid (acute) onset

Alert and strong

Slow onset

IDIOPATHIC

UPPER AIRWAY OBSTRUCTION (3)

(4) Anaesthetise
(6) Air sac cannula
(7) Endoscopic examination

(8) Tracheal wash, cytology, culture

FOREIGN BODY (seed, antibiotic tablet)

Extraction – retrieval, suction, tracheostomy

Steroid

NON-EMERGENCY

(11) Weight loss
Weakness
Depression

Anaesthetise **(4)**
Air sac

Ventilate

CBC

Radiograph **(5)**

LOWER RESPIRATORY

CHRONIC MALNUTRITION

AGONAL GASPING **(12)**

LEAD POISONING

TRACHEAL WORMS
Syngamus trachea
Cyathostoma spp.

Tracheal wash
Air sac wash

Air sac endoscopy

Serology (ELISA)

VIRAL PNEUMONIA

BACTERIAL PNEUMONIA

ASPERGILLOSIS
(Chronic, severe)
(see Flow Chart 3.2)

(9) GRANULOMA
(*Aspergillus* spp. typically)

(10) PLAQUE
(*Trichomonas* spp.)
(Hypovitaminosis A)

Surgical Excision

Medical Treatment

observation and handling prior to anaesthesia or provision of an air sac tube (see **(6)** if dyspnoea is severe).

(3) Acute blockage of the upper airways in an otherwise healthy bird is a true emergency. The respiratory difficulty that develops from chronic pulmonary disease can be life-threatening, but in most manageable presentations is not an emergency.

(4) Anaesthesia with isoflurane is not contraindicated. In many instances the state of unconsciousness and general relaxation results in an immediate amelioration of symptoms. Respiratory function can be maintained by tracheal intubation and/or air sac cannulation and mechanical ventilation. Oxygen flows of 1-1.5 litres per minute are recommended for birds 1kg in weight. Flow should be scaled up or down depending on the size of the bird (see Chapter 9).

(5) Ventrodorsal as well as lateral radiographs are necessary.

(6) Cannulation of the air sacs is a simple and remarkably effective technique for immediately relieving dyspnoea, administering oxygen and anaesthetics, and countering apnoea. Equipment required consists only of a scalpel, small forceps, plastic or rubber tube or a large metal needle, and suture material. Rubber urinary catheters and foreshortened endotracheal tubes (size 4-5mm for a 1kg bird) are particularly useful. The tube is placed in the flank area either in the last intercostal space, behind the last rib, or behind the leg in a sublumbar position; essentially the same sites as would be used for laparoscopic sexing. After a small skin incision is made, the opening is enlarged with a forceps and the tube placed through the opening. It may be sutured in place by attaching a tape around the tube and suturing it to the body wall. Tubes may be left in place for 3-5 days while conditions elsewhere are being managed. Though the potential for air sac contamination would appear great, in practice it has not proved to be problematic (Quesenberry and Hillyer, 1993) (see Chapter 9 for further details of technique).

(7) Endoscopic examination of the trachea with an appropriately sized endoscope (1.7-4.0mm) is an efficient, accurate and well-tolerated means of assessing the upper airways. If the endoscope has a sheath with an operating channel, a retriever may be introduced to recover a foreign body. Once an object has been located, some clinicians have recommended placing a needle tranversely through the trachea below the offending object to prevent further passage into the respiratory system (Quesenberry and Hillyer, 1993).

(8) If a lesion is encountered with an endoscope or if a diagnostic sample is desired independent of the endoscopic examination, recovery of material for examination may be accomplished by injection and subsequent withdrawal of sterile saline into the trachea (10ml/kg) using either a syringe and catheter via the glottis or syringe and needle between tracheal rings (see Chapter 18).

(9) Tracheal aspergillosis is characterised in the early stages by a change in voice.

(10) Tracheal plaques may be caused by trichomoniasis (Samour *et al*, 1995).

(11) In these circumstances, unless an otherwise ill bird has become simultaneously plagued with a problem listed on the left side of this Flow Chart, the respiratory embarrassment is secondary to another, typically chronic and debilitating, disease condition, of which lead poisoning and aspergillosis are the most frequent causes.

(12) Birds in agonal stages of lead poisoning or other conditions causing severe pulmonary congestion and interference with gas exchange display severe dyspnoea. The provision of oxygen in the atmosphere or via an air sac cannula may help in determining where the gas exchange/transport deficit is occurring.

SCREENING AND PREVENTION OF ASPERGILLOSIS (see Flow Chart 3.2).

(1) Aspergillosis is the commonest cause of death among wild birds undergoing medical care, and is a moderate threat to domesticated birds that have been injured or otherwise subjected to a significant change in their management. All individuals should be evaluated by history and a range of screening tests to determine their status with regard to this disease at the time of admission (Aguilar and Redig, 1994).

(2) Prophylactic treatment is indicated for certain species of birds that are undergoing change of management or have become ill or injured. Because of the propensity for individuals of these species to develop this disease, treatment is undertaken on a pre-emptive basis. The preferred drug is itraconazole (10mg/kg p/o bid for one week prior to or at the time of the stressful event, followed by 2-3 weeks at 10mg/kg p/o sid).

(3) The avian species and the specific clinical conditions warranting prophylactic treatment are listed.

(4) If preliminary diagnostic procedures indicate a diagnosis of clinical aspergillosis, further definition of the extent of the disease, a factor which will affect the decision to treat, can be derived from these two procedures.

(5) Recent attempts to treat advanced cases of this disease have been successful with the combination of drugs listed here:

● Itraconazole (15mg/kg p/o, sid or bid).
● Clotrimazole (1-2ml of a 10mg/ml solution in polyethylene glycol, by nebulisation for one hour per day).
● Amphotericin B (1.5mg/kg i/v tid through an indwelling catheter). The catheter is inserted into the basilic or jugular vein, capped off and sutured in place. It may be left in place for the duration of the therapy and is generally not interfered with by the bird.

Itraconazole is given bid for the first week followed by sid for the entire duration, including a month after the remission of signs. Clotrimazole is given for two

Flow Chart 3.2: *Aspergillosis diagnosis and prevention.*

SCREENING AND PREVENTION OF ASPERGILLOSIS

— History

— Clinical examination

— Observation

(1)

Screening
- ELISA
- Culture
- CBC
- Clinical suspicion

⊕ ──→ **(2)** **Prophylaxis**

(3)

Species	**Conditions**
- Gyr Falcon	- Lead poisoning
- Northern Goshawk	- Oil
- Juvenile Red-tailed Hawk	- Stress
- Golden Eagle	- Management changes
- Snowy Owl	
- Rough-legged Buzzard	
- Eider Ducks	
- Divers (Loons)	
- Swans	

⊖

Repeat two weeks after admission

(4) ⊕

⊖

Further diagnostic tests
- Radiography
- Endoscopy of air sacs

(5)

Treatment
See Chapter 18.

months. Amphotericin B is given for one week at the outset of treatment.

Direct injection of amphotericin B into the trachea or an air sac via a cannula or percutaneous, transcostal injection (1mg/kg diluted to 1ml in sterile water) is another frequently employed route. Whilst intravenous treatment is typically not used beyond the first 5-7 days, these other modes of installation are maintained for 2-3 weeks as needed.

Further information on aspergillosis can be found in Chapter 18.

TRAUMA (see Flow Chart 3.3)

* Triage is defined as 'a procedure that involves the sorting and classification of injured or acutely or severely ill patients, undertaken at a hospital emergency room or military advanced station hospital, or during other disaster situations, in order to determine the priority of need and proper place of treatment (Bennington, 1984).

(1) Seventy five per cent of admissions to a rehabilitation facility occur as a result of blunt trauma, the common causes being moving vehicles, windows and power line collisions, as well as shooting, trapping and a host of miscellaneous conditions. History is often obscure and the condition of the bird often dictates taking a generalised approach to treatment without anything more than a sketchy definition of the problems at hand. A range of diagnostic techniques applied at admission, in conjunction with the administration of basic stabilisation treatment, is effective in progressing the bird to the secondary stages of treatment and management.

(2) A traumatised bird is typically malnourished, anaemic, dehydrated, in pain and subject to maggot infestation and bacterial infection of open wounds.

(3) The generalised treatment protocol presented in Appendix 3.1 (Stabilisation Treatment) is recommended for all trauma cases (Redig, 1992).

(4) Anaesthesia with isoflurane does not compromise the bird. It reduces stress of handling at admission and renders the clinic staff capable of performing a more efficient and effective job of diagnosing and administering stabilisation treatment (Quesenberry and Hillyer, 1993).

Flow Chart 3.3: The traumatised avian patient.

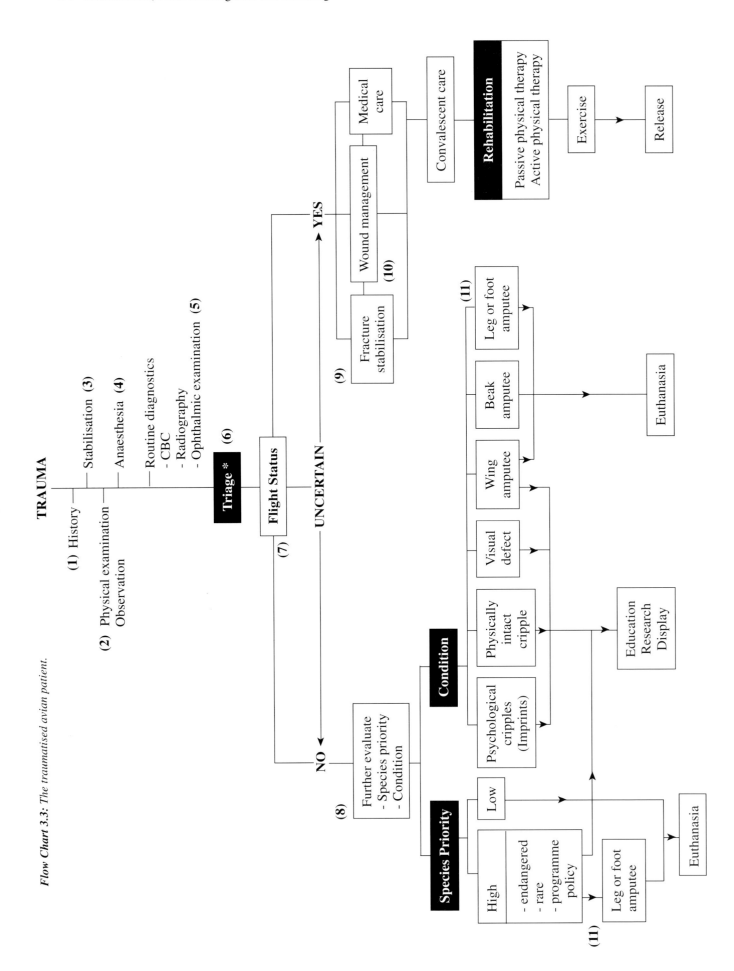

TRAUMA

(1) History

(2) Physical examination
Observation

Stabilisation **(3)**

Anaesthesia **(4)**

Routine diagnostics
- CBC
- Radiography
- Ophthalmic examination **(5)**

Triage * **(6)**

Flight Status

(7)

YES

UNCERTAIN

NO

Fracture stabilisation **(9)**

Wound management **(10)**

Medical care

Convalescent care

Rehabilitation
Passive physical therapy
Active physical therapy

Exercise

Release

(8) Further evaluate
- Species priority
- Condition

Condition

Psychological cripples (Imprints)

Physically intact cripple

Visual defect

Wing amputee

Beak amputee

Leg or foot amputee **(11)**

Education
Research
Display

Euthanasia

Species Priority

High
- endangered
- rare
- programme policy

Low

Leg or foot amputee **(11)**

Euthanasia

(5) An ophthalmic examination should be part of every trauma case examination. Detached retinas, which cause blindness, frequently occur in birds involved in vehicle collisions. Visual function is usually, but not always, lost in the affected eye(s). As noted later, such loss will render the bird unsuitable for release to the wild (Murphy *et al*, 1981) (see Chapter 15).

(6) Triage is essential when dealing with trauma cases and to some extent with other medical conditions. The future health, comfort, function and utility of the patient must be assessed at the outset. If release to the wild is a desired outcome, then extant conditions that would preclude normal function and survival in the wild may render the bird a candidate for euthanasia, the implementation of which should be undertaken as soon as it is realised that release is not a possibility. Loss of an eye or partial visual function, or loss of limbs or digits, are typical compromising factors in trauma cases with multiple injuries (Redig, 1987b). For birds destined to remain in captivity or domestic situations there is more latitude. The temperament of the bird, either at the species or individual level, is an important consideration in evaluating a bird for a life in captivity as a permanent cripple. Fractious species, such as the accipiters, and fractious individuals, especially American Bald Eagles, will predictably develop management related problems and injuries if held in captivity; these inevitably lead to debilitation, death or euthanasia. In many cases, euthanasia is a preferable choice at or near the time of admission if the severity of the aftermath of the injury precludes release. Further discussion of rehabilitation can be found in Chapter 23.

(7) In many instances, flight status may not be ascertained at the time of primary triage. As treatment progresses, continuous evaluations should be made regarding possible outcomes. If at any time the patient fails to meet the requirements for flight or suitability for one of the possible captive destinations, euthanasia should be considered.

(8) Retention in captivity must depend on the ability of the individual bird to be able to live comfortably. Fractious temperament and non-treatable orthopaedic problems may be factors in preventing a bird from being held long term.

(9) Stabilisation at this point is typically a bandage or splint, intended to suffice only until the patient has recovered sufficiently to be able to withstand the rigours of more complex procedures. However, if the injury is less severe, this first bandaging may be entirely adequate for longer-term management (Redig, 1987a).

(10) See Flow Chart 3.5 for further details of wound management.

(11) Foot and leg amputees should never be released into the wild, and their long-term survivability in captivity is poor except for very small (< 200g) individuals. In time, most one-footed birds develop untreatable bumblefoot in the remaining limb and must eventually be euthanased.

FLUID THERAPY (see Flow Chart 3.4)

(1) Injured or debilitated birds are assumed to be presented in a state of dehydration. If debilitation is severe, so also is the state of dehydration. Although no practical means exist to assess the exact level of dehydration, a presumption of 5-10% is a reasonable estimate. Fluids may be administered via the oral, subcutaneous, intravenous and intraosseous routes. However, rapid administration of fluids by the intravenous route is the single most important and effective procedure that may be undertaken in the management of a bird in shock, extreme debilitation or severe injury (Quesenberry and Hillyer, 1993; Murray, 1994).

(2) Given the common physiological status of injured and debilitated birds, extensive laboratory work is not necessary to initiate therapy. Packed cell volume (PCV) and total protein (TP) will have stabilised by movement of fluids from the interstitial space to the vascular compartment within 24-48 hours of injury, and these parameters, therefore, are a useful monitor of progress. Whilst it is accepted that the evaluation of TP using a refractometer is not accurate (see Chapter 7), it does give a rapid and useful prognostic indication in an emergency situation such as this. There is no need to wait for results of other laboratory tests such as haematology or serum biochemistry to initiate life-saving therapy.

(3) Appendix 3.1 (Stabilisation Protocol) contains the materials and dosages for the components of the standard stabilisation protocol to be used in avian species (Redig, 1992).

(4) Routes of fluid administration. Various authors present different viewpoints and opinions as to the amount and rate at which fluids may be given; most are conservative.

Intravenous route. This author has used rapid bolus intravenous injection over a period of ten years in over 6,000 individual raptors with great success. Bolus injection of fluids at the rate of 10ml/kg/minute through a 25G needle or catheter yields well tolerated and satisfactory results. The most frequently used site for intravenous injection is the ulnar vein which (albeit smaller) is more accessible than the basilic vein (see Figures 3.1, 3.2). Injecting into the ulnar vein is easier than some other sites as restraint of the bird in dorsal recumbency with the wing extended is readily achieved. Blood samples may be taken from this site using a 25G needle, provided the blood is withdrawn reasonably slowly. The jugular may be the only accessible vein in birds weighing less than 150g. The medial metatarsal vein is well developed in waterfowl and is an excellent site for fluid administration in these and other large species of birds. It lends itself to the placement of an indwelling butterfly catheter that allows the repeated administration of fluids and requires minimal restraint of the patient. The intravenous route is used repeatedly in the first 24-48 hours of replacement therapy, hence good venipuncture technique and vein management is essential (Redig, 1992).

Intraosseous route. In cases presenting with extreme debilitation, the peripheral veins may be too collapsed to permit venipuncture. Therefore, the use of the intraosseous route is required for the first stage of rapid fluid administration. This route may be accessed by placement of an appropriately sized spinal needle, eg. 21G in a 500-1,000g bird, in the marrow cavity of the ulna or tibiotarsus. The needle is inserted into the olecranon with the elbow flexed (see Figure 3.1). If the medial aspect of the olecranon is used there is little chance that the function of the humerotriceps or scapulotriceps muscles will be compromised. An intraosseous injection can be seen to enter the venous circulation directly when this site is used. In birds weighing less than 150g, a 25-27G hypodermic needle may suffice; however, problems with plugging of the needle bore with a core of bone may occur. Since the marrow cavity lacks the capacitance of the venous system, volumes and rates are limited, although the exact tolerances are un-known. A rate of 10ml/kg/hour has been proposed (Quesenberry and Hillyer, 1993). Fluid flow rate is controlled through an infusion pump or a simple gravity-fed fluid administration set. This route offers the advantage of requiring no further restraint for longer-term administration, but it is more complex and costly to administer than simple intravenous injection and some birds will pull the catheters or become entangled in the tubing.

Subcutaneous route. The subcutaneous route is used effectively for providing larger volumes of fluids on a maintenance basis. The inguinal region (see Figure 3.3) and the axillary regions are the sites typically used for administration. Using a small bore needle, eg. 27G, 8-10ml/kg can be injected on each side. This route is not effective for rehydration of birds with poor peripheral circulation or those which are severely hypoproteinaemic.

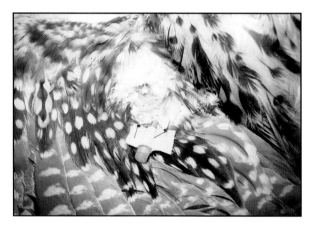

Figure 3.2. *Ventral aspect of the wing of a Lanner Falcon showing an indwelling intravenous catheter in the ulnar vein.*

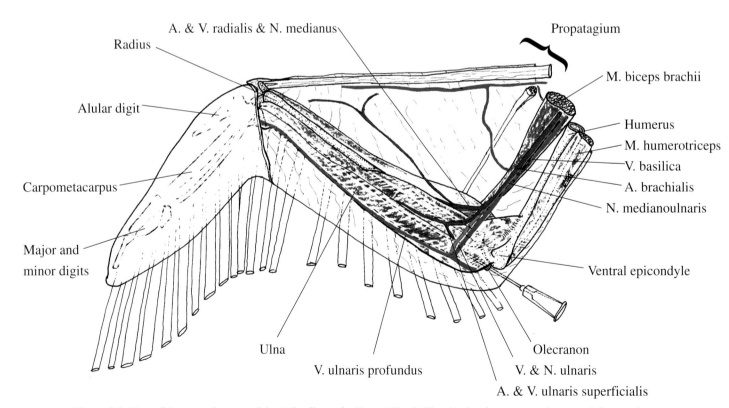

Figure 3.1. *View of the ventral aspect of the right elbow of a Harris' Hawk. The skin has been removed to reveal the muscles (shaded grey), and the arteries (red), veins (blue) and nerves (green). The bones are seen as broken lines where they are overlain by tissue. A site of needle insertion for intraosseous cannulation is shown. (Drawing by N H Harcourt-Brown)*

Flow Chart 3.4: *Fluid therapy.*

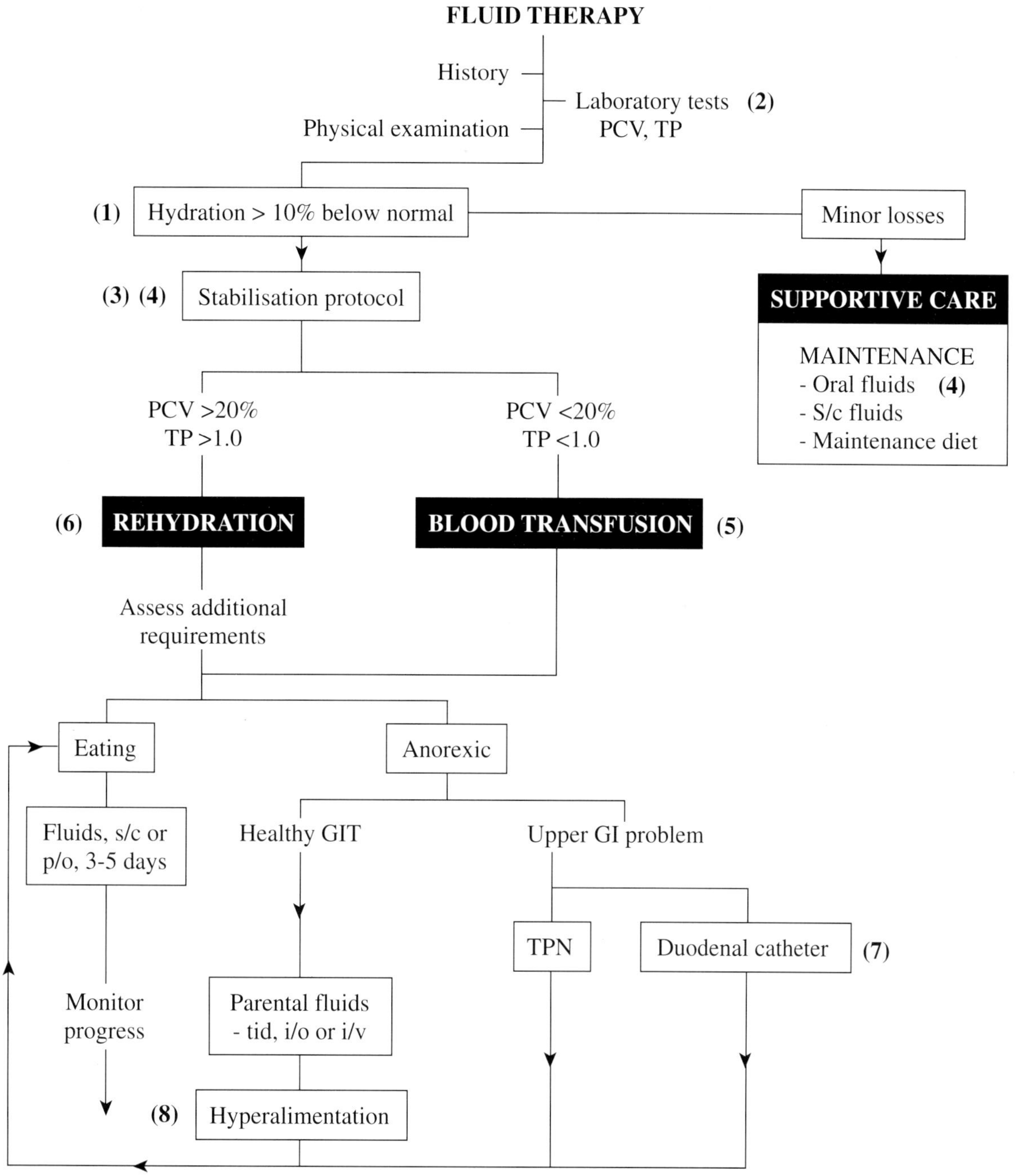
FLUID THERAPY
History
Physical examination
Laboratory tests (2)
PCV, TP
(1) Hydration > 10% below normal
Minor losses
(3) (4) Stabilisation protocol
SUPPORTIVE CARE
MAINTENANCE
- Oral fluids (4)
- S/c fluids
- Maintenance diet
PCV >20%
TP >1.0
PCV <20%
TP <1.0
(6) REHYDRATION
BLOOD TRANSFUSION (5)
Assess additional requirements
Eating
Anorexic
Fluids, s/c or p/o, 3-5 days
Healthy GIT
Upper GI problem
TPN
Duodenal catheter (7)
Monitor progress
Parental fluids - tid, i/o or i/v
(8) Hyperalimentation

Oral route. The oral route is used effectively for routine administration of fluids to mildly dehydrated individuals and for in-hospital maintenance. It is not effective for meeting the needs of the severely dehydrated or debilitated patient, nor may it be used in cases where the patient is vomiting or has decreased motility within the gastrointestinal tract. Soft rubber urinary catheters, giving sets or curved stainless steel feeding needles affixed to the hub of an appropriately sized syringe constitute the basic equipment needed. The bird is held in a vertical position with the beak held open with fingers, and the cannula is passed to the right of the glottis and into the crop (see Figures 3.4.1, 3.4.2).

(5) In view of the benefits derived from a single heterologous blood transfusion, they are recommended in cases where PCV at admission is below 15%. The greatest single benefit is derived in cases where PCV is between 5% and 10%. While cell life may actually be less than 24 hours (Murray, 1994), nevertheless, transfusions can be an effective first line of treatment to keep the patient alive until other forms of longer-term treatment may be instituted.

Blood transfusions need not be complicated. After checking the donor bird for an adequate PCV and total plasma protein, the desired amount of blood should be withdrawn through at least a 22G needle into a

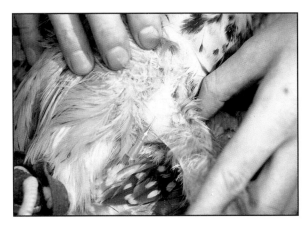

Figure 3.3. Inquinal region of a Lanner Falcon, showing a suitable site for subcutaneous injection.

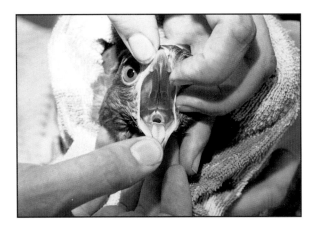

Figure 3.4.1. Harris' Hawk showing the clinicians finger in the commisure of the jaw acting as a 'gag'. Note the position of the glottis, which must be avoided when passing the crop tube.

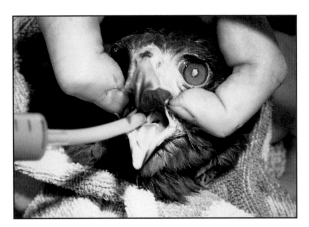

Figure 3.4.2. Harris' Hawk with a crop tube in place adjacent to the glottis.

heparinised syringe. The vein of the recipient must be cannulated immediately and the blood injected slowly so as not to damage the erythrocytes. It may be desirable to replace the volume removed from the donor with saline. Transfusion reactions occur only rarely even though blood from chickens or pigeons are frequently transfused into such distantly related species as parrots and raptors.

(**6**) Selection of rehydrating agents. Lactated Ringers Solution (LRS) is the agent of choice for parenteral administration. It is a mild alkalinising agent and will therefore mitigate the state of metabolic acidosis affecting debilitated and injured patients (Redig, 1984). Where extreme emaciation is present, a 1:1 mix of LRS with dextrose 5% provides an isotonic rehydrating solution with a utilisable energy source; however, it is a metabolic acidifying agent.

LRS, dextrose 5%, saline, commercial products such as Gatorade, and decarbonated cola-based soft drinks have all been used successfully as oral rehydrating fluids. A dextrose/glucose component to the solution appears to facilitate fluid uptake from the intestine (Lumeij, 1987).

While crystalloid agents such as LRS have been used to great advantage in the last two decades, they require frequent readministration in order to maintain circulatory volume. Colloidal agents, eg. Haemaccel (Hoechst), because of their large molecular size, have the potential to replace deficient plasma proteins, thereby preventing osmotic passage of fluids from the vascular compartment to the intracellular space. Hetastarch Colloidal Plasma Expander (Hespan, NPBL Emmer-Compascuum) is currently under investigation. Preliminary results have shown no undesirable side-effects and performance at least equal to that seen with crystalloid preparations. It is administered at a rate of 10ml/kg 2-4 times daily.

The objective of fluid therapy is to provide for deficit replacement and daily maintenance, as well as contemporaneous losses. Owing to the refractoriness of avian species towards haemorrhage, only the first two are of practical concern. The deficit is estimated from the percentage dehydration (taken as 10% for the typical trauma/debilitation case) and bodyweight according to the formula: estimated dehydration (%) x bodyweight (g) = fluid deficit (ml) (Redig, 1984). Maintenance is estimated at 50ml/kg/day. A clinically proven protocol replaces 50% of the deficit in the first 24 hours and the remainder over the next 48 hours while providing maintenance needs (see Appendix 3.2 for a sample problem).

(**7**) Total parenteral nutrition (TPN) and enteral nutrition (duodenal catheterisation) has not enjoyed widespread use. The former is rendered difficult because of lack of specific solutions for use in birds and the need for near continuous infusion (Quesenberry and Hillyer, 1993). The latter, though invasive, provides a more manageable route for administering commercially available enteric preparations (Goring *et al*, 1986), especially in larger species.

(**8**) Once the gastrointestinal tract is capable of processing solid or semi-solid food, hyperalimentation may be substituted with other forms of nutritional support. A slurry of chopped or pureed food items in sufficient diluent (usually an electrolyte solution) is injected in appropriate volume into the crop of the bird with a

Flow Chart 3.5: Wound management.

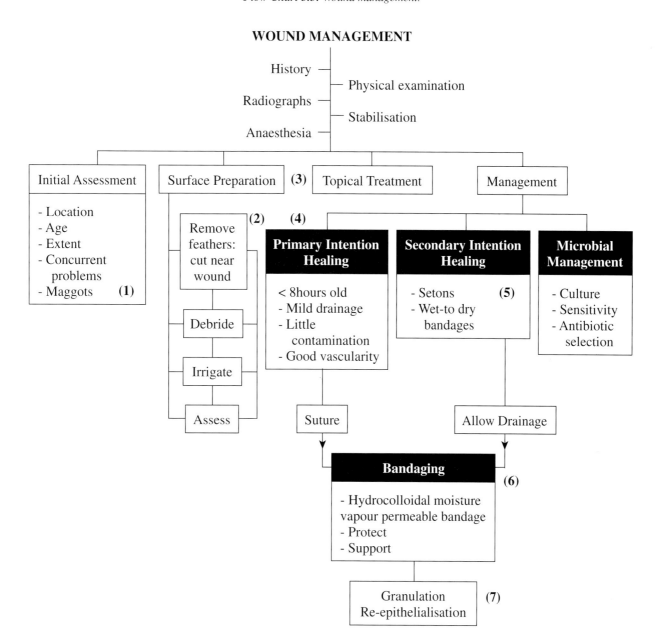

crop tube (see Figure 3.4.2) (comprising a syringe with either a curved stainless steel feeding needle or a rubber tube attached). A recipe and schedule for hyperalimentation is given in Chapter 4 (see Flow Charts 4.1 and 4.2). A commercially available alternative is the use of Hill's A/d convalescent diet. Other aspects of this procedure are available in the references (Quesenberry and Hillyer, 1993).

WOUND MANAGEMENT (see Flow Chart 3.5)

(1) It is extremely important during the warm months of the year to be especially diligent in examining wounds for any evidence of infestation with fly larvae. Due to the laying of live larvae by some species, the large numbers deposited and their fast rate of growth, large volumes of vital soft tissue can be consumed in a few hours.

(2) When removing the feathers in the vicinity of a wound, it is better to cut them right next to the skin rather than attempt to pluck them. Plucking feathers in this situation may well lead to tearing of the skin. Small, sharp-sharp, pointed iris scissors are effective.

(3) In general, application of topical wound treatment preparations is not recommended. In particular, nitro-furazone and gentamicin sulphate preparations retard wound healing. Bacitracin, neomycin and polymyxin preparations are used in avian wounds, and silver sulphadiazine is useful in managing burn wounds.

(4) The decision to manage a wound for primary intention healing is based upon the listed factors. For most body and wing wounds, debridement and

irrigation, along with surgical undermining of skin, will allow a primary closure or a delayed primary closure to be sought after a few days of cleaning. Wounds on the feet and toes are best managed by second intention healing.

(5) Open infected and severely contaminated wounds should be managed with wet-to-dry bandages for the first few days to facilitate the process of debridement. These consist of sterile gauze soaked in a sterile dilute povidone iodine/saline solution. Chlorhexidine may be used in place of the iodine. Exudates and debris cling to the gauze mesh, resulting in their removal as the bandages are changed. Setons (narrow gauze strips soaked in the above solution) should be packed into deeper wounds, especially those of the feet. In either application the gauze should be covered with a dry sterile layer of gauze, over which is wrapped a type of conforming bandage material, eg. Vetrap, (Degernes, 1993).

(6) Two types of wound dressing materials are available to cover a wound and promote granulation and epithelialisation after debridement is completed. Hydrocolloid or hydroactive dressings, eg. Duoderm or Granuflex, are spongy membrane materials that absorb fluid and exudate while retaining impermeability to moisture and oxygen. They adhere to normal skin but not wounds, and form a gelatinous mass over the wound which creates a very good environment for healing. Moisture vapour permeable dressings are clear polyurethane membranes with an adhesive backing, eg. BK Biodress. They are permeable to air, but not to water or bacteria. They, as well as hydrocolloid membranes, prevent scab formation and promote more rapid epithelialisation while preventing wound dessication.

(7) Once a clean wound site is established and granulation has begun, the application of topical ointments containing live yeast cell derivatives (LYCDs - haemorrhoid treatment products, eg. Preparation H) have been found to be effective in promoting rapid re-epithelialisation and collagen synthesis. Protective bandaging should be maintained until wounds are healed.

Acknowledgement

The author would like to acknowledge Dr Patricia Brown for her persistent efforts in preparing the Flow Charts through an extended series of revisions and for providing input and review of this material.

REFERENCES

Aguilar RA (1994) Shock, steroids and fluid therapy of the avian critical care patient. In: *Seminars in Avian and Exotic Animal Medicine and Surgery: Critical Care*. Eds A Fudge and JR Jenkins. WB Saunders, Philadelphia.

Aguilar RA and Redig PT (1995) Diagnosis and treatment of avian aspergillosis. In: *Current Veterinary Therapy XII*. Eds RW Kirk and JD Bonagura. WB Saunders, Philadelphia.

Bennington JL (1984) Ed *Saunders Dictionary and Encyclopedia of Laboratory Medicine and Technology*. WB Saunders, Philadelphia.

Degernes LA (1993) Trauma medicine. In: *Avian Medicine: Principles and Application*. Eds BW Ritchie, GJ Harrison and LR Harrison. Wingers, Lake Worth.

Goring RL, Goldman A, Kaufman KJ, Roberts C, Quesenberry KE and Kollias GV (1986) Needle catheter duodenostomy: a technique for duodenal alimentation of birds. *Journal of the American Veterinary Medical Association* **189**, 9.

Howard D and Redig PT (1993) Retrospective analysis of avian fracture repairs: implications for captive and wild birds. In: *Proceedings of the Association of Avian Veterinarians Annual Conference 1993*. AAV, Lake Worth.

Lumeij JT (1987) Plasma urea, creatinine and uric acid concentrations in response to dehydration in racing pigeons (*Columba livia domestica*). *Avian Pathology* **16**, 377.

Murphy CJ, Kern TJ, McKeever K, McKeever L and MacCoy D (1981) Ocular lesions in free-living raptors. *Journal of the American Veterinary Medical Association* **181**, 11.

Murray M (1994) Management of critical care avian trauma cases. In: *Seminars in Avian and Exotic Animal Medicine and Surgery: Critical Care*. Eds A Fudge and JR Jenkins. WB Saunders, Philadelphia.

Quesenberry KE and Hillyer EV (1993) Supportive care and emergency therapy. In: *Avian Medicine: Principles and Application*. Eds BW Ritchie, GJ Harrison and LR Harrison. Wingers, Lake Worth.

Redig PT (1984) Fluid therapy and acid-base balance in the critically ill avian patient. In: *Proceedings of the 1984 International Conference on Avian Medicine (sponsored by the Association of Avian Veterinarians)*. AAV, Lake Worth.

Redig PT (1987a) Radiographic review of orthopedic management of fractures in raptors. In: *Owl Rehabilitation*. 2nd Edn. Ed K McKeever. Vinland, Ontario.

Redig PT (1987b) The release of one-eyed, one-footed and other partially impaired raptors. In: *Proceedings of the International Wildlife Rehabilitator's Association Annual Symposium, Foster City Ca, 1987*. IWRA, Coconut Creek.

Redig PT (1992) Management of medical emergencies in raptors. In: *Current Veterinary Therapy XI*. Ed RW Kirk. WB Saunders, Philadelphia.

Samour JH, Bailey TA and Cooper JE (1995) Trichomoniasis in birds of prey (Order Falconiformes) in Bahrain. *Veterinary Record* **136**, 14.

Appendix 3.1. Stabilisation Protocol.

Agent	Dose schedules
Intravenous Lactated Ringers Solution (LRS)	10ml/kg bolus injection through a 22-27G catheter or needle may be given at a rate of 10ml/minute.
Dexamethasone (2mg/ml) or dexamethasone phosphate (4mg/ml)	2mg/kg, usually mixed with LRS as above.
Iron dextran	10mg/kg i/m.
B complex vitamins	Volume sufficient to provide 10mg/kg thiamine from preparation in use, i/m.
High calorific enteral preparation (see Flow Chart 4.1 for formulation recommendations)	10-15ml/kg. Stomach capacity of raptorial species is about 40ml/kg.
Enrofloxacin or other broad-spectrum antibiotic.	15mg/kg i/m or p/o, bid.

Appendix 3.2. Fluid Therapy: Sample Problem.

Patient:	Adult female Red-tailed Hawk with an open fracture of the humerus.
	Bodyweight: 1,040g.
	PCV: 28%
	TP: 2.6
	Hydration state: 10% dehydrated.
Fluid:	Fluid deficit: 1,040g x 0.10 = 104ml.
Requirements:	Maintenance: 50ml/kg/day.
Plan:	Replace 50% of deficit (+ maintenance) in the first 24 hours; the remainder (+ maintenance) over the next 48 hours.

Therapy	Administration
Day 1: 50% of deficit = 52ml Maintenance = 50ml Total = 102ml	Administer 25ml i/v qid = total of 100ml.
Day 2: 25% of deficit = 26ml Maintenance = 50ml Total = 76ml	Administer 25ml i/v tid = total of 75ml. Start oral alimentation.
Day 3: 50% of deficit = 26ml Maintenance = 50ml Total = 76ml	Administer 25ml i/v tid = total of 75ml
Day 4: Maintenance = 50ml	Provide maintenance fluids in two doses, ie. 25ml i/v bid. Oral alimentation as indicated. Increase solid intake to near normal levels.

CHAPTER FOUR

Nursing Avian Patients

Patrick T Redig

INTRODUCTION

In many respects it is the nursing of avian patients which differs greatly from other fields of small animal work. It is, however, the most important.

ACCOMMODATION

The hospital requirements of bird patients differ from those of cats and dogs. Many birds are already stressed and shocked (see Chapter 3) prior to presentation. Confinement, proximity to humans, dogs, cats or predatory birds all tend to increase that stress, although different species and individuals will be variably affected. With the exception of waterfowl, most birds are accustomed to being above man and other stressors in their surroundings or are able to flee threatening conditions; high cages help to maintain this height advantage which reduces stress. Unless habituated to man, birds benefit from being protected from the continual sight and sound of human activity. Unhabituated birds are best kept in a quiet, darkened environment, by hanging a clean blanket or similar on the inside of their cage door. Covers are useful; however, greater attention must be made to regular patient observation, as they are less easily observed by passing nurses or clinicians. Most birds benefit from subdued lighting, although sufficient light for regular feeding is essential (this is less important for raptors who naturally eat less often). Ideally, birds should be maintained in a separate ward, away from the sounds of cats and dogs. Although both pigeons and waterfowl (with the exception of aggressive or territorial waterfowl species - see Chapter 33) will frequently benefit from the sight of other similar birds, no bird of any group should ever be hospitalised within sight of any raptor.

When designing housing for birds, consideration should be made to the likelihood of the spread of infectious diseases between patients. Attention must be paid to airborne infections, especially zoonoses: for example, chlamydiosis which is a common infection in pigeons, sometimes occurs in waterfowl, and is occasionally seen in raptors. The room must be well ventilated, readily cleaned and with no dust traps. Local health and safety rules should be posted on the entrance to the avian ward and the avian treatment area warning staff of the potential risk. The public should be excluded from such areas (see Chapter 12). The cage materials should be impermeable and readily cleaned and disinfected. A removable floor tray may be used for ease of cleaning or, alternatively, a layer of disposable paper. Cage doors should consist of vertical bars only, as mesh doors cause considerable feather damage. Door cleaning is easiest if the doors are hung on bayonet hinges, so that they can be lifted off and immersed in cleansing and disinfectant solutions.

Perching

The tree and perching ducks, pigeons and raptors all naturally want to perch whenever they have the opportunity. Not only do they feel happier and more at home, but also the use of suitable perches lifts the wings and tail feathers off the floor of the cage, thereby reducing feather damage. All hospitalised raptors should have a tail guard applied in order to protect the tail whilst hospitalised (see Figure 14.4). Perches may be readily constructed of blocks of wood, or bricks covered in a towel, blanket, old carpet or Astroturf. Any such materials must be disposable or easily and completely cleaned. Perches for pigeons are easily prepared from natural wood branches. Clinics regularly dealing with raptors should equip themselves with standard 'block' and 'bow' perches (see Chapter 13). Bathing is essential for many birds, unless contraindicated as a consequence of their treatment. Baths should be no deeper than 2cm for smaller birds and up to 6cm for large raptors, eg. buteos and eagles, and they should be designed to prevent drowning. Wherever possible, baths should be supplied at the birds' body temperature (40-41°C), although they should not be maintained at that temperature. In waterfowl the opportunity to bathe not only stimulates preening but is essential for maintaining the waterproofing of the feathers. Keeping waterfowl away from water for even a few days can lead to permanent damage to that set of feathers. Regular access to water is also essential for the integrity of the feet of waterfowl. Waterfowl deprived of regular access to water may suffer 'vent gleet'. The latter is a localised cloacal infection, typically with *Pseudomonas* spp., which arises as a consequence of the bird not being able to defecate naturally into water whilst swimming.

Handling and Treatments

Handling of birds should always be kept to a minimum. If possible the same nurse should carry out all injections and gavage feeding, whilst a different nurse is responsible for observation and monitoring. If possible, either a closed-circuit television monitor (high tech approach) or a wide-angle lens viewer installed in the door of the room (low tech approach) should be used; this will allow observation without entering the room. Birds will frequently not relax when in view of a person whom they regard as a threat.

PHYSIOLOGICAL CONSIDERATIONS OF A HIGH METABOLIC RATE

Birds have a higher basal metabolic rate than the mammals commonly encountered in veterinary practice. The smaller the bird the higher the rate. This has a number of important implications. As the body surface area to body volume ratio increases, so does the rate of heat loss. This leads to increased utilisation of body energy reserves simply to maintain body temperature. For this reason, ill birds should be maintained at 25-30°C or, for a very sick bird, even at 35°C for an initial 24-48 hour period. By maintaining a high environmental temperature the patient utilises less

Flow Chart 4.1: Nursing care for debilitated avian patients.

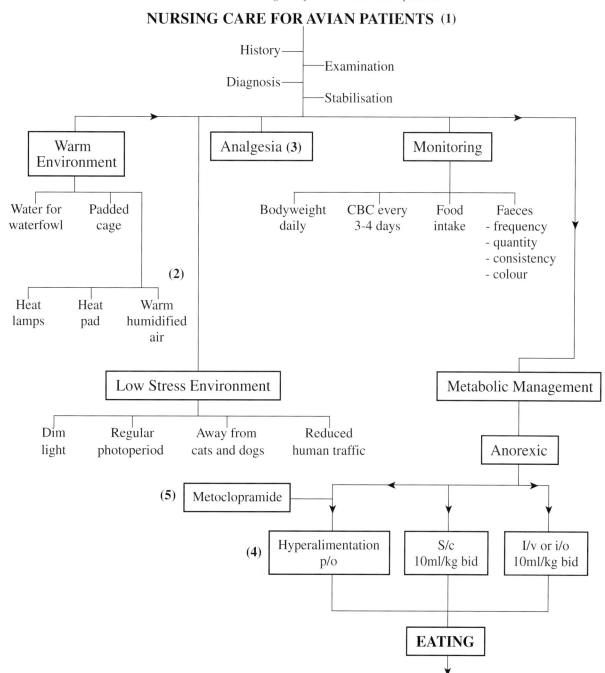

energy to counteract lost body heat. Birds which have lost feather integrity due to waterlogging, oiling, contamination, damage or feather loss will suffer greater heat loss.

A range of avian hospital cages is now available in which temperature and humidity can be controlled as well as allowing nebulisation medication and maintenance of an oxygen rich environment. Similar conditions can be provided by using a standard human baby incubator; as and when they become obsolete, baby incubators may be available from human hospitals. Circulated water heating pads, eg. K-pads, and infrared lamps can also be used. Infrared lamps, because they heat only the area on which they are directed, allow the bird to choose whether to stand under the heat or away from it depending on its personal comfort level. However, they should not be used in cases where the bird is unable to move.

NURSING CARE FOR AVIAN PATIENTS
(see Flow Chart 4.1)

(1) This protocol considers the general needs of all hospitalised avian patients and has a specific section on metabolic management, which addresses the management of extremely debilitated birds that require an intensive care approach in meeting their daily nutritional needs. The objective of this protocol is to establish the patient on a pathway of positive weight gain from the first day of hospitalisation.

(2) A relative humidity of 60-70% can be achieved by passing the incoming air through a nebuliser that contains either water or saline diluted 50:50 with sterile water.

(3) The true effects of analgesics in birds are unknown. Birds have apparently high thresholds for pain tolerance. The following agents have been used without adverse effect:
- Butorphanol (3-4mg/kg i/m).
- Flunixin meglumine (1-10mg/kg i/m) or ketoprofen (1-5mg/kg i/m bid).
- Acetylsalicylic acid (aspirin). No dosage recommendations are available, but 0.5 grains (30mg/200g bodyweight) has been used without adverse effect (Murray, 1994).

(4) Hyperalimentation may be provided with homemade concoctions or with any of a number of commercially available products, eg. Critical Care Formula (Vetark), Emeraide, Hill's A/d. Greater consistency in nutrient and calorific content may be attained with commercial products, but such inconsistency is not necessarily an overwhelming concern.

A recipe used by The Raptor Center at the University of Minnesota for hyperalimentation of raptors is shown below. It contains sufficient water, calories and protein to produce a weight gain in birds maintained on this programme.
- Prepare a 30% solution of Nutrical (Evsco Phar-

maceutical) in an electrolyte solution, ie. 70ml of electrolyte and 30ml of Nutrical. Make up 500-1,000ml and store in a refrigerator.
- Add two parts of human infant 'second food' series meat paste (beef, veal, chicken or turkey) to one part of the 30% solution. A convenient volume to make is 90ml, ie. one 60g jar of baby food plus 30ml of 30% Nutrical. Store in a refrigerator and make a new batch each day.
- Administer to the patient via a crop tube at a rate of 40ml/kg tid - monitor by weighing daily.

(5) Metoclopramide (2mg/kg i/m, administered at the time of feeding) is effective in overcoming crop stasis and ileus of the gastrointestinal tract.

NURSING CARE FOR RAPTORS IN LOW CONDITION
(see Flow Chart 4.2)

(1) Raptors affected with this condition typically present with a history of active use in the field for falconry over a period of 4-6 weeks or more during which time they have been maintained at their 'flying weight'. At this weight, most raptors have been dietarily managed so that they are in a lean body state, a state which is a motivation to pursue game. The immediate clinical condition appears to have had a very rapid onset, although the bird has actually been in a generalised state of catabolism for an extended period of time and now no longer has the energy to compensate. A sudden lowering of environmental temperature often precipitates the condition.

(2) The problem is most commonly seen in male birds during their first field season.

(3) The condition is seen most frequently 4-8 weeks into the bird's flying season.

(4) Immediate recognition of this problem is imperative as the birds usually have only a few hours to live when presented. Laboratory tests should consist of only those that can be conducted immediately and on site. A packed cell volume (typically < 20%, although it can be as high as 35%) and total proteins (by refractometer) (invariably < 10g/l) determination is sufficient to confirm the diagnosis based on history and signalment. Treatment must begin immediately.

(5) Sour crop is a fluctuating, fluid-filled, swollen crop accompanying low condition. It occurs as a result of crop stasis and subsequent bacterial proliferation. The problem may be exacerbated by the actions of the bird's owner; upon discovering the bird in an acutely weakened condition, the owner will often feed the bird a bulging crop full of food. Crop stasis ensues and endotoxins produced by bacterial action in the crop worsen the clinical condition of the bird, frequently leading to a rapid death.

(6) The disruption of gastrointestinal function and general stress associated with this condition, along with antibiotic therapy, renders the patient more susceptible

Flow Chart 4.2: Nursing care for raptors in low condition.

LOW CONDITION

to infections by *Candida* spp. and *Aspergillus* spp. Therefore, prophylactic therapy with antifungal agents is recommended (see Flow Chart 3.2).

(7) If a crop full of decaying meat is present, it is imperative that the meat is removed. Isoflurane anaesthesia is well tolerated, even by toxic birds. Following induction, the bird should be intubated in order to eliminate the risk of an iatrogenic inhalation pneumonia. The clinician may then retrieve the food by massaging it into the back of the mouth and removing it with a curved forceps. Alternatively, a midline incision may be made in the crop to allow direct access for removal. Once the food has been removed, flushing several times with 10ml volumes of warm saline or 0.1% chlorhexidine in warm saline will reduce the level of pathogens and endotoxins in the crop.

(8) Feeding and fluid regimens as recommended for treatment for an extremely sick bird should be implemented (see Flow Chart 3.4). It is necessary to monitor continuously the vital signs of a bird recovering from this condition.

(9) Treatment for endotoxic shock consists of the fluid and steroid regimens outlined in the stabilisation treatment protocol (see Appendix 3.1). It is advantageous, however, to use dexamethasone phosphate at twice the regular dose, ie. 4mg/kg i/v (Redig, 1992).

FOOD REQUIREMENTS FOR AVIAN PATIENTS

The smaller the bird the greater the percentage of its bodyweight it must eat daily in order to maintain body condition (see Table 4.1).

Although raptors are accustomed to filling their crop with a single large meal once daily, it is not advisable to give an ill raptor such a large volume at one time

Table 4.1. Feeding requirements of a bird in relation to its bodyweight.

Bodyweight (g)	Percentage of bodyweight required daily (%)
100-200	18-25
201-800	11-19
801-1,200	7-11
4,000-10,000	3.5-6

for fear of 'sour crop' (see Flow Chart 4.2).

If avian patients are not self-feeding, nourishment is required at least five times daily. Small birds (< 200g) require hourly feeding. Birds that are ill or shocked have an even greater energy requirement than normal, healthy birds. Wherever possible, hospitalised birds should be weighed at a regular time each day; this will give a rapid indication of the birds' progress. Hospitalised waterfowl should be offered clean, fresh green river or pond weed, as well as cereals (which should be offered both dry and submerged in water). Pigeons are easily fed on standard proprietary pigeon cereal mixes. Raptors are fed on day-old cockerels or mice, rats, pigeons, quail or rabbits (see Chapter 13). If a bird is not eating for itself, it is important that any convalescent food given by crop tube is similar in constitution, albeit more digestible, than its normal food. Raptors should receive an animal protein-based diet, whilst waterfowl and pigeons should receive a cereal-based diet. Although raptors normally ingest 'casting' material, ie. fur or feathers, which is regurgitated *per os* some 12-18 hours later, the administration of such material precludes additional food in the interim. No 'casting' should be given to sick raptors; they may then be fed as often as required in order to maintain or increase bodyweight.

The correct use of fluid therapy (see Chapter 3) and nutritional supplementation will save the lives of more birds than any other form of therapy (see Flow Charts 3.4, 4.1, 4.2).

REFERENCES

Redig PT (1992) Management of medical emergencies in raptors. In: *Current Veterinary Therapy XI*. Eds RW Kirk and JD Bonagura. WB Saunders, Philadelphia.

Murray M (1994) Management of critical avian trauma cases. In: *Seminars in Avian and Exotic Animal Medicine and Surgery: Critical Care*. Eds A Fudge and JR Jenkins. WB Saunders, Philadelphia.

CHAPTER FIVE

Principles of Therapy

Gerry M Dorrestein

INTRODUCTION

The knowledge of the principles of therapy in birds is rapidly expanding. Large interspecies differences in relation to metabolic elimination, anatomy and physiology of the digestive and respiratory system, and differences in drug distribution do exist. As in mammals, formulation of the dosage form and the presence of disease conditions may influence drug efficacy (Dorrestein, 1993).

Drug preparations licensed for use in raptors and waterfowl are generally not available. A few licensed preparations are available for pigeons. Formulations licensed for other species (including poultry, mammals and man) may be administered under the responsibility of the veterinarian who has the animal 'under his care' (Bishop, 1996). Preparations which have not been clinically tested can be dangerous to birds, even when highly effective against the isolated agent and compatible in other animals.

Although similar diseases and conditions may affect raptors, pigeons and waterfowl, methods of housing and rearing and whether the birds are kept for hunting or rehabilitation, for exhibition or racing, or for ornamental purposes or even for production, leads to varying treatment regimens.

The basis for the successful management of any avian patient is knowledge of the principles and techniques of supportive care and emergency medicine (Quesenberry and Hillyer, 1994). Although the basic concepts of therapy of small animal medicine apply to birds, adaptations must be made to compensate for their unique anatomy and physiology.

Stabilisation of the patient is essential, especially in a critically ill bird. It is not sufficient to start 'an antibacterial therapy'. Other major components might include additional medical and surgical components such as fluid therapy, tube feeding, debridement of inflammatory tissue or drainage of exudate. The physiology of metabolism, body temperature, temperature regulation, heat loss, heat stress and the role of water economy, eg. waterfowl are less economical with water than pigeons, are essential elements in understanding and correcting the derailments of normal functioning.

THE HIGH BODY TEMPERATURE OF BIRDS

Birds have a high metabolic rate. Flight and maintenance of high body temperature (endothermia) use large amounts of energy. In general, the rates of physiologic processes increase with temperature (Gill, 1994). However, the maintenance of high body temperatures through endothermia is energetically expensive; birds consume 20-30 times more energy than do similar sized reptiles. Both the circulatory and respiratory systems have evolved exceptional capacities for the delivery of energy and oxygen to the body's cells as well as rapid removal of poisonous metabolic waste products.

Birds regulate their body temperatures at 40-42°C by adjusting plumage insulation, by increasing heat production through shivering when cold, and by evaporative water loss through panting and gular fluttering when hot. Regulation of blood flow through the feet, particularly in Anseriformes (with special vessels), aids heat loss or retention. Heat production during flight can be lost quickly with little loss of water. However, birds have little latitude for higher body temperatures: 46°C is lethal.

LEVELS OF METABOLISM

Basal Metabolism

All birds have a high basal metabolic rate (BMR). For their various sizes, passerine birds have the highest rates of any group of vertebrate animals. The average BMR of a passerine bird is 50-60% higher than those of non-passerines of the same body size. There are, however, exceptions in both directions.

Basal metabolism relates directly to mass, although not in a 1:1 relationship. In most cases the relationship is given by the formula $BMR = K(WKg^{0.75})$. K = a theoretical constant for kcal required per 24 hours and varies with the species of bird. K is 129 for passerines and 78 for non-passerines.

The formula reflects the relationship between metabolism and mass in the context of the surface area from which heat is lost. This formula is essential for calculating the daily energy needs of a bird suffering from illness or stress and with a decreased nutritional intake. In addition, the BMR is sometimes used for extrapolating a drug dosage regimen from one species to another.

Activity Metabolism

Basal metabolism represents the expenditure of minimal energy. A bird usually spends only a fraction of its day at this low metabolic level. In clinical situations, the maintenance energy requirement (MER) is used. This is defined as the BMR plus additional energy (approximately 1.5 times the BMR in adult birds) needed for normal physiologic activity, digestion and absorption (Quesenberry and Hillyer, 1994).

Birds that are growing, diseased or stressed are in a hypermetabolic state with daily energy needs 1-3 times the normal requirement. Raptors which are not eating generally have no fluid intake, therefore food and water supplementation is essential for sick birds (see Chapter 3).

Flight is generally a more efficient form of locomotion than running. To fly one kilometre, a 10g bird uses less than 1% of the energy that a 10g mouse uses to run the same distance. Peak reproductive activities increase total daily energy expenditures by as much as 50%. Moulting draws significantly on protein and energy reserves to synthesise feather structure and also to offset the effects of poorer insulation and flight efficacy. The increase in daily metabolism during peak periods of feather production can be as high as 15-25%.

BASIC PRINCIPLES OF PHARMACOTHERAPY

Medication of birds is accomplished by the same methods of administration used in mammals, but with several special considerations (Dorrestein, 1993). In avian medicine, many dosage regimens have been designed largely on an empirical basis. However, as the knowledge of drug disposition and metabolism in various avian species expands, it is increasingly evident that differences exist in dosage, dosage interval and organ distribution, not only between birds and mammals but between individual avian species. It is not possible to speak of 'the bird' because of the large number of totally different species, even when we are 'only' dealing with raptors or waterfowl. Each group consists of many different species. In pigeons there is more experience and a substantial amount of pharmacokinetic data is available.

Optimal use of drugs, including the treatment of infectious diseases, depends on diagnosis, sensitivity to the drug, potential toxicity, pharmacokinetics and dynamics of the drug, husbandry practices, anatomical and physiological differences between the species and many other considerations. Furthermore, it should be realised that the pharmacokinetics of drugs can be substantially changed by disease, especially when organs that play a major role in the absorption, biotransformation and excretion of drugs, eg. intestine, liver and kidney, are involved. This becomes especially important when the excretion of drugs with a low therapeutic index is impaired. Another important point is that it is not only the plasma (blood) concentration which is clinically relevant but, especially, the concentration at the site of action.

The relationship between bacterial identification and the need for antibiotic therapy is a tenuous one. The identification and isolation of potential bacterial pathogens is not a 'green light' for the recommendation of antibiotic administration. Rather, it should act as a signal that further consideration is necessary to reach a therapeutic plan if it is deemed necessary (Worell, 1993). Also, the finding of coccidial organisms in a faecal sample does not necessarily indicate anticoccidial therapy. The clinical evaluation of the patient should, at least, support the laboratory findings.

Environmental evaluation and manipulation, coupled with good hygiene, husbandry and nutrition, should always be considered as part of a therapeutic plan to aid in correcting a potential infectious problem (Fudge et al, 1992).

SENSITIVITY TESTS AND INTERPRETATION

The decision whether or not to begin antibiotic therapy before culture and sensitivity test results are available depends on the clinical situation. Some antibiotics, such as chloramphenicol, (chlor)tetracycline and doxycycline, are known to suppress the immune system and may actually make the situation worse when a fungal infection rather than a bacterial infection is present. On the other hand, birds are often critically ill when they suffer from bacterial infections and postponing antibiotic therapy until culture results are available could be fatal. However, when appropriate samples are taken before treatment is started, this may help the practitioner to correct the therapy when remission of clinical signs does not occur.

Under optimal conditions the sensitivity test is important in selecting antimicrobial therapy. It is becoming more obvious that the breakpoints between sensitive and insensitive in avian medicine may be different from the accepted standard in human and mammalian medicine. A reason for this is that the attainable blood levels for many drugs might be lower in birds than in mammals. This is due to short elimination half-lives, different bioavailability and different administration routes (Dorrestein 1993; Flammer, 1994).

Treatment failure may occur even when the drugs are reported as sensitive in vitro. Reasons for this include inappropriate drugs, failure to reach the effective minimum inhibitory concentration (MIC) in blood or tissues, inadequate treatment intervals or length, compromised tissues, inadequate host immune system and persistent exposure to environmental sources of the organism. If no clinical response is seen within 48 hours, a change to an antibiotic from another group should be considered and, in addition, the diagnosis and therapeutic approach should be re-evaluated.

ROUTES AND METHODS OF ADMINISTRATION

Medication may be accomplished either by individual bolus dosing or by treating on an individual or flock basis by mixing the drug with feed or drinking water. Individual treatment of raptors requires special skill in handling the bird. Although the desired formulation of drugs for avian species is often dictated by the most practical or economical method of administration, the route of administration is often limited by the drug formulation available. In general, medicated food and drinking water are the traditionally favoured routes for poultry but they seldom achieve therapeutic drug concentrations in companion and aviary birds. Most virulent microbial infections must be treated by the direct oral route or a parenteral route (Flammer, 1994).

Factors influencing the route of administration and dosage regimen in birds are:
- Severity of the disease or infection.
- Flock versus individual treatment.
- Tame or domesticated versus wild birds.
- Large versus tiny birds.
- Seed-eating versus meat(fish)-eating birds.
- So-called food specialists.
- Anatomical differences.
- Behavioural or environmental differences.
- Availability of drug formulations.
- Frequency of administration.
- Ability of the owner to complete the treatment regimen.
- Economics (and registration demands).

The route of administration is also influenced by the drug chosen, eg. some drugs can be given only by one (or more) specified routes.

DOSE EXTRAPOLATION

The available dosage regimens for birds are based on information available from empirical and experimental data. For other drugs or other species the dosage regimen needs to be extrapolated from available data. Although species are sometimes considered to be similar in their metabolism of drugs, this belief may lead either to inadequate therapy or to toxicity. Therefore, when this information is not available, extrapolation is best based on metabolic extrapolation (allometric scaling). Allometric scaling is a method that can be used to predict dosages of pharmaceuticals for non-traditional animals (Sedgwick and Pokras, 1988). Basically, the metabolic rate rather than bodyweight is used for dose estimation. Allometric scaling allows the translation of a dosage regimen from mg/kg^{-1} to $mg/kcal^{-1}$ units.

The metabolic rate is more closely related to body surface than to body mass. The half-life of a drug that is metabolised and eliminated by the body will decrease as the metabolic rate increases. However, the BMR in birds (K=78) does not differ significantly from mammals (K=70) as a Class, with the exception of Passeriformes (K=129). Therefore, differences found in pharmacokinetics between endothermic animals are often predominantly related to differences in body surface or metabolic weight and sometimes to differences in metabolic pathways.

The fate of a drug in the body (protein binding, volume of distribution, biotransformation and excretion) can differ between species (sometimes strains of a species), since the relationship between transformation and excretion is determined by BMR and heredity (different metabolic pathways or metabolites). In general, there is minimal variation among species in the manner by which polar compounds (like gentamicin) are handled by the excretion mechanisms. This is in contrast with the wide interspecies variations and unpredictability associated with biotransformation of extensively metabolised drugs, eg. chloramphenicol and sulphonamides.

Chloramphenicol is an example of an antibiotic which is eliminated by biotransformation (conjugation with glucuronic acid and by reduction to inactive aryl amines). Differences in the rate of elimination (elimination half-life 0.4 hours in pigeons to 5.1 hours in cat) are most likely related to differences in rates of biotransformation existing among the various species (Davis *et al*, 1972; Clark *et al*, 1982).

In general, mammalian carnivorous species will conjugate xenobiotics more slowly or to a lesser extent than herbivorous species, whereas omnivorous species are in between. As in mammals, notable differences in half-life between Orders of birds are found. In raptors the concentration two hours after administration is unexpectedly high relative to the half-life, which could indicate a lower metabolic turnover as is found in mammalian carnivores.

Allometric scaling can be used to help tailor drug dosages to different body sizes; however, it does not take into account variations in metabolic pathways for drugs between species. However, these limitations are also generally valid for the direct extrapolation. Without using the current knowledge about pharmacokodynamics and allometric scaling, especially in raptors, treatment regimens can be inadequate and sometimes potentially dangerous (Cooper, 1993). Consequently, when enough information is available, the therapeutic regimens should be adapted for each species.

Flow Chart 5.1: Therapy of a sick bird.

COMPARATIVE ANATOMY IN RELATION TO DRUG ADMINISTRATION

The oral route is often used for administration of drugs to avian species. When the drug preparation is a suspension, capsule or tablet, release from the dosage form is frequently a rate-limiting step in the overall absorption process. Because of marked differences in the anatomy of the digestive system of birds, variations can be expected in both rate and extent of drug absorption from an oral formulation (Dorrestein, 1993). Availability and absorption are influenced by crop, crop-flora, crop pH, gizzard function and morphology, the presence of grit, form and function of the intestines, the presence of functional caeca and an indigenous microflora.

The differences between birds and mammals in their response to nebulisation are the result of the unique anatomy and physiology of the avian respiratory system. Anatomical differences in lung structure (neo-

and paleopulmo - see Chapter 18) and the lack of physical activity of the sick bird during treatment will, even under optimal technical conditions, reduce a drugs access to only 20% of the lung tissue in many bird species. The cranial air sacs will not be reached at all. At rest there is no air exchange in most of the respiratory tract. Nevertheless, therapeutic levels in the lungs and air sacs are reported after nebulisation in several birds (Locke and Bush, 1984). To establish local drug levels in the lungs and air sacs, the particles or drops should be between 1-3μm. In chickens, aerosolised particles between 3-7μm are generally deposited on the mucosal surface of the nasal cavity and trachea. The primary benefit of nebulisation is to humidify the air and treat locally any respiratory tract conditions. Nebulisation is an excellent method of preventing dehydration of a patient, which can occur when respiratory distress increases evaporative water loss in a heated hospitalisation cage.

Local therapeutic levels of drugs in the respiratory tract, eg. amphotericin B, can be attained by intratracheal application or by using an air sac tube (Quesenberry and Hillyer, 1994).

METHODS OF DRUG ADMINISTRATION

There are many routes for drug administration. The choice is dependent on many different factors. A short review of the different routes is given in Flow Chart 5.1.
(1) Parenteral: always work aseptically. Advantages: blood levels will be rapidly attained; can be used in uncooperative or unconscious birds. Disadvantages: should be carried out by the clinician (cost may be a factor); can cause muscle damage or haematoma; often large volumes required.
(2) Intraosseous: only use in emergencies or in neonates where other routes are impracticable. Advantages: simulates the i/v route; can be used for fluid replacement. Disadvantages: requires hospitalisation; risk of osteomyelitis.
(3) Subcutaneous: avian skin is non-elastic; small volumes may need to be given at differing sites.
(4) Intramuscular: can lead to haematoma/necrosis.
(5) Intravenous: may be difficult to locate and access a vein. Repeated doses may be administered by the use of an indwelling catheter. Risk of considerable haematoma.
(6) Intratracheal: mostly used for fungal infections. Advantage: topical therapy is often efficacious for fungal infections whilst parenteral therapy is of limited efficacy. Disadvantage: risk of aspiration pneumonia or suffocation.
(7) Nebulisation: used for local application to the upper respiratory tract (see Chapter 18). Advantages: drugs which are relatively toxic when given parenterally may often be given safely via this route; little stress involved in repeated medication; also humidifies inspired air. Disadvantages: no lower respiratory or blood levels; can lead to environmental contamination, with the risk of exposure of staff.
(8) Topical: skin, conjunctiva. Advantage: direct application to the site of the insult. Disadvantages: ingestion during preening may cause intoxication - always apply minimal amounts - steroid containing creams can cause polydipsia etc. if used excessively; any topical oil based product is likely to affect the feathers adversely - this is particularly significant in waterfowl.
(9) Capsule/tablet: preferably administer on an empty crop with small amounts of food or at beginning of feeding. Advantages: can be successfully administered by the owner; definite drug volume administered to specific bird, as long as vomiting of the capsule/tablet does not occur. Disadvantages: capsule or tablet may stick to the mucosa on administration causing mucosal damage; due to the storage effect of the crop the rate of release and absorption can be unpredictable; time consuming on a flock basis.

(10) Fluid/suspension: especially in a cooperative bird or by gavage; never in an unconscious or semi-conscious bird. Advantages: arrival in the gut within a few minutes; good absorption; easy to administer the correct dose. Disadvantages: often stressful as may require casting and forced gavage; risk of regurgitation and aspiration; time consuming in flocks.
(11) Medicated food: medication for raptors may be given hidden in meat. For whole grain eating birds, powder will adhere to seed when mixed with vegetable or olive oil. Advantages: self-administration; no stress; for seed eating birds, will self-medicate all day; useful in a flock situation; generally very reliable blood levels or gut concentrations. Disadvantages: seeds must be coated or the bird must eat a mash or pellet; taste may influence food intake; interaction between food and drug is not always predictable; raptors may pick through meat and discard medication.
(12) Medicated water: Advantages: easy to dose for individuals and flocks; can be used for local medication of the gut. Disadvantages: for systemic use, blood levels are often totally unreliable; often insufficient consumed because of taste; some drugs unstable in water; waterfowl cannot be maintained off water; raptors consume little or no water (although it must always be available).
(13) (14) Patient monitoring: must always be carried out for response to therapy.
(15) (16) Vomiting: some birds will vomit following oral administration of drugs. See Chapter 4 for nursing care of the vomiting bird.

Flock Versus Individual Treatment
Pigeons and waterfowl are mostly kept in flocks or large numbers of breeding couples confined to separate flight pens or ponds. Most raptors are housed individually or in couples. The approach to medication will depend on the situation presented at the time of treatment. While individual sick birds are often treated, a loft of pigeons should be considered as a colony (Debuf, 1994). Parasitic infections, for example, may only appear to affect some birds clinically, but most of the birds in the loft are likely to harbour the infection. Therefore, individual treatment is often given to sick birds, with simultaneous mass medication to the colony.

Flock treatment regimens for poultry have been fairly extensively researched and are often, but not always, applicable when treating flocks of pigeons or waterfowl. When a drug is to be used for the first time in a flock of birds, a small number of the birds should be treated first to assess possible toxic effects.

When dealing with individual birds the drug administration techniques might differ from those commonly used in individual mammals. Techniques differ when dealing with the individual tame bird or wild bird, a breeding flock or a hand-feeding bird. Since many drugs are rapidly eliminated in birds, the maintenance of therapeutic levels requires frequent dosage, which necessitates excessive handling of the birds. Individual handling and physical restraint are stressful and must be minimised. The value of frequent administration of drugs must then be weighed against the stress caused by handling.

Individual Oral Dosage Forms

Tablets
Tablets are not commonly used for the treatment of large numbers of birds because the administration can be both time-consuming and uncertain. However, in individual birds, especially raptors, it is an easy method and one that can be handled easily by the owner.

Tablets available for humans or other mammals can contain too much of the drug. Administering part of a tablet will make the dosage uncertain. Pigeons, as with many other seed-eating birds, have a crop that forms a storage organ for seeds or grains. The crop does not differentiate between a grain or a tablet. The unpredictable emptying time of the crop, the lack of a large volume of fluid and the relatively high pH make the crop incomparable to the mammalian stomach. Administration into an empty crop improves the uniformity of the pharmacokinetics. The problems can be overcome by grinding the tablet, making a suspension and feeding it by crop cannula (see Figure 3.4).

There are tablets licensed for pigeons. These are antiparasitic drugs (carnidazole, clazuril, levamisole and praziquantel). These drugs need to be dosed only once to be effective and the onset of activity after administration is less important. Most of these tablets do not need to be administered into an empty crop and will not disintegrate before arriving in the gizzard, resulting in a bolus delivery.

Capsules
Capsules are a good alternative dosage form to tablets. They are preferably administered into an empty crop. Capsules are specially useful for the treatment of individual raptors, pigeons and ducks. In avian medicine the capsule is used also as a container for drugs to be applied to the food or drinking water. It gives an exact measure for medication in a small amount of food or volume of water.

Solutions and Suspensions
Solutions and suspensions are seldom used on a large scale for direct administration to birds. If used, they should be administered directly into the empty crop by gavage using metal tubes, plastic catheters or syringes. A disadvantage of all liquid drug forms is that the administration may result in regurgitation or inhalation, especially when given into the upper oesophagus; some of the dose may be lost or aspiration pneumonia may occur. In raptors, regurgitation may be prevented by offering a small piece of meat after

administration of the drug. Alternatively, the medication can be given on an empty stomach and the bird not fed for at least two hours after administration. Solutions and suspensions can be mixed with food and administered by gavage, especially in handfed birds or sick birds requiring fluids and nutrients. In individual raptors the addition of drugs to a piece of meat increases the chance of acceptance. When possible the medication should be given in several portions during the day.

Cloacal Administration
The cloacal route is sometimes used as an alternative to non-parenteral administration.

Parenteral Dosage Forms
Parenteral administration is the most exact and effective method for administering drugs. This route is mainly used in individual birds that are difficult to handle, critically ill birds or birds that are unconscious. An exception to this is the treatment of chlamydiosis with doxycycline or long-acting oxytetracycline: these birds need be injected once weekly only. Aseptic procedures must be strictly adhered to with all parenteral applications.

Intramuscular (i/m) Injection
Parenteral preparations are most commonly administered into the caudal portion of the pectoral muscle close to the keel. With the bird restrained in ventral recumbency, the caudal edge of the sternum should be palpated and the needle introduced cranially into the pectoral muscle, parallel to the sternum. This places the bolus into the pectoral muscle without risking injection into the liver through either the medial fenestra or the lateral incisura, one or both of these being found in the sternum of many species. The venous plexus, which lies between the superficial and deep pectoral muscle, should not be punctured. A disadvantage is the relatively large volume that may have to be injected. Therefore, individual birds should be carefully weighed and appropriate dilutions and syringes should be used to enable accurate dosing. Repeated injections into the same side of the breast or the i/m use of irritating drugs may result in muscle necrosis or atrophy. I/m injection of irritating formulations increases the creatine phosphokinase (CK), alanine-aminotransferase (ASAT) and aspartate-aminotransferase (ALAT) activity. Drugs administered into the posterior pectoral muscle or legs may pass through the renal portal system prior to entering the general circulation. Sympathetic stimulation tends to open the valves in the renal portal system, resulting in a direct flow of the blood from the caudal part of the bird to the *vena cava caudalis* (Skadhauge, 1981).

Subcutaneous (s/c) Injection
The s/c route into the dorsal neck region or the groin

is often a preferable alternative, but because of minimal amounts of dermis and the low elasticity of the skin, part of the fluid may flow out. Irritating drugs may cause skin necrosis and ulceration. The dorsal neck region is also the site of choice for s/c fluid infusions (see Figure 3.3).

Intravenous (i/v) Injection
I/v injections into the right jugular or the ulnar vein should be reserved for emergencies, for one-time drug administration and for catheter placement for repeat administrations. In raptors the left jugular vein might sometimes be more accessible. Veins may also be needed for blood withdrawal for diagnostic tests (see Figures 3.1, 3.2).

Other Routes
If repeated drug administration is required, the intraosseous route (see Figure 3.1) allows stable access to the intravascular space (Flammer, 1994). Air spaces may be effectively reached by intratracheal or air sac injections. Joints and sinuses are other sites in which direct injection of drugs may be useful.

Topical Medications
Topical medications include skin application for local or systemic action, eye drops and ointments, nasal flushes, infraorbital sinus injections, intratracheal injections and administration directly into an air sac.

External applications should be applied carefully and sparingly because they will mat the feathers. If medications are ingested when the bird preens, they may cause toxicosis.

Medication in Feed or Water
The major methods of administering drugs to poultry and other birds are via feed and water. This is based largely on convenience and the difficulties associated with individual administration to large numbers of birds.

Feed Medication
Feed medication in avian medicine is a reliable way of medicating birds, as long as the birds are still eating normally. The total intake of drug with the food during the day should be equal to the desired day-dose calculated on an individual basis. Some birds may have a reduced feed intake and may require adjustment of the drug concentration in their feed. However, the interactions between a drug and food cannot be entirely predicted, and the dosage forms need to be evaluated. The only proof of bioavailability is pharmacokinetic study in various species.

Pigeons and most waterfowl are grain-eating or pellet-eating birds, a type of food that is not suitable for mixing homogeneously. In some cases, when large quantities are required, medicated pellets can be prepared. It may take time to get the feed mixed at a mill.

Because of the negative influence of calcium and magnesium on the bioavailabilty of tetracyclines, grit-mineral administration has to be stopped during treatment. During egg production and breeding this can result in the laying of soft-shelled eggs and the appearance of rickets in the chicks.

A practical method of adding drugs to a grain mixture is by coating a moist food which is then added to the mixture. Half of the estimated amount of the food to be consumed daily is placed in a small container and sprinkled with vegetable oil or buttermilk. This is thoroughly mixed into the feed and the appropriate amount of drug, in the form of oral powder or suspension, measured, added and likewise mixed. This method is often used for pigeons and backyard poultry. Sick birds should be isolated and medicated individually. When birds are medicated via the feed and/or water, they must be confined to prevent access to external sources, for example puddles.

In contrast to the situation with tablets, the storage of medicated food in the crop of many birds is an advantage; there is a continuous delivery of drug from this reservoir. Pharmacologically, food medication can simulate a slow-release system which provides decreased fluctuations in drug concentrations in tissues.

Drug concentrations for medicated feed cannot be extrapolated from one diet to another without knowing the energy content and palatability of the diets (Flammer, 1994). Both factors influence feed intake.

Water Medication
Water medication is controversial in avian medicine but is often the only practical means of drug administration. It is the least stressful method for medicating birds, especially for drugs that are palatable. Theoretically, the bird will frequently self-dose during the day. However, studies in pigeons and chickens have shown that therapeutic blood levels for many drugs are not attained via the drinking water, because of factors such as non-acceptance, poor solubility, weather conditions and daylength. Polydipsia may lead to overdosing. As a guide, the volume of water consumed by the bird needs to contain the calculated daily dose in mg/kg. In waterfowl, water medication might give additional complications when the birds are allowed to swim. They will not drink the medicated water.

Many drugs are stable in water for only a short time; this necessitates frequent changes (refreshing) of the medicated water.

While therapeutic blood levels may not be achieved with many drugs, levels in the intestine may be sufficient to control enteric infections. The use of medicated water can be valuable for reducing the spread of diseases which have arisen through contaminated water.

In breeding situations the male bird may consume large amounts of water in order to feed the female in the nest, resulting in toxic drug levels in the male. In addition, water intake may be increased in hot weather.

Squabs (young pigeons) are often fed greatly increased quantities of water at weaning time.

TOXICITY

Although limited information is available on toxic effects of drugs in birds, in general, drug administration should be avoided during the breeding season and during periods of feather growth.

● Fenbendazole and corticosteroids are known to interfere with normal feather development in pigeons.

● The benzimidazole endoparasiticides may lead to vomiting and death in nestlings when used in the breeding season.

● Fenbendazole is considered to be toxic in vultures.

● Oral levamisole may cause vomiting in severely infected birds.

● Pyrantel tartrate and mebendazole are considered toxic for pigeons, resulting in regurgitation and vomiting, and finally chronic kidney and liver damage.

● Haloxon is toxic for raptors and waterfowl.

● Corticosteroids can be toxic in doses over 1mg/kg bodyweight and skin applications of corticosteroids can result in necrosis.

● Anticoccidials such as monensin, narasin or salinomycin should not be administered concurrently with tiamulin, as toxic effects are often fatal.

● Erythromycin and sulphonamides have been reported to cause toxic effects when administered with monensin.

● In ducklings the use of the coccidiostatic drug arprinocid will interfere with cartilage and bone formation resulting in the 'Donald Duck-syndrome'.

● Furazolidone should be used with caution in wild mallard and ducks.

● The aminoglycoside antibacterials are potentially nephrotoxic. This is particularly so in dehydrated birds and is a real problem in inappetent raptors. It is important to ensure adequate fluid intake in all birds receiving medication.

● Sulphonamides may cause tissue haemorrhage and anaemia. They may induce feather changes (Curling effect) and other damage in the vanes and calmus when administered to young pigeons and pigeons which are moulting.

● Co-trimazine may cause gastrointestinal disturbances such as crop stasis or emesis.

● Enrofloxacin given i/v, i/m or p/o may cause emesis in raptors, especially if there is food in the crop or proventriculus. Marbofloxacin p/o does not cause emesis in the same situation and is therefore preferable to enrofloxacin.

● Dimetridazole is toxic for goslings and ducklings when administered in a drinking water concentration of 1g/l. Toxic nervous signs are seen when pigeons are feeding their squabs, as they drink too much of the medicated water. In male waterfowl and pigeons, dimetridazole will reduce spermatogenesis and motility.

● Ketoconazole and miconazole - used for the treatment of aspergillosis - are hepatotoxic with prolonged therapy.

● Amphoteracin B is hepatotoxic and nephrotoxic and should not be used in birds that are dehydrated or have renal impairment.

REFERENCES

Bishop YM (1996) *The Veterinary Formulary*. Pharmaceutical Press, London.

Clark CH, Thomas JE, Milton JL and Poolsby WD (1982) Plasma concentrations of chloramphenicol in birds. *American Journal of Veterinary Research* **43**, 1249.

Cooper JE (1993) Infectious and parasitic diseases of raptors. In: *Zoo and Wild Animal Medicine*. 3rd Edn. Ed ME Fowler. WB Saunders, Philadelphia.

Davis LE, Neff MS, Baggot JD and Powers TE (1972) Pharmacokinetics of chloramphenicol in domesticated animals. *American Journal of Veterinary Research* **33**, 2259.

Dorrestein GM (1993) Antimicrobial drug use in pet birds. In: *Antimicrobial Therapy in Veterinary Medicine*. 2nd Edn. Eds JF Prescott and JD Baggot. Iowa State University Press, Ames.

Flammer K (1994) Antimicrobial therapy. In: *Avian Medicine: Principles and Application*. Eds BW Ritchie, GJ Harrison and LR Harrison. Wingers, Lake Worth.

Fudge AM, Reavill DR and Rosskopf WJ (1992) Clinical aspects of avian *Pseudomonas* infections: a retrospective study. In: *Proceedings of the Association of Avian Veterinarians Annual Conference 1992*. AAV, Lake Worth.

Gill FB (1994) *Ornithology*. 2nd Edn. WH Freeman, New York.

Locke D and Bush M (1984) Tylosine aerosol therapy in quail and pigeons. *Journal of Zoo Animal Medicine* **15**, 67.

Quesenberry KE and Hillyer EV (1994) Supportive care and emergency therapy. In: *Avian Medicine: Principles and Application*. Eds BW Ritchie, GJ Harrison and LR Harrison. Wingers, Lake Worth.

Sedgwick CJ and Pokras MA (1988) Extrapolating rational drug doses and treatment periods by allometric scaling. In: *Proceedings of the 55th Annual Meeting of the American Animal Hospital Association*. AAHA.

Skadhauge E (1981) *Osmoregulation in Birds*. Springer Verlag, Berlin.

Spink RR (1986) Aerosol therapy. In: *Clinical Avian Medicine and Surgery, including Aviculture*. Eds GJ Harrison and LR Harrison. WB Saunders, Philadelphia.

Worell AB (1993) Pediatric bacterial diseases. *Seminars in Avian and Exotic Pet Medicine* **2**, 116.

CHAPTER SIX

Cytology

Gerry M Dorrestein

INTRODUCTION

Diagnostic cytology in avian medicine provides a means for better disease definition, which allows for a more specific therapeutic approach. Cytology can be used in the clinical patient and can provide microscopic information of many different disease processes. At *post mortem*, cytology is an invaluable tool for defining the presumptive diagnosis and starting treatment in the flock situation. It is important that cytologic specimens are taken from fresh sources, since cells degenerate rapidly following the death of the bird or the tissue. Cytologic evaluation is always an adjunct to other diagnostic procedures. A final diagnosis often requires information from the clinical history, physical examination, evaluation of samples obtained from the bird, radiographs, surgical investigations, *post-mortem* examination and histopathology. The avian patient often does not lend itself to all of the diagnostic aids that are available for mammals. The small body size and blood volume of many birds often limits the use of extensive biochemical and serodiagnostic evaluation. In pigeons and waterfowl, economics will sometimes prohibit an extensive clinical work-up.

In the clinic a cytologic examination of swellings, discharges of eyes, nostrils and wounds, fluids, crop and cloacal swabs, and faecal smears can give much additional information about the nature and aetiology of a process or symptom. The diagnosis of many protozoal infections, eg. *Plasmodium* spp., *Haemoproteus* spp., *Leucocytozoon* sp., *Sarcosporidia* spp. or *Trypanosoma* spp., depends on demonstrating these organisms in smears of peripheral blood or a selection of organs at *post mortem*. Cytologic samples of the alimentary tract of live birds can be obtained by using a cotton swab or crop aspiration.

At *post mortem*, cytology is an indispensable tool for rapid investigation of possible bacterial, mycotic or yeast infections. This technique is an invaluable aid for quick differentiation between tumour and inflammation. Samples are obtained by scraping any lesions with a cotton swab or spatula blade. The material can also be used for microbiologic culture and microscopic examination.

Cytology is a technique based on the study of individual cells. In disease situations it can give information about pathophysiologic changes caused by the disease. The technique provides a simple, rapid, inexpensive method of diagnosis that can be performed in any veterinary practice. Frequently, the aetiologic agent causing the lesion can be identified. However, the veterinarian should be aware of the limitations of diagnostic cytology. It does not give information concerning the architecture of the tissue (cells in the same smear may have originated from different areas of the organ or lesion), the size of the lesion or the invasiveness of a malignant lesion. The cells observed may not necessarily represent the true nature of the lesion. An example of this is the imprinting of the ulcerated surface of a neoplastic mass that reveals the cytologic features of inflammation and infection only.

Cytopathology should not compete with histopathology; the two should complement each other in achieving the final diagnosis. It is important to note that occasionally it is not possible to characterise the cells in a specimen and that a repeat smear or biopsy for histopathologic evaluation may be required to define the lesion.

SAMPLING TECHNIQUES AND SAMPLE PREPARATION

Blood for cytologic evaluation can be obtained by several methods as described in other chapters. Blood smears should be made with fresh, non-heparinised blood (heparin interferes with the proper staining of the blood cells). EDTA-treated blood can also be used.

Fine-needle aspiration biopsy often provides a good cytologic sample for a rapid presumptive diagnosis without radical tissue removal, and this can be performed in the examination room. Where an aspiration sample contains much fluid or blood, it is important to notice small lumps of cells or tissue and to use them for a smear. For more detailed information see Campbell (1984, 1988, 1994), Fudge (1988), Hawkey and Gulland (1989) and Ingh and Vos (1989).

A successful cytologic examination is only possible if the following four conditions are achieved:

- Representative sample.

- Good quality smear.
- Good staining technique.
- Correct evaluation of the cytologic findings.

Contact smears are made by imprinting the removed mass or the tissue obtained from the scraping of an exposed lesion *in situ* or at *post mortem*. During a routine *post-mortem* examination, impression smears should be made from liver, spleen and lungs, and also from a rectal scraping. All this material can be collected onto one slide. Extra impressions are made from macroscopically altered organs. Impressions of organs should be made from a freshly cut surface, which should be fairly dry and free of blood. This can be achieved by gently blotting the surface onto a clean paper towel. Imprint slides can then be made by gently touching the glass or by touching the microscope slide onto the surface of the mass. It is important not to use too much pressure and to air-dry the sample quickly. Several imprints of the same organ should be made on each slide.

If the imprints show poor cellularity, more cells may be obtained by scraping the mass with a scalpel blade to improve exfoliation of the cells. The imprinting procedure can be repeated or imprints can be made from the material remaining on the scalpel blade.

Direct smears should be made from aspirated fluids, eg. ascites or cyst contents. They can be made using the wedge method or the coverslip method commonly used for making blood smears. A 'squash-prep' procedure should be used to make smears from thick tenacious fluid or from fluid that contains solid tissue fragments. Fluids that have low cellularity require concentration methods to increase the smear cellularity. Sediment smears made after slow-speed centrifugation (500rpm for five minutes) of the fluid, or smears made with cytocentrifuge equipment, will usually provide adequate cytologic specimens.

Once a sample has been collected and a smear has been made, the specimen must be properly fixed to the slide. If smears are to be sent to a diagnostic laboratory, they must be air dried, well-packed (broken slides are fairly common) and accompanied by a distinct identification and case history.

The method of fixation depends upon which staining procedure is to be used. Fresh air-dried blood smears and cytology slides are adequate for Romanowsky stains, eg. Giemsa stain and many quick stains.

A variety of stains and staining methods, eg. acid-fast (*Mycobacterium* spp.), Giemsa (cells), Gram (microorganisms), modified Giminez (*Chlamydia* spp.), Stamp (*Chlamydia* spp.) and Sudan III (fat globules), are used by cytologists (Campbell, 1984, 1986, 1988, 1994a). Proper fixation must be applied if specific stains are used. To obtain this information the diagnostic service should be contacted.

The cytologic descriptions in this text are based primarily on slides stained with a modified quick Wright's stain (Hemacolor®, Merck). The great advantage of the quick stains is a short staining time (usually 20 seconds) which allows rapid examination of the specimen and provides satisfactory staining quality. These stains are suitable for use in private veterinary practice where a simple staining procedure is desirable. Many quick stains also provide permanent reference smears for comparison with other cytologic specimens.

Once the smears have been stained and dried they are ready for microscopic examination. For a reliable evaluation of the cellular changes in the sample it will often be necessary to consult a cytopathologist. The recognition of many aetiologic agents is often easier and can give a presumptive diagnosis.

Scanning and low magnifications (x100 or x250) are used initially to obtain a general impression of the smear quality. At these magnifications the examiner is able to estimate the smear cellularity, identify tissue structures or large infectious agents (that is, microfilariae and fungal elements) and determine the best locations for cellular examination. Oil immersion (x1000) magnification is used to examine cell structure, bacteria and other small objects.

In addition to viewing cellular structure, the cytologist should also determine background characteristics, the amount of peripheral blood or stain precipitation present, the thickness of different areas in the smear and the distribution of the cells. The background characteristics may be useful in defining the nature of the material being examined. Protein aggregates create a granular background with the quick stains. Bacteria, crystals, nuclear material from ruptured cells and exogenous material (for example, plant fibres, pollen and talcum or starch crystals from examination gloves) may be seen in the non-cellular background of the smear. Excessive peripheral blood contamination of a specimen will dilute and mask diagnostic cells; this will make interpretation difficult.

Stain precipitate on the smear should not be confused with bacteria or cellular inclusions. Stain precipitate varies in size and shape and will be more refractive than bacteria or most cellular inclusions. The thickness of the smear will affect the appearance of the cells and the quality of the smear. Thick areas do not allow the cells to expand on the slide, so they appear smaller and more dense when compared with the same cell type on thinner areas of the smear. Therefore, examination of the cells in thick smears should be avoided. The cellular distribution should also be noted.

GENERAL PRINCIPLES OF CYTOLOGIC INTERPRETATION

The cytologic appearance of many cells obtained from avian tissues and fluids is similar to those described for mammalian species. A cytologic classification divides body tissue into four groups: haemic, epithelial-glandular, connective and nervous.

Haemic Tissue (Blood and Blood-Forming Tissue)

Haemic tissue is composed of cells that are found in the peripheral blood, bone marrow and ectopic haemopoietic sites. Peripheral blood primarily contains the mature cells that are derived from cell lines located in the haematopoietic tissues. Blood cells are a common cell type in *post-mortem* impression smears of the lungs, and also as a component of most cytology preparations. The following blood cells can be recognised: erythrocytes, thrombocytes and leucocytes, granulocytes (heterophils or pseudo-eosinophils, eosinophils and basophils) and lymphocytes. Details plus illustrations of the morphologic characteristics and pathophysiologic conditions can be found in Chapter 8. Helpful references to the identification of avian leucocytes together with beautiful illustrations are also found in (Lucas and Jamroz, 1961; Campbell, 1994). The common blood parasites are described later (Internal Organs - Lungs).

Differentiation of the heterophil from the eosinophil can be a problem. The diverse granular morphology of the eosinophil in raptors and waterfowl contributes to this problem (Lind *et al*, 1990). The principal differences are:
● Heterophil: the cytoplasm is colourless, the nucleus is lobed and usually stains lighter than the eosinophil nucleus; the granules are rod-shaped and eosinophilic in colour.
● Eosinophil: the cytoplasm is light blue or of a bluish tinge, the nucleus is lobed and stains darker than the heterophil nucleus; the granules are evenly distributed and granular morphology will be consistent on an individual slide, but colour, shape and size of granules can vary from species to species.

Epithelial (including Glandular) Tissue

Epithelial cells tend to exfoliate in clumps or sheets. Apart from mature squamous epithelium, they are usually round or oval with abundant cytoplasm and have round or oval nuclei. The nuclear chromatin is generally smooth and a prominent nucleolus may be visible. The cytoplasmic borders of epithelial cells are usually distinct, except for the liver. Normal epithelial cells are uniform in appearance.

Connective Tissue

Connective tissue cells tend to exfoliate poorly and provide cytologic specimens with few cells. Traumatic exfoliation is often required to obtain significant numbers of cells for evaluation. Depending on their origin, connective tissue cells tend to vary in the amount of cytoplasm and nuclear shape.

Nervous Tissue

Nervous tissue cells are rarely seen on cytological specimens, unless the specimens were made from central or peripheral nervous tissue. Nervous tissue cells may be present in smears from other tissues, but are of little significance.

The goal of cytology is to identify the cellular message and classify the cell response into one of the basic cytodiagnostic groups. These groups include inflammation, tissue hyperplasia or benign neoplasia, malignant neoplasia and normal cellularity. The smears or impressions can give information about the possible aetiology of the pathologic changes.

Inflammation

Inflammation may be caused by living agents (microorganisms) or non-living agents (traumatic, thermal, toxic or chemical agents). The cytology of inflammatory lesions may be classified into purulent and proliferative (including granulomatous) inflammatory reactions. Inflammatory cells include heterophils, eosinophils, macrophages, lymphocytes, plasma cells, multinucleated giant cells and (angio)fibroblasts.

Purulent Inflammation

The purulent reaction is characterised by a predominance of heterophilic granulocytes. Overwhelming bacterial infections commonly cause degenerative changes to the heterophils, eg. pyknosis, karyolysis, karyorrhexis, loss of granules, basophilic cytoplasm with phagocytic vacuolisation. The agent may be phagocytosed within the macrophages (see Figure 6.1).

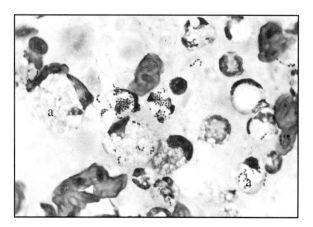

Figure 6.1: Lung - cocci-pneumonia. (Hemacolor® - Oil Immersion x 1000). a. cocci in macrophages.

Proliferative Inflammation

The cytology of proliferative inflammation shows many lymphocytes mixed with various numbers of plasma cells and macrophages. Occasionally, heterophils tend to be non-degenerate in appearance. This reaction becomes more granulomatous as evidenced by a predominance of mononuclear cells (macrophages and lymphocytes). A granulomatous reaction can also be represented by giant cell formation, eg. acute aspergillosis, or by macrophages coalescing into net-like sheets, eg. atypical tuberculous granulomata in the lungs.

The inflammatory response can also be classified as either heterophilic (acute inflammatory response), mixed-cell (an established, active inflammation) or macrophagic inflammation (common in avian tuberculosis, chlamydiosis, foreign body reaction, mycotic infections and cutaneous xanthomatosis).

(Malignant) Neoplasia

In the practical situation, cytodiagnosis of swellings should differentiate between inflammation and neoplasms. Certain criteria are required for the cytologic diagnosis of neoplasia. In many cases, however, the differentiation between inflammation, hypertrophy and neoplasia is not so clear cut. The main cytopathologic criteria for the diagnosis of neoplasia can be divided into several categories: general cellular, nuclear or cytoplasmic.

General Cellular

The general cellular features refer to the cell population on the smear. The neoplastic cells may appear related (have common origin) but can exhibit pleomorphism (variation in shape).

Nuclear

Sometimes, the nuclei are different from the nuclei of the normal tissue cells. The changes in the nucleus include nuclear hypertrophy, variations in size and shape of the nuclei and in the ratio of nuclei to cytoplasm, changes in the nucleoli, multinucleation, irregularity of the chromatin and nuclear membrane, and abnormal mitotic figures.

Cytoplasmic

The cytoplasm can also be different, eg. a different cytoplasmic volume, variations in the shape of the cytoplasmic borders, basophilia, vacuolation and

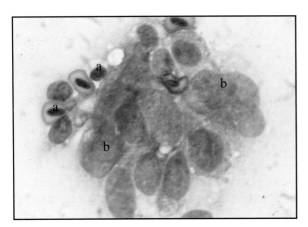

Figure 6.2: Swollen wing - sarcoma. (Hemacolor® - Oil Immersion x1000). a. erythrocyte; b. tumour cell.

inclusions bodies. Based on cytology only, it will be very difficult and often impossible to classify the neoplasm as a carcinoma (= epithelial), sarcoma (= mesothelial) (see Figure 6.2) or discrete cell (eg. lymphoid leucosis) tumour. The presence of cell types that are foreign to the tissue being examined (ectopic cells) may indicate a metastatic neoplasm.

SPECIFIC ORGAN SYSTEMS

Each organ system has its specific approach and normal cytology. Basically, pathologic changes need classification as inflammation or neoplasm. In many cases the demonstration of an aetiologic agent will make this technique worth trying.

CONJUNCTIVA AND CORNEA

Samples can be obtained using a sterile moist swab or a metal or plastic spatula and gently scraping the margins of the cornea or conjunctiva. Local ophthalmic anaesthetic agents should not be used; they can be toxic to cells. Normal conjunctival cytology shows a few epithelial cells occurring singly or in sheets, often with brown or black pigmented granules in the cytoplasm. These granules should not be confused with bacteria. Corneal cells are non-keratinised, squamous epithelial cells with a central vesicular nucleus. A few extracellular bacteria are present on normal smears. Many inflammatory cells and cell debris can be seen with bacterial conjunctivitis and corneal infections. Chlamydial or mycoplasmal infections of the eye may show inflammatory cells, cell debris and epithelial cells or macrophages containing intracytoplasmic inclusions.

SKIN AND SUBCUTIS

The skin is composed of keratinised, stratified squamous epithelium and exfoliation produces primary cornified squamous epithelial cells. Bacterial infections are represented by large numbers of inflammatory cells, cell debris and bacteria. Fungal infections may reveal fungal elements on cytologic examination. Foreign bodies produce granulomatous reactions with macrophages, giant cell formation and a variable number of heterophils.

Cutaneous and subcutaneous masses should be examined cytologically. Pox lesions frequently produce cytologic features of inflammation and swollen epithelial cells with small, round, pale eosinophilic inclusions (Borrel and Bollinger bodies) when stained with Wright's stain. A needle aspirate of a subcutaneous lipoma reveals numerous background fat droplets and a variable number of fat cells. Subcutaneous lymphosarcoma (lymphoid leucosis) is characterised by a marked number of immature lymphocytes with variable nucleus size.

FLUIDS

Accumulation of fluid in avian species is confined mainly to the abdominal cavity (ascites, peritonitis, haemoperitoneum), but is also encountered in isolated air sacs and cysts, or as synovial fluid in the joints. Effusions can be classified as transudate, exudate, synovia, or haemorrhage.

The normal cytology of abdominal fluid, which is usually not present, occasionally shows mesothelial cells and macrophages. Mesothelial cells are round or oval and variable in size, and have a homogenous basophilic cytoplasm and a centrally positioned round nucleus. Reactive mesothelial cells may show cytoplasmic vacuolisation and eventually may contain phagocytosed material. It is difficult to differentiate transformed mesothelial cells, active histiocytes and monocyte-derived macrophages.

Transudate and Exudate

Transudate fluids are characterised by low cellularity; exudate is characterised by high cellularity. Purulent exudate may demonstrate bacteria or degenerated heterophils. Plasma cells frequently occur in chronic inflammatory lesions. They are lymphoid cells with an eccentric nucleus, dark blue cytoplasm and a prominent Golgi apparatus. An egg-related peritonitis (yolk peritonitis) can be recognised by the presence of yolk drops, which are homogeneous, round, highly variable in size and deeply basophilic in smears stained with quick stains (see Figure 6.3). The same basophilic droplets can often be found in macrophages within the spleen, liver or lung.

Synovia

Most normal avian joints contain a fluid volume that is too small for aspiration. Normal synovial fluid has poor cellularity; the majority of the cells are mononuclear. Septic joints usually have an increased synovial fluid volume. Cytology reveals large numbers of heterophils and bacteria. The eosinophilic granules in the heterophils have often disappeared, eg.

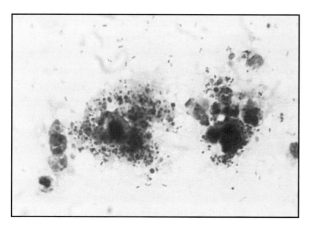

Figure 6.3: Peritoneal material - yolk peritonitis. (Hemacolor® - Oil Immersion x1000).

salmonellosis in pigeons (see Figure 6.4). Chronic traumatic arthritis demonstrates many macrophages and erythrophagocytosis. Articular gout is often diagnosed by the gross appearance of the affected joint. The fluid is dense, white or yellow in colour, and cloudy. Large numbers of inflammatory cells are present. Urate crystals are birefringent, needle-like crystals and are best seen under polarised light in a wet-mount.

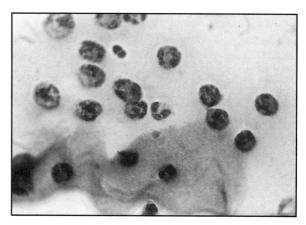

Figure 6.4: Synovial fluid - Salmonella arthritis; activated heterophils. (Hemacolor® - Oil Immersion x1000).

Haemorrhage

Acute haemorrhagic effusions resemble peripheral blood smears.

DIGESTIVE TRACT

Oral Cavity, Oesophagus and Crop

Examination of the oral cavity is part of the routine physical examination of a bird. White or yellow plaques, nodules or ulcers may be found. Cytologic examination of these lesions will aid in the diagnosis of candidiasis, trichomoniasis, capillariasis, poxvirus, bacterial infections, abscesses and squamous metaplasia due to hypovitaminosis A.

Wet-mount slides will aid the identification of live *Trichomonas* spp. or other flagellates. At *post mortem* these flagellate protozoa can be identified, after staining, by their undulating membrane, their axostyle and their anterior flagella. Some other species of flagellates, without axostyle or membrane, may also be present.

The oesophageal and crop lumina are lined by stratified squamous epithelium. These cells are polygonal with varying degrees of keratinisation and possess a condense nucleus. Many extracellular bacteria (a variety of morphological types) are visible and are often found in association with squamous cells.

Bacterial infections are indicated by leucocytes. Smears with a large number of bacteria of one morphologic type should be considered abnormal and an indication for bacterial culture. Candidiasis can be detected by demonstration of the oval, thin-walled yeasts (3-6μm). They stain dark blue with quick stain and Gram-positive (purple) with Gram stain.

Cloaca

Cloacal cytology in a live bird is indicated when inflammation, prolapse or masses are detected. Wet-mount preparations will aid in the detection of helminth eggs, coccidial oocysts or protozoa.

Normal cloacal cytology reveals a variable number of squamous cells that have varying degrees of keratinisation, but most cells appear non-keratinised and have a central vesicular nucleus. The normal mucosal cells of the intestinal lining are of the columnar type, often arranged in multicellular rows. In smears, the same changes may be found at *post mortem* (see later).

Stomach, Intestinal Tract and Cloaca at *Post Mortem*

A dilated ventriculus may be seen in many species of birds. So-called 'megabacteria' can often be demonstrated in mucosal scrapings. Candidiasis may be a cause of gastric ulceration.

At *post mortem*, a mucosal scraping (mostly from the rectum) is prepared for cytologic evaluation. A variable amount of bacteria (rods, cocci, *Campylobacter* spp., *Vibrio*-forms, 'megabacteria', spores), fungi and yeasts, protozoa (coccidial schizonts, macro- and microgamonts, intra- and extracellular trophozoites, *Microsporidia* spp., flagellates) (see Figure 6.5), inflammatory cells, spermatozoa, starch or amylum particles, brown-black denatured haemoglobin, and debris (plant material, chitin-skeletons of insects, urates) may be present. *Chlamydia* spp. may be demonstrated with a Stamp or Macchiavello's stain; *Mycobacterium* spp. with a Ziehl-Neelsen stain.

RESPIRATORY TRACT

A sinus aspirate is indicated in avian patients with sinusitis. Cytology demonstrates a moderate amount of background debris and a variable number of inflammatory cells, depending on the severity of the inflammation. Sometimes, the aetiologic agent can be detected phagocytosed by leucocytes. An initial

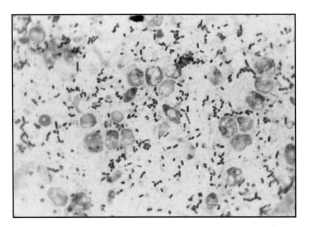

Figure 6.5: Intestine - Hexamita columbae. (Hemacolor® - Oil Immersion x1000). A mixture of bacteria and flagellates.

examination with a magnification of x100 is essential to detect fungal elements.

Transtracheal aspiration is one method for evaluating upper respiratory disease in birds. The procedure is simple, but requires general anaesthesia. A large-bore hypodermic needle can be inserted into an air sac to aid respiration during the procedure if the bird is severely dyspnoeic (see Chapter 9). Tracheal swab samples can be obtained by passing a small cotton swab directly into the trachea. The trachea and primary bronchi are lined by pseudostratified, ciliated columnar epithelium with goblet cells, whereas the syrinx (located at the junction of the trachea and bronchi) consists of either bistratified squamous cells or columnar epithelial cells.

Tracheal material exhibiting large numbers of heterophils and macrophages suggests tracheo-bronchitis even in asymptomatic birds. Mycotic tracheal or bronchial (or syringeal) lesions may be confirmed by the presence of fungal elements in a tracheal wash or *post-mortem* scrapings.

Air sac samples can be obtained in a live bird using an endoscopic laparotomy technique such as that used for surgical sexing of birds. At *post mortem*, scrapings can be made from the epithelial surface. The air sacs are lined by simple squamous epithelium. Air sacculitis is indicated by many inflammatory cells and a variable amount of background debris. Intracellular bacteria indicate a bacterial aetiology and fungal hyphae or elements confirm mycotic involvement. Special stains are required to confirm chlamydial infections.

INTERNAL ORGANS

Lungs

At *post mortem*, the lungs are removed from the thoracic cavity and a freshly cut surface is blotted dry on a clean paper towel. A microscope slide is touched gently several times onto this dry surface. The impression smear should be as thin as possible.

The impression smear of normal lung tissue consists mainly of blood cells mixed with columnar epithelial cells, ciliated cells, isolated cilia, pieces of striated muscle fibres and an occasional macrophage or lymphocyte.

Pneumonia is characterised by the presence of many heterophils and vacuolated macrophages, often in an eosinophilic background due to oedema and/or protein-containing fluids (exudate) within the respiratory tissue. The impression smear will give information on chlamydial, fungal, cryptococcal, bacterial respiratory or neoplastic disorders. With severe anthracosis, macrophages containing black phagocytosed particles may be found. Lung tissue smears will also give an impression of the composition of the blood cells. In anaemic conditions, many immature erythrocytes or their precursor cells may be recognised with a basophilic cytoplasm and a large round and vesiculated nucleus. Extracellular blood parasites (*Trypanosoma* spp., *Microfilaria* spp.) and intracellular schizonts (*Plasmodium* spp.) are easily seen under low power magnification. Under high power magnification, intracellular blood parasites can be seen within erythrocytes - *Plasmodium* spp., *Haemoproteus* spp. (both with brown pigment), *Leucocytozoon* spp. (without pigment) - and within leucocytes - *Leucocytozoon* spp., (see Figure 6.6) *(A)toxoplasma* spp., *Toxoplasma*-pseudocysts.

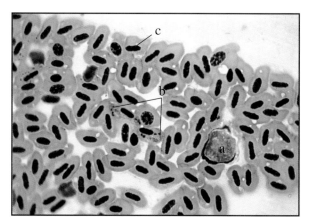

Figure 6.6: Lung. (Hemacolor® - Oil Immersion x1000). a. Leucocytozoon infection; b. Plasmodium infection; c. erythrocyte.

Spleen

The avian spleen is a blood forming and blood destroying organ; it also contains lymphoid tissue. Impressions of the normal spleen show a significant amount of blood cells and heavy background cellular debris. Frequently, groups of lymphocytes in various stages of maturity can be seen. Macrophages showing varying degrees of erythrophagocytosis and iron accumulation are common. Large clusters of brown pigment are seen in *Plasmodium* spp. infections. Cells with a variable amount of pale blue cytoplasm and indistinct cytoplasmic borders are present. These cells have an eccentric round or oval nucleus with coarse granular chromatin. Splenic impressions are good samples for the detection of bacterial infections, intracellular and extracellular blood parasites, and chlamydial inclusions.

Liver

Liver cytology can be examined from smears or imprints made from aspiration biopsy or excisional biopsy. At *post mortem*, the freshly cut surface should be blotted very thoroughly until almost no cells are exfoliated. Liver specimens tend to provide a smear which is too cellular with an abundance of circulating blood cells. Background material is thick and basophilic (hepatocyte cytoplasm with many mitochondria) with a marked amount of cell fragments and free hepatocyte nuclei. Normal hepatocytes occur singly, in sheets or in clusters. They are large and have

abundant basophilic cytoplasm with coarse granulation (mitochondria). Fine eosinophilic granulation and iron particles can be detected in most cells. The nuclei are round or oval, slightly eccentric in location, contain coarse chromatin and have a single prominent nucleolus. The nuclei are uniform in appearance; an occasional binucleated cell can be seen. Occasionally, spindle-shaped stromal cells, lymphocytes, plasma cells and macrophages are present.

Macrophages often contain iron pigment or phagocytosed material. Lymphoid aggregates may be found in most normal avian livers. These consist primarily of small mature lymphocytes. Reactive lymphoid aggregates contain a large number of plasma cells and often also heterophils. Lymphoid neoplasia is indicated by large numbers of immature lymphocytes. Microfilarial larvae are sometimes found in liver cytology in birds without peripheral blood microfilarial infection. *Mycobacterium* spp. may be seen (sometimes even in birds without conspicuous macroscopic alterations) as empty, non-coloured, rod-shaped ghosts, often grouped together in the basophilic background. An acid fast staining technique will confirm the diagnosis. In raptors and pigeons, liver necrosis can sometimes be caused by *Trichomonas* spp. (see Figure 6.7).

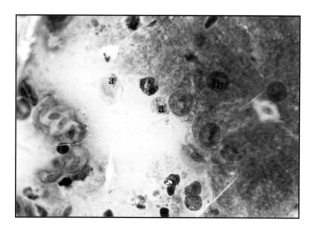

Figure 6.7: Liver. (Hemacolor® - Oil Immersion x1000). a. Trichomonas columbae; b. liver cell nucleus.

Degenerated hepatocytes are seen with *post-mortem* autolysis or hepatic disease. Fatty livers show swollen hepatocytes with intracellular and extracellular lipid droplets. Inflammatory hepatic lesions are characterised by degenerate hepatocytes and marked inflammatory cell infiltration. Bacterial infections are recognised by intra- and/or extracellular bacteria; some viral infections may show intracytoplasmic or intranuclear inclusion bodies. Neoplastic lesions contain cells with cytologic features of neoplasia.

REFERENCES

Campbell TW (1984) Diagnostic cytology in avian medicine. *Veterinary Clinics of North America: Small Animal Practice* **14**, 317.

Campbell TW (1986) Cytology. In: *Clinical Avian Medicine and Surgery, including Aviculture*. Eds GJ Harrison and LR Harrison. WB Saunders, Philadelphia.

Campbell TW (1988) *Avian Hematology and Cytology*. Iowa State University Press, Ames.

Campbell TW (1994a) Hematology. In: *Avian Medicine: Principles and Application*. Eds BW Ritchie, GJ Harrison and LR Harrison. Wingers, Lake Worth.

Campbell TW (1994b) Cytology. In: *Avian Medicine: Principles and Application*. Eds BW Ritchie, GJ Harrison and LR Harrison. Wingers, Lake Worth.

Fudge AM (1988) Avian clinical cytology. In: *Proceedings of the Association of Avian Veterinarians Annual Conference 1988*. AAV, Lake Worth.

Hawkey C and Gulland F (1989) Clinical haematology. In: *Manual of Parrots, Budgerigars and Other Psittacine Birds*. Ed CJ Price. BSAVA, Cheltenham.

Ingh TSGAM van den and Vos JH (1989) Technical aspects of fine-needle aspiration cytology. *Tijdschrift voor Diergeneeskunde* **114**, 713.

Lind PJ, Wolff PL, Petrini, KR, Keyler CW, Olson DE and Redig PT (1990) Morphology of the eosinophil in raptors. *Journal of the Association of Avian Veterinarians* **4**, 33.

Lucas AJ and Jamroz C (1961) *Atlas of Avian Hematology*. United States Department of Agriculture, Monograph 25, Washington DC.

CHAPTER SEVEN

Biochemistry and Sampling

J (Sjeng) T Lumeij

INTRODUCTION

Plasma biochemistry is an important diagnostic tool in helping to establish a clinical diagnosis of diseases of the gastrointestinal, hepatic, renal, cardiovascular, musculoskeletal and endocrine systems. The value of the results is highly dependent on the blood collection and processing techniques. The most important investigative methods and the associated pitfalls will be discussed. Table 7.1 summarises the main clinical significance of various plasma biochemical variables. Plasma biochemistry reference values for pigeons are given in Chapter 8 (Appendix 8.1). Conversion factors from conventional units to SI units and some discussion on the International System of Units can be found in Appendix 7.1. The reader is referred to other sources for more detailed information on interpretation of plasma biochemistry (Lumeij, 1987c, 1987d, 1994a,b,c,d; Lumeij and Ritchie 1994).

BLOOD COLLECTING METHODS AND ANTICOAGULANTS

In most avian species the right jugular vein is the preferred site for blood sampling. In the racing pigeon the jugular vein is not readily accessible and the medial metatarsal vein is used. The medial metatarsal vein is also a good site for blood sampling in raptors. In ducks and geese the venous occipital sinus is the preferred site for blood sampling (Vuillaume, 1983). It is located within the cranium at the junction of the base of the skull and the first cervical vertebra. The use of a vacuum system greatly facilitates blood sampling from all sites. Although the ulnar vein ('wing vein') can be located in all avian species, this site is not recommended as a first choice since it is very prone to the formation of a haematoma. When a toenail is clipped to obtain a blood sample, contamination of the sample with urates from the droppings may give false high readings.

Generally, 1% of bodyweight appears a safe limit for the amount of blood that can be collected for diagnostic purposes. Lithium heparin is the anticoagulant of choice when dealing with avian blood samples; serum should not be used.

It is not necessary to prevent glycolysis for reliable glucose determinations as long as the blood is not stored for more than two hours (Lumeij, 1987b). Avian erythrocytes consume very little, if any, glucose and depend on fatty acid metabolism. Plasma and cells should be separated by centrifuging immediately after obtaining the sample. Any delay may cause decreases of plasma potassium concentrations due to a shift of potassium ions from the plasma into the red blood cells (Lumeij, 1985a).

For the determination of lead, which is the most widely reported and clinically described poison in ducks and raptors, whole unclotted blood should be sent to the laboratory, since more than 90% of the lead in whole blood is associated with the red blood cells (Lumeij, 1985b).

REFERENCE VALUES

Reference values of plasma biochemical variables are highly dependent on materials and methods used and can be different between laboratories. Blood samples should only be sent to laboratories which can supply reference values established in their own laboratory for the species and variables concerned. There are many laboratory tests which have not been validated for birds and which may give erroneous results when used indiscriminately on avian plasma samples. In order for the clinician to evaluate the results from the laboratory it is essential that reference values from a clearly defined reference population of the species concerned are available. These values should be established by the same methods. When using published reference values the avian clinician should take into consideration the materials and methods used, and discuss these with the laboratory to avoid errors due to differences in methodology. Many references do not give the methodology of their test or running temperature etc.

Since many biological variables do not show a normal distribution, non-parametric statistics have to be used to establish reference values. Therefore, it is recommended to use the inner limits of the percentiles P2.5 and P97.5 with a probability of 90% if reference values are published for clinical use, and not mean

Table 7.1. Plasma biochemical variables and their significance for the diagnosis of internal diseases in birds.

Variable	Interpretation of abnormal values
Urea	Elevated values post-prandially or in dehydrated birds.
Uric acid	Elevated values post-prandially, in renal function disorders or in dehydrated birds .
Glucose	Elevated values in diabetes mellitus or after corticosteroid injection. Prolonged starvation tends to cause hyperglycaemia.
Potassium	Artificially low values are often seen when plasma and cells are not separated immediately. Elevated values are seen with renal function disorders and mineralocorticoid deficiency.
Calcium	Should be interpreted together with total protein values. Hypercalcaemia is physiological in female birds before egg laying. Hypocalcaemia is seen in nutritional secondary hyperparathyroidism.
Aspartate aminotransferase (AST)	An enzyme which occurs in many tissues, eg. liver/muscle. Elevated activities indicate organ damage.
Alanine aminotransferase (ALT)	An enzyme which occurs in many tissues, eg. liver/muscle. Elevated activities indicate organ damage. Because of its long half-life (12 hours), ALAT activity from muscle origin may be elevated for a prolonged period after i/m injection (up to 10 days).
Lactate dehydrogenase	An enzyme which occurs in many tissues, eg. liver/muscle. Despite high tissue concentrations, its clinical importance is not so great because of its short half-life in plasma (30-40 min).
Gamma glutamyl transferase (GGT)	Elevated activities in plasma are seen in cholestatic liver disorders.
Glutamate dehydrogenase	An enzyme which occurs in the mitochondria of liver cells. Elevated activities of this enzyme in plasma are indicative of liver cell necrosis.
Cholinesterase	Low activity of this enzyme in plasma is seen in intoxications with cholinesterase inhibitors, eg. organophosphates.
Creatine phosphokinase	An enzyme which is specific for muscle. Elevated concentrations indicate muscle damage. Because of its relatively short half-life (three hours), activities return to reference values well before AST or ALT activities return to normal. Differentiation between creatine phosphokinase of skeletal muscle and cardiac muscle origin in birds is possible.
Alkaline phosphatase (ALP)	Elevated activities may be physiological or pathological and indicate increased osteoblastic activity.
Bile acids	Elevated concentrations of bile acids are seen post-prandially and with liver function disorders. Sensitive and specific variable for liver function disorders.
Total protein and protein electrophoresis	Non-specific, but useful adjuncts to diagnosis of gastrointestinal, hepatic and renal disorders, inflammatory conditions and dehydrated birds. Sequential samples may be used to assess response to therapy and prognosis.

plus or minus two times standard deviation (Rümke and Bezemer, 1972).

STARVATION AND POST-PRANDIAL EFFECTS ON PLASMA BIOCHEMISTRY, AND CIRCADIAN AND CIRCANNUAL RHYTHMS

Interestingly, starvation in pigeons for up to 96 hours induces starvation hyperglycaemia within 73 hours after food withdrawal, rather than starvation hypoglycaemia (Lumeij, 1987b).

Plasma glucose concentrations in fasted birds are subject to a circadian rhythm. A rise in plasma glucose concentration starts during the scotophase, reaching peak values early during the photophase. Subsequently, a gradual increase can be observed with the lowest values at the end of the photophase. Afternoon plasma glucose concentrations in birds which are fed early during the photophase are significantly higher compared to fasted birds (Lumeij, 1987b).

When performing research in avian species it should be borne in mind that other blood biochemical variables may also show a circadian rhythm, eg. plasma corticosterone (Joseph and Meier, 1973) or even a circannual rhythm, eg. plasma thyroxine (Lumeij and Westerhof, 1988). To prevent erroneous conclusions, appropriate controls should always be included in experimental or clinical studies.

Food consumption can also result in elevated concentrations of plasma bile acids (Lumeij, 1991; Lumeij and Remple, 1992) and plasma uric acid concentrations (Lumeij and Remple, 1991). A post-prandial effect should always be ruled out when these variables are elevated in a plasma sample. In carnivorous birds, blood for uric acid analysis should not be taken until 24 hours after the last meal. Clinicians should be aware that starvation of ill birds, especially small birds, can be deleterious.

PLASMA PROTEINS

Plasma proteins can be considered as important complementary variables in the diagnosis of avian diseases. Although determination of plasma proteins seldom leads to a specific diagnosis, it will help the clinician to evaluate the severity and progress of a disease (Lumeij, 1987d).

Methodology
The total protein (TP) in a plasma sample should be measured using the biuret method with human protein as a standard, and the albumin and globulin concentrations (and the A:G ratio) from the results of TP and cellulose acetate electrophoresis in heparinised plasma samples. The refractometric method is unreliable for determination of total protein in birds. It should be stressed that albumin determinations performed with dry methods, eg. Kodak Ektachem, are not validated for use in birds and give unreliable albumin values and hence an unreliable A:G ratio.

Various diseases are accompanied by a decreased albumin concentration and an elevated globulin concentration, while the TP concentration remains in the normal range. Examples of diseases with a decrease in the A:G ratio are egg-related peritonitis and chronic infectious diseases such as aspergillosis, chlamydiosis and tuberculosis. In liver failure, extremely low plasma protein concentrations can occur in combination with a decreased A:G ratio. Gastrointestinal and renal diseases can also lead to severe hypoproteinaemia. Elevated TP concentrations with a normal A:G ratio can be expected in dehydrated birds.

Physiological Variation in Female Birds
In female birds a considerable increase in plasma TP concentration occurs just prior to egg laying. This can be attributed to an oestrogen-induced increase in the globulin fractions. The proteins are the yolk precursors, eg. vitellogenin and lipoproteins, which are synthesised in the liver and transported via the plasma to the ovary, where they are incorporated in the oocyte.

REFERENCES

Andreasen CB, Latimer KS, Kirchner IM and Brown J (1989) Determination of chicken and turkey plasma and serum protein concentrations by refractometry and the biuret method. *Avian Diseases* **33**, 93.

Ekstrom DD and Degernes L (1989) Avian gout. In: *Proceedings of the Association of Avian Veterinarians Annual Conference 1989*. AAV, Lake Worth.

Joseph MM and Meier AH (1973) Daily rhythms of plasma corticosterone in the common pigeon, *Columba livia. General and Comparative Endocrinology* **20**, 326.

Lumeij JT (1985a) The influence of blood sample treatment on plasma potassium concentrations in avian blood. *Avian Pathology* **14**, 257.

Lumeij JT (1985b) Clinicopathological aspects of lead poisoning in birds: a review. *The Veterinary Quarterly* **7**, 133.

Lumeij JT (1987a) Avian clinical pathology: general considerations. *The Veterinary Quarterly* **9**, 249.

Lumeij JT (1987b) The influence of blood sample treatment, feeding and starvation on plasma glucose concentrations in racing pigeons. In: *A contribution to clinical investigative methods for birds with special reference to the racing pigeon*. JT Lumeij, PhD Thesis, Utrecht University.

Lumeij JT (1987c) Plasma urea, creatinine and uric acid concentrations in response to dehydration in racing pigeons *(Columba livia domestica). Avian Pathology* **16**, 377.

Lumeij JT (1987d) The diagnostic value of plasma proteins and non-protein nitrogen substances in birds. *The Veterinary Quarterly* **9**, 262.

Lumeij JT (1991) Fasting and post-prandial plasma bile acid concentrations in racing pigeons (*Columba livia domestica*) and mallards (*Anas platyrhynchos*). *Journal of the Association of Avian Veterinarians* **5**, 197.

Lumeij (1994a) Avian clinical enzymology. *Seminars in Avian and Exotic Pet Medicine* **3**, 14.

Lumeij JT (1994b) Gastroenterology. In: *Avian Medicine: Principles and Application*. Eds BW Ritchie, GJ Harrison and LR Harrison. Wingers, Lake Worth.

Lumeij JT (1994c) Hepatology. In: *Avian Medicine: Principles and Application*. Eds BW Ritchie, GJ Harrison and LR Harrison. Wingers, Lake Worth.

Lumeij JT (1994d) Nephrology. In: *Avian Medicine: Principles and Application*. Eds BW Ritchie, GJ Harrison and LR Harrison. Wingers, Lake Worth.

Lumeij JT and DeBruijne JJ (1985a) Evaluation of the refractometric method for the determination of total protein in avian plasma or serum. *Avian Pathology* **14**, 441.

Lumeij JT, DeBruijne JJ and Kwant M (1990) Comparison of different methods of measuring protein and albumin in pigeon sera. *Avian Pathology* **19**, 255.

Lumeij JT and Remple JD (1991) Plasma urea, creatinine and uric acid concentrations in relation to feeding in peregrine falcons (*Falco peregrinus*). *Avian Pathology* **20**, 79.

Lumeij JT and Remple JD (1992) Plasma bile acid concentrations in response to feeding in peregrine falcons (*Falco peregrinus*). *Avian Diseases* **36**, 1060.

Lumeij JT and Ritchie BW (1994) Cardiology. In: *Avian Medicine: Principles and Application*. Eds BW Ritchie, GJ Harrison and LR Harrison. Wingers, Lake Worth.

Lumeij JT and Westerhof I (1988) Clinical evaluation of thyroid function in racing pigeons (*Columba livia domestica*). *Avian Pathology* **17**, 63.

Rümke CL and Bezemer PD (1972) Methoden voor de bepaling van referentiewaarden II. Nieuwe methoden. [Methods for the determination of normal values II. New methods.] *Nederlands Tijdschrift voor Geneeskunde* **116**, 1559.

Vuillaume A (1983) A new technique for taking blood samples from ducks and geese. *Avian Pathology* **12**, 389.

Appendix 7.1. The International System of Units (SI) (JT Lumeij and N Mauroo).

With the increasing exchange of knowledge between the USA and Europe with regard to avian clinical biochemistry, it is imperative that a uniform system of units is used to avoid confusion. The World Health Assembly recommended the International System of Units (SI, Système International d'Unites) for the health professions in 1977. The SI is the result of many decades of international efforts to develop a universally acceptable system. In many countries and many scientific journals the use of the SI is mandatory. It seems that the SI has gained more acceptance in European countries than in the USA. Many American veterinary journals still use conventional units (*Journal of the Association of Avian Veterinarians*) or a mixture of conventional and SI units (*Avian Diseases*), while European journals use the SI (*Avian Pathology*). Until the SI is used in all scientific papers and handbooks, conversion factors are indispensable.

This Appendix is not complete and further information may be obtained from: *Units, Symbols and Abbreviations* (Royal Society of Medicine Services, London, 1988).

Analyte	Conventional units	International system of units (SI)	Conversion factor to SI
Albumin	g/dl	g/l	10
Ammonia	μg/dl	μmol/l	0.5871
Bile acids	mg/l	μmol/l	2.547
Bilirubin	mg/dl	μmol/l	17.1
Calcium	mg/dl	mmol/l	0.25
Chloride	mEq/l	mmol/l	1
Chloride	mg/dl	mmol/l	0.272
Cholesterol	mg/dl	mmol/l	0.02586
Corticosterone	μg/dl	nmol/l	28.9
Cortisol	μg/dl	nmol/l	27.59
Creatinine	mg/dl	μmol/l	88.4
Globulin	mg/dl	g/l	10
Glucose	mg/dl	mmol/l	0.05551
Insulin	μU/ml	pmol/l	7.175
Iron	μg/dl	μmol/l	0.1791
Lead	μg/dl	μmo/l	0.04826
Magnesium	mEq/l	mmol/l	0.5
Magnesium	mg/dl	mmol/l	0.4114
Phosphate (inorganic)	mg/dl	mmol/l	0.3229
Potassium	mEq/l	mmol/l	1
Progesterone	ng/dl	nmol/l	0.032
Protein	g/dl	g/l	10
Sodium	mEq/l	mmol/l	1
Thyroxine	μg/dl	nmol/l	12.87
Triglycerides	mg/dl	mmol/l	0.01129
Urea	mg/dl	mmol/l	0.167
Urea nitrogen (BUN)	mg/dl	mmol/l	0.7140
Urea nitrogen (BUN)	mg/dl	mmol urea /l	0.3670
Uric acid	mg/dl	mmol/l	59.48

CHAPTER EIGHT

Haematology

Ivan B Jennings

INTRODUCTION

The use of clinical haematology as an aid to differential diagnosis, monitoring of disease and response to treatment is well established within mammalian species and is now becoming more widely used in avians. Whilst there are many similarities between avian and mammalian blood cells, there are many fundamental differences that effect the techniques involved. Avian blood differs from mammalian blood mainly in the morphology of the red cells and thrombocytes, both of which are nucleated, and the appearance of the heterophil. The term 'neutrophil' is not appropriate in avian haematology as the cytoplasm contains many eosinophilic granules: the term 'heterophil' is used.

It is not possible within the limitations of this chapter to cover avian haematology in any great depth; instead, however, it describes briefly avian blood cells and parasites, the routine techniques used in haematology and how they can be adapted for use in avians. A knowledge of mammalian haematological techniques has been assumed and the emphasis placed on the modifications.

COLLECTION OF THE BLOOD SAMPLE

Blood taken for haematological examination should be taken into ethylenediaminetetra-acetic acid (EDTA) (1.5mg/ml blood) anticoagulant and ideally be of venous origin. Puncture of the ulnar vein, or of the right jugular vein, should be possible in birds over 100g bodyweight. Heparin as an anticoagulant is not ideal as the affinity of the cells to Romanosky stains is affected, leucocytes often show clumping and the estimation of fibrinogen becomes unreliable.

Only 0.3-0.5ml of blood is required to perform a full blood count and this should be taken with the minimum of suction being applied to the syringe. The blood volume in birds varies from 5-13% of the total mass. One percent of total mass, ie. 10ml/kg, can be collected safely from any healthy bird; lesser volumes may be advisable in sick birds.

AVIAN BLOOD CELLS AND PARASITES

Any clinician embarking on avian blood film examinations is advised to obtain those references listed at the end of this chapter and, although the *Atlas of Avian Hematology* is now out of print, it will prove very useful if it can be obtained.

A brief description of avian blood cells and common blood parasites is given in Tables 8.1 and 8.2.

Reticulocytes
Most avian red cells stained by standard mammalian procedures, such as methylene blue (Dacie and Lewis, 1991), show some evidence of residual cytoplasmic ribonucleic acid (RNA). This ranges from non-aggregated reticulum to large numbers of reticulum aggregates showing a distinct ring around the cell nucleus. This latter form shows good correlation to the numbers of polychromatic cells present.

Blood Parasites
The occurrence of avian blood parasites, although rare, has increased significantly in the UK since 1994. They are seen predominantly in young birds.

LABORATORY TECHNIQUES

Blood Smear Preparation
Blood smears should always be prepared from fresh non-anticoagulated blood or as soon as possible from the EDTA sample.

Avian blood cells appear more fragile than mammalian cells and, as such, are more prone to 'smearing' during spreading of the blood film. The standard two-slide wedge method used in mammalian haematology is suitable if high quality, pre-cleaned and bevel edged microscope slides are used. However, a gentle touch and practice is required if 'smearing' is to be minimised and high quality blood films obtained.

Blood Film Examination
Any of the Romanowsky stains formulated for use in mammalian haematology are suitable, and those commonly used include Wright's, Wright's-Giemsa and

Table 8.1. Avian blood cells.

Cell type	Main distinguishing features
Erythrocyte (see Figure 8.1)	Oval cell. Clear orange/pink cytoplasm. Central oval nucleus showing clumped chromatin becoming more condensed as the cell ages.
Immature erythrocyte	Round to slightly oval cell. Clear light blue cytoplasm. Central round to slightly oval nucleus showing clumped chromatin. Up to 5% in adults; more common in immature birds.
Heterophil (see Figure 8.2)	Round cell. Colourless or pale pink cytoplasm. Lobed nucleus (average 2-3). *Rod shaped or oval granules that usually stain brick red.
Eosinophil (see Figure 8.3)	Round cell but has a tendency to irregularity. Clear blue cytoplasm. Bilobed nucleus with coarse clumped chromatin that stains more intense than in the heterophil. *Granules usually round (or oval) and usually stain bright red.
Lymphocyte (see Figure 8.4), monocyte (see Figure 8.5) and basophil (see Figure 8.6)	Similar to those seen in mammals.
Thrombocyte (see Figure 8.1)	Oval cell, more rounded and smaller than erythrocyte. Clear reticulated cytoplasm which may contain small red granules. Dense nuclear chromatin. Often seen in clumps and average 2-3 per field on oil immersion in normal avians.

* Granules range from round to rod shape and bright red to brick red within heterophils and eosinophils depending on the species, making differentiation difficult. The heterophil, however, is usually the more numerous of the two cells and will show a consistent but different stain affinity within the individual. This is a useful guide when dealing with an unfamiliar species.

Table 8.2. Common avian blood parasites.

Genus	Main distinguishing feature	Frequency and pathogenicity
Haemoproteus	Halter-shaped intraerythrocytic gametocytes that partially encircle the nucleus, appear pigmented and occupy more than 50% of the cytoplasm.	An avian parasite with generally low pathogenicity, but may be pathogenic in pigeons.
Plasmodium	Elongated or round intraerythrocytic gametocytes that often displace the nucleus, appear pigmented and occupy less that 25% of the cytoplasm. Small round intraerythrocytic trophozoites with a 'signet ring' appearance. Round intraerythrocytic schizonts containing darkly stained merozoites.	A parasite with a worldwide distribution causing avian malaria. May be pathogenic in some raptors, pigeons and waterfowl, whilst others could be asymptomatic carriers.
Leucocytozoon	Elongated intraerythrocytic gametocytes that grossly deform the host cell.	May be pathogenic in waterfowl and young raptors.
Trypanosoma, Microflaria	Similar to those found in other species.	Pathogenic only if organisms very numerous.

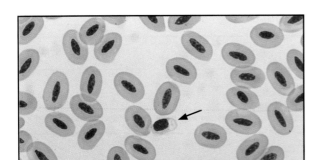

Figure 8.1: *Erythrocytes plus a thrombocyte (arrowed) (Red-tailed Hawk). (Modified Wright's Stain x660)*

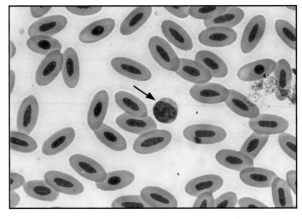

Figure 8.4: *Lymphocyte (arrowed) (Golden Eagle). (Modified Wright's Stain x660)*

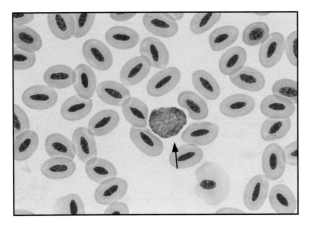

Figure 8.2: *Heterophil (arrowed) (Red-tailed Hawk). (Modified Wright's Stain x660)*

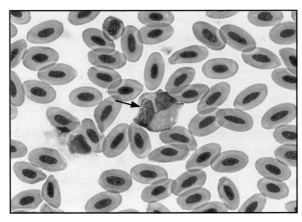

Figure 8.5: *Monocyte (arrowed) (Golden Eagle). (Modified Wright's Stain x660)*

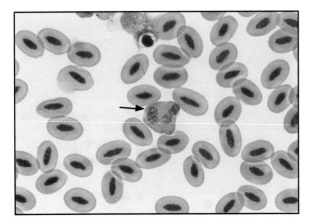

Figure 8.3: *Eosinophil (arrowed) (Red-tailed Hawk). (Modified Wright's Stain x660)*

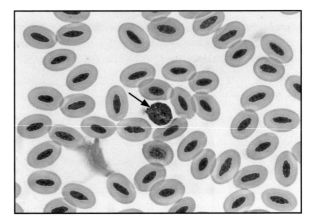

Figure 8.6: *Basophil (arrowed) (Red-tailed Hawk). (Wright's Stain x660)*

May-Grunwald-Giemsa. Rapid stains, eg. Diff Quik, give variable results, making cell identification very difficult, and so they are not recommended.

Examination of a stained avian blood film can be the single most important procedure to be performed, especially when only a small volume of blood is available. Whilst a rapid examination may be necessary, referring fresh smears to an experienced avian haematologist is advisable if the maximum information is to be obtained. Several unstained smears should be submitted.

PACKED CELL VOLUME (PCV)

The determination of PCV is a quick and simple way of assessing subjectively the erythrocyte numbers. The standard manual procedure using microhaematocrit capillary tubes centrifuged between 10,000g and 12,000g for five minutes can be used. Where only a very small sample is obtained, microhaematocrit centrifuges are available (Stat Spin) which require only 10μl of blood to perform the estimation.

Blood for PCV can be collected directly from the needle hub or lancet prick into a heparinised or, where fibrinogen is to be estimated, a full sized EDTA haematocrit tube. As automated PCVs are not direct measurements, but calculations derived from the red blood cell (RBC) count and the mean cell volume (MCV), both of which (in particular the MCV) may be inaccurate, the results obtained are often unreliable. In adult birds, PCV values below 0.32l/l suggest anaemia and values above 0.58l/l suggest dehydration or primary/secondary polycythaemia (respiratory or cardiac disease).

Examination of the plasma and buffy coat should be carried out following centrifugation (see Table 8.3).

FIBRINOGEN

Although fibrinogen is essential for normal blood coagulation, it is also one of the acute phase proteins and as such is often increased in acute inflammation and infectious diseases. Estimation of fibrinogen levels uses the fact that it can be selectively denatured in EDTA plasma at 56°C and, therefore, can be carried out on the haematocrit tube used in the estimation of the PCV.

Method of Estimation

The microhaematocrit tube should be incubated by immersion in a water bath thermostatically controlled at 56°C for three minutes, ensuring that it is immersed to above the plasma column. The temperature and time are critical if non-specific denaturation is to be avoided. The microhaematocrit should be recentrifuged as for PCV determination.

The height of both the precipitate (B) and the plasma (C) from the buffy coat/precipitate interface (A) is measured (see Figure 8.7). The concentration of fibrinogen can be calculated as follows:

$$\frac{B}{C} \times 100 = \text{fibrinogen (g/l)}$$

Levels greater than 4g/l are usually considered to be elevated: however, certain species of owl often show slightly higher values.

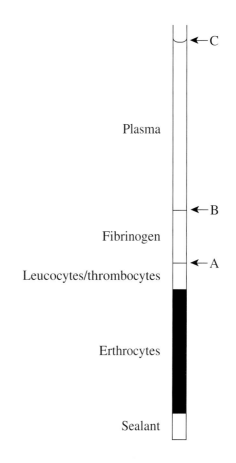

Figure 8.7: *Fibrinogen estimation. Diagrammatic representation of a microhaematocrit tube following incubation and recentrifugation.*

Table 8.3. Examination of the microhaematocrit capillary tube.

Appearance	**Possible cause**	**Effect**
Red plasma	Haemolysis due to poor sampling or an aged sample.	PCV and RBC results invalidated.
Cloudy plasma	Lipaemia due to a diet rich in fatty foods.	Haemoglobin result invalidated.
Yellow plasma	Jaundiced. Diet supplementation.	Raised bilirubin. Normal bilirubin.
Buffy coat > 1%	Raised white cell count. Raised thrombocyte count.	WBC/thrombocyte count indicated.

TOTAL RBC COUNT

Most electronic particle counters used in mammalian haematology can be used for avian RBC counts. However, adjustments may be required to compensate for the larger average size of avian cells. Different threshold and aperture currents may be required for each species depending on the MCV. Most manufacturers will have a technical support team who will advise on how to establish the optimum settings.

Diluting fluids used for mammalian haematology counts are suitable for avians and do not require any specific modifications.

Manual Procedure

A 1:200 dilution is prepared by adding 20μl of blood into 4ml of formal citrate solution (1ml of 40% formaldehyde plus 99ml of 31.3g/l trisodium citrate solution) using an automatic pipette. The use of Thoma pipettes and suction tubes, or any other form of mouth pipetting, is no longer an acceptable procedure in haematology.

Alternatively, the Unopette 5851 (Becton Dickinson) system may be used: this provides an easy method of obtaining accurate dilutions (10μl of blood into 1.99ml diluting fluid).

After the blood and diluting fluid have been well mixed, a metallised improved Neubauer haemocytometer can be charged, either directly from the Unopette or by using a plain microhaematocrit capillary tube, taking care not to overfill. The haemocytometer is placed into a damp chamber for five minutes to allow the cells to settle. This minimises the need for continual focal adjustments during counting: a Petri dish containing damp filter paper is ideal for this purpose.

The total number of erythrocytes in 10 groups of 16 small squares within the centre large square of the counting chamber should be determined using the high-dry objective. Ideally, the four corner squares and the centre square on each side of the chamber should be used (see Figure 8.8).

The RBC count can be calculated as follows:

Number of RBCs in 10 squares (160 small squares)
x 5,000 = RBC/μl

$$\frac{RBC/\mu l}{1,000,000} = RBC \times 10^{12}/l$$

HAEMOGLOBIN ESTIMATION

The measurement of haemoglobin in birds is complicated by the presence of red cell nuclei after haemolysis and conversion of the haemoglobin to cyanmethaemoglobin. It is necessary, therefore, to centrifuge the sample to remove the red cell nuclei before reading spectrophotometrically at 540nm, as

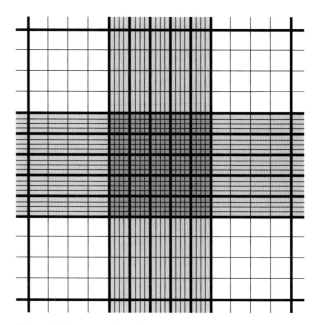

Figure 8.8: *Improved Neubauer haemocytometer. The central area consists of 25 groups of 16 small squares separated by closely ruled triple lines (thick lines in this diagram).*

for mammalian haemoglobin. It has been reported that a small amount of haemoglobin is bound to the nucleus and falsely low results may be obtained by this method. As an alternative the measurement of oxyhaemoglobin has been suggested by some authors (Hawkey *et al*, 1987).

The effect of the red cell nuclei on the haemoglobin can be minimised by measuring haemoglobin bichromatically. This principal is utilised by the haemoglobinometer manufactured by HemoCue AB, where haemoglobin is measured at 570 and 880nm.

Whilst there is some species variation, haemoglobin levels between 120-180g/l are commonly found in healthy adult birds, with slightly lower values in immature individuals.

RBC ABSOLUTE VALUES

Calculation of the MCV can be of value, where normal ranges are known, in determining whether the individual is microcytic (as found in chronic haemorrhage), macrocytic or normocytic, and can be calculated as follows:

$$\frac{PCV \ (l/l)}{RBC \times 10^{12}/l} \times 1,000 = MCV \ (fl)$$

Calculation of the mean cell haemoglobin concentration (MCHC) can be of value in determining whether the individual is hypochromic. Most birds show an MCHC range of 290-360g/l. However, lower values are often found in immature birds. MCHC can be calculated as follows:

$$\frac{Hb\ (g/l)}{PCV\ (l/l)} = MCHC\ (g/l)$$

TOTAL WBC AND DIFFERENTIAL COUNT

There are no selective lysing agents that can remove erythrocyte nuclei and leave leucocyte nuclei intact. Because of this, automated WBC counting is not yet possible.

Manual Procedures
Many manual procedures have been described for the estimation of WBC counts in avians, two of which are described below.

Indirect
This is the simplest procedure in which the number of leucocytes relative to the number of erythrocytes are estimated from a stained blood smear. The use of a graticule within the microscope eyepiece is an advantage for speed and accuracy. The WBC count can then be calculated using either a mean average RBC count for that species or, preferably, from an accurate RBC count obtained from the same blood sample. The WBC count can be calculated as follows:

$$\frac{\text{Number of leucocytes counted}}{\text{Number of erythrocytes counted}} \times RBC/\mu l = WBC/\mu l$$

$$\frac{WBC/\mu l}{1,000} = WBC \times 10^9/l$$

Where an accurate RBC count is not available and the PCV is outside the normal range, the WBC count should be corrected using the following formula:

$$Estimated\ WBC/\mu l \times \frac{Observed\ PCV}{Average\ PCV}$$

$$= Corrected\ WBC/\mu l$$

(The average PCV for most avians is 0.42l/l.)

The indirect method is often the method chosen. However, the accuracy diminishes when counts exceed 15 x 10^9/l and/or average RBC counts and PCV values are used. A well-made, well-stained blood smear with an even distribution of cells is essential if this method is used.

Semi-indirect
This method uses a combination of an absolute heterophil and eosinophil count obtained using an improved Neubauer haemocytometer, and a correction factor for the percentage of other white cell lines present obtained by performing a differential count.

One of the most convenient methods available involves the use of the Unopette 5877 (Becton Dickinson) as described below:
- The pipette is filled with blood (25μl).
- The blood is mixed with the diluent (phloxine B), giving a dilution of 1:32, and the haemocytometer is charged (as for RBC count). To avoid overstaining this should be carried out within a few minutes of mixing.
- The haemocytometer is placed into a damp chamber for five minutes.
- All the granulocytes that fall within the ruled area on both sides of the haemocytometer (18 large squares) are counted (see Figure 18.8). These cells appear round, stain distinctly red-orange and are refractile.

After performing a differential the WBC count is calculated as follows:

$$\frac{\text{Number of cells counted in the chamber} \times 1.1 \times 16 \times 100}{\text{Percentage of heterophils and eosinophils}}$$
$$= WBC/\mu l$$

With experience the semi-direct method can be an accurate procedure. However, care should be taken not to overstain the cells as this will make granulocyte identification more difficult.

Whilst direct methods for estimating WBC counts are available using Natt and Herricks solution (Campbell, 1988) or toluene blue, identification of the different cell types is difficult and is not recommended for the inexperienced.

Standard mammalian procedures can be used to perform a differential count (%) and conversion into an absolute count can be achieved as follows:

$$\frac{\text{Total WBC} \times 10^9/l \times \text{cell count \%}}{100}$$
$$= Absolute\ count \times 10^9/l$$

SUMMARY

Primary haematological diseases are rare in birds. More commonly, abnormal results are obtained secondary to infections and inflammation or as a result of poor management and diet. Many other factors may affect the results obtained from the individual bird under examination, as well as from those birds used to establish normal ranges. These factors include age, sex, season, diet, reproductive status and stress, as well as the effect of the sedative used. Whilst some work has been carried out to investigate these effects, it has been limited and is still far from complete. This lack of knowledge should not deter the clinician from using avian haematology as a diagnostic tool. However, the limitations should be noted. Where ranges are not available for a specific species, the wider avian range, or that obtained from a similar species, should be used.

Sample haematology (and clinical biochemistry) values are listed in Appendix 8.1.

If this situation is to improve, any data obtained in avian haematology should be published, or at least made available, thus increasing the pool of data available.

Acknowledgement

The values supplied by IBJ and NH-B to help compile the Appendix of haematological and biochemistry values were supported by a generous donation from the British Falconry Club.

REFERENCES AND FURTHER READING

Campbell TW and Dien FJ (1984) Avian hematology. *Veterinary Clinics of North America: Small Animal Practice* **14**, 233.

Campbell TW (1988) *Avian Hematology and Cytology*. Iowa State University Press, Ames.

Dacie JW and Lewis SM (1991) *Practical Hematology*. 7th Edn. Churchill Livingstone, New York.

Hawkey CM and Samour HJ (1987) The value of clinical hematology in exotic birds. In: *Disorders of Exotic Animals*. Eds DE Jacobson and G Kolias. Contempory Issues in Small Animal Practice. Churchill Livingstone, New York.

Jain NC (1986) *Veterinary Hematology*. 4th Edn. Lea and Febiger, Philadelphia.

Lind EJ, Wolff PL, Petrini KR, Keyler CW, Olson DE and Redig PT (1990) Morphology of the eosinophil in raptors. *Journal of the Association of Avian Veterinarians* **4(1)**, 33.

Lucas AM and Jamroz C (1961) *Atlas of Avian Hematology*. United States Department of Agriculture, Monograph No 25, Washington DC.

Lumeij JT (1987) The influence of blood sample treatment, feeding and starvation on plasma glucose concentrations in racing pigeons. In: *A contribution to clinical investigative methods for birds with special reference to the racing pigeon*. JT Lumeij, PhD Thesis, Utrecht University.

Rosskopf WJ and Worple RW (1984) Clinical experience with avian laboratory diagnostics. *Veterinary Clinics of North America: Small Animal Practice* **14**, 249.

Appendix 8.1. Haematology and Clinical Biochemistry Values.

The ranges for raptors and waterfowl are the results of observations by the author and one of the scientific editors (NAF) on apparently normal healthy individuals, performed at two separate laboratories. These levels are not intended to be used as 'normal ranges' as the birds sampled were of both sexes and of all (non-juvenile) ages, and the methods used and the results obtained will vary between laboratories. Clinicians are advised to use a laboratory which can provide normal reference ranges, for their laboratory, for the species being tested. The values for pigeons are from Lumeij (1987).

Species	Lanner Falcon	Lagger Falcon	Merlin	Peregrine Falcon	Saker Falcon
	n = 42	n = 13	n = 33	n = 70	n = 50
RBC (x10^{12}/l)	2.63-3.98	2.65-3.63	2.85-4.1	2.95-3.94	2.54-3.96
PCV(l/l)	0.37-0.53	0.39-0.51	0.39-0.51	0.37-0.53	0.38-0.49
Hb (g/l)	122-171	128-163	132-179	118-188	115-165
MCV (fl)	127-150	123-145	105-130	118-146	124-147
MCH (pg)	42.3-48.8	38-47.7	36-45.9	40-48.4	41.4-45.4
MCHC (g/l)	317-353	312-350	340-360	319-352	304-349
WBC (x10^9/l)	3.5-11	5-9	4-9.5	3.3-11	3.8-11.5
Heterophils (x10^9/l)	1.65-8.8	3.5-6.57	3.2-4.03	1.4-8.55	2.6-5.85
Lymphocytes (x10^9/l)	1.1-5.13	1.7-4	1.2-1.56	1.1-3.3	0.8-4.25
Monocytes (x10^9/l)	0-0.9	0-0.85	0-0.5	0.1-0.86	0-0.8
Eosinophils (x10^9/l)	0-0.2	0-0.2	0-0.15	0-0.3	0-0.2
Basophils (x10^9/l)	0-0.45	0.17-0.83	0-0.15	0-0.6	0-0.45
Thrombocytes (x10^9/l)	5-40	12-35		6-46	12-25
Fibrinogen (g/l)	<4	< 4	<4	<4.2	<3.5
	n = 26		n = 39	n = 55	n = 38
Total protein (g/l)	33-42		27.5-39	25-40	27-36
Albumin (g/l)	9.6-16		8.6-16.1	8.3-12.5	9-12.3
Globulin (g/l)	21.2-28.8		17.2-25	16-28	18-28
A:G ratio	0.44-0.57		0.47-0.58	0.4-0.55	0.45-0.57
Urea (mmol/l)	1.3-2.7			0.9-2.8	0.5-2.6
Creatinine (μmol/l)	37-75		16-50	41-91	23-75
Uric acid (μmol/l)	318-709		174-800	326-675	320-785
Bile acids (μmol/l)				20-118	20-90
ALT (SGPT) (u/l)				15-51	36-55
ALP (u/l)	180-510		54-310	97-350	285-450
GGT (u/l)				0-7	0.8-5.9
AST (SGOT) (u/l)	30-118		50-125	50-105	45-95
CK (u/l)	350-650		521-807	357-850	355-651
LDH (u/l)	434-897		320-630	625-1210	551-765
Glucose (mmol/l)	11-15		9-12	11-16	12-14
Cholesterol (mmol/l)	3-8.8		3-7.8	3.9-10.5	4.5-8.6
Inorg phosphate (mmol/l)	0.68-2		0.95-1.79	0.77-2.1	0.72-2.16
Calcium (mmol/l)	2.07-2.45		2-2.45	2.1-2.56	2.15-2.61
Sodium (mmol/l)	152-164		155-170	153-164	154-161
Potassium (mmol/l)	1-2.1		1-1.8	0.9-1.7	0.8-2.3
Chloride (mmol/l)				117-127	114-125

Species	Ferruginous Hawk	Red-tailed Hawk	Harris' Hawk	Eurasian Buzzard	Northern Goshawk
	n = 18	n = 15	n = 53	n = 26	n = 43
RBC (x10^{12}/l)	2.41-3.59	2.2-3.35	2.63-3.5	2.13-2.76	2.6-3.48
PCV(l/l)	0.37-0.48	0.35-0.53	0.4-0.55	0.32-0.44	0.43-0.53
Hb (g/l)	107-166	123-175	121-171	101-167	121-177
MCV (fl)	150-178	157-168	147-163	151-165	141-156
MCH (pg)	46-57.4	43-50.4	45.4-51.1	48-53	44.5-51.6
MCHC (g/l)	297-345	312-350	301-330	307-339	305-343
WBC (x10^9/l)	4.5-6.8	3.4-7.5	4.8-10	5-13	4-11
Heterophils (x10^9/l)	1.89-3.76	1.9-3.5	2.3-6.71	3.2-11	3.5-6.97
Lymphocytes (x10^9/l)	0.78-1.74	1.3-1.1	0.6-2.36	0.3-3.1	1.38-1.93
Monocytes (x10^9/l)	0.24-1.5	0.12-1.2	0.2-1.49	0.2-0.68	0-0.1
Eosinophils (x10^9/l)	0.3-0.7	0.1-0.9	0-0.75	0.1-0.8	0-0.65
Basophils (x10^9/l)	0.15-0.6	0-0.5	0-1.55	0-0.9	0-0.35
Thrombocytes (x10^9/l)	8-47	4-33	10-59	8-46	15-35
Fibrinogen (g/l)	<3.5	<3	<4.3	<3.6	<3.5
			n = 17		n = 24
Total protein (g/l)			31-45.7		26.3-42
Albumin (g/l)			13.9-17		8.8-12.4
Globulin (g/l)			21-29.4		18-29.2
A:G ratio			0.46-0.55		0.4-0.57
Urea (mmol/l)			0.7-1.9		
Creatinine (μmol/l)			20-59		41-94
Uric acid (μmol/l)			535-785		511-854
Bile acids (μmol/l)					
ALT (SGPT) (u/l)					
ALP (u/l)			20-96		15.6-87.5
GGT (u/l)			2-6.9		3-7.6
AST (SGOT) (u/l)			160-348		176-409
CK (u/l)			224-650		218-775
LDH (u/l)			160-563		120-906
Glucose (mmol/l)			12.2-15.7		11.5-15.9
Cholesterol (mmol/l)			6.6-13.1		4-11.5
Inorg phosphate (mmol/l)			0.8-2.14		0.8-1.97
Calcium (mmol/l)			2.1-2.66		2.15-2.69
Sodium (mmol/l)			155-171		
Potassium (mmol/l)			0.8-2.3		
Chloride (mmol/l)			113-119		

Species	Golden Eagle	Tawny Eagle	Northern Eagle Owl	Pigeon*
	n = 16	**n = 29**	**n = 20**	**n = 507**
RBC (x10^{12}/l)	1.69-3.21	2.32-2.83	1.65-2.35	3.1-4.5
PCV(l/l)	0.31-0.52	0.37-0.47	0.36-0.52	0.425
Hb (g/l)	112-173	108-175	107-180	81-99
MCV (fl)	165-186	163-188	189-204	
MCH (pg)	53.8-67.7	54-62	64.6-76	
MCHC (g/l)	326-364	296-360	325-376	
WBC (x10^9/l)	6.2-17	5-9.5	3.5-12.1	13-22.3
Heterophils (x10^9/l)	4.5-15.2	3.58-6.45	2.2-9.23	4.3-6.2
Lymphocytes (x10^9/l)	0.75-3.37	0.51-2.72	1.5-5.07	10.9-12.2
Monocytes (x10^9/l)	0-0.63	0.2-1.07	0-0.48	0.4-1.1
Eosinophils (x10^9/l)	0.1-0.6	0.3-2.1	0-0.48	0.1-0.3
Basophils (x10^9/l)	0-0.16	0-0.4	0-0.35	0.1-0.5
Thrombocytes (x10^9/l)	7-45	19-25	1-29	7-27
Fibrinogen (g/l)	<4.5	<3.5	<4.5	
		n = 13	**n = 20**	**n = 507**
Total protein (g/l)		29-41.4	30.1-34.5	21-35
Albumin (g/l)		11.5-18	11.1-13.5	
Globulin (g/l)		25.3-28.4	18.7-22.4	
A:G ratio		0.44-0.55		1.5-3.6
Urea (mmol/l)		0.8-2.7	0.9-2.9	0.4-0.7
Creatinine (μmol/l)		31-59	31-49	23-36**
Uric acid (μmol/l)		413-576	475-832	150-765
Bile acids (μmol/l)				22-60
ALT (SGPT) (u/l)				19-48**
ALP (u/l)		17.1-69.7		
GGT (u/l)		1-2.7		0-2.9**
AST (SGOT) (u/l)		124-226		45-123**
CK (u/l)				110-480**
LDH (u/l)		211-369		30-205**
Glucose (mmol/l)		10.2-14.5	13.5-21.7	12.9-20.5
Cholesterol (mmol/l)		7.9-10.7	3.9-7.1	
Inorg phosphate (mmol/l)		1.2-1.78	1.15-1.94	
Calcium (mmol/l)		2.21-2.66	2.16-2.61	1.9-2.6
Sodium (mmol/l)		153-157		141-149
Potassium (mmol/l)		1.5-3.1		3.9-4.7
Chloride (mmol/l)		114-123		

* Pigeon haematology values and plasma biochemistry reference values (as established and used at the Utrecht University Department of Clinical Sciences of Companion Animals) are from Lumeij (1987).

** Enzyme estimations for pigeons carried out at 30°C. All other estimations carried out at 37°C.

Species	White-winged Wood Duck	Hawaiian Goose	Canada Goose	Swan	Flamingos
	n = 30	n = 10	n = 15	n = 50	n = 25
RBC (x10^{12}/l)	2.6-3.48	2.35-2.89	2.25-3.35	1.96-2.9	2.25-3.45
PCV(l/l)	0.46-0.57	0.38-0.45	0.35-0.49	0.32-0.5	0.4-0.53
Hb (g/l)	122-181	129-170	122-172	110-165	143-193
MCV (fl)	163-177	156-161	162-178	164-200	141-207
MCH (pg)	46.6-51.9	54.9-59.3	47-58.7	52.9-65.5	53-65
MCHC (g/l)	270-321	340-380	342-363	290-365	290-360
WBC (x10^9/l)	4.7-9.4	6.2-13.4	3-5.15	6.3-22	3.5-13.3
Heterophils (x10^9/l)	2.7-5.6	0-5.57	0.5-2.7	3.33-14.67	0-4.2
Lymphocytes (x10^9/l)	0.65-4	0-7.74	0.8-3.8	0.9-9.77	0-6.35
Monocytes (x10^9/l)	0.15-0.76	0-0.28	0.15-0.8	0.05-1.39	0-0.17
Eosinophils (x10^9/l)	0-0.3	0-0.6	0-0.5	0.11-3.5	0-0.45
Basophils (x10^9/l)	0.1-0.9	0-0.6	0-0.25	0-0.82	
Thrombocytes (x10^9/l)					
Fibrinogen (g/l)		<3.5			<3.6
	n = 18		n = 10	n = 50	n = 25
Total protein (g/l)	34-54		37.3-56.3	35.5-54.5	34-40
Albumin (g/l)	10-25		17.5-23.6	12-21.5	15.2-25.4
Globulin (g/l)	26.4-29.1		20.3-42.6	23-35.5	18.5-36
A:G ratio				0.43-0.65	0.45-0.56
Urea (mmol/l)	0.76-1.05		0.8-3.56	0.1-2.4	0.35-1.25
Creatinine (μmol/l)	6-14		4-11	18-89	44-91
Uric acid (μmol/l)	165-691			126-700	183-685
Bile acids (μmol/l)					
ALT (SGPT) (u/l)	0-67.5			10-59	0-55
ALP (u/l)	0-198		0-149		11-95
GGT (u/l)	0-14		1-10.5	4-26	1-5.8
AST (SGOT) (u/l)	9.8-43.2			17-112	61-154
CK (u/l)				124-894	155-750
LDH (u/l)			145-435	165-724	125-685
Glucose (mmol/l)	8-13.4			6.2-12.6	9.5-13.2
Cholesterol (mmol/l)				3-7.8	3.6-8.2
Inorg phosphate (mmol/l)	0.55-1.66			0.7-2.36	0.65-1.72
Calcium (mmol/l)	2.01-2.52			2.19-2.89	2.2-2.85
Sodium (mmol/l)				132-150	149-158
Potassium (mmol/l)			3.9-4.7	3-5	2.5-3.8
Chloride (mmol/l)			101-133		

The following reference values for Peregrine Falcons and pigeons are from Lumeij, Remple and Riddle (unpublished data) and Lumeij (1987) respectively.

	Peregrine Falcon	Pigeon
	n = 79	n = 507
Urea/uric acid ratio	1.7-6.4	1.8 ± 1.8*
GLDH (u/l)	<8	<8
Osmolality (mOsmol/kg)	322-356	297-317
Thyroxine (nmol/l) before and 16 hours after stimulation with 2 IU/kg TSH	6-35	100-300
Corticosterone (nmol/l) before and 90 minutes after stimulation with 250g/kg ACTH	0.2-1.24	2.22-11.2
Argenine vasotonine (AVT) (pg/ml) before and after 24 hours water deprivation	1.7 ± 1.4	6.3 ± 2.2*

* mean ± standard deviation

CHAPTER NINE

Anaesthesia

Martin P C Lawton

INTRODUCTION

Raptors have previously been considered difficult patients to anaesthetise and poor anaesthetic risks (Paddleford, 1986) mainly due to problems associated with shock, improper handling or regurgitation. With the advances brought about by the newer, safer anaesthetic agents, eg. isoflurane, there is now no reason why birds may not be successfully anaesthetised, providing the basic principles of anaesthesiology are followed. The rapid avian metabolism, the peculiarity of their respiratory system and the physical size of the avian patient are all factors that must be assessed in the approach to anaesthesia. An approach to anaesthetising birds is outlined in Figure 9.1.

REQUIREMENTS OF SEDATION/ ANAESTHESIA

The aims of anaesthesia should be to provide a smooth, reliable induction with adequate restraint, muscle relaxation and analgesia, followed by a fast, but full, uneventful recovery.

Restraint
The degree of restraint required depends upon the purpose for which the bird is being sedated or anaesthetised. Sedatives or low doses of injectable anaesthetics may be sufficient to immobilise a bird for a brief but thorough clinical examination or to obtain laboratory samples. Heavier sedation or a light plane of anaesthesia may, however, be required for radiography, laparoscopy, biopsy or minor surgery. Total restraint with moderate to deep anaesthesia is required for most surgery. The choice of anaesthetic or sedative agent depends upon the degree of restraint that is required.

Muscle Relaxation
The requirements for muscular relaxation depend on the procedure or investigation to be performed. Radiography requires only sufficient relaxation to allow correct positioning of the patient. More relaxation will be required when abdominal or orthopaedic surgery is contemplated, and this will therefore affect the choice and depth of anaesthetic.

Analgesia
All birds undergoing surgery require analgesia both intra- and postoperatively. In many cases the correct choice of anaesthetic agent(s) will provide all the analgesia that is required. The use of reversible injectable anaesthetics, such as medetomidine and xylazine, should be carefully considered, especially if the analgesia may be compromised by the antagonists. Choosing anaesthetic agents which provide a good degree of analgesia will often allow better restraint and muscle relaxation, as well as proving safer by allowing the anaesthetist to maintain the bird on a lower plane of anaesthesia.

PRE-ANAESTHETIC CONSIDERATIONS

Handling
Handling should be as gentle and stress free as possible. Experience of handling the type of bird about to be anaesthetised will help achieve this aim. Handling most diurnal birds in an environment that has subdued lighting will reduce the degree of stress. Raptors that are trained to the 'hood' may be hooded; this will help reduce the degree of stress. Although the bird has to be handled for a full clinical examination, ideally this should be done some time before the anaesthetic is given, to allow time for recovery from any stress. Handling of all birds should be kept as short as possible prior to induction of the anaesthetic. Preparations for anaesthetising the bird should be made well in advance.

Clinical Examination
The importance and techniques of a full clinical examination have been covered elsewhere (see Chapter 2). Assessment of the health status of birds prior to an anaesthetic is mandatory. Birds should be in as fit a state of health as is possible prior to being anaesthetised. Dehydration should be corrected before the anaesthetic is administered. Some thought should be given to performing routine biochemical examination for liver and kidney function in older birds. Birds with kidney disease should not be given ketamine, as elimination relies on renal excretion. Halothane is contraindicated in birds with hepatic dysfunction or debilitated

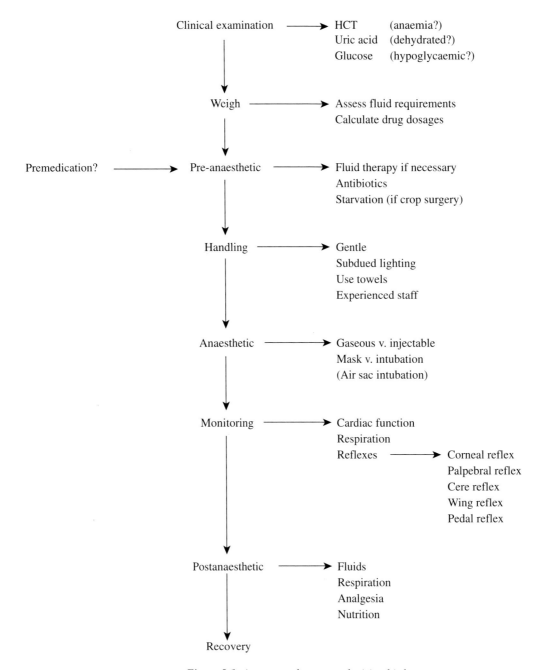

Figure 9.1: An approach to anaesthetising birds.

birds due to the risk of cardiac arrest. All surgical patients should at the very least have an HCT (PCV) and blood glucose estimation performed. Birds with an HCT above 55% require fluid therapy prior to the anaesthetic, whilst birds with hypoglycaemia (<16mmol/l) should be given intravenous glucose 5% before, during and after surgery (Altman, 1991).

Weight

Birds should always be accurately weighed. Good falconers will know the weight of their bird and will be feeding to maintain a fixed weight depending on the season. It is impossible to work out an accurate and safe dosage of an injectable agent (anaesthetic, analgesic or antibiotic) unless an exact weight is known.

Knowing the exact weight is not so important if a gaseous anaesthetic agent is to be used, but will be required for administration of medications or fluid therapy. In these cases, birds can be weighed once they are anaesthetised.

Warmth

Warmth should be provided before induction, during anaesthesia and in the recovery period. The high metabolic rate of birds causes a high core body temperature (CBT). A sick or anaesthetised bird is often unable to maintain its CBT adequately. Hypothermic birds may become hypoglycaemic in an attempt to maintain body temperature; this may be fatal. Anaesthetising a bird and placing it onto a cold operating table is deleterious to the bird and may result in a rapid fall in body temperature. Excessive removal of feathers at the site of surgery will result in lost insulation and lead to heat loss. An anaesthetised bird should be placed onto a towel, a Vetbed or a heating pad. The use of Opsite (Smith and Nephew) will help to minimise the area to be prepared for surgery, yet maintain an adequately clear surgical site. Surgical spirit or other wetting agents should be used sparingly to reduce further heat loss. Cold anaesthetic gases will also have a chilling effect on the bird, but there is little that can be done about this.

Fluid Therapy

Birds, like reptiles, are uricotelic. Uric acid is extremely insoluble and even a slight degree of dehydration may result in uricaemia and renal damage and/or gout. The blood concentration of uric acid will be highest in the kidneys and the liver. Tophii (microcrystals of urates) formation will therefore affect particularly the kidneys and liver. Dehydration should be corrected before anaesthesia, unless isoflurane is available, in which case it is less stressful to administer fluids immediately after induction. Fluids may be administered by the intravenous, intramuscular, intraosseus (see Chapter 3) or subcutaneous route. If the bird is showing signs of severe dehydration or gout, allopurinol or colchicine should be administered in addition to essential fluid therapy.

Starvation

Pre-anaesthetic starvation, although normal for dogs and cats, should be considered more carefully for avian patients. Starvation in smaller birds may result in hypoglycaemia and an increased anaesthetic risk. Cooper (1989) stated that small birds should never be deprived of food for longer than three hours. Pigeons or waterfowl should not be routinely starved; however, anaesthesia may be delayed if the crop is full (unless the bird has an impacted crop requiring surgery). Raptors are not continuous feeders, allowing anaesthetics to be scheduled after the crop is empty, which usually takes a maximum of 4-6 hours.

Premedication

Premedication is not usually advised due to the additional handling and stresses involved. If sedatives or tranquillisers are used, they should not delay the recovery from anaesthesia or cause more disorientation of the bird and increased flapping than is experienced with the anaesthetic itself. The use of atropine (0.04-0.1mg/kg) is debatable. Altman (1991) considered that there was an advantage in reducing respiratory secretions, although Sinn (1994) stated that atropine thickens respiratory secretions, which could cause complications and increased anaesthetic risk, especially in smaller birds. The use of atropine is best

avoided, unless there is excessive oral secretions.

ANALGESIA

Mention of analgesia being provided with anaesthesia has been made earlier. Postoperative analgesia can be provided by the use of buprenorphine (0.01-0.05mg/kg i/m), ketoprofen (5-10mg/kg i/m) or carprofen (5-10mg/kg i/m).

ANATOMICAL CONSIDERATIONS

On inspiration, air passes through the nares, into the nasal cavity and out of the choana into the pharynx. It travels down the trachea (which contains complete rings of cartilage) to the syrinx where the trachea divides into the two primary bronchi which extend to the caudal border of the lungs. When intubating a bird, it is important that the cuff is not overinflated or these tracheal cartilage rings will be damaged.

Avian respiratory anatomy has been reviewed by McLelland (1990). There is some debate about whether or not inspired air passes over the lung tissue twice (James et al, 1976; Haigh, 1981; Paddleford, 1986) or only once (Scheid and Piiper, 1971; Fitzgerald and Blais, 1993). Inspired gases pass twice through the neopulmonic tissue of the lungs, which has only a minimum gaseous exchange and absorption. Inspired air passes only once through the paleopulmonic part of the lungs, which is responsible for gaseous exchange (Scheid and Piiper, 1971; Fitzgerald and Blais, 1993). Much of the inspired air passes through the lungs and directly into the caudal air sacs, without gaseous exchange (see Figure 18.2). There is no dead space in avian lungs, as in the mammalian alveolus, therefore the air is continually circulated past the flowing blood.

There are usually eight air sacs: the unpaired cervical, unpaired clavicular, paired cranial thoracic, paired caudal thoracic and paired abdominal sacs (McLelland, 1990). The air sacs themselves have very poor vascularity so gaseous exchange does not take place other than in the lungs.

The air sacs extend into some of the long bones (pneumatised bones) and the skull sinuses. The sternum and humeri are always pneumatised; this reduces their overall weight, thus aiding flight. Depending on the species, some or all of the following are also pneumatised: cervical vertebrae, thoracic vertebrae, synsacrum, ribs, sternum, scapula, coracoid, femur and/or pelvis.

Birds have no diaphragm. Muscular contractions, mainly of the abdomen, cause the air sacs to act as a bellows, blowing the air back into and through the lungs. A deeply anaesthetised bird may not be generating sufficient muscular contractions to allow adequate 'pumping' of air back into the lungs. Sinn (1994) advised the routine use of intermittent positive pressure ventilation (20-40/minute at 15mmHg) to overcome any possibility of hypocapnoea and maintain adequate oxygenation; the author has also found this helpful. The air sacs hold 80% of the volumetric capacity of the respiratory system. There is some recirculating of air between the abdominal and posterior thoracic air sacs and then into the anterior and clavicular air sacs, as well as the connections with the pneumatised bones. This bellows system will act as a reservoir for anaesthetic gases within the bird, and may result in increasing depth of anaesthesia following induction with high concentrations of certain anaesthetics such as halothane, even when the vaporiser concentration is reduced. The air sacs may be compromised in their bellows action if birds are positioned on their backs. The weight of the viscera on the sternum and abdominal muscles normally helps inspiration. If birds are positioned on their backs, gravity cannot have such an effect, thus reducing the minute volume.

It is during the passage through the paleopulmonic portion of the lungs that the majority of gaseous exchange occurs. The avian lungs are fixed and unexpandable; they are not divided into lobes as seen in mammals. The capillary blood supply to the lungs is, however, greater than that found in mammals. Air diffuses into the air capillaries in the opposite direction to the arterial blood flow, thus producing crosscurrents and resulting in an extremely effective gaseous exchange system (McLelland, 1990). Avian lungs are considered to be ten times more effective than mammalian lungs (James *et al*, 1976). The avian lung is therefore more sensitive to smaller changes in the concentration of gaseous anaesthetics.

CHOICE OF ANAESTHETIC CIRCUITS

In the majority of birds (other than diving waterfowl) the relative ease of induction by face mask with isoflurane reduces many of the complications of handling and injecting the bird (see Figure 9.2). The subsequent fast recovery eliminates the complications of trauma due to unsteadiness, falling off the perch or wing flapping. Therefore, the most basic anaesthetic circuit consists of a vaporiser, a source of carrier gas (usually oxygen) and a face mask. There is no advantage in the use of nitrous oxide when isoflurane is being used.

A face mask does have disadvantages, especially if examining or operating around the head. Other than for the shortest procedure, the author advises the intubation of birds and maintaining them via a Bethune, Ayre's T piece or, for larger birds, a mini Bain system. Care has to be taken with small birds to prevent the risk of blockage of the small diameter tube with mucus. Intubation has the advantages of facilitating ventilation should this prove necessary, and allowing scavenging of waste gases (see Figure 9.3). Scavenging of waste gases is difficult with an open face mask

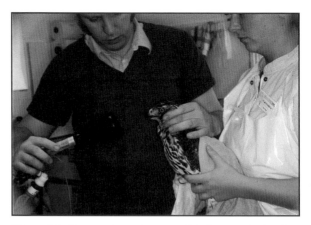

Figure 9.2: Preparation prior to mask induction of a hawk.

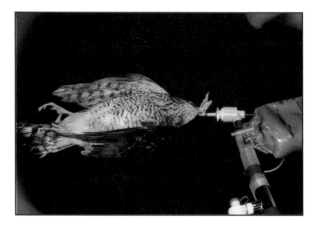

Figure 9.3: Intubation of a Northern Sparrow Hawk. The circuit is a mini Bain which allows active scavenging of waste gases.

unless a more expensive active scavenging system, such as the Fluvac (designed for a face mask), is used.

Intubation of birds can be via the glottis or, if necessary, through a small incision into an abdominal air sac. Uncuffed paediatric endotracheal tubes (diameter is dependent on the size of the bird) are most commonly used, as they are easily placed due to the forward placement of the glottis. In small birds it may be helpful to have forceps ready to gently pull the tongue and, therefore, the glottis forward. The use of a cuffed tube is only recommended for water birds (see Figure 9.4). This prevents inhalation of any fluids in the crop after induction. If cuffed tubes are used, they should not be overinflated (see Anatomical Considerations).

AIR SAC INTUBATION (See also Chapters 3 and 18)

There are often occasions when the use of a face mask or endotracheal tube is not possible. Surgery around the head makes the use of a face mask difficult. Surgery in the mouth or of the beak, or in cases of tracheal obstruction, requires alternative techniques. The presence of air sacs and the unique air flow from the abdominal and caudal thoracic air sacs into the lungs mean that, when a tube is placed into one of these air

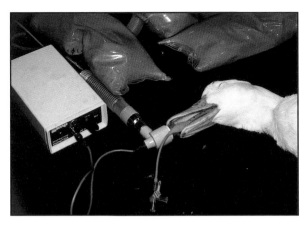

Figure 9.4: Anaesthetised duck with a cuffed incubation tube to prevent the inhalation of any regurgitated fluid. Note the respiratory monitor.

sacs, anaesthetic gases (or just oxygen where there is an airway obstruction) can be introduced. The placement of the air sac tube is usually performed once a bird is induced by injectable or gaseous anaesthetic agents (see Figure 9.5). In cases of airway obstruction it is possible to place the tube in a restrained bird. In emergency situations the author restrains the bird with its head in a mask delivering 100% oxygen in an attempt to reduce the risks that are associated with handling a dyspnoeic bird. The placement of the tube in a conscious bird is quick and appears to cause no discomfort or distress.

The site for placement of an air sac tube is similar to the site for endoscopic examination. Traditionally, this is the left side and just behind the ribs, although Sinn (1994) has suggested the use of short endotracheal tube or rubber tubes into the clavicular or caudal thoracic air sacs. It is also possible to position the tube behind the left leg and run the tube in a cranial direction to the correct position; this reduces the risk of kinking when the bird is conscious. However, any available approach to an appropriate air sac can be used (Dustin, 1993). To gain access to the air sac, the leg is extended and the skin over the sternal notch is incised using a stab incision. The underlying muscles

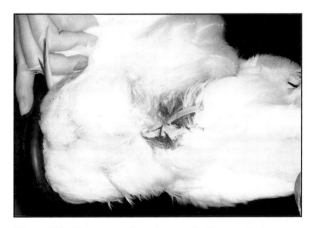

Figure 9.5: Placement of an air sac tube in a masked anaesthetised owl.

are spread with haemostats (or a trocar can be used) to gain entry into an air sac. As large a tube as possible (French 14G) of inert material, such as silastic tubing, should be used. The author's experience is that the flexibility of silastic tubing makes it less likely to kink. The tube is placed into the air sac to a depth of no greater than 1cm to reduce the risk of damage to the liver or spleen (especially if enlarged). The tube is then sutured in place with a purse string suture which should transfix the tube and the musculature and skin to reduce the risk of displacement. The end of the tube is attached to the anaesthetic circuit. It is best to intermittently positive pressure ventilate the bird at a higher flow rate via the placed tube while under anaesthesia. Korbel *et al* (1993) reported that following ventilation birds will stop breathing due to the expulsion of all the carbon dioxide from the respiratory system. Ventilated birds will not breath again spontaneously until after perfusion via the air sac is terminated and the blood carbon dioxide levels rise. Postoperatively, the tube can be removed, or left *in situ* in cases of dyspnoea (such as after surgery to the neck or in cases of aspergillous plugs of the syrinx).

CHOICE OF ANAESTHETIC DRUGS

Injectable Anaesthetics
A list of suggested dose rates for anaesthetics and related drugs is given in Table 9.1. Before the introduction of isoflurane as a reliable and safe gaseous anaesthetic, injectable agents were routinely used. Although Olsen (1994) reported the use of isoflurane by mask for the induction and maintenance of anaesthesia in Anseriformes, injectable agents are generally used for induction in waterfowl or in the 'field' where gaseous anaesthesia is not available. Where gaseous anaesthesia is available, it is still advantageous to induce with ketamine and then maintain with isoflurane or halothane.

Volatile Anaesthetics
The use of gaseous anaesthesia in birds allows more control of anaesthesia than the use of injectable agents. There are three volatile anaesthetics that may be found in veterinary practice. Although halothane is the volatile anaesthetic most commonly used in small animal practice, it is not the most suitable for avian anaesthesia. The three anaesthetic agents that can be used in birds are described and compared in Table 9.2.

The combination of safety and rapid induction and recovery makes isoflurane the anaesthetic agent of choice. Rapid induction with isoflurane (within 4-5 breaths) is substantially less stressful for a bird than continued restraint with a mask over its face, as occurs with methoxyflurane. Although halothane induction could also be almost as fast as isoflurane, the decreased safety margin requires a lower concentration (3%) for induction, compared to isoflurane (5%),

Table 9.1. Injectable anaesthetic agents.

Agent	Dose and route	Comments
Alphaxalone/ alphadalone	5-10mg/kg i/v; 36mg/kg i/m or intracoelomic. The i/v route is favoured in view of the high volume required for i/m use.	Alphaxalone/alphadalone is a relatively good anaesthetic, although there is often a transient apnoea following intravenous administration (Cooper and Frank, 1973), which can be alarming. When compared with other anaesthetic agents, this is a major disadvantage. There are reports of deaths when used in Red-tailed Hawks (Cooper and Redig, 1975). Despite this, there is considered to be a wide safety margin but only a short length of action (10-20 minutes). Intracoelomic or intramuscular routes produce immobilisation but poor analgesia. In all water birds there is a thick area of subcutaneous fat which could affect intramuscular injections and absorption. For this reason, Humphreys (1985) advised the use of the thigh muscle rather than the pectoral muscle.
Ketamine	20-50mg/kg s/c, i/m or i/v (higher doses are required for smaller birds than for larger ones – see end of comments).	Ketamine used to be considered one of the drugs of choice; it is now used less often in avian practice, although it is useful for reducing stress when handling larger species such as swans. Ketamine by itself is a good sedative but a poor anaesthetic, with poor muscle relaxation and little analgesia, although there is little respiratory or cardiovascular depression (Flammer, 1989). Ketamine may give up to 30 minutes anaesthesia with full recovery taking up to three hours (Ensley, 1979), although these are dose dependent. There is often wing flapping during recovery, even when used in combination with tranquillisers: this may continue for several minutes. Ketamine has been used orally (Garner, 1988) as a means of immobilising a captive-bred Harris' Hawk which had flown off and was avoiding recapture. The dose used was 100mg/kg in a 30g piece of meat, although it took up to two hours to have the desired effects. This route may also be used for catching ducks on a pond or free ranging peacocks etc. Ketamine is eliminated by the kidneys. Toxicity may be noted in debilitated or dehydrated birds, or in those with renal dysfunction. Intravenous fluids can hasten recovery from ketamine by causing diuresis. The use of ketamine in waterfowl was reported at a dose of 18mg/kg; where necessary a further 9mg/kg given five minutes later produced good immobilisation (Borzio, 1973). The sleep time was directly proportional to the dosage given and the size of the bird. Large birds tend to recover slower than other birds due to their decreased metabolism. Doses of 35mg/kg i/v may cause immediate cardiac arrest, or prolonged apnoea followed by cardiac arrest, in a number of raptors, with others that survive having convulsions after induction (Redig and Duke, 1976). This was considered to be due to overrapid injection of high dosages. Forbes (1991) recommended weight related dosages of ketamine for raptors: 30mg/kg for birds up to 150g bodyweight; 20mg/kg up to 200-400g; 10mg/kg up to 1kg; 5mg/kg for birds over 2kg.
Ketamine/ diazepam	Ketamine 10-30mg/kg i/v and diazepam 1-1.5mg/kg i/m.	Diazepam gives a smoother induction and recovery when compared with ketamine by itself.
Ketamine/ medetomidine	1.5-2mg/kg ketamine + 60-85µg/kg medetomidine. (Reversed by atipamazole [250-380µg/kg i/m]).	Medetomidine has sedative and analgesic properties, but it also has hypotensive, bradycardic and hypothermic effects. Medetomidine and ketamine combination provides deep sedation and good muscle relaxation with no arrhythmias or respiratory depression. This combination is particularly good in waterfowl or when working with birds in the 'field'.

Table 9.1. Continued.

Agent	Dose and route	Comments
Ketamine/ xylazine	4.4mg/kg ketamine + 2.2mg/kg xylazine i/v (then reversed by yohimbine 0.1mg). (Atipamezole can be used to reverse the effects of xylazine).	The synergistic action of the combination of xylazine with ketamine produces a smooth induction and improved muscle relaxation, without difficulties in recovery due to residual ketamine effect (Degernes *et al*, 1988). Petruzzi *et al* (1988) found 18.5mg/kg ketamine and 1.5mg/kg xylazine to be effective in raptors. However, they were not reversing the xylazine and therefore not worried about the continual effect of ketamine, as recovery was more prolonged due to non-reversal of xylazine. Unreversed, there is a prolonged recovery and postoperative depression that may result in the bird being unable to perch properly or unable to feed, leading to hypothermia, hypoglycaemia and even death (Lawton, 1984). Lumeij (1993) also reported two deaths postoperatively (24 hours and 50 hours) in Northern Goshawks, which were attributed to severe sinus bradycardia.
Propofol	1.33mg/kg i/v.	Propofol is metabolised far too quickly in birds to be of realistic use as an induction agent. This is especially a disadvantage if isoflurane is to be the maintenance gaseous anaesthetic. The combination of these two agents may lead to difficulties keeping the bird anaesthetised long enough to intubate, other than re-inducing with isoflurane by way of mask.
Tiletamine/ zolazepam	5-10mg/kg i/m.	Tiletamine is a phencyclidine derivative which is more potent than ketamine. It causes convulsions unless given with a sedative, thus the manufactured combination. It provides good immobilisation and is considered safe (Kreeger *et al*, 1993).
Xylazine	1-20mg/kg i/m or i/v. (Reversed with yohimbine hydrochloride, 0.1-0.2mg/kg i/v).	Xylazine by itself is unreliable, causes bradycardia and A/V block, and is extremely respiratory depressant. The bradycardic effects can be reduced if atropine is used. Raptors may show a hypersensitivity to external stimuli, including increased trembling, vocalisation and laboured respiration, and higher dosages do not increase the depth of sedation (Freed and Baker, 1989).

thus making safe halothane induction much slower.

The cost of isoflurane and the need for a dedicated vaporiser may dissuade veterinary surgeons from its use. Isoflurane can be used in a halothane vaporiser (Harvey, 1990) and, although the concentration settings are not entirely correct, the difference is probably of minimal significance (Werner, 1987). Isoflurane cannot, however, be used in a vaporiser that has contained halothane, unless it has been serviced and cleaned. The preservatives that maintain the stability of halothane and methoxyflurane will make the vaporiser sticky and affect the accuracy if isoflurane is subsequently used. Servicing or several flushes with ether is required before using a halothane vaporiser for isoflurane anaesthesia.

For the veterinarian who does not have access to isoflurane and will only be anaesthetising a very small number of birds each year, it would probably be safer to weigh the birds and use only injectable agents, such as ketamine and medetomidine (see Table 9.1); this would be safer than using halothane. Oxygen must be available at all times, as should doxapram, in case apnoea occurs.

MONITORING OF ANAESTHESIA

Avian anaesthesia, especially with isoflurane, is now considered a very safe and routine procedure. However, there is no excuse for complacency over anaesthetic monitoring. Fatalities may and will occur in the absence of adequate monitoring of the anaesthetised bird. The depth of anaesthesia may only be controlled if the bird is carefully and continuously monitored. The monitoring of birds should be approached in exactly the same way as the monitoring of any mammalian species.

Reflexes
As the bird becomes more deeply anaesthetised the standard reflexes usually slow-down or decrease in strength, or eventually disappear. The toe, cere and wing reflexes disappear as the bird enters a medium

Table 9.2. Volatile anaesthetics.

	Isoflurane	Halothane	Methoxyflurane
Safety margins The ratio of lethal dose to anaesthetising dose.	5.7 Rosskopf *et al* (1992) considered this safety margin alone made other agents obsolete.	3.0	3.7
Blood gas partition coefficient This reflects the solubility in blood and the potential for tissue distribution and, more importantly, retention.	·1.4 at 37°C Very low solubility allows rapid induction and rapid recovery.	2.3 at 37°C Potential for more redistribution from the body compartments back into the circulation after induction.	12.0 at 37°C High solubility means a slower induction and recovery.
Metabolism	0.3% Virtually no metabolism means that excretion solely on expiration and, therefore, no residue. Excretion is not dependent on liver or kidney function.	15-20% Due to distribution in body tissues and metabolism, there is a slower recovery than with isoflurane. Metabolism and recovery is impaired where there is liver disease.	50% High level of metabolites leads to 'hang-over' effect and depression.
Muscular relaxation	Very good.	Poor.	Moderate to good.
Analgesia	Good.	Poor.	Good.
Respiratory effects	Little respiratory depression.	Markedly respiratory depressive.	Markedly respiratory depressive.
Cardiac effects	Slight myocardial depression which often results in little or no changes in the heart rate (Jenkins, 1993).	Moderate myocardial depression. Causes catecholamine sensitisation of the myocardium which occasionally results in arrhythmias.	Moderate myocardial depression.
Contraindications	None reported.	Hepatic dysfunction, cardiovascular disease or an excited bird at time of induction.	Hepatic dysfunction or cardiovascular disease.
Overdose	Apnoea before cardiac arrest. Prompt artificial ventilation should lead to full recovery as it will remove the excess isoflurane while the heart is still functioning.	Apnoea and cardiac arrest, usually simultaneously.	Apnoea and cardiac arrest, usually simultaneously.

plane. The corneal reflex is usually the last reflex to be abolished and shows that the bird is very deeply anaesthetised. The tone of the jaw should also be assessed; it becomes less tense as the bird enters a medium plane of anaesthesia.

Respiration

Respiration is the best indicator of the depth and stability of anaesthesia. Both the respiratory rate and depth should be monitored, electronically if possible (such as Imp or Apalert). The pattern of respiration is also important and should be stable during anaesthesia. Sudden change in pattern, especially in the depth of respiration from shallow to deep, may indicate that the bird is becoming light or feeling pain. As the bird enters a deeper plane of anaesthesia the rate and depth usually decrease. The respiratory rate should not fall below 25-50 per minute for birds weighing less than 500g, or below 12-15 for large birds such as swans. Below these rates there is a risk of hypercapnoea. The respiratory rate of any anaesthetised bird should never fall below half its normal resting rate (see Chapter 18).

Heart Rate

The routine use of cardiac monitors is recommended, although an oesophageal stethoscope can be of use (Lawton, 1993). The heart rate is affected dramatically by pain and, therefore, it is the best indicator of analgesia and the adequacy of the depth of anaesthesia. The use of a cardiac monitor is reassuring to show there are no abnormalities, such as AV blocks that may occur with xylazine. The standard placement of leads are over the distal lateral tarsometatarsus and the carpal joints of each wing (Burtnick and Degernes, 1993), using atraumatic clamps or silver needles (see Figure 9.6). Careful monitoring of respiration and heart rate will allow immediate resuscitation and administration of drugs, such as doxapram, should this be required.

Temperature

The high metabolic rate of birds results in their temperature fluctuating while under anaesthesia, often with considerable heat loss of many degrees, depending upon the ambient temperature and exposure of tissues. The core body temperature of birds is usually between 40-44°C (smaller birds being 41°C). The cloacal temperature should be monitored during anaesthesia (see Figure 9.6). The temperature drop is particularly noted if the bird is placed directly onto an operating table. It is advisable to keep an anaesthetised bird on a towel, Vetbed or other insulatory layer, eg. heated pad, heat lamp, exposure blanket or bubble wrap. The use of a heated water ripple blanket to maintain body core temperatures during prolonged anaesthesia has been used (Clutton, 1986). Cold anaesthetic gases may also cool the bird, but dealing with this effect is difficult. Although body temperature rapidly returns to normal postoperatively, usually within 10-20 minutes (Altman,

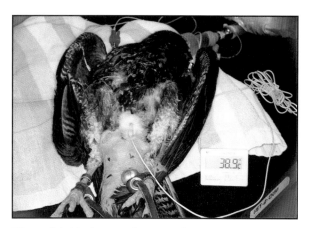

Figure 9.6: Monitoring of an anaesthetised hawk. Note the placement of the ECG lead and the cloacal temperature probe.

1991), the stress or shock involved in reduced body temperatures during surgery can cause fatalities. It is also advisable to provide additional heat in the recovery cage.

Fluid Balance

The control of haemorrhage during surgery is important; however, some loss may be unavoidable. If haemorrhage or surgical shock is anticipated, fluid therapy should be started prior to surgery but after induction (see Chapter 3).

POSTOPERATIVE CARE OF BIRDS

Birds should be carefully monitored not only during anaesthesia but in the recovery phase, in particular the depth of respiration. If an anaesthetic regime other than isoflurane is used, the bird should be wrapped in a towel when recovering from the anaesthetic. Wrapping allows body temperature to be maintained, prevents damage from excess wing flapping, and is required especially when ketamine anaesthesia has been used. When the bird is able to crawl out of its wrappings, it is usually recovered enough to perch. When isoflurane has been used, the bird should be held until a full recovery is made and then placed straight back onto its perch (Lawton, 1993). Additional heating should be maintained for several hours after recovery from anaesthesia.

If smaller birds are not eating within a very short time of recovery from anaesthesia, they should be crop tubed with fluids and nutrients. The time interval from pre-anaesthetic starvation to eating postoperatively should not exceed three hours. Small birds may become hypoglycaemic and die. Fluid intake is also important.

REFERENCES

Altman RB (1991) Avian anesthesia. In: *Exotic Animal Medicine in Practice. Vol. 1*. Ed DE Johnston. Veterinary Learning Systems, New Jersey.

Borzio F (1973) Ketamine hydrochloride as an anesthetic for wildfowl. *Veterinary Medicine/Small Animal Clinician* **35**, 1364.

Burtnick NL and Degernes LA (1993) Electrocardiography on fifty-nine anesthetized convalescing raptors. In: *Raptor Biomedicine*. Eds PT Redig, JE Cooper, JD Remple and DB Hunter. University of Minnesota Press, Minneapolis.

Clutton RE (1986) Prolonged isoflurane anesthesia in the Golden Eagle. *Zoo Animal Medicine* **17**, 103.

Cooper JE (1989) Anaesthesia of exotic species. In: *Manual of Anaesthesia for Small Animal Practice*. 3rd Edn. Eds ADR Hilbery, AE Waterman and GJ Brouwer. BSAVA, Cheltenham.

Cooper JE and Frank LG (1973) The use of the steroid anaesthetic CT 1341 in birds. *Veterinary Record* **92**, 474.

Cooper JE and Redig PT (1975) Unexpected reactions to the use of CT1341 in Red-tailed Hawks. *Veterinary Record* **97**, 352.

Degernes LA, Kreeger TJ, Mandsager R and Redig PT (1988) Ketamine-xylazine anesthesia in Red-tailed Hawks with antagonism by yohimbine. *Journal of Wildlife Diseases* **24(2)**, 322.

Dustin LR (1993) Surgery of the avian respiratory system. *Seminars in Avian and Exotic Pet Medicine* **2(2)**, 83.

Ensley P (1979) Cage bird medicine and husbandry. *Veterinary Clinics of North America: Small Animal Practice*. Ed WJ Boever. **9(3)**, 391.

Fitzgerald G and Blais D (1993) Inhalation anesthesia in birds of prey. In: *Raptor Biomedicine*. Eds PT Redig, JE Cooper, JD Remple and DB Hunter. University of Minnesota Press, Minneapolis.

Flammer K (1989) Update on avian anesthesia. In: *Current Veterinary Therapy X*. Eds RW Kirk and JD Bonagura. WB Saunders, Philadelphia.

Forbes NA (1991) Birds of prey. In: *Manual of Exotic Pets*. New Edn. Eds PH Beynon and JE Cooper. BSAVA, Cheltenham.

Freed D and Baker B (1989) Antagonism of xylazine hydrochloride sedation in raptors by yohimbine hydrochloride. *Journal of Wildlife Disease* **25(1)**, 136.

Garner MM (1988) Use of an oral immobilizing agent to capture a Harris' Hawk (*Parabuteo unicinctus*). *Journal of Raptor Research* **22(2)**, 70.

Haigh JC (1981) Part II: surgery and anaesthesia. In: *Recent Advances in the Study of Raptor Diseases*. Eds JE Cooper and AG Greenwood. Chiron Publications, Keighley.

Harvey RC (1990) Isoflurane anaesthesia in small animal practice. *Veterinary Technician* **11(2)**, 97.

Humphreys PN (1985) Water birds. In: *Manual of Exotic Pets*. Eds JE Cooper, MF Hutchison, OF Jackson and RJ Maurice. BSAVA, Cheltenham.

James AE, Hutchings G, Bush M, Natarajan TK and Burns B (1976) How birds breathe: correlation of radiographic with anatomical and pathological studies. *Journal of the American Radiological Society* **17**, 77.

Jenkins JR (1993) Postoperative care of the avian patient. *Seminars in Avian and Exotic Pet Medicine* **2(2)**, 97.

Korbel TJ, Milovanovic A, Erhardt W, Burike J and Henke J (1993) Aerosaccular perfusion with isoflurane - an anaesthetic procedure for head surgery in birds. In: *Proceedings of the Association of Avian Veterinarians European Conference, Utrecht, 1993*. AAV, Lake Worth.

Kreeger TJ, Degernes LA, Kreeger JS and Redig PT (1993) Immobilization of raptors with tiletamine and zolazepam (Telazol). In: *Raptor Biomedicine*. Eds PT Redig, JE Cooper, JD Remple and DB Hunter. University of Minnesota Press, Minneapolis.

Lawton MPC (1984). Avian anaesthesia. *Veterinary Record* **115(3)**, 71.

Lawton MPC (1993) Monitoring the anaesthetised bird. In: *Proceedings of the Association of Avian Veterinarians European Conference, Utrecht, 1993*. AAV, Lake Worth.

Lumeij JT (1993) Effects of ketamine-xylazine anesthesia on adrenal function and cardiac conduction in goshawks and pigeons. In: *Raptor Biomedicine*. Eds PT Redig, JE Cooper, JD Remple and DB Hunter. University of Minnesota Press, Minneapolis.

McLelland J (1990) *A Colour Atlas of Avian Anatomy*. Wolfe Publishing, London.

Olsen JH (1994) Anseriformes. In: *Avian Medicine: Principles and Application*. Eds BW Ritchie, GJ Harrison and LR Harrison. Wingers, Lake Worth.

Paddleford R (1986) Anesthetic management for birds of prey. In: *Zoo and Wild Animal Medicine*. 2nd Edn. Ed ME Fowler. WB Saunders, Philadelphia.

Petruzzi V, Coda S, Ximenes LA and Naitana P (1988) L'associazione ketamina-xilazina nell'anestesia generale dei rapaci. Valutazione di alcuni parametri vitali. *Documenti Veterinari* **6**, 59.

Redig PT and Duke GE (1976) Intravenously administered ketamine HCl and diazepam for anesthesia of raptors. *Journal of the American Veterinary Medical Association* **169(9)**, 886.

Rosskopf WJ, Woerpel RW, Reed S, Snider K and Dispirito T (1992) Part 1. Anesthetic agents: anesthesia administration for pet birds. *Veterinary Practice Staff* **4 (2)**, 34.

Scheid P and Piiper J (1971) Direct measurement of the pathway of respired gas in duck lungs. *Respiratory Physiology* **11**, 308.

Sinn LC (1994) Anesthesiology. In: *Avian Medicine: Principals and Application*. Eds BW Ritchie, GJ Harrison and LR Harrison. Wingers, Lake Worth.

Werner RE (1987). Isoflurane anaesthesia: a guide for practitioners. *Compendium on Continuing Education for the Practicing Veterinarian* **9(6)**, 603.

CHAPTER TEN

Radiology

Nigel H Harcourt-Brown

INTRODUCTION

Radiology is a routine diagnostic procedure that is used in all branches of clinical veterinary science. A large proportion of the techniques that are used for dogs and cats are applicable to birds. Because of the relatively small size of most birds, and their pneumatisation, radiology is often even more revealing in birds than in dogs and cats. However, the radiographic details that are necessary for diagnosis are often critical and a challenge to obtain.

X-RAY GENERATION

Any X-ray machine suitable for small animal practice will be able to produce good avian radiographs. It is very uncommon to use more than 65kV. The majority of birds seen in general practice will require 50 or 55kV to give good contrast. A large mA is useful as it will allow fast exposure times, but perfectly adequate radiographs can be produced with 20mA and exposure times of 0.05-0.2 seconds, provided modern intensifying screens are used.

SCREENS AND CASSETTES

The use of non-screen film in general practice has been superceded by the introduction of 'fine definition' screens in cassettes. Fine definition screens are used to show the detail of the extremities in man and are very useful for birds. Fine definition screens are slower and therefore require more mAS than fast screens, but a lot less mAS than non-screen film. They produce far more fine detail than fast screens. Fast screens usually lose too much fine detail to be useful for avian radiography.

Increasing the kV will allow a reduction of the mAS required. It may also be useful to decrease the distance from the tube head to film. This has the same effect as an increase in the kV without increasing the radiation dose to the radiographer. The closer the tube head is to the film the less the mAS required to give an adequate exposure. A drawback to this technique is that the area that can be examined is also reduced. This is usually irrelevant in the majority of avian patients because of their small size and also because the area to be examined is usually small as well.

FILMS AND PROCESSING

The choice of film and processing chemicals is decided by the type of screen to be used in the cassette. Regular changing of developer and fixer is important where manual processing is used: fresh chemicals give the best contrast. This is extremely important. Many birds are so small that good contrast is vital to allow differentiation of the various structures. Fixer deteriorates within a few weeks and can cause a dramatic loss of contrast even when the radiograph has been correctly exposed.

ANATOMY

It is impossible to interpret avian radiographs reliably without a reasonable knowledge of avian anatomy. Avian anatomy can vary greatly from Family to Family. Help will be gained from the texts at the end of this article, but radiography of *post-mortem* specimens, followed by dissection, will provide the necessary anatomical expertise and will give in-house testing of interpretive skill.

The three Families (Falconiformes, Columbiformes and Anseriformes) have some significant differences that are not obvious from external examination (see Figures 10.1.1, 10.1.2, 10.2.1, 10.2.2, 10.3, 10.4, 10.5.)

Raptors have a smaller intestinal tract than pigeons and waterfowl. The gizzard in Columbiformes and Anseriformes usually contains grit; Falconiformes do not normally eat grit.

The male members of the sub-Family Anatini, ie. the typical ducks, except stifftails (Oxyurini), have a syringeal bulla which is seen radiographically at the thoracic inlet. Swans and geese (Anserini), tree ducks (Dendrocygnini) and the Magpie Goose do not have a syringeal bulla, neither do pigeons or raptors. The Ruddy Duck has an inflatable tracheal sac. In swans and cranes (Gruidae) the males, and sometimes the females, have a loop of their trachea coiled into an excavation in the sternum. In Anseriformes the thoracic vertebrae are separate; in Columbiformes and

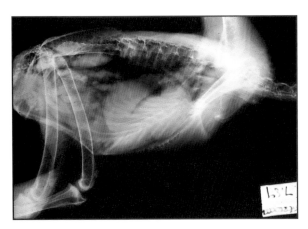

Figure 10.1.1: *Lateral view of the body of a normal Harris' Hawk. The bird was starved for 12 hours prior to radiography.*

Falconiformes they are fused to form the notarium and there are only two intervertebral joints between the notarium and synsacrum.

POSITIONING

Nearly every radiographic view of the patient can be complemented by a second view taken at 90° from the first. This technique attempts to make up for the distortion produced by reducing three dimensions down to two. Perfect positioning is vital to produce a diagnostic radiograph. Poor positioning can be at best useless and at worst misleading.

For the ventrodorsal view the aim should be to

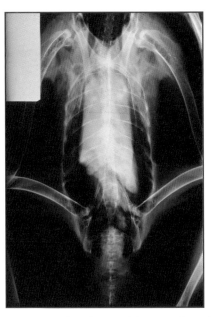

Figure 10.2.1: *Ventrodorsal view of the same Harris' Hawk as in Figure 10.1.1.*

superimpose the keel over the vertebral column. For the lateral view the hip joints should be superimposed, as should the shoulder joints; the legs should be extended caudally and the wings dorsally. The legs can be held in extension with ties and the wings with a light sandbag, which can also be positioned to stop the body rotating. For radiography of the limbs, zinc oxide tape and foam wedges are necessary to position the limbs correctly.

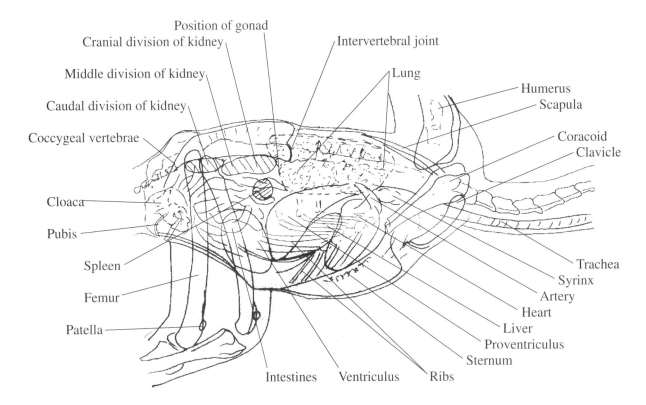

Figure 10.1.2: *The major internal organs that are to be seen in the lateral view of a Harris' Hawk (see Figure 10.1.1).*

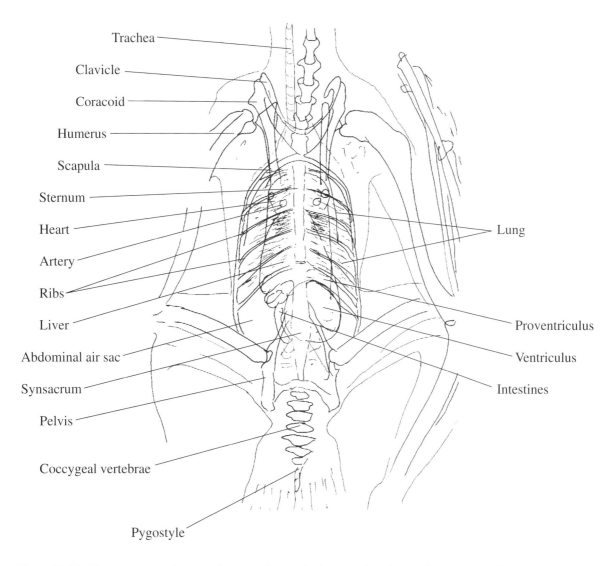

Trachea

Clavicle

Coracoid

Humerus

Scapula

Sternum

Heart

Artery

Ribs

Liver

Abdominal air sac

Synsacrum

Pelvis

Coccygeal vertebrae

Pygostyle

Lung

Proventriculus

Ventriculus

Intestines

Figure 10.2.2: The major internal organs that are to be seen in the ventrodorsal view of a Harris' Hawk (see Figure 10.2.1)

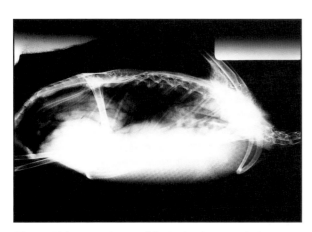

Figure 10.3: Lateral view of the body of a normal Blue-winged Teal. The bird had been starved for 12 hours prior to radiography. The syringeal bulla is visible at the thoracic inlet. Two radiographs at 5kV difference will reveal a greater amount of detail in radiographs of a large bird.

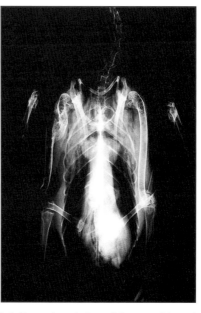

Figure 10.4: Ventrodorsal view of the same Blue-winged Teal as in Figure 10.3. The gizzard contains grit.

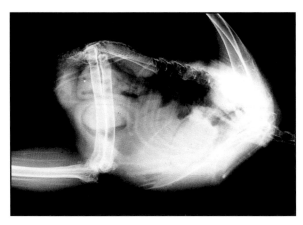

Figure 10.5: Lateral radiograph of a Eurasian Tawny Owl with a bacterial hepatitis and septicaemia. There were abnormal noises associated with the heart sounds and the pericardium seems to contain gas. The liver shadow is larger than normal. Intramuscular ossifications in the tibial region are normal in Strigiformes.

To allow perfect positioning and to keep within the Health and Safety at Work Act, restraint with a general anaesthetic is mandatory in nearly every case. There are special positioning devices, such as Plexiglas screens, that 'pin' the conscious bird to the cassette, but the author prefers to anaesthetise nearly every bird presented for radiography using isoflurane. The patient is usually intubated and maintained on an Ayre's T-piece or Magill circuit (see Chapter 9). Very ill or dyspnoeic birds can be more safely restrained under anaesthesia than if they are held manually; this is beneficial to both the bird and the radiographer. The only exception to this rule are cases that have an oral bolus of barium. It is possible to construct a box with a single perch and a clear front. The cassette is positioned behind the rear wall of the box, so that the bird, stands on the perch in front of the cassette. Repeated exposures may be taken without handling the bird, as the barium goes through the alimentary tract. It is possible to anaesthetise a bird repeatedly using isoflurane, without affecting the passage of barium. However, inhalation of the barium by regurgitation from the crop is a possibility and great care must be taken to guard against this during induction and recovery as well as whilst radiographing the bird.

Whole body radiographs should be used as part of the routine examination of most ill birds.

INTERPRETATION OF RADIOGRAPHS

The lateral and ventrodorsal views of the whole body of the bird are very useful. They are used as a general overview of the body and are often the next step towards a diagnosis after a clinical examination. It is important to take both views and also to use two different kV values for each view. This will give the best set of radiographs for accurate diagnosis.

Respiratory System

The trachea can be seen arising from the larynx and running in the cervical region. It may be dorsal as well as lateral to the cervical vertebrae as it runs along the neck. In cranes, swans and Magpie Geese the trachea is convoluted. The trachea enters the body through the thoracic inlet and terminates as the syrinx, which can be seen in many birds. Many male ducks have a syringeal bulla which can be seen at the thoracic inlet. The syrinx can be identified and it leads into the primary bronchi, which are not seen. The lungs are visible on both views in a normal bird. Laterally, the normal lung looks like a sponge due to the parabronchi being viewed end-on. The lungs overlie each other on a lateral view. The ventrodorsal view shows each lung on either side of the vertebral column. In this position the lungs have the appearance of a fingerprint, as the parabronchi tend to run laterally across the lung on this view. The air sacs are visible surrounding the heart and abdominal viscera, as dark, air-filled spaces. The clavicular air sac can be seen just caudal to the shoulder joint on the ventrodorsal view, again dark against the denser surrounding muscle because of the air it contains.

Pneumonia and air sacculitis can be seen on both views. The fine detail of the lung is lost and the organ becomes blurred. It is possible to see abscesses in the lung as areas of increased density. The air sacs become more dense and, when there is gross pathology, they appear locular. The walls of the air sacs thicken visibly (see Figure 18.5). This loculation is typical of aspergillosis. The clavicular air sac is not easy to see if it is filled with fluid or pus. Congestive heart failure and some tumours, causing effusion, will produce huge amounts of fluid in the air sacs.

Cardiovascular System

The heart is visible on both views. The main arteries appear as a pair of twin dots cranial and lateral to the heart on the ventrodorsal view. On the lateral view these blood vessels are much more recognisable. Enlargement of the heart, calcification of the major arteries and oedema within the air sacs can be seen when present. Oedema due to congestive heart failure is impossible to differentiate radiographically from effusion caused by a visceral tumour, purulent air sacculitis or, occasionally, an enlarged liver.

Digestive System

The liver is visible on both views, but its size is best assessed on the ventrodorsal view. In raptors a recent meal will fill the proventriculus and gizzard and spread the liver shadow so that the liver will appear larger. This must be differentiated from pathological enlargement of the liver. Barium or air can be used to outline the alimentary tract in this area and therefore differentiate liver from proventriculus.

The proventriculus is seen most clearly on the lateral

view. It can be distended normally with food, but can enlarge and overdistend in waterfowl or in any case of heavy metal poisoning. Again, barium is useful.

The gizzard is visible on both lateral and ventro-dorsal views. The muscular, grinding gizzard normally contains grit in pigeons and waterfowl, but not in raptors. Grit will show very clearly on plain radiography. Grit can reflux into the proventriculus in a normal anaesthetised bird. Lead is frequently ingested by waterfowl and occasionally by raptors and pigeons. The lead will collect in the gizzard. Birds which have lead in their gizzard will **always** be suffering from lead poisoning and should be treated (see Chapter 38). Lead is much more radiopaque than grit.

The intestines are seen as a mass in which only small amounts of detail are visible. The cloaca can be demonstrated most obviously on the lateral view and can be seen to contain urates in some individuals. Occasionally, a urolith can be confirmed as present in the cloaca. The spleen is usually only visible on the lateral view, but it can also be seen on the ventrodorsal view if very enlarged. A slightly oblique ventrodorsal view is often useful. Avian tuberculosis, lymphoma and chlamydial infection will all dramatically enlarge the spleen.

The kidneys are seen very easily on a lateral radiograph, but they overlie each other. They appear relatively smaller in pigeons and waterfowl than in raptors. The kidneys can be differentiated into their various divisions on the ventrodorsal view, but are overlain and somewhat obscured by the intestines. Sometimes, the kidneys are very distinct on the ventrodorsal view and they may well be enlarged and more dense in these cases.

Occasionally, the gonads of either sex are obvious just ventrocranial to the kidney on the lateral view.

Extremities

The head and neck, and the thoracic and pelvic limbs should all be evaluated separately. It is very useful to radiograph and compare both the normal and abnormal limbs. Although the whole wing or leg can be examined on a single radiograph, the necessary detail will be revealed more clearly if the affected area is viewed with the beam coned down and at an appropriate exposure (see Figures 10.6.1, 10.6.2). The exposure will vary for different areas of the limb in the same bird. Positioning is all important. The area under examination should be held in position using sandbags or tape, eg. 1.25cm Paragon zinc-oxide tape - it sticks well, but is easy to remove and is cheap (see Figure 10.7).

Because of the use of fine definition screens there is a lot of useful soft tissue detail visible on limb radiographs. Soft tissue swellings are frequently apparent and it is important to decide whether the swelling involves the bones, joints or muscle masses. This is often difficult to appreciate at clinical examination.

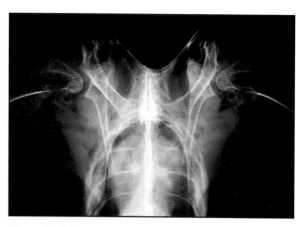
Figure 10.6.1: *Ventrodorsal view of the shoulders of a normal female Saker Falcon. The positioning is correct and the humeri, scapulae, coracoids and clavicles are all visible.*

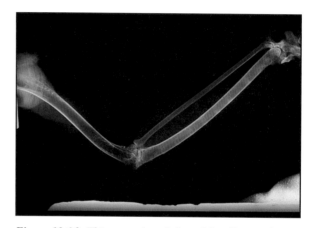
Figure 10.6.2: *This ventrodorsal view of the elbow and carpal joints of a Northern Goshawk was taken with an exposure of 5kV less but the same mAS as 10.6.1. The humerus is less radiodense than the ulna due to pneumatisation of the humeral medullary cavity.*

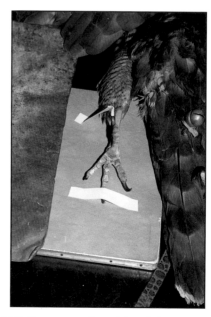
Figure 10.7: *For a correctly positioned plantarodorsal view this female Northern Goshawk has been anaesthetised and zinc oxide tape used to position the foot precisely. The tape is almost completely radiolucent*

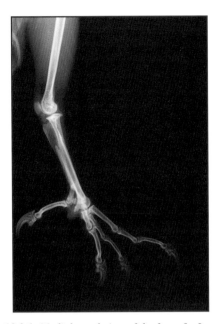

Figure 10.8.1: Mediolateral view of the foot of a Lanner Falcon showing various ossifications in tendons, ligaments and cartilages. This combination of these structures is typical of all Falco spp., but most of them do not appear in accipiters. A knowledge of the normal anatomy of the species that is being radiographed is very helpful.

With radiography it is possible to see changes in soft tissue density, distortion of fascial planes, soft tissue masses and foreign bodies. Soft tissue masses are also able to distort the shape of the bone by external pressure (see Figures 10.8.1, 10.8.2).

OSTEOPATHOLOGY

There are several changes that occur in bone that are specific to certain diagnoses.

Osteomyelitis

Osteomyelitis usually arises in the medullary cavity of the long bones. Pus in birds is caseous and does not flow as it does in mammals. As the abscess enlarges it causes distortion of the cortex and the bone appears to bulge and dissolve (see Figure 10.9). The cortex is usually thinner where the bone bulges. Osteolysis is nearly always due to infection. Increased medullary bone density is always significant. If medullary bone is laid down in a well formed manner it is often due to reaction to infection; the new bone is produced in an attempt to 'wall off' the infected area.

Septic arthritis and osteomyelitis are sometimes seen

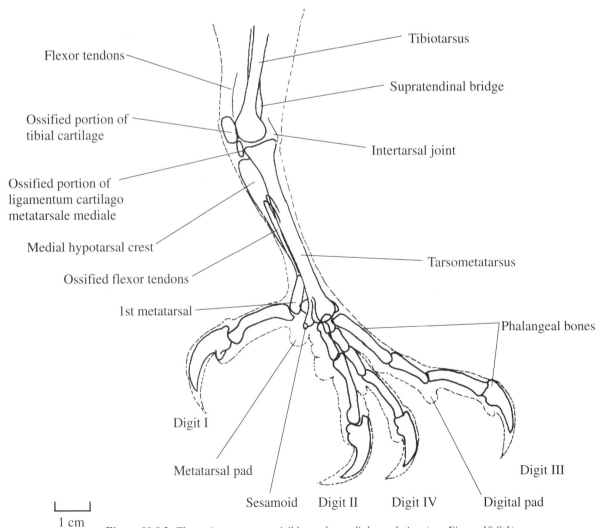

1 cm

Figure 10.8.2: The major structures visible on the mediolateral view (see Figure 10.8.1).

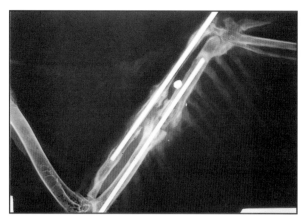

Figure 10.9: *Ventrodorsal view of a wing with a compound fracture, supported by two intramedullary pins, which has developed osteomyelitis. The typical bubbling of the cortical bone is especially visible in the proximal radius. The distal ulna has a thinning of the cortex and a walling-off process around the distal pin. The callus is involved in the infection and a bony sequestrum is forming at the fracture site. A piece of lead shot is also present.*

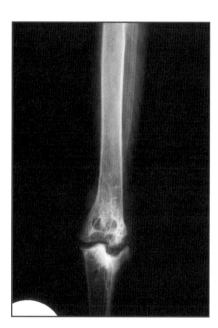

Figure 10.10: *A small wound over the intertarsal joint of this Saker Falcon allowed a septic arthritis to develop. The joint surface of the medial aspect of the tarsometatarsus has eroded and the bone surrounding it has become more dense.*

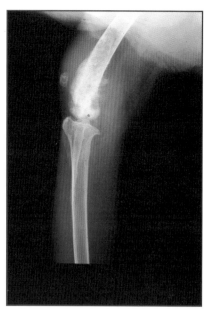

Figure 10.11: *The typical changes of a bone tumour are seen in the femur of this Red-tailed Hawk. The pneumatisation has been lost, radiating periosteal proliferation is present, cortical definition is lost, and osteolysis is present in two areas. The changes have not crossed the joint.*

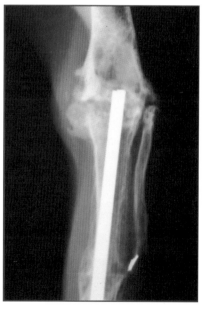

Figure 10.12: *Osteoarthritis in the femorotibial joint of a Tawny Eagle. Osteophytes have been laid down on the lateral and medial aspects of the joint. The cortex of the bone and the medullary cavity are not involved in these changes.*

in joints, especially the phalangeal or carpal joints. The articular surface and usually some of the bone is lost, but the edge of the lesion is not clear cut and it has a more roughened outline (see Figure 10.10). There is lysis of bone. Radiographic changes are diagnostic, but joint fluid with a heterophilia can also be a useful adjunct to the diagnosis.

Neoplasia

Bone tumours are uncommon, usually malignant and cause bone lysis. These tumours give a hazy radiographic outline in the bone caused by gradual osteolysis as they infiltrate. There is always periosteal proliferation; malignant bone tumours can show a 'sun burst' appearance due to the aggressive periosteal proliferation. As with dogs and cats the tumour does not cross the joint (see Figure 10.11).

Osteoarthritis

This is less common in birds than in mammals, but gives similar periarticular changes. It is usually seen as a sequela to joint injury, with or without infection (see Figure 10.12).

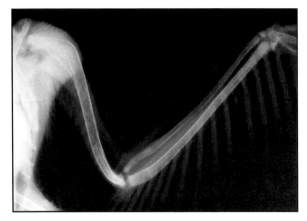

Figure 10.13: Ventrodorsal view of the wing of a young Barn Owl with osteodystrophy. There is a folding fracture of the proximal humerus. The elbow joint is normal, the proximal radius is bent and the whole bone deviates from the normal appearance. The proximal ulna has also bent. In the areas of maximum deviation the cortical bone is of variable thickness.

Osteodystrophy and Osteoporosis

Advanced osteodystrophy is obvious: the bones are less dense than normal and the cortices are usually thin and uneven. In young growing birds, osteodystrophy is usually accompanied by folding fractures. In older growing birds, osteodystrophy shows as misshapen bones, especially of the pelvic limb, with an increased tendency to fracture (see Figure 10.13).

In adult birds, osteoporosis due to malnutrition or excessive egg production causes loss of bone density, gross irregularity of the cortices of long bones and multiple fractures.

In both these conditions there is thinning of cortical bone, but there is no loss of the normal line of the cortex, which differentiates the condition from osteomyelitis.

Early or mild osteoporosis is much more difficult to diagnose with certainty. Comparison with the surrounding soft tissue and great confidence in both the

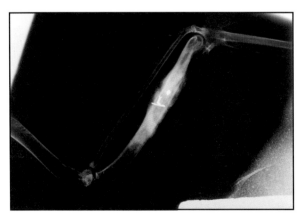

Figure 10.14: The fractured ulna of this Peregrine Falcon has been healing for four weeks after reduction of the fracture with a single wire suture. There is normal callus, with no signs of infection in spite of a piece of lead shot in the medullary cavity.

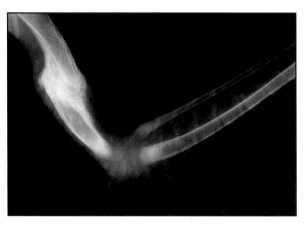

Figure 10.15: Normal mature callus is stabilising the fracture of the humerus in this 42-day-old Harris' Hawk. The elbow joint is normal: growing avian bones do not have a calcified epiphysis.

radiographic technique and the processing are required to make the diagnosis.

Callus Formation

Smooth and well defined masses of new bone are seen in healed fractures (see Figure 10.14), often with signs of parallel periosteal response. Early callus formation has a more regular periosteal appearance (see Figure 10.15).

Malunion

Malunion of fractures is usually atrophic and shows as rounding of the ends of the fracture and no periosteal proliferation.

Pneumatisation of Bone

A variable number of the bones have a medullary cavity that is pneumatised in adults of most species of birds. Pneumatisation varies from species to species and even between individuals, but is usually visible on radiography. The pneumatised bones are connected with the air sacs. The medullary cavity of non-pneumatised bones is filled with marrow. These bones appear more dense on radiography.

CONTRAST TECHNIQUES

Air

Air is rarely used as a contrast medium because it is often present normally. Air can be seen in some areas, such as the clavicular air sac or the abdominal cavity, in healthy birds. In some cases of pathology, eg. rupture of the cervicocephalic air sac or compound fractures, air can be found in abnormal situations. Air can be introduced into the alimentary tract with a piece of tubing or an endoscope and will show the extent of the crop, proventriculus or gizzard. It is also possible, using an endoscope, to introduce air into the uterus and the rectum and ileum via the cloaca, with similar results.

Barium

Barium is very useful when given orally, either as a diluted liquid or mixed with food such as liquid baby food. Both these preparations should be given, using a cannula, directly into the crop. For giving a barium meal to a Peregrine Falcon the following procedure would be adopted. Take a piece of Steriflex tubing approximately 10cm long. A standard liquid barium preparation is diluted half and half with water and about 3ml is given directly into the crop with a crop tube. It is ideal if the bird has been starved for a sufficient time to allow the gut to empty. If the bird is well, this could be overnight; if the bird is ill it may not need starving at all because its gut will be nearly empty already and further starvation could be fatal. Lateral and ventrodorsal views are taken five minutes later, by which time a normal bird should have barium in its crop, proventriculus, gizzard and even the small in-

testine. The barium will outline the alimentary tract and will give an indication of the rate of passage of ingesta, which can be seen with sequential radiographs. Obstruction of the alimentary tract is seen and is caused by tumours, intussusception and foreign bodies. It is impossible to differentiate liver enlargement from alimentary tract enlargement without a barium meal. Because barium will outline the bowel, it is possible to show the displacement or enlargement of the viscera, thereby differentiating the enlarged liver-bowel outline. This technique is also very useful for showing tumours of the kidney or gonad and differentiating the other causes of abdominal distension.

Iohexol

Intravenous iohexol (Omnipaque, Nycomed) will safely give an arteriogram or venogram, or outline the heart internally. It is also safe for producing an intravenous pyelogram (IVP). An IVP will increase the contrast of the kidneys with the surrounding tissue as well as filling the ureters. One millilitre of the 340 product given intravenously to a male Peregrine Falcon will give a good flow of contrast through the ureters within 5-10 minutes of administration (see Figure 10.16).

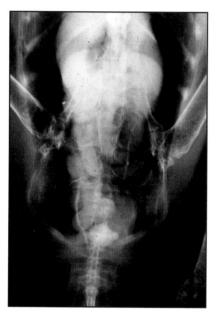

Figure 10.16: Ventrodorsal view of the kidneys of a Peregrine Falcon. The bird had been given 1ml of iohexol intravenously 10 minutes previously. The kidneys are revealed as they are more radiodense. Both ureters can be seen and are normal.

REFERENCES AND FURTHER READING

Rubel G, Isenbugel E and Wolvekamp P (1991) *Atlas of Diagnostic Radiology of Exotic Pets*. Wolfe, London.

Harcourt-Brown NH (1994) Radiology. In: *Diseases of the Pelvic Limb of Birds of Prey*. FRCVS Thesis. Royal College of Veterinary Surgeons, London.

Smith SA and Smith BJ (1992) *An Atlas of Radiographic Anatomy*. WB Saunders, Philadelphia.

Walsh M (1986) Radiology. In: *Clinical Avian Medicine and Surgery, including Aviculture*. Eds GJ Harrison and LR Harrison. WB Saunders, Philadelphia.

CHAPTER ELEVEN

Post-Mortem Examination Technique

Jason C Waine

INTRODUCTION

Post-mortem examination, including associated laboratory techniques, is the single most powerful diagnostic tool available to the avian clinician. It may be used to define a flock or loft problem, thus enabling preventive measures to be recommended; it may be necessary forensically in either civil or criminal court cases; it can be useful as a retrospective diagnostic aid in difficult cases or to satisfy a client's curiosity following the death of their bird; and it may also be useful in giving timely warning of a zoonotic risk to the client or to the general public.

The fresher the material examined at autopsy, the greater the quantity and quality of information that can be gained. Ideally, the subject should be a sacrificed bird that has been killed immediately prior to examination. If there is to be any delay, the carcase should be cooled rapidly by soaking in cold water, stored in a sealed plastic bag with all the surplus air removed, and placed in a fridge until required. Plucking may also help in cooling the body, although in so doing, important detail may be lost. When the delay is in excess of 24 hours, deep freezing in a sealed plastic bag is recommended. This process may damage the tissues for histological examination and may adversely affect the recovery of microorganisms, but much useful information can still be gained.

EQUIPMENT

A full set of equipment should be stored separately and be available only for *post-mortem* examinations. After use, the equipment should be washed in a disinfectant, dried, oiled where appropriate, and housed in a suitable, marked container. A list of basic equipment is given in Appendix 11.1.

HISTORY

A full history is essential. This is best taken by the clinician, but it may be helpful to have preprinted forms for the client to complete, perhaps with the help of a nurse. Information on the sheet will save the veterinarian time by providing accurate details that the client may feel should be common knowledge, eg. the bird's species. A suggested format for such a sheet is shown in Appendix 11.2.

In cases which may proceed to court, formal identification procedures must be carried out. The carcase must be identified by the submitter in the presence of the veterinary surgeon who will undertake the examination, and a note made of the time. When this is not possible, each additional person in the chain must identify the evidence and note the time when it is received.

Any ambiguities in the history should be clarified with the client before the carcase is examined. It may also be prudent at this stage to discuss the likely costs involved in the various stages of the diagnostic procedure.

SAFETY

Avian zoonoses are numerous and common. They include such important pathogens as *Chlamydia psittaci*, *Salmonella* spp., *Erysipelis* spp., *Yersinia* spp. and *Aspergillus* spp. Many of these are spread as aerosols or from feather dust. A face mask should be worn throughout the course of the examination and, if possible, the autopsy should be carried out in a fume cupboard. COSHH regulations should be observed and the necessary steps taken to prevent any possible contagion to staff, clients or patients (see Chapter 12). Disposable latex gloves should be used and replaced immediately if they become damaged. At the conclusion of the autopsy, any unwanted material should be wrapped and sealed in a plastic container and disposed of as for clinical waste.

AUTOPSY

Little reference will be made here to specific lesions or conditions that can be found at *post-mortem* examination. A Table giving a summary of such information can be found at the end of this chapter (see Table 11.1), and for greater detail, reference should be made to the relevant systematic chapter. An example of an Autopsy Check List is shown in Appendix 11.3.

Collection of Samples

It is much easier to discard tissue samples, swabs, etc. than to collect them later after possible contamination. For this reason the following items must be at hand at the start of the *post-mortem* examination: at least six microbiology swabs; two containers (one with formol-saline and one with 70% alcohol); three empty, sterile containers; virus transport medium; and clean, grease-free microscope slides.

During the examination swabs should be taken from relevant tissues before they are contaminated. Two small, representative samples of each organ, including any lesions, should be collected, one for histology (to be put in formol-saline) and one for virology (to be put in virus transport medium which has previously been warmed to room temperature). Samples of fat, muscle, kidney and liver from wild raptors can be frozen and sent to The Institute of Terrestrial Ecology at Monks Wood Experimental Station, Abbots Ripton, Huntingdon, Cambs PE17 2LS, where they may be examined for levels of environmental poisons (polychlorinated biphenol residues, mercury, DDE - a by-product of the insecticide DDT - and HEOD - a by-product from the insecticides aldrin and dieldrin). This laboratory will not normally examine for other toxins. If poisoning is suspected, the case should be referred to the Ministry of Agriculture, Fisheries and Food (MAFF), with a full history, as a suspected wildlife incident.

Where histology is desired, it is worth noting that some laboratories will examine any number of tissues from one subject under a single covering charge.

Metazoan parasites are best stored in 70% alcohol (or failing that, methylated spirits) for future identification. The Department of Zoology (Entomology or Parasitic Worms Division) at the Natural History Museum, Cromwell Road, London SW7 5BD will undertake such identification, although a charge may be made for this service.

Fresh samples of duodenal, ileal and caecal contents, and scrapings from the mucosa can be retained for microscopic examination for parasitic ova and coccidial oocysts, and for making smears for Gram staining. Impression smears can be made from virtually any surface or lesion. By using a rapid stain, these can provide a quick technique for help with diagnosis (see Chapter 6). In freshly killed subjects, blood smears can also be made. The mucosal surface of the oesophagus and/or crop can be sampled for microscopic examination (this is particularly useful in the diagnosis of trichomoniasis and candidiasis).

It is sensible to re-read the history before proceeding to the next stage of the examination.

External Examination

1. Examine the container in which the body arrived - ectoparasites may have migrated from the bird into the corners of the plastic bag.

2. Note any identification marks: rings, including colour; which leg the ring is on and ring type (BTO metal; Darvik - the large, plastic, coloured, identification rings used on some wildfowl; DoE rings; owner's or breeder's own identification rings); microchip implants; information stamped in ink on the flight feathers (commonly used in pigeons to identify the owner's name and address). Rings should be retained for reference - disputes commonly occur over ownership or ancestry and may be easily resolved if the rings are still accessible.

3. Make any relevant measurements - weight (see Figure 11.1); tarsal length (see Figure 11.2); maximum chordal length (tip of the longest primary feather to the carpal joint) (see Figure 11.3); beak length using the distance from the tip of the beak to the craniofacial hinge (see Figure 11.4); head length, which is the longest distance between the tip of the beak and the back of the cranium (see Figure 11.5). At least one measurement other than weight should be recorded and the carcase should be condition scored (1-5 from thin to fat) based on the state of the pectoral muscles.

4. Radiography may be indicated at this point. In addition to assisting with the diagnosis of metabolic bone disease, shooting and lead poisoning, radiography of dead birds can provide helpful experience in improving avian X-ray technique.

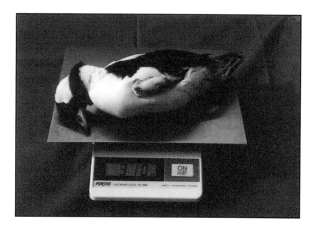

Figure 11.1: *Weighing a male Bufflehead.*

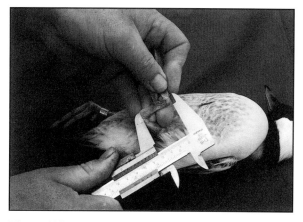

Figure 11.2: *Measuring the tarsal length of a male Bufflehead.*

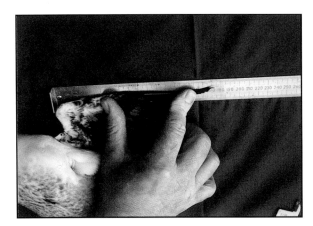

Figure 11.3: *Measuring the maximum chordal length of a male Bufflehead.*

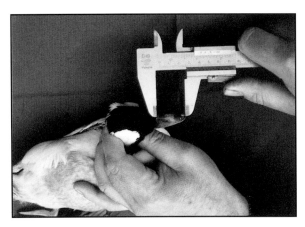

Figure 11.4: *Measuring the beak length of a male Bufflehead.*

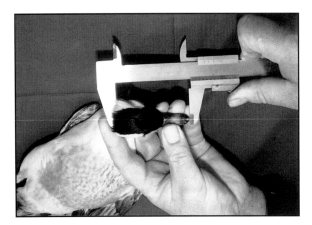

Figure 11.5: *Measuring the head length of a male Bufflehead.*

Endoscopy can also be performed at this stage. This may reveal parasites or lesions of aspergillosis in the bronchi, syrinx and trachea, or avian tuberculosis in the liver and kidney.
5. Examine the bones, palpating each joint and long bone for any fractures, dislocations or joint effusions, and at the same time check the integument for signs of ectoparasites or injury. Puncture wounds may result

from collision, fighting, predation or shooting. A shotgun or air rifle wound will usually have a significant plug of skin and feather debris carried deep into the wound. Injury from a high velocity bullet will result in a small entry wound with debris carried deep along a track of significant damage culminating in a very much larger exit wound free of skin and feather debris.

Evidence of pinioning or wing clipping should also be noted at this stage.
6. Examine the feathers for signs of abnormal wear, fractured vanes, discolouration, abnormal development, cysts, stress (fret) marks and ectoparasites. A note may be made of stages of moult. Plumage colour may help with ageing or sexing of the bird.
7. Check the uropygial (preen) gland at the base of the tail for neoplasia, impaction, infection or atrophy.
8. Note any discharges from the nares, buccal cavity, eyes, ears, vent or wounds. Swellings around or just below the eyes may indicate infraorbital sinusitis, especially in raptors. Look for abnormalities of the eyes, including hyphema and other signs of injury.
9. Examine the legs, feet and cere for encrustations or papillomata which may indicate parasitic, fungal or viral disease. Swellings of the feet may be a sign of bumblefoot or articular gout. Inspect for abnormalities in the growth or shape of the beak and claws. Look for signs of frostbite of the feet, especially in waterfowl, and for foreign bodies in the buccal cavity, eg. fishing hooks in ducks. Waterfowl may show signs of traumatic injury caused by discarded fishing line at the commisures of the beak. Avian pox lesions may be evident at the commisures of the beak in raptors and Columbiformes (but not waterfowl).

Internal Examination

A discussion on avian anatomy is not within the scope of this chapter, but useful references include King and McLelland (1984) and McLelland (1990).

Preparation and Initial Incision
1. Smaller birds or chicks: pin out on a cork board in dorsal recumbency and with the limbs outstretched and tense.
2. Soak the whole bird by immersion in a disinfectant detergent, eg. Florafree - Deb Group Limited, and part the feathers down the ventral midline in preparation for the initial incision (see Figure 11.6).
3. Incise through the skin along the midline from the gonys (the symphysis of the rami of the lower mandibles) to the vent.
4. Separate the skin from the underlying muscles of the thorax and abdomen (see Figure 11.7). Examine these muscles for abnormalities, eg. sarcocysts. Gentle traction should result in easy separation of the muscles and the skin, but in cases where dehydration has occured, either through disease or storage, the skin will detach only with difficulty and may require blunt dissection.

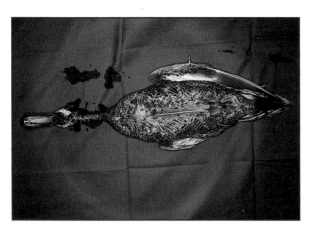

Figure 11.6: Feathers wetted and parted in preparation for the initial incision.

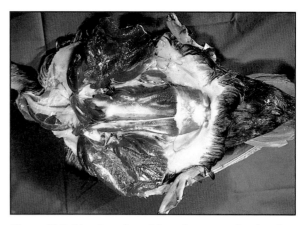

Figure 11.8: Muscles reflected from the sternum leaving the abdominal tunic intact.

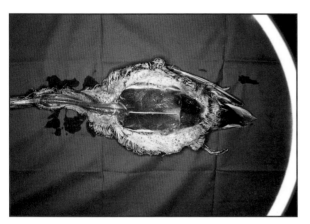

Figure 11.7: Primary midline incision with skin reflected.

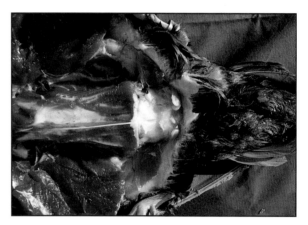

Figure 11.9: Abdominal tunic removed revealing the post-hepatic septum.

Removal of the Superficial Muscles and Examination of the Buccal Cavity

5. The buccal cavity can be opened either by incising through the skin just medial to one of the lower mandibular rami and then cutting through the hyoid bone on that side, or by cutting through the oral commissure and the angular process of the lower mandible on one side, thus allowing the lower mandible to be reflected. Examine the buccal cavity and the infraorbital sinuses.

6. Reflect the pectoral muscles away from the sternum and ribs (see Figure 11.8).

7. Dissect down the length of the throat, liberating the trachea and oesophagus but taking care not to incise the crop at this stage or watery crop contents may flood the visual field.

8. Incise the midline of the abdominal muscles and cut the insertion of the muscles to the rib cage. Examine the abdominal contents and air sacs *in situ* prior to any disturbance. Reflect the abdominal tunic using blunt dissection to separate the attachments to the underlying post-hepatic septum (see Figure 11.9).

Removal of the Sternum and Examination of the Viscera *In Situ*

9. The ribs should now be clear of overlying muscle and they can be cut along the line of angulation. Carefully lift the sternum using its caudal edge and dissect away the attachments to the thoracic air sacs and the pericardium. Using a scalpel blade, dislocate the joints between the coracoid bones and the edge of the sternum (alternatively, the coracoids and clavicles can be cut - this is difficult in larger birds). Remove the sternum and lower part of the rib cage, dissecting away the soft tissue attachments at the thoracic inlet and cutting through the clavicles (see Figure 11.10). Note any damage to the sternum (collision or shooting injuries frequently involve the sternum because of its large size and prominent position).

10. The base of the heart is visible protruding from the cranial aspect of the left and right hepatic lobes which occupy much of the exposed area. Caudal to the liver is a relatively thick sheet of tissue called the post-hepatic septum. In a well-fed bird this will be fat filled (see Figure 11.11). Remove this septum by cutting its lateral attachments and using blunt dissection to separate it from the viscera (see Figure 11.12). The liver still occupies much of the exposed field. Examine the air sacs and organs thus exposed and record any visible abnormalities, eg. pericardial or hepatic urates; pericarditis; abdominal or thoracic haemorrhage; size,

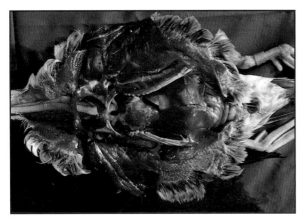

Figure 11.10: Sternum removed revealing thoracic and some abdominal viscera.

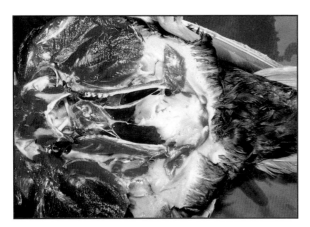

Figure 11.11: Compare the fat bird illustrated here with the thin bird in Figure 11.10.

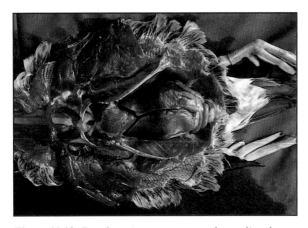

Figure 11.12: Post-hepatic septum removed revealing the abdominal viscera.

colour and shape of liver; gross hepatic lesions; cloudiness of the air sacs; presence of abnormal fluids, adhesions or parasites in the air sacs. At this point take a liver swab. Sterilise the surface of the liver with a red hot scalpel blade before making a small incision through the capsule.

Examination of the Upper Alimentary and Respiratory Tracts

11. Careful blunt dissection will be needed to free the crop and oesophagus (this is not so difficult in wildfowl and raptors, which have a poorly defined crop). After incision of these structures, store any parasites present and note the quantity, quality and make-up of the crop contents. Impression smears of the mucosal surface of the crop can be made for staining with a general purpose cytology stain, eg. Diff Quik or Gram stain.

12. Remove the trachea, syrinx and primary bronchi and hold them up to a light source to reveal any foreign matter or parasites within. Bisect the trachea, syrinx and primary bronchi using an incision down each side - a single cut is inadequate as the tracheal rings in birds are complete and strongly sprung, so the trachea will not stay open.

Removal of Liver and Alimentary Tract and Examination of Exposed Viscera *In Situ*

13. Remove the liver and gastrointestinal tract for separate examination. Gently lift the rectum, free the intestinal tract from the left and right abdominal air sacs, and cut the mesenteric attachment to the dorsal abdominal wall taking care not to damage the gonads, kidneys and adrenal glands. The proventriculus passes dorsal to the heart and through the arch made by the left and right brachiocephalic trunks. Use blunt dissection to free the proventriculus without damaging the arteries or the heart. The upper alimentary tract can now be drawn through the thorax. It may be necessary to ligate the rectum before cutting it to prevent contamination of the rest of the carcase. Leave a short length of rectum with the cloaca in the abdominal cavity. Lay aside the structures dissected out for further examination.

14. This is a convenient point to examine the brachial plexus which is now well exposed. It is formed by the ventral rami of four or five spinal nerves and supplies the nerves of the wings.

15. Examine the heart, lungs, kidneys, adrenals and gonads *in situ*. The sex and sexual state of the bird should be noted. The testes lie at the cranial pole of the kidneys just caudal and ventral to the adrenal glands. They are similar to each other in size, are smooth and shiny, and can vary in colour from black to grey to white. The single (left) ovary is lobular and resembles a bunch of grapes in shape. Occasionally, two ovaries may be present, especially in raptors. Most birds have seasonal sexual activity which is reflected in the development of the gonads. During the non-breeding season, and when the bird is unwell, the gonads may be small, whilst in the breeding season the testes will swell to five or six times their resting size and the ovary will show dramatic follicular development together with enlargement of the oviduct.

Detailed Examination of the Heart and Lungs

16. Remove and examine the heart and lungs. The

source of any haemorrhage in the thoracic air sacs should be identified remembering that, with the absence of a diaphragm, damage to organs such as the liver can result in blood in the thoracic air sacs. Open the pericardial sac and perform a transverse section below the left ventricle to assess the state of the cardiac muscle. Open up the heart in the usual manner (following the course of the blood via first the vena cava, then the right atrium, right ventricle, pulmonary artery, pulmonary vein, left atrium, left ventricle and finally the aorta) and inspect for endocardial lesions, filarial nematodes and arteriosclerosis. Lift the lungs away from the ribs and look at all surfaces for lesions of tuberculosis, salmonellosis, colibacillosis or aspergillosis. Any unusual pattern of congestion should be noted and lesions swabbed and sampled for histology. If the bird has been dead for several hours, hypostatic congestion will occur as a normal *post-mortem* change. If drowning is suspected (a surprisingly common occurrence in waterfowl), look for air sacs and lungs full of water. If there is any significant delay between drowning and autopsy, water in the air sac may have already drained away leaving an apparently normal state. The lungs, however, will remain full of water. In some cases of liver or heart disease, large quantities of transudate may give the appearance of drowning, but such fluid should also be present in the pericardial sac, unlike water from drowning.

Detailed Examination of the Kidneys and Gonads

17. Dissect away and section the kidneys and gonads. Note any abnormally large pockets of urates in the kidneys. Examine the ischiadic nerve and the rest of the lumbosacral plexus which are exposed following removal of the kidneys.

18. Examine the terminal rectum, oviduct and cloaca for tumours, physical trauma and prolapses. Check the oviduct and uterus for maturity, signs of enlargement that would suggest previous breeding history, and the presence of normal, damaged or diseased eggs.

Detailed Examination of the Liver, Spleen and Gall-Bladder

19. Separate the liver from the duodenum taking care not to damage the gall-bladder, which is present in raptors and waterfowl, but absent in many Columbiformes. The gall-bladder may be enlarged in birds which have eaten little or no food for a significant period, and grossly enlarged in cases of lead poisoning. After inspecting the liver for serosal or subserosal lesions, it can be sectioned and impression smears taken (see Chapter 6).

20. Remove, examine and section the spleen which is located on the right side of the junction between the ventriculus and proventriculus. Make smears for cytology. The spleen varies in shape between different groups of birds. It may be grossly enlarged in cases of septicaemia, especially chlamydiosis.

Detailed Examination of the Lower Alimentary Tract

21. Open the proventriculus using a longitudinal incision. Note any parasites and lesions, after first cleaning away any food and excess mucus. Section and inspect the duodenum and at the same time check the pancreas for abnormalities. Now cut open the ileum, colon and caeca (if present). In large waterfowl these structures are best left folded and representative lengths from each fold sectioned and examined. Care must be taken in interpreting the presence of blood-stained fluid in the intestinal lumen as agonal bleeding or *post-mortem* leakage can occur.

22. Cut open the gizzard and examine the contents. In waterfowl, these should be flushed out with tap water into a white enamel dish and the *cuticula gastrica* (the gizzard cuticle) examined for particles of lead. Gently flush the gizzard contents using running water to remove the bulk of the less dense material, and inspect the remaining grit for lead shot and other foreign bodies, eg. fish hooks. This is made much easier by using an illuminated magnifying glass.

Examination of the Joints

23. Cut into the major limb joints and investigate the joint spaces for urates, purulent material, physical damage and parasites. Microfilaria are commonly found in the joint spaces.

Examination of the Brain and Eyes

24. Remove the brain by carefully cutting the cranium laterally, removing the dorsal cranium and then dissecting out the brain together with the roots of the twelve pairs of cranial nerves. If histology of the brain is considered desirable, the brain should be stored in neutral buffered formalin. The eyes can also be removed, but special fixatives, eg. Zenker's solution or Bouin's fluid, are required. The clinician should be guided by advice from the histopathologist, who may have a preferential fixative for eyes. Agonal bleeding is common and typically has the appearance of apparent meningeal haemorrhage. It is, however, not significant if the blood is present within the substance of the bone rather than in the meninges or brain.

Table 11.1. Some common *post-mortem* findings.

This is not an exhaustive list and reference should be made to the relevant chapters. In the 'species affected' column, where no initials are present all three groups are equally affected, otherwise the initials of the susceptible groups are put in descending order of importance.   W - Wildfowl;   R - Raptors;   P - Pigeons

Stage of examination	Some common findings	Possible causes	Species affected
Container	Lice, mites, ticks, fleas.	Debilitation from illness. Inability to groom.	WPR
Radiography	Fractures, dislocations.	Trauma.	
	Osteoporosis.	Dietary management.	
	Arthritis.	Articular gout, osteoarthritis, filariasis.	
	Foreign bodies, eg. airgun pellet.	Trauma or ingested.	
	Proventricular impaction.	Lead poisoning. Proventricular dilatation syndrome.	W
	Eggbinding.	Hypocalcaemia, management.	
Endoscopy	Caseous or fungal lesions in airway.	Aspergillosis.	RWP
	Caseous lesions in pharynx and oesophagus.	Trichomoniasis.	PR
	'Cotton wool' lesions in pharynx and/or crop.	Candidiasis.	
	Small red nematodes in trachea.	Syngamiasis (gapeworm) or *Cyathostoma* spp.	
	Tracheal mucosal inflammation.	Bacterial or viral infections.	
Bones and integument	Ectoparasites.	Debility or inability to groom.	
	Flesh wounds/fractures.	Predation, bullying, shooting, collision.	
Feathers	Damaged feathers.	Poor housing, night fright, trauma, ectoparasites.	
	Abnormal feathers.	Disease, drug toxicity, poor feeding during moult.	
Uropygial gland	Swollen with/without purulent exudate.	Abscess, neoplasia, blocked duct.	
Head	Swelling below eyes.	Sinusitis, mucocele, ruptured cervical air sac.	
	Hyphema.	Trauma.	
	Keratitis.	Trauma, parasites, infection.	
	Exophthalmos.	Periorbital haemorrhage, tumours, sinusitis.	
	Scabs and hyperkeratosis.	Dermatophytes, trichomoniasis, avipoxvirus.	

Chapter Eleven **105**

Table 11.1 Continued.

Stage of examination	Some common findings	Possible causes	Species affected
Head (continued)	Yellow or brown papules on skin of head.	Pox lesions.	RP
	Subcutaneous haemorrhages on beak.	Lead poisoning, prolonged treatment for lead.	W
	Abrasions to crown.	Night fright, poor aviary design.	
	Foreign bodies in mouth.	Fishing hooks, line, etc.	
Sinuses	Abscess - infraorbital.	Bacterial, chlamydial, trichomonal or mycoplasmal infection.	
	Abscess - postorbital development of infraorbital abscess.	Bacterial or mycoplasmal infection leading to CNS signs and death.	
Legs, feet, cere	Swellings on plantar surface of feet.	Bumblefoot.	RWP
	Plaques on webs.	Pox lesions.	W
	Swollen, scabbed cere.	Trauma or *Cnemidocoptes* spp.	R
	Trauma to cere (or crown of head).	Wire netting injury.	R
	Missing digits.	Frostbite, trauma, ischaemia from other causes.	
Separation of skin	Difficulty in peeling away skin.	Dehydration.	
Buccal cavity	Mucopurulent material in choanae.	Sinusitis, upper respiratory tract infection.	
	Foreign bodies in choanae.		
	Foreign bodies caught in or over tongue.		
	Ulceration of tongue.	Infection, trauma, oiling.	
	White lesions in oropharynx.	Trichomoniasis, candidiasis, capillariasis, avitaminosis A, owl herpesvirus.	PRW
Pectoral muscles	Atrophy.	Inanition, lack of exercise.	
Sternum	Depression or deviation.	Neonatal hypocalcaemia (or osteomalacia) or osteoporosis.	PRW
Air sacs	Thickened +/− granulomatous lesions.	Aspergillosis, chlamydiosis, tuberculosis, collibacillosis, salmonellosis.	
	Ascarid worms.	*Serrataspiculum* spp., *Cyathostoma* spp.	
	Full of water.	Drowning.	W

Table 11.1 Continued.

Stage of examination	Some common findings	Possible causes	Species affected
Liver	Swollen + focal lesions + adhesions.	Chlamydiosis, leucosis, yersiniosis, tuberculosis, anthrax.	
		Bacterial septicaemia.	
		Duck viral hepatitis.	W
		Goose viral hepatitis.	W
		Pasteurella anatipestifer.	W
		Herpesvirus (inclusion body hepatitis).	RP
	White, powdery film on serosal surface.	Visceral gout.	
	Liver small, hard and gritty to cut.	Cirrhosis.	
	Liver swollen and pale.	Amyloidosis, leucosis.	
Oesophagus and crop	Yellow/white cheesy lesions.	Trichomoniasis, capillariasis, candidiasis.	PRW
	Diphtheresis of oesophageal mucosa.	Duck viral enteritis (diagnostic).	W
	Penetrating foreign bodies.	Fish hooks, thorns, splinters.	
	Accumulation of foul liquid.	Candidiasis, sour crop (bacterial infection), lead poisoning.	
	Impaction with food.	Lead poisoning, sour crop, proventricular dilatation syndrome.	WR
	Oesophagitis.	Ingestion of caustics, eg. oil from pollution.	
Trachea	As for endoscopy.		
Brachial plexus	Thickening of nerves.	Marek's disease.	
	Oedema and haemorrhage.	Brachial plexus avulsion.	
Testes	Small.	Immature or sexually inactive adult.	
	Large - both testes equal in size.	Sexually active.	
	Testis or testes large and/or irregular in shape.	Tumours or orchitis.	
Ovary	Small.	Immature or sexually inactive adult.	
	Large with different sized follicles.	Sexually active.	
	Active with irregular or abnormal ova.	Viraemia/toxaemia.	

Table 11.1 Continued.

Stage of examination	Some common findings	Possible causes	Species affected
Oviduct	Inflammation plus free yolk in abdomen.	Egg peritonitis.	
	Swollen and containing egg(s).	Normal point of lay.	
Heart	Fibrinous pericarditis.	Chlamydiosis.	
		Pasteurella anatipestifer.	W
	Echymoses and/or petechiae.	Septicaemia.	
	Rupture of right atrium.	Severe shock following collision or electrocution.	
	White, powdery film on epi- or pericardium.	Visceral gout.	
	Thickening and fibrosis of major arteries.	Arteriosclerosis.	RW
Lungs	Caseous/granulomatous lesions.	Aspergillosis, tuberculosis, colibacillosis, salmonellosis.	
	Regular congestion.	Hypostatic congestion (floats in water).	
	Irregular congestion.	Infections (including protozoal) (sinks in water).	
	Fluid filled.	Drowning (natural).	WR
		Drowning (incorrect administration of fluids).	
Kidneys	Pockets of purulent material.	Pyelonephritis.	
	Excess urates.	Visceral gout.	
	Swollen and irregular.	Tumour, eg. lymphoma, nephritis, amyloidosis.	
	Enlarged with white specks.	Renal coccidiosis, drug induced nephritis.	W
Proventriculus	Excess mucus with small nematodes.	*Echinura uncinata* infestation.	W
	Impaction.	Lead poisoning.	W
	Dilation and impaction.	Proventricular dilatation syndrome.	W

Table 11.1 Continued.

Stage of examination	Some common findings	Possible causes	Species affected
Duodenum/ileum	Bloody contents (fresh carcase).	Haemorrhagic enteritis (bacterial or viral).	
		Agonal bleeding.	
		Clostridial enterotoxaemia.	
	Bloody contents (old carcase).	*Post-mortem* leakage of blood.	
	Bloody contents plus annular mucosal lesions.	Duck viral hepatitis.	W
	Catarrhal intestinal inflammation.	Hexamitiasis.	P
	Congestion, haemorrhage and excess mucus.	Intestinal coccidiosis.	
	White spots on intestinal wall.	Intestinal coccidiosis.	
Spleen	Enlarged.	Infection, eg. falcon herpesvirus, chlamydiosis.	
Caeca	Congestion, haemorrhage and excess mucus.	Caecal coccidiosis, salmonellosis.	
Gizzard	Severe impaction + green stained cuticle.	Lead poisoning.	
	Presence of lead shot.	Lead poisoning.	
	Haemorrhage under cuticle.	Paramyxovirus-1 disease (notifiable in UK).	
	Small, fine nematodes.	*Amidostomum* spp. (gizzard worms).	
Joints	Purulent material.	Septic or mycoplasmal arthritis.	
	Swollen (chicks).	Calcium deficiency.	
	Urates.	Articular gout.	
Brain	Haemorrhage in cranium.	Agonal bleeding - not significant.	
	Haemorrhage in brain or meninges.	Concussion.	
	Inflamed meninges.	Meningitis.	
	Depressed cranial fracture with haemorrhage.	*Ante-mortem* trauma.	
	Depressed cranial fracture - no haemorrhage.	*Post-mortem* trauma.	

EXAMINATION OF UNHATCHED EGGS

The clinician may periodically be asked to identify the reasons for failure of eggs to hatch.

History
History is important and the following factors should be considered:
- Are the eggs artificially or naturally incubated?
- What is the percentage of hatch failures in the clutch or batch?
- What is the previous breeding history of the adult birds?
- If the eggs were naturally brooded, were there any disturbances during incubation, eg. territorial disputes, dog or fox attacks, which may have resulted in temporary abandonment of the nest?
- If artificially brooded, examine the incubator records which should include data on temperature, humidity, rates of turning, length of time over which the eggs were collected prior to incubation, egg weight during incubation and candling records.

Candling
Candling will reveal at what stage the egg died (for candling techniques refer to Anderson-Brown 1979 or Cooper, 1987):
- Clear with no blood ring or embryonic development indicates an infertile egg which may be the result of male sterility, mismating, overlong storage of eggs prior to incubation or infection.
- Clear with blood ring or early embryonic development indicates early embryonic death which can be caused by excessive length of storage, disturbance to incubation causing chilling, incubation temperature too high or damage to egg.
- Advanced development or full term but with failure to pip may be caused by hereditary factors, malposition of the chick, incorrect or fluctuating incubator temperature, wrong turning time or infection from damaged egg (see Chapter 40).

Examination of the Exterior of the Egg
- Measure and weigh the egg. Is the egg abnormally small? If so, it may be caused by inflammation of the oviduct. If the egg is abnormally large or double yolked it may be caused by slow passage through the oviduct.
- Note the degree of contamination or discolouration of the shell.
- Has it pipped (commonly known as 'dead-in-shell')?
- If it has pipped, is the beak protruding through a single hole - probably due to excessive moisture in the early stages of incubation.
- Does the egg have a row of chips around it but with the internal membrane intact? This can be caused by inadequate moisture, particularly towards the end of incubation.
- Are there any cracks in the shell not associated with pipping? If so, these may be the result of damage and can allow the contents of the egg to become infected.

Examination of the Interior of the Egg
- Remove the top of the egg (blunt end) with scissors. Wash and retain the shell fragment. Note the thickness of the shell.
- Examine the air cell - the chick's beak should be positioned in the air cell; if not, the chick is malpositioned and may have been unable to breathe.
- Note the odour and quality of any fluid in the egg. Infected chicks will often smell unpleasant and be surrounded by a foul liquid. This is not an infallible finding with infection. If no other cause of the chick's death can be found, culture of swabs taken from the yolk sac and the chick's liver and heart may reveal pathogenic bacteria. Similarly, swabs can be taken from the contents of clear eggs to see if infection may be the cause of the infertility. Secondary infection in aged eggs is common, so interpretation of bacteriological findings must be made with care. If the infection is primary, a pure, heavy culture of one or two organisms can be expected, whilst secondary infections will result in multiple bacterial cultures. Retain and freeze some of the egg contents for possible future viral or toxicological analysis.
- Finally, wash and weigh the shell fragments and measure the thickness of the shell at the pipping site (the air cell at the larger pole). Thin shells may be due to toxins or problems with the reproductive system of the female.

REFERENCES AND FURTHER READING

Anderson-Brown AF (1979) *The Incubation Book*. The World Pheasant Association, Reading.

Baker K (1993) *Identification Guide to European Non-Passerines*. British Trust for Ornithology, Thetford.

Beer JV (1988) *Diseases of Gamebirds and Wildfowl*. The Game Conservancy, Fordingbridge.

Coles BH (1985) *Avian Medicine and Surgery*. Blackwell Scientific Publications, Oxford.

Cooper JE (1987) Investigation of mortality in embryos and newly hatched chicks. In: *Breeding and Management of Birds of Prey*. Ed DJ Hill. University of Bristol Press, Bristol.

King AS and McLelland J (1979) *Form and Function in Birds. Vols. 1 to 4*. Academic Press, London.

King AS and McLelland J (1984) *Birds: Their Structure and Function*. 2nd Edn. Baillière Tindall, London.

Lowenstine LJ (1986) Necropsy procedures. In: *Clinical Avian Medicine and Surgery, including*

Aviculture. Eds GJ Harrison and LR Harrison. WB Saunders, Philadelphia.

McLelland J (1990) *A Colour Atlas of Avian Anatomy*. Wolfe Publishing, London.

Ochiai K, Jin K, Itakura C, Goryo M, Yamashita K,

Mizuno N, Fujinaga T and Tsuzuke T (1992) Pathological study of lead poisoning in Whooper Swans (*Cygnus cygnus*) in Japan. *Avian Diseases* **36**, 313.

Wobeser GA (1981) *Diseases of Wild Waterfowl*. Plenum Press, New York and London.

Appendix 11.1. Basic Equipment.

Table with an impermeable and washable surface.
Cork board (cork notice boards available from stationers are useful).
Clean plastic sheeting (discarded after each case) to cover the board.
Table lamp with magnifying glass (several types are available from lighting shops).
Variety of pins for securing the limbs (hypodermic needles are suitable, cheap and convenient).
White enamel dish (useful for searching for lead in gizzard contents).
Size 4 scalpel handle.
Size 3 scalpel handle.
Size 22 scalpel blades.
Size 15 scalpel blades.
Pair of 2 into 1 tooth dissecting forceps, eg. Treves.
Pair of fine dissecting forceps, eg. Gillies.
Pair of straight, fine-pointed surgical scissors size 6".
Pair of straight, fine-pointed surgical scissors size 3".
Pair of 6" Mayo scissors.
Pair of Liston bone cutters.
Screw top specimen containers filled with 10% formol-saline.
Sterile screw top specimen containers.
Sterile swabs with and without transport medium.
Two or three clean, dry, microscope slides that have been stored in methylated spirits.
Spirit lamp or bunsen burner.
Sterile gauze swabs.
Kitchen towel or tissues.
Protective clothing.
Face mask.
Disposable plastic gloves.
Fume cupboard (ideally).

Appendix 11.2. Sample Autopsy Submission Form.

Autopsy Submission Form

Name of owner: ....

Address of owner: ....

Post code: ....

Telephone number (day): ....

Telephone number (evening): ....

Bird: English name: ....

Latin name: ....

Sex: ....

Age: ....

Identification, eg. ring number: ....

Date of bird's death: ....

Date purchased or hatched: ....

What signs have been seen: ....

Has appetite been good? ....

Have there been any changes in the droppings? ....

Have there been any breathing problems? ....

Have there been any nervous signs? ....

What breeding history is there for this bird? ....

Have there been any recent purchases? ....

What birds have recently been in contact? ....

Details of any other recent deaths or illnesses: ....

Details of housing: ....

Details of diet: ....

Have you any other comments? ....

NB. The carcase of this bird cannot be returned to you following autopsy examination.

Appendix 11.3. Post-Mortem Check List.

PM No: .... Date: .... Owner: ....

Order: .... Family: ....

Species: .... Latin name: ....

Ring number: .... Sex: .... Age: .... Weight: ....

PM interval: .... Condition: .... X-ray: ....

External   Body length: ....

    Eyes: .... Maximum chordal length: ....

    Nares: .... Beak (culmen) length: ....

    Beak/mouth: .... Beak width: ....

    Vent: .... Beak depth: ....

    Feathering: .... Head length: ....

    Wings: .... Tarsus: ....

    Legs/feet: .... Tail length: ....

    Ectoparasites: .... Middle toe + claw: ....

Internal   Photos: ....

    Subcutis: ....

    Musculoskeletal: ....

    Trachea: ....

    Syrinx/bronchi: ....

    Crop/gullet: ....

    Thyroid: ....

    Air sacs: ....

    Liver: ....

    Gall-bladder: ....

    Spleen: ....

    Proventriculus: ....

    Gizzard: ....

    Ileum: ....

    Caeca: ....

    Pancreas: ....

    Testes/ovary: ....

    Kidneys: ....

    Heart: ....

    Lungs: ....

    Cranium: ....

    Endoparasites: ....

Samples taken: ....

Tentative Diagnosis: ....

CHAPTER TWELVE

Zoonoses and Health Implications Including COSHH

David A R Hannam

INTRODUCTION

Zoonoses have been defined as 'infectious diseases naturally transmissible between vertebrates and man' (Bell *et al*, 1988). The infectious agent is likely to be present in animal body products and may be transferred by direct contact, fomites or aerosols. Human infection with the pathogen can occur in several ways: ingestion or inhalation; contact with mucous membranes; or by injection via cuts, scratches or puncture by needle.

The Control of Substances Hazardous to Health (COSHH) Regulations 1988 require risk assessments to be made whenever activities are undertaken in the workplace which may result in a health risk. The possibility of exposure to microorganisms which might cause human infection is addressed in these Regulations, as well as contact with other harmful substances, such as drugs and disinfectants, and other chemicals.

COSHH ASSESSMENT

Before a raptor, pigeon or waterfowl is handled, the clinician should have made an assessment of the hazard of possible zoonoses. Many of the exotic viral diseases are unlikely to be present in birds which have been resident in the UK for a long while, whereas birds which become ill, or die, whilst in quarantine are more likely to be harbouring exotic disease. *Post-mortem* examination of birds which have died in quarantine should not pose a risk to the clinician because these cases should be submitted under the Import of Birds and Hatching Eggs Order 1979 to the nearest Veterinary Laboratories Agency (VLA) Veterinary Investigation Centre (VIC) for examination. However, a risk is present during the clinical examination of such cases and in the transportation of their carcases to the VIC.

The risk of zoonotic disease depends on several factors:
● The prevalence of disease in the population. Chlamydiosis is more common than, for instance, flavivirus (Togaviridae) infection.
● The route of transmission. Are the procedures which are to be carried out likely to increase the risk

of aerosol formation, contact with body fluids or accidental injection?
● The infectivity of the organism and the vulnerability of the victim. People with concurrent disease conditions or depressed immune status are more likely to succumb to a lower infective dose than are healthy individuals. Drug therapy may increase the likelihood of infection, eg. antibiotic treatment may increase susceptibility to *Salmonella* spp. infection. Pregnancy may also increase the individual's risk of infection and the severity of the consequences.
● The severity of the disease. Some zoonoses are fatal; others are mild and self-limiting. Some diseases are easily diagnosed and treated and are completely cured; others develop into chronic ill-health. If the risk of infection may be a fatal illness, this should be taken into account when assessing control measures.

PREVENTION AND CONTROL

In controlled domestic animal populations, prevention of zoonoses may be achieved by disease eradication programmes, eg. brucellosis and bovine tuberculosis. Similar disease control measures might be feasible in restricted populations of birds, eg. salmonellosis and chlamydiosis in pigeon lofts and waterfowl flocks, but wildlife reservoirs of infection make control breakdown highly probable. Prevention and control of human disease must, therefore, rest with correct techniques and personal and general hygiene.

HEALTH SURVEILLANCE

Regulation 11 of COSHH requires the health surveillance of workers where there is a probability that a disease may arise from occupational exposure. Surveillance should include information about the previous job(s) and sickness history of staff in case earlier illness might be significant. Records should be kept of the present health status of employees, and these should be reviewed at regular intervals by examination of sickness absences and symptoms. Whenever staff are receiving medical treatment, especially antibiotic therapy, they should inform their employers. This will allow any increase in risk to be assessed and appropriate steps taken to avoid exposing the employee to extra hazard.

INFORMATION TO EMPLOYEES

Employees should be informed about health risks from zoonotic infections, together with likely symptoms. They should also be given a medical contact card describing their work and the possibility of zoonotic infection for the benefit of doctors who might be investigating or treating any unexplained illness.

An assessment should also be made of the risk of infection to non-employees. This is especially important in veterinary premises where members of the public are present either as owners of birds being examined or attending with other pets.

POST-MORTEM EXAMINATION FACILITIES

Ideally, avian *post-mortem* examinations should be carried out in a suitable safety cabinet, but this probably cannot be justified in the majority of practices. However, a designated area should be provided for *post-mortem* examination with sampling, cleansing and disinfection, and waste disposal facilities all readily available. A separate *post-mortem* room encourages sound, careful techniques which reduce the risk of inadvertent cuts and stabs from instruments and the sharp ends of broken bones. Access to the room should be restricted to authorised personnel only; this reduces the numbers of people exposed to possible infection to a minimum. Correct preparation of the carcase can reduce considerably the risk of aerosol and feather dust (fomite) production. Before opening the carcase, it should be thoroughly wetted by lowering it tail first into a bath of detergent solution and spreading the wings and feathers. Care should be taken to avoid contaminating the beak, nares and eyes before examination. This technique prevents stray feathers and dander floating about.

Post-mortem room staff should always wear appropriate protective clothing. This should be either easily cleaned and disinfected apron and gloves dedicated to *post-mortem* work or, alternatively, single use disposable garments. Food and drink should not be consumed within the *post-mortem* room and no smoking should be allowed. Members of the public must be excluded from this area.

ZOONOTIC INFECTIONS

There are very few epidemiological data on potential zoonotic diseases in raptors, pigeons and waterfowl. It is therefore extremely difficult to make specific risk assessments. A full list of possible zoonotic infections may be obtained from suitable textbooks, eg. Bell *et al* (1988). Nevertheless, it is appropriate to mention the commonest diseases so that veterinarians are aware of their hazards.

Bacterial Zoonoses

Campylobacter spp.
The hazard of infection with these organisms is difficult to assess because many birds are symptomless intestinal carriers. Human infection is usually with *C. jejuni*; symptoms may be acute with fever, abdominal pain and bloodstained diarrhoea. Alternatively, incubation may take from 5-10 days. Recovery can take up to 10 days.

Chlamydia psittaci
Chlamydial infections are common in pigeons and ducks and have been reported in raptors. Human disease can be variable: headaches, joint and muscle pains, swollen lymph glands, influenza-like symptoms, non-productive cough and pyrexia may last for only a few days, although there may be frequent relapses. The severity of the disease tends to be greater in people over 45 years of age. Alternatively, there may be an atypical pneumonia with endocarditis and hepatitis which may persist for several weeks.

Salmonella spp.
Raptors, pigeons and waterfowl are all susceptible to salmonellosis or can be carriers of *Salmonella* spp. The human incubation period is up to three days; symptoms include watery diarrhoea and colic for about 10 days. There is a low grade pyrexia and dehydration may occur. Abscess formation is possible but rare, as is septicaemia. The severity of human symptoms depends on the infective dose and, as has been mentioned earlier, people already taking antibiotics are more susceptible to infection with fewer organisms than are healthy individuals. Symptoms are more severe in the very young and very old and in already debilitated people. Salmonellosis can be fatal in humans.

Mycobacterium avium
The human incubation period is unknown. Symptoms resemble tuberculosis, with lymphadenitis and respiratory signs. Infection is commonest in immune suppressed individuals.

Pasteurella multocida
This organism is ubiquitous and can cause localised wound infections following pecks or scratches.

Yersinia pseudotuberculosis
The risk assessment of this organism is similar to *Campylobacter* spp. because many birds are carriers. In humans the incubation period is 3-7 days. There is acute pyrexia followed by abdominal pain and diarrhoea for up to three weeks. Pharyngitis is also common.

Viral Zoonoses

Many of the viral zoonoses require an insect or other arthropod vector to complete natural infection. In the UK, such vectors, apart from ticks and mites, are probably rare. However, human infection is still feasible during clinical examination of birds and whilst carrying out *post-mortem* examination. Many of the viral zoonoses belong to the Family Togaviridae. It should be noted that, despite the low risk of infection, viruses of this Family have the potential to cause meningoencephalitis in humans. Viral infections endemic to the UK include:

Influenza

Orthomyxoviridae viruses are prone to antigenic reassortment and drift. Specific viruses often cross species barriers because of this antigenic shift and human infection can result. Typical influenza symptoms are described.

Louping Ill

The virus causing louping ill is a member of the Family Togaviridae. Human symptoms include pyrexia, muscle and joint pains, severe headaches, conjunctivitis and possible neurological signs.

Newcastle Disease

Paramyxovirus 1 (PMV-1) infection can cause a painful but short lasting conjunctivitis, although influenza-like symptoms and fever have also been described. Therefore, special precautions must be taken when administering live PMV-1 vaccine.

Miscellaneous Zoonoses

Cryptosporidiosis

Cryptosporidia infections cause a mucoid diarrhoea which can last for up to two weeks and may be accompanied by vomiting, colic and headaches.

Histoplasmosis

Infection with the fungus *Histoplasma capsulatum* can cause acute influenza-like symptoms in man. In heavy infections or reinfections these early symptoms can progress to pericarditis and endocarditis, miliary lung lesions and hepatomegaly and splenomegaly. Chronic meningitis may also occur.

Strongyloidiasis

Ducks are reservoir hosts of *Strongyloides stercoralis*. Infection in man is by skin penetration by larvae. Inflammation and pruritus at the penetration site occurs for up to four weeks, followed by fever, coughing, haemoptysis, mucoid diarrhoea and abdominal pain.

CLINICAL EXAMINATION AND HOSPITALISATION

COSHH assessments should be made for both clinical examination and hospitalisation of birds. All staff dealing with raptors, pigeons and waterfowl should be instructed on the correct and safe handling of these species. Many of the potential hazards have already been discussed, but it is worth reiterating the hazards of cuts and scratches when birds are handled by veterinarians and nursing staff and by the birds' owners. Obvious contact contaminants, such as blood and faeces, can be rapidly and safely contained using spill kits. These kits should contain absorbent cotton wool, disposable plastic gloves and a suitable disinfectant, and they must always be readily available. Aerosol production and contamination is not so obvious: handling birds creates a high risk of aerosol and feather dust formation, and these dangers cannot be overemphasised. Good, bird-proof ventilation should be maintained in order to reduce the potential aerosol loading and contamination of the environment.

Care should also be taken to make COSHH assessments of other substances in use such as drugs and disinfectants.

REFERENCE

Bell JC, Palmer SR and Payne JM (1988) *The Zoonoses: Infections Transmitted from Animals to Man*. Edward Arnold, London.

CHAPTER THIRTEEN

Management and Husbandry

Neil A Forbes and Jemima Parry-Jones

INTRODUCTION

Although for many centuries raptors were kept almost solely for falconry, they are now kept for a variety of reasons. Falconry, according to the purists, is the art of taking wild quarry with a trained bird of prey. It is one of the oldest sports, vying with coursing, and both claiming a history of 4,000 years. Although known in the Middle Ages as the Sport of Kings, ironically, these days it is more a sport of the unemployed or partially employed (by choice or necessity) as a great deal of time and commitment is required to train birds adequately.

In view of the age of the sport, many names and terms have arisen. A working knowledge of these terms will greatly assist the clinician, and help instil confidence in the owner's mind. A glossary of some of the (traditional) terms commonly used by falconers is given in Appendix 13.1 - Glossary.

In the last decade the interest in keeping raptors and owls has increased enormously. At the time of writing there are approximately 16,000 diurnal raptors registered with the Department of the Environment (DoE) belonging to 9,700 keepers. This does not include any of the vultures (of which there are only small numbers in UK) nor does it include any of the owls, which may well outnumber the diurnal raptors.

> Department of the Environment
> Wildlife Division,
> Tollgate House,
> Houlton Street,
> Bristol BS2 9DJ
> Tel. 01179.218811

There are more captive registered raptors in the UK than in any other country (other than the Middle East), including the USA. Non-indigenous raptors, plus kestrels, sparrow hawks and buzzards, no longer require to be ringed or registered, although they cannot be sold (except under special licence) unless they are ringed with a seamless closed ring as supplied by AC Hughes (Tel: 0181.979.1366) or the British Bird Council (see Figure 13.1). Vultures have never required ringing or registration; most owls are now required to be close

ringed to be sold and vultures may require rings. All birds held in captivity for whatever reason should either be ringed or have some method of proof that they are being held legally. Sensitive indigenous species, such as the Golden Eagle, Peregrine Falcon, Merlin, harriers, Hobby and Northern Goshawk, have to be ringed with an individually marked, government supplied ring, and registered.

Some birds, which were ringed as adults, will be wearing a cable tie ring with DoE markings (see Figure 13.2). They may be injured wild birds, imported birds, birds that were in the UK prior to the Wildlife and Countryside Act 1981, or those whose rings became illegible and were replaced. In future it is hoped that electronic identification microchips will be used

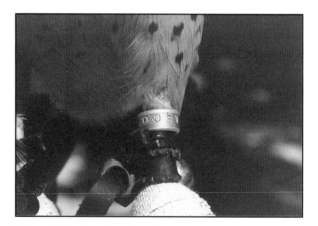

Figure 13.1: Seamless closed ring.

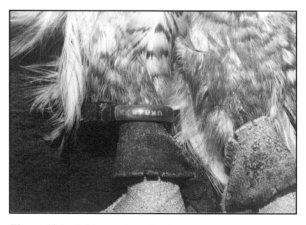

Figure 13.2: Cable tie ring with DoE markings.

either in combination with rings or in place of them. It is currently too easy to steal a bird, remove its ring, especially if it is a species which is not obliged to have one, and then keep or 'unofficially' sell the bird. All raptors are protected by law and none may be killed, taken or otherwise interfered with in any way. However, as the public's interest in wildlife increases, more injured wild raptors are brought to veterinary surgeons or centres specialising in keeping raptors. A bird may be taken from the wild if this is done solely in order to treat an injury, but every effort must be made to return the bird to the wild as soon as it is fit and the conditions are suitable. If these birds are treated by veterinary surgeons, they should, wherever possible, pass the bird, once treated, on to an experienced person for rehabilitation back to the wild. If birds are not fit for release, the veterinary surgeon must confirm the reason in writing, should the finder wish to retain the bird.

In the interest of aiding the uninformed but well meaning person, as well as assisting in controlling those intent on breaking the law, veterinary surgeons treating raptors should make themselves fully conversant with the current legislation.

Differences between members of the Family Falconiformes generally recognised as raptors have been described in the Introduction to this manual. Some further details on members of this Family likely to be kept in captivity are given below. The morphological differences are described.

FALCONS

Falcons are active searchers and hunters. Generally, they catch their prey by climbing high and stooping down at a fast speed (maximum 140mph). A few of the falcons can hover with varying degrees of success - kestrels are the best known for hovering and are often seen by roadsides hunting from a hovering position. Bumblefoot is found more often in the falcon group of raptors than in any other. In 99% of cases, bumblefoot (see Chapter 16) is caused by poor perching either in aviaries or on blocks for tethered working birds. Occasionally, a bird will puncture its own foot while hunting.

HAWKS

Hawks are the sprinters of the raptor world. They are very highly strung and use up their energy reserves quickly, especially if stressed. Historically, this group have frequently suffered from 'fits'. However, there is now greater understanding of the correct nutritional requirements of hawks and the incidence of fits has reduced (see Chapter 20). Northern Sparrow Hawks have quite fine skin and may suffer from bumblefoot if kept in unsuitable conditions. Hawks hunt from trees, or occasionally from a soaring position. They make a mad dash after quarry, either catching the intended prey

quickly or losing it in cover and giving up. Northern Sparrow Hawks often come into built-up areas in periods of hard weather and hunt in gardens. They are not universally popular when using the bird table as a source of food. They also have a tendency to fly into windows in the excitement of the chase: they have thin skulls, but will occasionally escape with only a headache and can be released almost immediately; others are less fortunate (see Chapter 15). In view of their nervous disposition, Northern Sparrow Hawks are difficult to manage in captivity, especially wild adult birds. They are very common in the wild and are frequently presented to veterinary surgeons with serious injuries. Some cases warrant treatment and release: those unlikely to be released should, in the authors' opinion, be euthanased, if possible when first examined. As Northern Goshawks become more common they may be presented as injured birds, usually because of road traffic accidents or shotgun injuries.

BUZZARDS

Buzzards are generally large soaring birds with small feet in comparison to their body size. They are predominately scavengers. Only Red-tailed Hawks have good sized feet and that makes them the most popular of the true buzzards. Buzzards hunt either by soaring or are stationary hunters like hawks. However, they are not as fast as hawks so prefer slower quarry and often eat carrion if the opportunity arises. The Harris' Hawk is the only species used for hunting where one can safely fly numbers (a cast) of birds together. They are bright, intelligent birds with the dash of the hawk and the more phlegmatic temperament of the buzzard. If put in the old fashioned 'skylight and seclusion' aviaries (four solid walls and only a wire or net roof for any view), or tethered in a quiet place, they may become bored and feather pluck. This is the only species of raptor which shows psychological feather plucking; it is probably also the most intelligent. Buzzards are generally robust, which is why they have been recommended in recent years as beginners' birds.

EAGLES

Eagles are usually medium sized to very large birds. The Tawny Eagle is probably the most commonly flown eagle in the UK, although other species are gaining in popularity. Normally found on open plains or mountains, eagles hunt by still hunting or by soaring. They can build up tremendous speed in a stoop, just like a falcon, but being heavier have greater difficulty stopping. They have very powerful feet, of which handlers should beware. Although the beak can give a nasty bite, the feet of a large eagle can be difficult to disengage once they have grabbed and 'bound' to an arm or other part of the body. Although generally robust like buzzards, to which they are closely related, eagles that have become accustomed to one home for a long period can suffer tremendous stress if moved to a new home. This often causes illness and may lead to the bird dying.

OWLS

Owls vary greatly in size and nature. They appear to cope better with captivity than many of the raptors. They settle in captivity quickly and some breed readily. They can be very large and powerful - a female European Eagle Owl can weigh as much as 4.5kg, ie. the same size as a male Golden Eagle: in contrast, some of the Scops Owls are only 90-120g.

BIRDS KEPT IN CAPTIVITY

All of the Family groups described earlier are kept in captivity for a number of reasons. Those trained and flown by their owners will have the closest relationship with the falconer, and must be kept feather perfect whenever handled or treated. They may be trained for hunting or demonstration, or for educational purposes, the latter being perhaps the most important role served by captive raptors (vital for the future well being of our countryside and wildlife). They may be used for feral bird clearance from airfields, rubbish dumps, churchyards, town centres, etc.

Birds may be kept for displaying as pairs to the public (caged in zoos), or they may be kept as breeding pairs, producing young each year. Some are bred for research or release schemes. Breeding of raptors has increased tremendously in recent years. On average, 2,500 diurnal raptors have been bred and registered in the UK annually in the period 1991-1993. Not only is falconry self-sufficient for the supply of birds required for the sport, but it has also contributed greatly in developing breeding projects for rare species such as the Mauritius Kestrel. Some birds are kept individually as pets. As no licence or qualification is required in order to keep a raptor, owners may require informed advice from their veterinary surgeon. In addition, owners should be encouraged to join one of the recognised clubs where they can receive training in the management and husbandry of raptors (see Appendix 13.2 - Useful Addresses).

HOUSING TRAINED BIRDS

Raptors are kept under many different conditions, varying from good to not so good. Trained birds tend to be kept tethered, although many falconers are now keeping trained birds loose in aviaries and flying them straight from the aviary; this is to be encouraged. However, all but hand-reared birds need to be tethered initially for training. This can be for a short period (10-14 days) up to an average of about one month, and sometimes longer for true accipiters and eagles.

Tethered birds wear leather straps, called jesses, which must be attached to both the birds' legs and be the same length. The jesses are threaded through a specially made swivel which in turn is attached to a leash (see Figure 13.3). The free length of the leash is kept short, otherwise excessive speed may be built up by a bird leaping from one side of the perch to the other. On occasions, sufficient force is generated to cause injuries to the legs.

Tethered birds should be looked after with more care than free lofted aviary birds. They must be kept out of extreme weather conditions (excessive heat is a particular risk). Most Falconiformes gain their total daily fluid intake with their food: however, they should have daily access to water. Young birds and those that are ill will have greater fluid requirements. Tethered birds should receive daily exercise. Most birds should not be tethered outside in the winter and they must not be left tethered near ground level during days or nights when temperatures may be close to freezing (see Chapter 17). Working birds tethered on blocks and receiving daily exercise should be placed in 'weatherings' to give some protection.

Weatherings are permanent shelters that have an open front and may have a sand or pea gravel floor; they should only be used from April-October. Falcons and very small hawks need an area 2.5m x 2.0m; larger

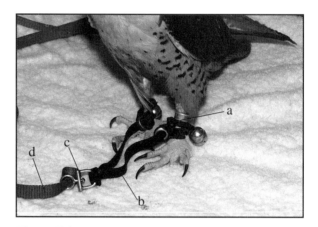

Figure 13.3: Aylmeri (a), jesses (b), swivel (c) and leash (d).

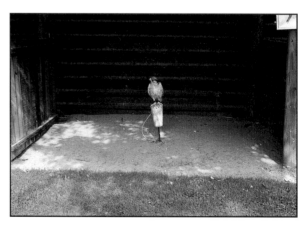

Figure 13.4: Lanner Falcon tethered on a block in a weathering.

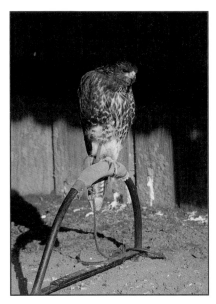

Figure 13.5: Harris' Hawk tethered on a bow perch.

birds an area 3.5m x 2.5m. In good weather, birds may be put out in the sun and allowed access to a bath. However, on hot days birds should be protected under shade netting. Birds outside should be under supervision at all times; while tethered, all but the largest of eagles are vulnerable to predation by foxes, cats, dogs, badgers and humans.

Falcons tend to sit on block perches (see Figure 13.4), whilst most of the other species sit on bow perches (see Figure 13.5). The perches should not have a smooth perching surface. Materials used include Astroturf (a commercially available, plastic artificial grass or door mat material), roughened cork, carpet, concrete or natural stone. Poor perch design is responsible for the majority of bumblefoot cases. Sadly, there is no one material which is suitable for all species. Falcons suffer from bumblefoot disproportionately. All 'blocked' birds should have the plantar aspect of their feet checked 2-3 times a week for early signs of this serious condition (see Chapter 16). If birds do have to be tethered during the colder months of the year, this may be done with a flat Astroturf-covered ledge, with a tubular heater placed underneath in order to prevent the effects of ground frost. The 'screen perch' is a more dangerous type of perch in which the bird is tethered to a perch some 1.25m from the ground. This type of perch is no longer recommended.

Under no circumstances should tethered birds be put on perches that are so far from the ground that the bird is left hanging, unable to reach the ground, if it flies off the perch.

AVIARIES

Aviary designs vary greatly: one should be aware that most raptors do not appreciate company from other raptors. Aviaries should be designed to give protection from predation, nuisance or weather, to prevent escape and to be readily cleaned. Ideally, the floor should be sloped, with a concrete underlayer covered over with sand or gravel (which can be washed through or removed if necessary). The aviaries currently used at the National Bird of Prey Centre are constructed with three solid sides, a solid roof and one open (wire mesh) side. They have a built-in bath which can be filled and cleaned from outside, and food is placed in the aviary from outside in a removable drawer, so that any excess food which is not taken is removed at the next feeding. Aviaries should have double entrance safety doors, one of which should always be closed. Aviaries should have a strong structure that will withstand strong winds and snow and keep the birds safe and warm. The aviary can be roofed with Onduline (tarred cardboard) or Eternit (concrete fibre); there is no condensation in cold weather and no overheating in hot weather. Steel or plastic roofs are not suitable. Birds should be approached only from one side. Where nervous or excitable species are housed, the open side (mesh) may need lining with hesian or soft netlon, so that the birds see the barrier and turn from it, rather than flying into the mesh. Aviaries should be easy to clean and maintain and have enough shelter to protect birds from all climatic extremes. If the 'skylight seclusion' type aviary is used, ie. four solid sides and a nylon mesh roof, the roof mesh should be lined with horizontal batons; this will prevent the birds scalping themselves on the mesh roof. Sizes of aviaries will vary. However, in practice the bigger the better, providing the birds can still be caught without causing undue stress, should they require treatment.

Veterinary surgeons should be aware of the accommodation used by their clients for their birds. Occasionally, the wrong situation, poor design or, for example, proximity to a compost heap (aspergillosis risk), may lead to recurrent problems.

HOUSING AND HANDLING OF SICK AND INJURED BIRDS

Although raptors enjoy good longevity in captivity, they do get ill and injured. When this happens birds need to be housed so that they will not traumatise themselves (skeletal, soft tissues or plumage) any further. At the start of treatment most birds should be kept in small quarters so that they can be caught easily and monitored. Large eagles and vultures may do better in a small room-type compartment rather than in the more usual box-type cupboard. Windows should be opaque and have vertical bars on the inside, or have a blind that can be pulled down over the glass. If birds accidentally get loose, they will fly straight for the light and impact injuries may occur. Raptors behave in a more settled fashion in subdued light. Removal of birds from cages or boxes, especially untrained birds from travelling boxes, should be carried out in a darkened room. Birds wearing jesses can usually be caught quickly by grabbing the jesses and removing the bird from the container. Alternatively, a towel may be dropped over the bird to restrain it and prevent it causing damage to the handler or clinician (see Figure 2.5).

CATCHING AVIARY BIRDS

Birds flying free in the aviary, if not currently trained to come to the fist, should be caught in a deep, soft-mesh fishing net, with an extending handle if necessary. As the bird is caught in the net, it will instinctively contract its claws and catch the netting, rather than damage either itself or the handler. Once caught the claws may be blunted by clipping, unless the bird is being flown at game at the time. This will help reduce the chance and severity of damage to either bird or handler.

NUTRITION OF RAPTORS

General Aims

The ideal diet is one that is as similar to the natural prey species that the bird would eat in the wild, whilst at the same time ensuring the correct food quantity, quality, wholesomeness and storage methods. Good raptor keepers should be feeding a mixed diet. This may consist of day-old chicks, quail, 'grown ons', rabbits, rats, mice and beef or horse meat. Over 50% of keepers feed day-old chicks alone. This is an unsatisfactory diet which should be discouraged unless it is supplemented.

The diet will differ depending on the size and type of bird being fed. For example, feeding mice to eagles is uneconomic as they will need large numbers; eagles should be fed rats. It is quite feasible to feed day-old chicks (with yolks removed) on 4-5 days of the week as long as other food is given on the remaining days. Whole carcases should always be given (even for young chicks, although the bones may need to be ground up so that small chicks are able to ingest them). Feeding should be to demand; excess should be avoided. Excess food will decay and may lead to a build-up of pathogens in the aviary. If, on a temporary basis, the normal varied diet cannot be maintained, vitamin and mineral additives should be administered.

Problems Encountered with Feeding Raptors

Irrespective of food type, one should be certain as to the quality, source, method of killing, freezing and storage of the food. Any ex-wild source of food, eg. pigeon, game, etc, must be considered to be potentially infected. Such birds can carry bacterial infections, eg. tuberculosis or *Salmonella* spp.; virus infections, eg. paramyxovirus, adenovirus or rotavirus; or they may have been poisoned, eg. alphachloralose, mercury, lead or pesticide. Any wild-sourced food should be in good body condition, have been caught and killed by identifiable physical means and, on examination of the carcase, should appear wholesome and free of disease. It is crucial that the abdomen of such birds is opened and the surface of the liver checked. If any small white spots are present on or in the liver (often indicative of avian tuberculosis), the whole carcase must be rejected.

The falconer should be wary of feeding road traffic casualties as these individuals have already failed the 'fitness' test. Non-avian foods, eg. rats, mice, squirrels or foxes, are less likely to carry diseases pathogenic to raptors. Conversely, feeding any avian derived foodstuff is a potential risk.

Raptors, Hygiene and Eating

The hygiene of the food supply, its preparation, storage and the manner in which it is offered is very important. However, many falconers are blasé about their own hygiene when in the presence of their birds. Infections such as *Salmonella enteridis* are common and may be present in day-old chicks. Avian tuberculosis is common in feral birds. These organisms can constitute serious risks. Raptors' furniture should not be held in or pulled using the teeth. Knives used in food preparation, as well as the occasional footing injuries to the hand, may introduce tetanus. Falconers and veterinary surgeons should ensure that their tetanus protection is up to date.

Pigeons are a special risk to raptors due to their high incidence of trichomoniasis (frounce). Even feeding pigeon breast alone will not avoid the risk of infection. Young, old or ill raptors are most susceptible to *Trichomonas* spp. infection. Pigeons should be frozen completely and thawed before feeding.

Many falconers feed ferreted, rifle or shotgun killed rabbits, or pigeons. Shotgun killed quarry should never be fed to raptors. Some falconers have fed such food for many years, and by feeding an increased level of casting material have avoided lead poisoning. Keepers should be aware that 'rifled' or 'ferreted' rabbit meat may still contain lead from previous, non-fatal, shotgun wounds and may therefore be a source of lead. The risk is low and the food source is good, but keepers should be aware of the possible risk and be alert for any presenting neurological signs (see Chapter 20).

Rabbit or hare can occasionally cause problems if the whole femur is swallowed intact. Usually the bird will cope with this. However, occasionally it will lodge transversely in the crop or proventriculus and may cause a perforation of the gut lining or an obstruction. The femurs of carcases should be broken before they are fed to birds of 1kg or less in weight.

Virus Infection

In recent years, outbreaks of virus disease, eg. adenovirus and rotavirus, have been encountered by the authors. Apparently healthy, commercially sourced quails, day-old chicks, turkey poults, etc. have been fed to healthy raptors, and these birds have then succumbed to disease and, in several cases, died. Many viruses can be carried subclinically by day-old chicks etc; but be pathogenic to raptors who eat them. The feeding of avian derived food should be avoided if at all possible.

Atherosclerosis

Atherosclerosis is a common cause of death in many caged birds. The condition is seen predominantly in overfed aviary birds, who have not benefited from exercise. There is no indication that the bird is ill: it is simply found dead in the aviary. A high blood cholesterol level indicates an increased likelihood of a bird being affected. The condition is commoner in older female birds, particularly after the breeding season, due to the high level of fats which are mobilised in order to complete the egg yolks (El-Sayed and Brackenbury, 1988). Susceptibility to atherosclerosis is hereditary (Shih *et al*, 1983; Marks and Washburn, 1991). The lesions of atherosclerosis are totally reversible by exercise and a reduced dietary fat content, provided the disease can be predicted or detected prior to death. The condition is best avoided by not feeding excessively fatty food. Old spent laying quails, mature fat laboratory rats/mice and egg yolks are the main sources of excess dietary fat. It is important that birds are not overfed. Aviary birds are generally fatter than wild or trained birds. When feeding in a breeding aviary, food is best supplied in a drawer system, rather than a shute. In this way, if excess food is given, it can be removed at the next feeding rather than remaining on the aviary floor. The positioning of the food drawer in the aviary is also important. It should not be in direct sunlight as this encourages putrefaction. When birds are fed, their reaction should be watched. They should come straight down to feed. If they do not, they are not very hungry and less food should be given that day.

Exercise is important. If possible, breeding birds should be taken out and flown after the end of the breeding season.

Feeding Birds in Low Condition

Birds in low condition are often inappetent or vomiting. This can be a significant management problem (see Chapters 3 and 19).

Dietary Supplements

Many supplements are available, but if a good varied diet is fed, these should not be necessary. However, there are certain situations where additional supplements are advantageous. Hatching chicks have a naive alimentary immune system. Hand-reared chicks should receive a good quality avian probiotic. This will reduce the incidence of enteritis and septicaemia in neonates.

A bird which is stressed or which has additional energy requirements, eg. breeding or moulting birds, will benefit from additional essential amino acids and vitamins. A good quality avian preparation should be administered, eg. Arkvits (Vetark). In some species, eg. the Secretary Bird, breeding females have a greater dietary calcium requirement and these, together with females which are likely to lay more than one clutch of eggs, should receive a calcium/vitamin D_3 supplement. Display birds flying in front of the public on a daily basis, who are rewarded with beef after flying each day, may suffer calcium deficiency and should also receive supplements. Several suitable preparations are available, eg. Nutrobal (Vetark), A1 Raptor (Butterworth), SA37 (Intervet).

Dehydration

Raptors, especially if young, ill or on medication, should be offered water on a daily basis. **Although many raptors do not drink often, they should be able to reach clean fresh water at all times**. Raptors will often need to drink when being medicated.

Feeding Baby Raptors (see Chapter 22)

IMPRINTING (see also Chapter 22)

To avoid hand rearing, many breeders place young birds back with their parents or foster parents at about 10-12 days old. The main reason for returning chicks to avian parents is to avoid adverse imprinting. This occurs when a young bird which has been reared by hand grows up thinking it is human. Initially, the chick will scream at the human on whom it has imprinted whenever he or she comes into sight, thinking that it will receive food or attention. When the bird becomes sexually mature it may present itself as a mate to the handler. In the case of injured or orphan raptor or owl chicks, it is crucial that they are left if possible where they are found, or, if this is not possible, they should be reared with other youngsters of similar breeding (crèche rearing). If a chick has to be reared singly it must be prevented from seeing the handler and fed with a gloved (or puppet) hand. Birds that become imprinted and are later mistakenly released may, once they become sexually mature, seek out humans, particularly children, in their search for a mate.

Conversely, there are situations where experienced bird keepers may imprint birds deliberately. This is most commonly carried out for the purpose of semen collection or receipt in artificial breeding projects.

INTERSEX AGGRESSION

This is a major problem which occurs in certain species (particularly Merlins and Northern Goshawks) as a consequence of changing sex hormone levels before, during and after laying. The most frequent outcome is that the larger, more aggressive female bird kills her spouse (see Chapter 21).

BIRD WEIGHTS

Many raptor species show sexual dimorphism. In many species, female birds are approximately 30% heavier than male birds. In consequence, males and females may often be differentiated by weight alone. However, there is considerable overlap between the sexes in some species. Many species occur as subspecies or races, each of which may have differing weights: this further complicates the situation. Chromosomal sexing by

DNA analysis is currently not commercially available for raptors. However, surgical sexing techniques may be used in the few cases in which the sex is indeterminate.

Falconers should know the current weight of their birds as well as the 'flying' and 'fat weight'. Wild birds should be weighed prior to drug administration. Small birds have a high metabolic weight and, therefore, higher food and drug requirements. Table 13.1 shows the daily food requirement of raptors of varying weights.

The daily requirements will increase by a factor of at least 1.2 at times of stress such as after injury or illness.

Table 13.1. Daily food requirements for raptors.

Weight of bird (g)	Percentage of weight required as food daily (%)
100-200	18-25
200-800	11-19
800-1,200	7-11
4,000-10,000	3.5-6

NUTRITIONAL MANAGEMENT OF THE HOSPITALISED RAPTOR

Most raptors being hospitalised are either wild birds who are stressed and not used to the food being offered, or are sick captive birds which may not be inclined to eat. Special consideration is required for the nutritional requirements of such patients (see Chapter 3).

FEEDING BIRDS BEFORE TRAVELLING

Birds should not be fed directly before travelling. Experienced flying birds accustomed to travelling may not suffer from travel sickness. However, many unseasoned travellers will regurgitate and are at risk of choking (this is a particular risk if a bird is hooded at the time). For a bird such as a Peregrine Falcon, it is advisable to give a cast-free meal 8-12 hours before travelling.

REFERENCES

El-Sayed MS and Brackenbury JH (1988) Sexual maturity and physical exercise alter fibrinolytic activity in birds (chickens). *Comparative Biochemistry and Physiology* **90A(3)**.

Marks HL and Washburn KW (1991) Plasma and yolk cholesterol levels in Japanese Quail divergently selected for plasma chlolesterol response to adrenocorticotropin. *Poultry Science* **70(3)**.

Shih JCH, Pullman EP and Kao KJ (1983) Genetic selection: general characteristics and histology of atherosclerosis susceptible and resistant Japanese Quail (*Coturnix coturnix japonica*). Atherosclerosis. *Biologcal Abstracts* **49(1)**, 77.

USEFUL READING

The Falconers and Raptor Conservation Magazine
20 Bridle Road, Burton Latimer, Kettering, Northants NN15 5QP. Tel: 01536.722794

Appendix 13.1. Glossary of Falconry Terms.

Accipiters	Often referred to as 'true' hawks; comprises sparrow hawks and goshawks, characterised by short rounded wings, long tails and light coloured eyes.
Aylmeri	A loop of leather which is placed around the tarsometatarsus and stapled with a brass eyelet through which a leather jess is run (see Figure 13.3). A mews jess has a knot on the end that prevents the jess pulling through. The mews jess is replaced with a hunting jess, a strip of leather that is pulled out as the bird is flown off the fist. As there is no strap trailing when flying, the bird has less chance of becoming tangled in a tree.
Bate, to	An attempt by the bird to fly off the glove or its perch, either at lure or quarry or away from an alarming object. The bird may hang from its jesses, beating its wings frantically. (Derived from the French *battre*: to beat frantically.)
Bell	Audible brass bells are generally attached to hunting birds to allow the falconer to locate a bird in flight or sitting still. Falcons tend to have bells on their legs; hawks tend to have the bells on their tails.
Bewit	Thin leather strap used to attach the bell to a bird's leg.
Bind, to	The action of a raptor hitting and holding prey with its feet.
Blain	Carpal bursitis, presenting as a watery swelling about the carpal joint. Caused by trauma to the carpus, often by repeated bating (see Chapter 17).
Block perch	Cylindrical or inverted cone shaped perch made of wood, stone or concrete, the flat top surface covered with cork, carpet or astroturf. There is a spike at the base of the block to allow the block to be stuck into the ground, or the spike can be fixed to a permanent mount. Around the spike is a swivel ring to which a falcon may be tethered (see Figure 13.4).
Block, to	To keep a bird on a block by tying its leash to the ring.
Blood feathers	New feathers, not yet fully grown, whose shaft still contains a blood supply.
Bow perch	Perch fashioned in the shape of a capital 'D' with the flat side against the ground. The top, curved surface of the bow, on which the bird stands, is padded with leather, rope, carpet or astroturf. The ends of the perch are spiked and embedded in the ground. Used for tethering short and broad wings and eagles (see Figure 13.5).
Broad (or Bay) wing	Term used to describe *Buteo* spp., eg. Eurasian Buzzard, and *Parabuteo* spp., eg. Harris' Hawk.
Cable tie	A plastic cable bearing the bird's identification number, placed around the (distal) tarsometatarsus (see Figure 13.2).
Cadge	A portable rectangular frame of perches with padded edges for carrying hooded long wings onto the hunting field. Allows several birds to be carried by one person. Traditionally suspended from the shoulders by a leather strap.
Cast, a	Two or more raptors flown together.
Cast, to	To hold a bird around its shoulders, place it on a table and restrain it.
Cast, to	To bring up a 'casting'.
Cast off, to	To launch a bird from the fist.

Casting	Fibrous material (fur or feather) in the diet that will be eaten by the bird and turned into a pellet within the gizzard. Brought back up 12-20 hours after ingestion.
Cope, to	To file or clip the beak or talons (claws) of a bird.
Crab, to	One raptor 'footing' another.
Cramps	Extensor rigidity or flaccid paralysis of a bird's legs.
Creance	A length of fine, strong line that is attached to the bird when flying during the later stages of training. This allows the bird to fly some distance but still be restrained by the falconer.
Crop	Food storage organ cranial to the thoracic inlet (absent in owls).
Crop tube	Syringe with 10-15cm of giving set tubing attached, used to administer fluid, liquidised food or medication.
Day-olds	Day-old cockerel chicks, sold dead, either fresh or frozen.
Deck feathers	The central two tail feathers, usually the first to be moulted. On occasions, a bell is attached to these feathers at their base. A telemetry transmitter can also be mounted here.
Diurnal	Daytime hunting.
Enter, to	When a bird makes its first kill.
Eyass	Nestling or first year hawk.
Falcon	Term used by falconers to describe female falcons (see below).
Falcons	Refers to all members of the Family Falconidae, otherwise known as long wings.
Fat weight	Maximum expected weight when fed *ad libitum* and not exercised.
Fed up	A bird being allowed a full or partial crop of food as a reward after it has flown at quarry or for display.
Feed on the fist	During training the bird is allowed to feed, whilst restrained by jesses, only on the falconer's gloved fist. This is done to strengthen the bond between bird and man by making the bird regard the falconer as the sole source of food.
Flights	Primary and secondary feathers, ie. flight feathers.
Flown, being	When a bird is allowed to fly either on a creance or free.
Flying weight	A weight less than the bird's full weight, at which it will be eager to hunt.
Foot, to	To strike or grab with the feet.
Fret mark	Line of weakness horizontally across the feather. Caused by a break in nutrition, illness or stress whilst the feather was growing (see Figure 14.2).
Frounce	Trichomoniasis; also known as 'canker' by pigeon fanciers.
Furniture	Collective term for the accoutrements of falconry, eg. jesses, hoods, bells, telemetry, etc.
Gauntlet	Traditional glove used in falconry on the left hand (unless left handed, when it is on the right hand).

Grown ons	Poultry or turkey chicks grown on to three weeks of age; more nutritious than day-old chicks.
Hack, to	Allow eyasses to fly free for a few weeks before starting training.
Hack back	To hack a bird back to the wild.
Haggard, a	A wild caught, adult raptor.
Hard penned	The feathers and the bird are said to be hard penned once a young bird has become fully feathered or, in an older bird, once the moult is completed and the blood supply to the quill has dried up.
Hawk	Otherwise known as a short wing; member of the Family Accipitridae.
Hood	A complete covering for the head that allows only the beak and nostrils to protrude. The hood is made of leather in several traditional patterns. To work correctly it should prevent the bird from seeing anything (hoodwink it).
Hood, to	Place a hood over the head of a falcon. Usually done single-handed with the bird on the falconer's fist. It is usual to hood falcons but not hawks, although hawks are sometimes hooded. When the bird is completely in the dark it relaxes and is usually tractable.
Hood, made to the	The training process in which a bird is trained to accept a hood.
Hunger traces	Synonymous with fret marks or fret lines (see earlier).
Imp	The replacement of a damaged feather by glueing a new tip onto the old stem in order to allow normal flight.
Imprinting	A lesson that is learnt and remembered, usually throughout the life of the bird, from a brief and well defined period during the growing stage of the chick. Situations, animals and objects may all be imprinted upon the chick with desirable or undesirable consequences.
Jack	Male Merlin.
Jerkin	Male Gyr Falcon.
Jessed up	A bird that has jesses attached to its pelvic limbs to facilitate restraint.
Jess	Length of leather which is looped around the tarsometatarsus and left long whilst the bird is flown. There is a danger of the bird getting the jess entangled in a branch etc.
Keen, to be	When a bird's weight is reduced a little, it responds well and is eager to hunt.
Lanneret	Male Lanner Falcon.
Leash	Cord or rope used to attach the bird's jesses via the swivel to the guantlet or perch.
Long wings	Otherwise known as 'falcons': members of the Family Falconidae.
Lure	A piece of fur or feathers that resembles the quarry, or an imitation bird made of leather. Used during training.
Make in, to	To approach a hawk on a lure or kill in order to pick it up.
Man, to	To tame a bird so it will accept handling and training.

Mantle, to	Action taken by a bird to cover its kill; the wings are raised like a cloak to prevent the kill being taken by another bird or rival.
Mantle, to	When a bird stretches out one leg and wing.
Mews	Building where trained, tethered birds are kept inside at night or in bad weather, or outside under shelter. Traditionally, it only referred to the building in which birds were placed whilst they were moulting.
Musket	Male Northern Sparrow Hawk.
Mutes	Faeces.
Mute, to	Action of defecation by a bird.
Nares, naris	Nostril of a falcon.
Pellet	The casting material after regurgitation.
Pull, to	Birds eat by holding food in their talons (claws) and 'pulling off' pieces of flesh that are small enough to swallow. This can be a very violent procedure.
Put in	When a bird dives into cover after quarry.
Put over	Action of food being passed over from the crop to the proventriculus ('to put the crop over'). The peristaltic movement of the crop is a visible muscular activity.
Rouse, to	To raise the feathers slightly before shaking them back into position.
Sakret	Male Saker Falcon.
Screamer	An imprinted bird who screams to its handler for food or attention, especially when hungry.
Screen perch	A perch, usually about 1.25m from the ground, with a weighted canvas screen hanging from it which reaches almost to the ground. The bird's leash is attached to the perch and the bird is prevented from wrapping itself around the perch by flying under it repeatedly. This perch is no longer recommended because some birds have difficulty regaining the perch and can hang by their leash with fatal consequences.
Set down	A bird is 'set down' to moult at the end of the flying season.
Sharp set	A bird which has been reduced to flying weight and is therefore eager for food and keen to hunt, and will return to the falconer to feed.
Short wings	Otherwise known as 'hawks'; members of the Family Accipitridae.
Slicing	The manner in which short wings defecate, often projecting the faeces several feet away from their body.
Spar	A female Northern Sparrow Hawk.
Sour crop	Toxaemia and bacteraemia following putrefaction of food in the crop.
Still hunting	A form of hunting used by many wild hawks. They sit still on a post or other vantage point waiting for prey to pass close enough for the bird to swoop down on it.
Stoop	The attack method used by falcons; a steep, fast descent onto prey or lure.

Strike the hood   To pull the short ends behind the hood and loosen the ties around the neck ready to remove it.

Swivel   Two metal rings, connected in a figure of eight fashion by a bolt or rivet, used for joining the jesses and the leash.

Take, to   The catching and, usually, killing of quarry by a bird.

Take up, to   To recover a lost bird or, more commonly, to restart 'manning' after a moult ready for flying.

Talon   Claw or *unguis*.

Telemetry   Radiotracking equipment often used when flying birds in case they become lost.

Tiercel   Special term for a male falcon. (Sometimes restricted to male Peregrine Falcons.)

Top weight   Maximum weight (as for 'fat weight').

Train, a   Alternative name for the tail feathers.

Train, to   Train or 'man' a bird prior to flying.

Wait on   Falcons circling over the falconer, often very high up, waiting for game to be flushed.

Weather, to   To place or keep a bird in a weathering.

Weathering   A sheltered but open air pen where birds are tethered when not in the mews.

Appendix 13.2. Useful Addresses.

London Hawking and Owl Club
c/o Paul Barham
4 Navenby Walk
Fairfoot Road
Bow London E3 4EZ
0171.515.7754/0171.639.9087

Southern Counties Raptor Club
c/o Terry Pearce
01273.542971

South Eastern Raptors Association
1 Sepham Farm Cottage
Filston Lane
Shoreham
Kent TN14 5JT

Welsh Hawking Club
c/o Adrian Williams
Maendy Farmhouse
Church Village
South Wales CF38 1SY
01443.206333

South East Falconry Group
c/o The Secretary
Tilbury Community Association
The Civic Square
Tilbury Essex
0124.522.6057

Bedfordshire Falconry Club
c/o Malcolm Forrest-Hazel
01582.451341/619883

New Forest Falconry Club
c/o Chris Hopkins
3 Southey Road
Christchurch
Dorset BH23 3EQ
01202.478862

Scottish Hawking Club
c/o Andrew Knowles-Brown
Crookedstone Elvanfoot
By Biggar
Lanarkshire ML12 6RL
01864.505245

East London Falconry Club
c/o Gary Leadley
Bretons Club The Manor House
411 Rainham Road
Rainham Essex RM13 7LP
0181.517.9362/01708.520160

Cumbrian Falconry Club
c/o Colin Taylor
20 Queens Avenue
Seaton
Workington
Cumbria CA14 1DL
01900.68063

Hampshire Falconry Club
c/o Peter Tudor
18 Green Mead Avenue
Everton
Nr Lymington
Hampshire SO41 0UF
01590.645225

Home Counties Hawking Club
Surrey/Berkshire
01344.423988/01276.23429

Heart of England Falconry Club
c/o Jenny Wray
184 Warwick Road
Kennilworth
Warickshire CV8 1HU
01926.50000

Northern England Falconry Club
c/o A Barnard
32 Well Grove
Hove Edge
Brighouse
Yorkshire HD6 2LT
01246.825209

Raptor Breeding Association
c/o Robin Pote
2 Old Bell Cottages
Ludford Ludlow
Shropshire SY8 1PP
01584.874874 9

Avon and Somerset Raptor Group
c/o Guy Whitmarsh
22 Reymend Walk
Bedminster
Bristol BS2 5AP
01179.660770

British Hawking Association
c/o George Roach
Kennel Farm Cottage
Old Kennel Lane
Annesley Park Annesley
Notts NG15 0AU
01623.751339

Central Falconry and Raptor Club
c/o Kim Oakshott
42 Larkrise
Woodfield
Northampton
Northants NN3 4QT
01604.414155

North Avon and West Wilts Raptor Club
c/o Phil 01225.891964
c/o Keith 01454.315810

British Falconry Club
c/o John Fairclough
Home Farm
Hints Tamworth
Staffordshire
01543.481737

Cheshire Hawking Club
c/o George Edwards
35 Sandbach Road
Salemoor
Cheshire M33 2SF
0161.976.1037/01204.523622
01706.845731

CHAPTER FOURTEEN

The Integument

A Dermod Malley and Trevor J Whitbread

INTRODUCTION

The avian integument has many similarities to that of mammals and has similar functions. The epidermis is layered, producing keratin squames with a continual turnover of cells. Beneath this there is the dermis which contains the connective tissue, feather follicles, feather erecting muscles, sensory nerve endings (Herbst corpuscles) and blood vessels. The subcutis contains fat, the quantity of which varies in indirect proportion to the number of feathers in the area (see Figure 14.1), and is arranged in a layer as discrete bodies attached to the underlying muscles.

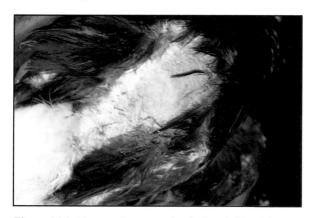

Figure 14.1: *The apterium ventrale of a female Harris' Hawk. The central area has subcutaneous fat, decreasing in quantity towards the margin with the pterylae. (Photo courtesy N H Harcourt-Brown).*

The outstanding features distinguishing avian from mammalian integument are the production of feathers and the virtual absence of specialised adnexal glands. There are no sweat glands. Lipid is produced in the transitional layers of the epidermis by cells (sebokeratinocytes) which eventually die to form the stratum corneum. As the cells die they exude their lipid content and this covers the skin. Lipid is also secreted by a small number of specialised glands (the uropygial gland at the base of the tail, the cloacal glands around the vent and the aural glands around the base of the ear).

It is thought that this lipid content and the relatively few portals of entry on the surface of the skin are the major factors contributing to the low incidence of infectious dermatoses in birds. Because lipid is the major factor in the defence of the skin, diet and intercurrent disease profoundly influence the health of the avian integument.

FEATHERS

Feathers are tough, keratinised cellular derivatives of the epidermis, formed in follicles which penetrate deep into the deep dermis (Spearman and Hardy, 1985) (see Chapter 35 for illustrations of normal feathers). Feather follicles are distributed in pterylae or feather tracts which follow species-specific patterns. There are no glands and in adults the follicles are compressed and inaccessible to parasites and bacteria.

Feather Colour
The colour of the feathers of raptors is supplied by pigments, mostly melanin and carotenoids. Feathers show coloured bars in many raptor species.

Moulting
Moulting is the shedding and replacement of plumage and the stratum corneum. The latter is shed as large segments amongst the feathers and helps to remove surface bacteria and fungi. Raptors moult once a year, usually after breeding, and the process takes three to seven months, although in some species, eg. Old World vultures, moulting may extend over a longer period (up to 2-3 years) with only some of the feathers changing each year. Pruritus may occur during moulting: in addition, calcium is resorbed from the Haversian systems and bones become more fragile. Feathers are pulled by the bird or fall out naturally.

Sequence of Moulting
The sequence of moulting of the feathers of raptors is:
● Inner to outer primary wing feathers.
● Inner to outer secondary wing feathers
● Central to lateral deck (tail) feathers

Factors Affecting Normal Moulting Patterns
Normal moulting patterns are affected by:
● Photoperiod.

● Nutrition, especially avitaminoses (protein deficiencies, which are uncommon in raptors, affect feather replacement rather than moult).

● Stress or fear - feathers are lost following withdrawal of the stress factor (Angel, 1982; Spearman and Hardy, 1985).

● Egg laying.

● Ambient temperature - increased ambient temperature results in a faster moult in hawks (Cooper, 1985).

● Illness - a protracted illness may delay a moult. After health is regained, the ensuing moult may be more rapid than expected.

● Corticosteroids can retard the progression of a moult (Cooper, 1985). They may cause the formation of feathers which appear to have a deformity once erupted. Feathers already formed and erupted are not affected.

● A trained raptor which is flown into the moulting season may moult late or not at all.

As a result of a combination of some or all of the above factors, many raptors do not undergo a complete moult each year.

Control of Moulting

The natural stimulation for the shedding of a feather is the growth of its successor. Moult may be induced by influencing feather growth by the following methods:

● Reduction of the photoperiod: fluctuation of light falling on the retina and the pineal body (gland) leads to neural stimulation of the hypothalamus and subsequent release of gonadotrophins from the hypophysis. This provides control of egg production, spermatogenesis and the production of new feathers.

● The effect of sex hormones in raptors is unknown, but in other species oestrogens depress the growth of the new feathers, whereas progesterone stimulates the feather papillae and feather growth.

● Thyroxine will stimulate feather growth: the feathers will usually erupt as the hormone is withdrawn. The dose recommended for a 1.4kg Red-tailed Hawk is 25μg thyroxine daily for a week, followed by 50μg daily for a week, then 75μg daily for a week, then 50μg daily for a week and finally back to 25μg daily for a week (Harcourt-Brown, personal communication).

Abnormal Feather Growth

Overexertion and diseases, including ecto- and endo-parasitism, can affect the regrowth of feathers. Damage to feather follicles by trauma, burning or infection may lead to future feathers being distorted. The use of pharmaceutical agents during feather replacement can also cause abnormalities. Particular attention should be given to nutrition during the moult as the diet will be responsible for the plumage of the ensuing twelve months. Physical damage caused by poor housing may

be avoided by maintaining the moulting bird in a skylight seclusion aviary.

Brood Patch

The brood patch (incubation patch) is a physiological area situated between the caudal border of the sternum and the pubic bones. The patch is present in both sexes if the incubation is shared, but is absent from the male if he does not share the incubation duties. Feather loss from this site is seasonal and is often accompanied by thickening, oedema and an increased blood supply useful for incubating eggs.

Feather Deformities

The presence of feather deformities indicates a history of physiological compromise (due to the effect of endogenous or exogenous corticosteroids). They may arise due to stress induced by starvation, infection or injury, but may not reflect the current health status of the bird. The clinician should always remember that the plumage reflects the health status of the bird at the time the feather was being formed.

Nutrition

Various feather deformities are encountered from time to time. Some are referred to as 'stress lines' or 'hunger traces' and are manifested as translucent lines on the vane of contour feathers perpendicular to the rachis (Figure 14.2). Both these and the 'pinched off' phenomenon (constriction at the base of the feather shaft) are ascribed by Cooper (1985) to non-specific nutritional deficiencies. It is difficult to condemn particular amino-acids in this respect, but stress lines and notches have been reported due to methionine deficiency in raptors (Lowenstine, 1986). Cystine is required for maintenance of the beta-fibrils which give strength to feather keratin; deficiency can lead to weak and broken feathers.

Drugs

As far as the authors are aware, the effect of drugs on plumage has not been recorded in raptors as it has been in other species, but drug related causes should be considered in the event of feather pathology. Many feather dyscrasias are blamed on the use of drugs in birds. The incidence is probably exaggerated, but there is always a possibility of feather dyscrasias following the use of benzimidazoles and trimethoprim-potentiated sulphonamides.

BASIC EXAMINATION OF THE RAPTOR INTEGUMENTARY SYSTEM

Clinical Examination

The clinical examination of raptor skin should follow the same lines as for birds presented for any other reason (see Chapter 2). When birds are scarred and no feathers grow, the exposed skin commonly

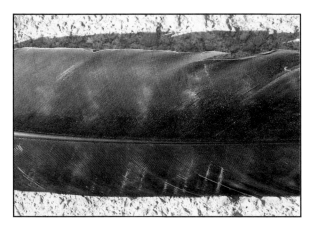

Figure 14.2: Fret marks on the feathers of a Golden Eagle. (Photo courtesy N A Forbes)

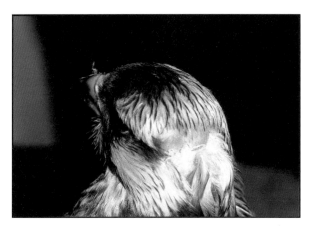

Figure 14.3: This area of subcutaneous fat in a Lanner Falcon developed at the site of an old injury where the feathers had failed to grow. (Photo courtesy N H Harcourt-Brown)

overlies an increased layer of fat (see Figure 14.3). Abnormalities of the skin may indicate primary skin disease or could reflect underlying systemic diseases. Laboratory investigations should follow the routine detailed in Chapter 7.

NURSING AND THE CARE OF FEATHERS

Plumage Contaminants
The plumage of raptors may become soiled with man-made and refined chemicals. In addition, Peregrine Falcons which nest on sea cliffs often suffer from contamination with fish oil regurgitated by Northern Fulmars during attack. The oil destroys the waterproofing qualities of the plumage and reduces or totally prevents flight capabilities and heat insulation (Mearns, 1983).

Removal of Contaminants
There is a standard procedure for dealing with all plumage contamination. This is described in detail in Chapter 35.

Prevention of Feather Damage

Tail Guard
Every hospitalised raptor should have an effective tail guard applied. This can be made from a strong manila envelope, thick plastic (eg. an autoclave bag), cardboard or radiography film cut to size as shown in Figure 14.4. It is necessary to cover only the distal two-thirds of the tail. The material is cut to size, folded around the tail, sealed with tape or staples, and kept in place by means of a cable tie which may be fastened to a tail mount (often already present in trained birds - see Figure 14.5) or around the two central 'deck' feathers, or with a single strip of 2.5 cm Elastoplast as shown in Figure 14.4.

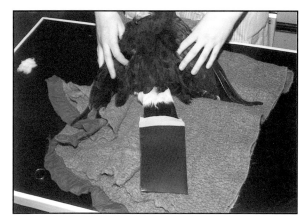

Figure 14.4: Tail guard made from X-ray film to protect the tail feathers of a hospitalised wild bird. (Photo courtesy N A Forbes)

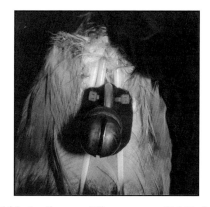

Figure 14.5: A tail mount. (Photo courtesy N A Forbes)

Hospital Cages
Hospitalised birds provided with a suitable perch or block will keep their tails clear of the floor and suffer little or no damage to their feathers. As cage fronts made from wire mesh cause damage to the tails of raptors, only those with vertical wires or battens are suitable; it might be better to use a cardboard box. Temporary measures include covering existing doors on the inside with a blanket or towel to prevent damage. Birds that are kept in the dark are less likely to damage feathers.

Remigeal Haemorrhage

Feathers grow from the vascularised dermal papillae. The dermal papilla can bleed if the feather is pulled out or the calamus is broken. The haemorrhage can be arrested only by 'casting' the bird and removing the broken feather by gentle torsion and traction, followed by digital pressure on the follicle for 5-10 minutes to encourage haemostasis. Before attempting this procedure the clinician should warn the owner that the dermal papilla may be damaged and that the new feather may not grow or may grow at an angle. The clinician may have to reassure ill-informed falconers that the growth of the next feather is not dependent on the follicle remaining patent and that the colouration and pattern of the feather will be that of the next plumage. The application of household white pepper to the bleeding follicle is, in the authors' hands, a useful haemostat in an emergency.

Imping

Imping is a procedure that the experienced falconer is unlikely to request of a practising veterinarian, but the clinician should understand the principle involved. Ford (1992) described the technique which has been used since medieval times to salvage a broken feather, usually a primary wing or tail feather. The shaft of the broken feather is cut off obliquely. The donor feather (preferably one from the same species and position, collected from the previous moult) is similarly cut across its shaft. An 'imping needle' (a soft metal, bamboo or carbon fibre pin of triangular cross-section, measuring 3-4cm in length in the case of a Peregrine Falcon) is inserted. The imping needle may be dipped in butylcyanoacrylate (Vet-Bond, 3M Animal Care Products; Isobond, Ellman International) before insertion in the feather shafts. Care must be taken that the vane of the implanted feather overlaps its neighbour in the same way as the previous feather and that the glue does not soil the vanes of any of the feathers on the bird.

CONDITIONS AFFECTING THE SPECIALISED AREAS OF RAPTOR SKIN

Uropygial or Preen Gland

The uropygial (preen) gland is a bilobed holocrine gland situated craniodorsally to the base of the tail (see Figure 14.6). This gland produces sebum which provides an antimicrobial veneer on top of the intrinsic epidermal and feather lipid. The incidence of infection in this gland is rare, but treatment with prolonged (three weeks) courses of antimicrobial agents can be undertaken following culture and determination of antibiotic sensitivities. As in other species, both adenocarcinoma and blockage of the duct of the preen gland can occur in raptors.

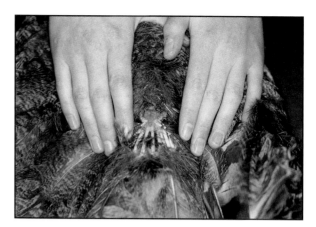

Figure 14.6: *The uropygial gland is clearly seen in this Ural Owl.*

Scales (or Scutes)

Scales are raised areas of highly specialised skin separated by less keratinised folds of skin. They are found on the podotheca or non-feathered part of the foot. Scales can be affected by *Cnemidocoptes* spp. The preferred treatment is the parenteral use of ivermectin (200mcg/kg i/m, s/c or percutaneous).

In Northern Goshawks and Red-tailed Hawks in particular, the larger scales located on the dorsal and plantar aspects of the tarsometarsal region have evolved to form a protective shield which serves as a 'shin guard'. The protective function of this area predisposes it to trauma as the heavy bird flies through undergrowth. Ideally, the scale is only 2-3mm thick, but on occasions, especially in older birds, the scale becomes thickened and more rigid. Trauma can lead to a break in the scale and, therefore, the skin underneath, allowing access to bacteria. As there is limited or no drainage, cellulitis develops. The resultant subcutaneous infection forms pus which must be removed and, therefore, must be treated by debridement until healthy pink skin is exposed. The growth of new skin is stimulated by repeated application of Preparation H (Whitehall Laboratories) (Forbes, personal communication).

Northern Goshawks are commonly affected by trauma which involves full-thickness skin. Crusts appear under the furniture, eg. jesses, during the hunting season and if allowed to develop they can form a subcutaneous abscess (see Figure 14.7.1). The crust should be picked off whilst the bird is cast in a towel. Removal of the crust exposes the subcutaneous tissues (see Figure 14.7.2). Parenteral antibiotic therapy and a covering of Granuflex (Squibb) to hydrate and stabilise the wound will allow healing over a period of a few weeks.

Oil of proflavine cream or Dermisol (Pfizer) have been used with equal success to remove infection and stimulate granulation. Dry gangrene of the skin can be a problem if a jess becomes tightly wrapped around the leg (see Figure 14.8.1). The wound should be debrided to healthy granulation tissue (see Figure 14.8.2)

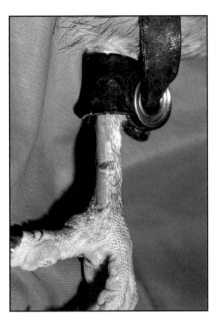

Figure 14.7.1: Northern Goshawk with a crust involving the skin of the leg. (Photo courtesy N H Harcourt-Brown)

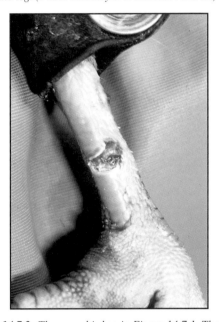

Figure 14.7.2: The same bird as in Figure 14.7.1. The crust has been removed exposing the subcutaneous tissue beneath. (Photo courtesy N H Harcourt-Brown)

and covered at first with oil of proflavine under a non-adherent bandage. A ball bandage can be applied to prevent injury (see Figure 14.8.3). Once epithelialisation has commenced the wound can be protected with Granuflex until the process is complete (see Figure 14.8.4). This has the added effect of immobilising the skin above and below the wound and also preventing reinfection of the area (Harcourt-Brown, 1994).

Many birds become affected with crusts between the claw and the digital pad (see Figure 14.9.1). These must be softened by the use of daily applications of Fucidin Gel (Leo) to allow them to heal (see Figure 14.9.2, 14.9.3).

Dry Skin

Seborrhoea sicca is encountered in eagles; topical application of Oil of Evening Primrose Hand Cream (Efamol) is efficacious (Harcourt-Brown, 1994). Although atopy has not been definitively diagnosed in raptor species, some cases of pruritic dermatosis have been observed to respond to essential fatty acids, eg. Dermplus (C-Vet) (0.5ml/kg p/o daily), and have relapsed when the therapy has been withdrawn (Forbes, personal communication).

Birds that are maintained on a diet composed predominantly of rodents often present with pale, dry feet

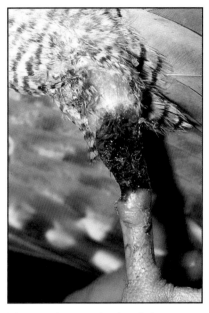

Figure 14.8.1: Northern Goshawk with dry gangrene seven days after a jess becoming tightly wrapped around the leg. (Photo courtesy N H Harcourt-Brown)

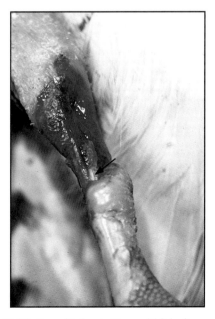

Figure 14.8.2: Same bird as in Figure 14.8.1 after debridement. Note that the flexor hallucis longus tendon (arrow) has been sectioned as a result of the necrosis. (Photo courtesy N H Harcourt-Brown)

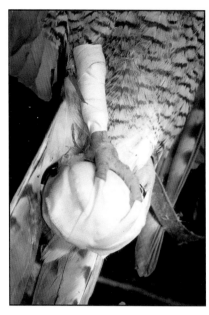

Figure 14.8.3: The same bird with a ball bandage applied to prevent injury to the dorsal aspect of the first digit. (Photo courtesy N H Harcourt-Brown)

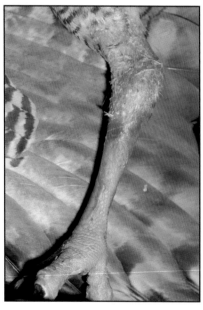

Figure 14.8.4: The same bird six weeks later when the skin injury had healed. The tendon was repaired and the bird made a complete recovery (see Chapter 16). (Photo courtesy N H Harcourt-Brown)

and cere. The dry feet may be treated with a lanolin/ oil of evening primrose hand cream. Beta-carotenes may be provided in vitamin supplements, eg. Spirulina (Lanes), or with the yolk sac from day-old chicks.

TREATMENT OF WOUNDS IN RAPTORS

Minor cuts and abrasions are usually treated simply by cleansing thoroughly with broad-spectrum antiseptics such as povidone-iodine or chlorhexidine (see

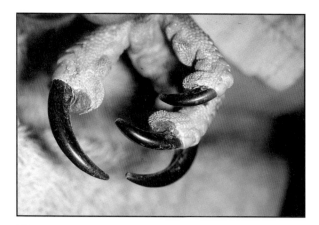

Figure 14.9.1: Harris' Hawk with crusty toes (see Chapter 16). (Photo courtesy N H Harcourt-Brown)

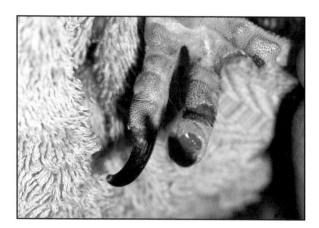

Figure 14.9.2: Same bird with the crusts softened and bleeding. (Photo courtesy N H Harcourt-Brown)

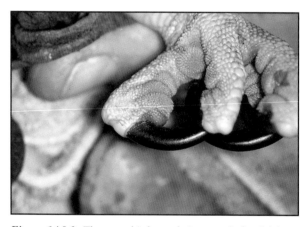

Figure 14.9.3: The same bird greatly improved after 14 days treatment with sodium fusidate ointment. (Photo courtesy N H Harcourt-Brown)

Chapter 3, Flow Chart 3.5). Small wounds with minimum tissue damage (such as those that occur in badly designed sky-light seclusion aviaries - see Chapter 13) respond well to topical applications of Orabase (Convatec) once or twice daily (or as often as the bird will allow!). Fucidin Gel can also be used. **Wound powders intended for mammals may contain benzocaine (eg. Aureomycin Topical Powder,**

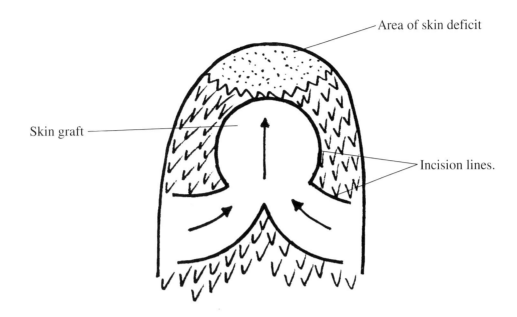

Figure 14.10: Diagram of a skin flap from the dorsal cervical area to cover skin loss from the crown of the head. (Drawing courtesy N A Forbes)

Cyanamid), propoxur or coumaphos (eg. Negasunt, Bayer), or other agents which should be avoided in avian species due to the risk of toxicity.

Wounds, which may be severely lacerated, are often found in the crural fold. There may be considerable loss of tissue. To effect a satisfactory repair, the surgeon may have to resort to drawing skin from the sides of the wound. It may be necessary to perforate the mobilised skin to enable it to stretch adequately, applying the principle that 15-20 small deficits, each with a diameter of less than 3mm, will heal by secondary intention much more quickly and efficiently than one single large deficit. Alternatively, if there is a large dead space under the skin, abscess formation can be prevented by leaving the wound unsutured. The wound will granulate, but any pus must be removed every 2-3 days otherwise healing is prevented.

Wounds involving loss of tissue on the head are frequently encountered in Northern Goshawks and are particularly difficult to manage. They are usually badly 'degloved' with considerable tissue loss and, if closure is attempted by simple traction, the upper eyelid may become elevated and its mobility compromised; this predisposes to exposure keratitis. The surgeon must be prepared to execute a sliding pedicle graft from the back of the neck, but should be aware that because of the different structure of the feathers in this area it is not acceptable to rotate a pedicle from the base of the neck. Forbes (personal communication) has had some success with the mobilisation of skin flaps from the sides of the neck by means of a bilateral Z-plasty technique. This results in a more acceptable, aesthetic appearance. A skin flap with lateral connections conserved is shown in Figure 14.10. **However much care**

is taken in performing these techniques, in a number of cases the skin that has been grafted or sutured can die and dry gangrene ensues. This can be a real problem and can make the injury considerably worse.

Underweight, chronically thin birds, eg. birds with bumblefoot, are often unable or unwilling to perch. They lie in sternal recumbency and split the skin over the keel bone. Healthy, flying birds colliding with lure or quarry may also damage the skin over the keel bone. Treatment includes adequate debridement with due control of sepsis and apposition of the edges of the wound by means of mattress sutures, finally suturing Granuflex over the incision. This protects and cushions the keelbone. Removal of the Granuflex after two weeks usually gives satisfactory results.

Infection can sometimes invade the sternum. In these cases the muscles must be reflected and the infected bone removed. The pectoral masses can be sutured together and the skin closed over them. If the infected bone is not removed these cases will prove intractable.

Caustic burns of apterylae are rare in raptors, but should be considered amongst the differential diagnoses in the event of erythematous dermatoses of the face and feet. Birds that are flown at landfill sites can sustain thermal injuries when they fly through methane flames. The use of silver sulphadiazine (Flamazine, Smith and Nephew) appears to be the treatment of choice (Perry, 1987).

ECTOPARASITES

Clinically significant infestations with ectoparasites are encountered occasionally in raptors. Ectoparasites cause feather loss only if there is pruritus. Signs of ectoparasitism in birds include restlessness, excessive and frantic preening, poor condition of the feathers (broken, rough or soiled), and feather plucking (Greve, 1986). The presence of large numbers of ectoparasites in raptors is usually related to debilitation due to other causes. The underlying cause of debilitation must always be addressed and, although the eradication of the ectoparasites may not always be of primary concern, in many cases they may have to be treated before the underlying condition will respond.

Great care should be taken in the treatment of ectoparasites of birds, particularly raptors, because of the danger of toxicity to these species from pesticides.

Red (or Roost) Mite

Dermanyssus gallinae is a periodic parasite found occasionally on birds housed in wooden mews or aviaries. The mites are usually visible on the birds only at night. They generally do not produce many lesions in normal healthy adults, but are known to be the cause of broken feathers in some individuals, eg. juveniles and Saker Falcon/Peregrine Falcon hybrids. The presence of red mites may be suspected when damaged plumage is observed, especially when other birds in the same premises are seen to be well feathered. Feather loss may be observed on the breast, overlying the crop, on the anterior aspect of the proximal metatarsus, just distal to the intertarsal joint (an examination should rule out feather loss in this area due the rubbing action of jesses or rings - see Figure 14.11), or at the top of the neck near the ventral surface of the mandible.

Treatment

The preferred treatment involves the use of ivermectin percutaneously, keeping the dose below 200mcg/kg. The aviary or mews should be sprayed with insecticide. Sprays useful for the treatment of premises include cypermethrin, eg. Dy-Sect (Deosan), diluted to 2% (this product stimulates the nerve endings in the skin and causes some discomfort, so care should be taken that the product does not contact bare skin) and malathion, eg. Duramitex (Harkers), diluted to 0.93% and painted on perches and walls of aviaries.

Cnemidocoptes spp.

This burrowing mite has been recorded in a Great Horned Owl (Schulz, 1989) and in three Northern Sparrow Hawks (see Figure 14.12). The life cycle is completed entirely on the host and typical honeycombed skin lesions are produced. The parasites may be demonstrated in skin scrapings.

Treatment

The use of ivermectin (200mcg/kg i/m, s/c or percutaneously, repeated after 14 days) is recommended.

Lice

All avian lice belong to the Order Mallophaga: members of this order have mouth parts which are adapted for chewing. The life cycle lasts 3-4 weeks and the parasites are very host-specific (Philips, 1990). The occurrence of lice on a hunting bird may be due to acquisition from a prey species, especially rooks, and may, therefore, not be of clinical significance. Damage due to lice may be seen as pin holes in the feathers and irregular edges to the feathers (see Figure 14.13).

Treatment

Treatment includes the use of piperonyl butoxide blended with pyrethrins, eg. Ridmite Powder (Johnson). Treatment should be repeated at or after three weeks to eliminate new generations hatching from the nits (eggs). The premises should be treated with cypermethrin as described earlier for red mite.

Louse Flies ('Flat Flies')

Louse flies (Hippoboscidae) cause irritation and may transmit blood disease, eg. *Haemoproteus* spp. (Keymer, 1969) and *Leucocytozoon* spp. (Forbes,

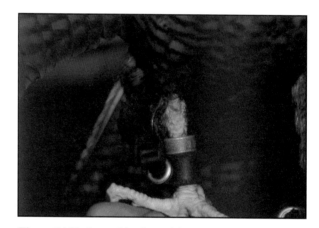

Figure 14.11: Loss of feathers of the anterior aspect of the proximal metatarsus of a Peregrine Falcon due to infestation with Dermanyssus spp. (Photo courtesy N A Forbes)

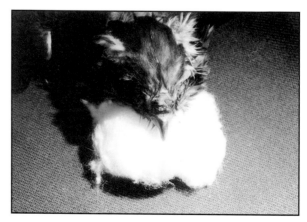

Figure 14.12: Northern Sparrow Hawk infested with Cnemidocoptes spp. (Photo courtesy N A Forbes)

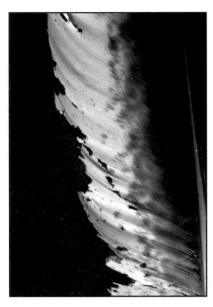

Figure 14.13: *Feather damage typical of louse infestation. (Photo courtesy N A Forbes)*

personal communication). The adult louse flies are winged, but immature flies are unable to fly. They are capable of causing significant blood loss in very young birds.

Treatment
Treatment is by dusting the feathers with piperonyl butoxide blended with pyrethrins to eliminate the adult parasites. The nests should be cleaned every 2-3 weeks and dusted similarly to eliminate the pupae.

Mosquitoes
Mosquitoes (Culicidae) constitute a biting nuisance but also transmit avipoxvirus and blood parasites, particularly in some warm countries, eg. USA and Middle East. Treatment and prevention involve the elimination of breeding sites near mews and aviaries and the dusting of birds with suitable insecticides before flying in 'risk' areas.

Gnats
Gnats (Simulidiae) transmit *Leucocytozoon* infection. Treatment and prevention is as for mosquitoes (see earlier).

Blow Flies
Myiasis caused by blow flies (Tachinidae) was reported as a problem in the USA by Ward (1986) and appears to be associated with infestations of nestlings in wet nests. In Europe, birds usually nest and fledge prior to the blow-fly season, so cutaneous myiasis is a problem only in very severely debilitated birds after traumatic injuries.

Treatment
Treatment involves physical removal of larvae and the institution of improved methods of hygiene. Affected birds may be sprayed with 0.0005% ivermectin (ie. 0.5ml Ivomec 1% Injection for Cattle in one litre of water) prior to removing the maggots, taking care not to exceed a total dose to each bird of 200mcg/kg. Products containing coumaphos, eg. Negasunt (Bayer), should not be used due to the risk of toxicity.

Ticks
Argasidae (soft ticks - lair parasites) and Ixodidae (hard ticks - ubiquitous) are occasionally found on raptors, sometimes with fatal consequences (Forbes and Simpson, 1993), possibly due to tick-borne toxins (Gothe *et al*, 1979).

VIRAL DISEASES

Viral diseases of the skin of raptors are relatively uncommon in the UK.

Poxvirus
Avipoxvirus has been reported in all avian species except owls (Graham and Halliwell, 1986). Species-specific antigenic strains are transmitted by mosquitoes and may cross the 'species barrier', but the resultant syndrome is usually far less pathogenic. Usually, only the dry form of the disease is seen in raptors. Following the abolition of border inspections within the European Union, it is important for clinicians to be alert to the possible introduction of this disease into countries in which it may not have been encountered before.

The clinical signs of raptor pox are nodular lesions distributed on the cere, eyelids and feet, which progress through papules, vesicles and pustules to scab formation. The lesions are pruritic and prone to secondary infection. Establishment of infection requires a breach of the integument.

Diagnosis
Diagnosis is by viral culture or histological demonstration of the typical proliferation of epithelial cells which become ballooned and show intracytoplasmic inclusion (Bollinger) bodies.

Treatment
Treatment involves the removal of the virus lipid envelope by means of lipid solvents (dilute quaternary ammonium compounds) or application of an eye spray made up by mixing 6ml Tylan 50 Injection (Elanco), 1.5ml Betadine (Napp Laboratories) and 100ml Water for Injection (2-4 times daily until the lesions have resolved). Nutritional, antibiotic and physical supportive treatment should also be given. The reader is referred to the paper by Samour and Cooper (1993).

BACTERIAL INFECTIONS

The avian skin is fairly resistant to primary bacterial

infections, but bacterial folliculitis often arises following infection of an open or damaged feather follicle. Feather base culture and antibiotic sensitivity testing is recommended. Treatment with the indicated antibiotic should be maintained for at least three weeks. The special considerations of oral administration of antibiotics in raptors should not be overlooked (see Chapter 5). Pododermatitis is frequently encountered in raptors (see Chapter 16).

FUNGAL INFECTIONS

Fungal infections are uncommon. Diagnosis is made on Cotton Blue or Diff Quick stained skin scrapings or on culture.

Candida spp.

The authors have encountered cases of candidiasis as secondary infection following bacterial pododermatitis. Chronic dermatitis in a Harris' Hawk has been treated with topical enilconazole (1:10 dilution). Systemic antifungal agents do not appear to be efficacious in this situation.

Aspergillus spp.

According to Richard (1991) cutaneous manifestations of aspergillosis in birds are rare, but Forbes (personal communication) reports the occasional occurrence of cutaneous aspergillosis in raptors (see Figure 14.14) and recommends vigorous surgical debridement and the use of daily topical applications of a 1:10 aqueous solution of enilconazole for 5-6 weeks.

NEOPLASIA

With the possible exception of **lipomata** and **virally induced neoplasms**, birds have a much lower general incidence of cutaneous neoplasia than mammals, and the incidence in raptors is particularly low. The only neoplastic condition of the skin of raptors encountered by the authors during an extensive literature search was **a malignant melanoma** recorded in a Red-tailed

Hawk by Kufuor-Mensah and Watson (1992). The primary tumour occurred in the upper beak and secondaries were found in the pancreas, adrenals, lungs and skeletal muscles. Forbes (personal communication) has recorded three cases of **squamous cell carcimomata** - two in Peregrine Falcons and one in a Lanner Falcon (see Figure 14.15) - and five **spindle cell tumours**, always in the wing tips - two in Northern Goshawks, one in a Common Kestrel, one in a Lanner Falcon and one in a Peregrine Falcon (see Figure 14.16).

Non-neoplastic disturbances are also rare. Proliferative lesions on the feet can be seen in response to infection and one author (TJW) has seen a very mature fibrovascular proliferation on the foot of an Eagle Owl. This involved large tortuous blood vessels with a rather scant fibrous stroma and it was not possible to conclude whether this was a congenital hamartomatous lesion or a reaction to some previous trauma.

BEHAVIOURAL DISTURBANCES AFFECTING THE SKIN

Psychotic Feather Plucking

This is not encountered as frequently in raptors as in other avian species, but the more excitable and

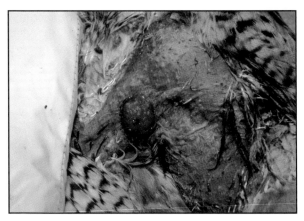

Figure 14.15: *Squamous cell carcinoma in the wing of a Lanner Falcon. (Photo courtesy N A Forbes)*

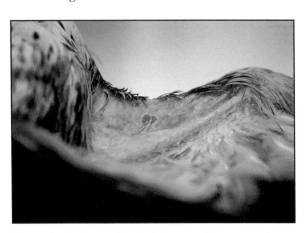

Figure 14.14: *Aspergillosis of the skin of the propatagium. (Photo courtesy N A Forbes)*

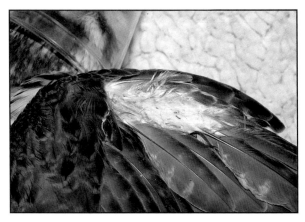

Figure 14.16: *Spindle cell tumour in the wing tip of a Northern Goshawk. (Photo courtesy N A Forbes)*

'intelligent' hawks, such as Harris' Hawks, especially those used for public display, are prone to this vice and often pluck at the underside of the breast and the medial aspects of the legs when bored. Darkness often acts as a deterrent, but Forbes (personal communication) has recorded at least one individual which continued to pluck even when hooded. The provision of toys, such as tennis balls, can control such vices.

Treatment

Recently, the use of behaviour-modifying drugs such as clomipramine, as used in psittacines (Ramsay and Grindlinger, 1992), has been attempted with equivocal results in the treatment of the neurogenic aspect of this condition. Secondary infections may develop in the intertrigial areas leading to feather loss and a yellow, waxy appearance of the skin without erythema. The skin is seldom thickened unless the condition is chronic and advanced. Microscopic examination of an exfoliative preparation from the affected area will invariably show the presence of budding yeasts (*Candida* spp.) which may be difficult to confirm on culture. Treatment involves the use of a topical antifungal agent, eg. dilute enilconazole. However, systemic antifungals, eg. itraconazole or ketoconazole, have not proved effective (Forbes, personal communication).

Failure to Preen

This might be attributable to other illnesses and conditions and investigative profiles and radiography should be instituted to elucidate the cause(s).

Acknowledgement

The authors are grateful for the help and encouragement of colleagues, particularly the scientific editors of this manual, whose personal communications have been incorporated into this chapter.

REFERENCES AND FURTHER READING

Angel S, Hyams M and Levinger IM (1982) Loosening of the feather follicle attachment by subcutaneous application of crude papain. *British Poultry Science* **23**, 251.

Cooper JE (1972) Feather conditions in birds of prey. *Journal of the North American Falconers' Association* **11**, 39.

Cooper JE (1985) Miscellaneous and emerging diseases. In: *Veterinary Aspects of Birds of Prey*. 2nd Edn. Ed JE Cooper. Standfast Press, Saul.

Forbes NA and Simpson GN (1993) Pathogenicity of ticks on aviary birds. *Veterinary Record* **133**, 532.

Ford E (1992) *Falconry Art and Practice*. Blandford, London.

Gothe R, Kunze K and Hoogstraal H (1979) The mechanisms of pathogenicity in the tick paralyses. *Journal of Medical Entomology* **16(5)**, 357.

Graham DL and Halliwell WH (1986) Viral diseases of birds of prey. In: *Zoo and Wildlife Medicine*. 2nd Edn. Ed ME Fowler. WB Saunders, Philadelphia.

Greve JH (1986) Parasitic diseases (of birds). In: *Zoo and Wildlife Medicine*. 2nd Edn. Ed ME Fowler. WB Saunders, Philadelphia.

Harcourt-Brown NH (1994) *Diseases of the Pelvic Limb of Birds of Prey*. FRCVS Thesis. Royal College of Veterinary Surgeons, London.

Keymer IF (1982) Parasitic diseases. In: *Diseases of Cage and Aviary Birds*. 2nd Edn. Ed M Petrak. Lea and Febiger, Philadelphia.

King AS and McLelland J (1984) *Birds: Their Structure and Function*. 2nd Edn. Baillière Tindall, London.

Kufour-Mensah E and Watson GL (1992) Malignant melanomas in a penguin (*Eudyptes chrysolphus*) and a Red-tailed Hawk (*Buteo jamaicensis*). *Veterinary Pathology* **29(4)**, 354.

Lowenstine LJ (1986) Nutritional disorders of birds. In: *Zoo and Wildlife Medicine*. 2nd Edn. Ed ME Fowler. WB Saunders, Philadelphia.

Lucas AM and Stettenheim PR (1972) *Avian Anatomy: Integument, Parts I and II. Agriculture Handbook 362*. US Department of Agriculture, Washington DC.

Mearns R (1983) Breeding peregrines oiled by fulmars. *Bird Study* **30**, 243.

Perry RA (1987) Avian dermatology. In *Companion Bird Medicine*. Ed EW Burr. Iowa State University Press, Ames.

Philips JR (1990) What's bugging your birds? Avian parasitic arthropods. *Wildlife Rehabilitation* **8**, 155.

Ramsay EC and Grindlinger HW (1992) Treatment of feather picking with clomipramine. In: *Proceedings of the Association of Avian Veterinarians Annual Conference 1992*. AAV, Lake Worth.

Richard JL (1991) Aspergillosis. In: *Diseases of Poultry*. 9th Edn. Ed BW Calnek. Iowa State University Press, Ames.

Samour JH and Cooper JE (1993) Avian pox in birds of prey (Order Falconiformes) in Bahrain. *Veterinary Record* **132**, 343.

Schulz TA, Stewart JS and Fowler ME (1989) *Knemidocoptes mutans acari* (Knemidocoptidae) in a Great Horned Owl (*Bubo virginianus*). *Journal of Wildlife Disease* **25(3)**, 430.

Smith SA and Smith BJ (1988) Lice in birds of prey. *Companion Animal Practice* **2(9)**, 35.

Spearman RIC and Hardy JA (1985) Integument. In: *Form and Function in Birds. Vol. 3*. Eds AS King and J McLelland. Academic Press, London.

Ward FP (1986) Parasites and their treatment in birds of prey. In: *Zoo and Wildlife Medicine*. 2nd Edn. Ed ME Fowler. WB Saunders, Philadelphia.

CHAPTER FIFTEEN

Diseases of the Head (including the Eyes)

Ian P Boydell and Neil A Forbes

INTRODUCTION

The head and its contents should be systematically examined as part of any physical examination of an avian patient. This generally requires restraint of the patient by an assistant so that both hands are available. The avian eye is a very important structure within the head and is particularly well developed in raptors. It is impossible to cover all aspects of ophthalmic disease within the limits of this manual, but the main points are described.

OCULAR ANATOMY

Raptors have a visual acuity 2-2.6 times as great as humans (Shlaer, 1972: Fox, 1976). The eyes are large and virtually fill the orbit, and are separated only by a thin bony, or even fibrous, septum in the midline. There is minimal movement of the globe within the orbit. The eye comprises a small anterior chamber with a larger posterior chamber, giving a characteristic shape which, when seen in cross-section, is globular in diurnal species and tubular in nocturnal species. The anterior part of the wall of the eye is supported by a bony skeleton made up of scleral ossicles which support the globe and provide some protection for intraocular tissues. The eyelids are thin, the lower one being the more mobile. The third eyelid is highly developed and under control of the abducens nerve. It sweeps from dorsomedial to ventrolateral (more ventral in owls). Lacrimation derives principally from the Harderian gland (situated on the 3rd eyelid).

Iris colour varies with species and age. Both smooth and striated muscle is present and the pupillary light reflex can be very fast. All optic nerve fibres cross at the optic chiasma, therefore there is no consensual light reflex, although there may be some illumination of the contralateral eye through the median wall of the globe. This reflex may be significantly affected by the voluntary muscle influence, in addition to the effects of stress causing mydriasis. The striated component complicates examination of the posterior segment as mydriasis cannot be achieved by the use of topical parasympatholytic agents (as in mammals). The topical application of the muscle relaxant vecuronium (4mg/ml solution - one drop topically three times at five minute intervals) allows safe mydriasis (Mikaelian *et al*,1994) and is preferred to other methods of intraocular drug administration for both examination and treatment. Wild and non-imprinted birds tend to be more nervous when handled and may not require pharmacological mydriasis. The avian lens is soft, facilitating rapid refractive change. It is supported by an annular pad which assists accommodation and nutrition.

The retina follows the typical vertebrate pattern, both nocturnal and diurnal birds possessing rods and cones. There is a higher concentration of cones in the fovea. These are single in owls, but Falconiformes have two foveae permitting high visual acuity for both binocular and monocular vision. The foveae act like a telephoto lens to further improve acuity (Snyder and Miller, 1978). The retina is avascular and derives its nutrition from choroidal vessels and the pecten (Williams, 1994), a pigmented sail-like structure situated on the optic disc and protruding into the vitreous (see Figure 15.1).

ASSESSMENT OF VISION

This is of particular importance in wild birds destined for rehabilitation, as a visual deficit may prevent a bird from finding and killing sufficient prey to sustain itself once released. Observation of normal behaviour is of prime significance both in the aviary and in flight,

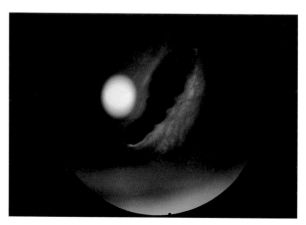

Figure 15.1: *Eye of a Tawny Owl with a normal pecten.*

and preferably during finding and killing prey using falconry techniques.

CONGENITAL LESIONS

Many conditions have been reported affecting the eyes and beak and these may be referred to in more complete texts. An increase in the number of raptors bred from a limited genetic pool, frequently utilising close inbreeding, may be responsible for an increased incidence of some of these conditions. The authors have noted an increased incidence of corneal abnormalities, cataract, micropthalmia, eyelid agenesis and retinal dysplasia.

CONDITIONS AFFECTING THE HEAD

The main conditions effecting the head of raptors are listed in Table 15.1.

TRAUMA

Trauma is the commonest reason for the presentation of a wild raptor to a veterinary or rescue centre. Many raptors are prone to collision which can be at high speed. Northern Goshawks, in particular, are renowned for their attempts to go through obstructions (rather than around them) while hunting. Porter (1990) estimated that about 80% of owls brought to a wildlife centre were the victims of road traffic accidents.

The head, in terms of volume, comprises predominantly the eyes; penetrating wounds some considerable distance from the eyelids may enter the anterior or posterior chambers. Penetrations caused by another raptor's claws characteristically have a small wound, sometimes with great depth. The bird should receive antibiosis and drainage should be encouraged. Captive raptors, in particular accipiters, eg. Northern Goshawks or Northern Sparrow Hawks, are easily startled

Table 15.1. Conditions affecting the head of raptors.

Site	Condition and cause	Diagnostic protocol	Action
General	Superficial soft tissue injury, self-trauma in flight, or attack by predator (bird, cat, fox, etc.).	Examination.	Wound management. Antibiosis. Skin graft.
Skeletal structures	Bone damage by penetrating wound or impact.	Radiography.	Conservative. External or internal fixation.
Hyoid apparatus of neonates.	Occasional problem in calcium deficient chicks 0-5 days of age. As the bird swallows, the ceratobranchial bones, instead of holding the tongue forward in a cranial direction, bend caudally so that the tongue is vertically or caudally aligned.	Clinical examination	If necessary, a single stay suture is applied to hold the tongue in an anterior direction. Bird is handfed with a calcium and vitamin D_3 supplement, eg. Nutrobal (Vetark), for three days, then the suture is removed.
Beak/cere (see Figures 15.6, 15.7 for normal falcon and hawk beak shape).	Cracks, typically on the upper beak. Overgrowth or trauma.	Examination.	Paring to remove crack (see later) or support of crack by tension wire and/or resin.
	Cere damage, trauma or parasitic (see Chapter 14 for illustration and further discussion).	Examination/skin scrape.	Husbandry change. Ivermectin for mites. If the proximal one third of the upper beak is damaged or lost, regrowth may not occur.
	Encrustation, eruptions, swellings of cere/eyelids caused by avipoxvirus, or other virus infections (see Figure 15.9).	Examination or histopathology.	Covering antibiosis, control of direct or fomite (insect) spread between birds. Not currently in UK. Vaccination may be useful.
Auditory canals.	Neoplasia or bacterial infections.	Examination.	Biopsy, antibiosis.

Table 15.1. Continued.

Site	Condition and cause	Diagnostic protocol	Action
Oral cavity (see Chapter 19)	White lesions in mouth/tongue.	Smear.	
	a) *Capillaria* spp.	Bi-operculate ascarid egg.	Fenbendazole (100mg/kg p/o once or 20mg/kg p/o daily for five days).
	b) *Candida* spp.	Budding yeast, readily visible on Diff Quik stained smears.	Nystatin 300,000 units (ie. 3ml)/kg p/o bid for seven days); ketoconazole (10mg/kg p/o bid for seven days); itraconazole (10mg/kg p/o bid for seven days).
	c) *Trichomonas* spp. (Samour *et al*, 1995) (see Figure 15.8).	Motile protozoa. Fresh wet prep or hanging drop.	Metronidazole (50mg/kg p/o daily for five days) or carnidazole (25mg/kg p/o once).
	d) Bacterial (see Figure 15.9).	Sensitivity test.	Antibiosis.
	e) Viral (see Figures 15.9, 15.10) (Gough *et al*, 1995).	Smear, virus isolation.	Covering antibiosis.
	Swelling of hard palate.	Examination.	See sinusitis below.
Rhinitis, sinusitis, conjunctivitis (see Chapter 18)	Bacterial, *Trichomonas* spp., mycoplasmal, fungal, foreign body. Swellings around eyes, below nares or in hard palate.	Aspirate, smear and wet prep. Culture from site of swelling or from discharge.	Rhinitis, sinusitis and conjunctivitis form a 'disease complex' and are commonly treated as one condition. Sinus flushing via nares is generally effective.
	Discharges from eyes, nares or choana. Chlamydiosis can occasionally cause severe conjunctivitis: this should always be eliminated as a possible cause.	ELISA or polymerase chain reaction (PCR) test.	Peri-ocular swellings benefit from local infusion with anti-inflammatory (steroid) + antibiotic (eg. enrofloxacin) cocktail.
Eye	Corneal wound (see Figures 15.2, 15.3).	Examination.	Surgical repair.
	Hyphema (traumatic - see Figure 15.4). Penetrating wounds or inflammatory disease may leave a residual iris bombé (see Figure 15.5).	Ophthalmoscopy.	Conservative. Mydriasis, flush anterior chamber.
	Cataract (see Figure 15.11).	Ophthalmoscopy.	Surgery.
	Retinopathy.	Ophthalmoscopy.	Usually none.

and, if kept in mesh topped aviaries, frequently damage their scalp. Small wounds heal spontaneously; larger wounds may require skin grafting. A bipedicle graft derived from the back of the neck is used: this allows the skin graft to be moved up whilst maintaining the correct feather orientation (see Figure 14.10). Simple apposition of wound edges may cause traction on the upper eyelids, with a consequent exposure keratitis. Appropriate husbandry changes should prevent recurrence (see Chapter 13). Although ocular disease is common in raptors presented to clinicians, many of these birds are already blind and the visual defect might have been responsible for the incident which permitted capture of the bird. Many birds will be presented with severe chronic changes. Some of these may be treated medically (as in other species) but in some, enucleation will be indicated. The relative size of the globe necessitates an extensive lateral canthotomy, often as far as the internal aspect of the auditory canal. Access for enucleation is also improved by removing the portion of the prefrontal bone directly beneath the upper eyelid. Removal of the prefrontal bone also allows easy wound closure without tension on this point. The globe should be removed intact (in particular, if histopathology is required or infection is feared); however, if necessary it may be removed piecemeal. Care should be taken to avoid excessive traction to the optic nerve (which is shorter in comparison with mammals) as this can damage the opposite optic nerve and lead to temporary or permanent total blindness. The technique for enucleation is fully described by Murphy *et al* (1983).

Ocular wounds, eg. corneal scratches (see Figure 15.2) and penetrations (see Figure 15.3), are common, with hyphema (see Figure 15.4), anterior synechia and iris bombé (see Figure 15.5) being frequent sequelae to trauma of the anterior chamber.

Secondary uveitis may be a blinding sequela and should be treated aggressively with anti-inflamatory (Ocufen), antibiotic (tobramycin) and mydriatic (atropine drops) agents. Flushing of organised haematoma from the anterior chamber may reduce the extent of the membranes and adhesions which are likely to persist on recovery. Corneal and scleral wounds should

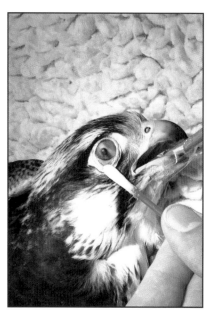

Figure 15.3: Male Lanner Falcon with a healed corneal wound following corneal rupture and iris prolapse.

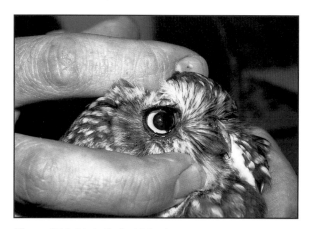

Figure 15.4: Little Owl with hyphema.

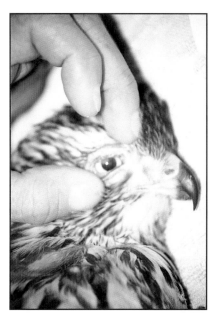

Figure 15.2: Juvenile male Northern Goshawk with a flourescein stained corneal scratch.

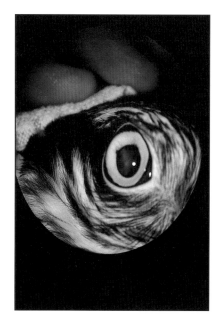

Figure 15.5: Northern Sparrow Hawk with iris bombé.

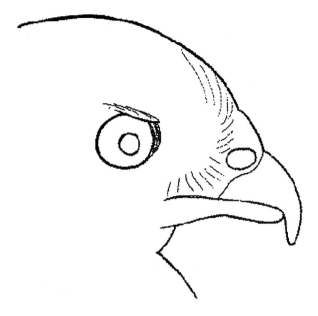

Figure 15.6: Short wing/broad wing (hawk) beak.

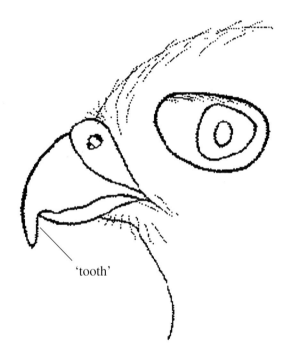

Figure 15.7: Long wing (falcon) beak.

be repaired using the appropriate microsurgical technique. If there is any disruption of the lens capsule, such as may be caused by trauma or mature cataract, severe uveitis may develop and removal of the lens may be necessary at an early stage of treatment.

Most retinal pathology is also considered to be due to trauma. Haemorrhage in the vitreous is generally associated with severe damage to the wall of the globe or to the pecten. Some retinal degenerative lesions are thought to result from blunt trauma to the head causing a contrecoup injury.

BEAK AND CERE

Experienced falconers will pare ('cope') their birds' beaks when they become overlong. However, some novice falconers may seek veterinary assistance. Coping' is carried out using clippers on the point, a round file inside the curve of the upper beak and a flat file elsewhere. Short wings and broad wings (hawks and buzzards) have an entirely different beak shape to that of long wings (falcons) (see Figures 15.6, 15.7). The normal 'tooth' behind the tip of the upper beak of long wings should be noted (see Figure 15.7). If cracks appear in the beak, these should be filed back above the start of the crack. If the upper beak is damaged or lost, repeated filing of the lower beak is required to prevent overgrowth.

Loss of the upper beak or damage to the proximal one third will typically cause damage to the germinal epithelium and underlying bone (*rostrum maxillare*). Damage to the bone can preclude normal regrowth. Prostheses can be applied, but they will eventually work loose. Coepack (Coe Laboratories, Chicago) has been used with success; when applied as a prothesis it prevents dehiscence of the germinal epithelium. The beak may eventually regrow after 3-4 months. Failure of a beak to regrow will necessitate an unnatural diet of soft food, or euthanasia. Beak deformities may be congenital or consequent to calcium deficient diets. Deformities can often be repaired using dental acrylics, together with K-wires and tension bands. Fractures of the mandible are not uncommon and respond well to intramedullary fixation techniques.

MOUTH

Oral lesions are a common cause of presentation of raptors. Typically, the bird has a poor appetite and may demonstrate head or food flicking. The main causes and appropriate treatments are listed in Table 15.1. The common mouth lesions appear white (see Figure 15.8), although primary viral infections with concurrent bacterial infection may present with encrustation (see Figure 15.9) or erythema (see Figure 15.10). Diagnosis should not be made on clinical signs alone. The causative agent must be demonstrated on wet prep and/or stained smears collected from the lesions. Viral stomatitis is most commonly caused by herpesvirus (Gough *et al*, 1995) or avipoxvirus (see Chapter 14).

RHINITIS/SINUSITIS/ CONJUNCTIVITIS

The three anatomical regions of the nasal cavity, sinuses and conjunctivae are intimately related; commonly, pathology of one affects all three. These conditions should be considered as a single syndrome and treated accordingly. Aspirates, smears and culture and sensitivity testing should be carried out. Systemic

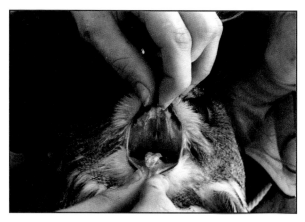

Figure 15.8: Indian Eagle Owl with trichomoniasis. (Compare with Figure 23.11.)

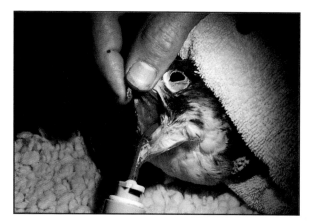

Figure 15.10: Male Peregrine Falcon with erythematous viral stomatitis.

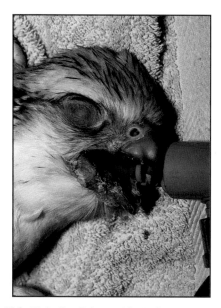

Figure 15.9: Male Gyr Falcon with viral stomatitis and secondary bacterial infection.

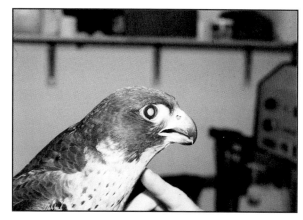

Figure 15.11: Peregrine Falcon with mature cataract.

doxycycline (50mg/kg p/o bid for 45 days), although total elimination of the organism from a collection is unrealistic. Post-treatment serological monitoring of the collection is recommended (Forbes, 1995).

CRANIAL NEMATODES

Nematodes, eg. *Cyathostoma* spp., may be found within the orbit of the eye or in any periocular or sinus region. Infection occurs after larvae are coughed up from the trachea. Clinical signs will vary dependent on the exact site of the worm (Simpson and Harris, 1992).

CATARACT

Lens opacity is a common finding (see Figure 15.11). The condition may be congenital, inherited, senile (metabolic) or a sequela to trauma or uveitis. Small incision surgery using phacoemulsification and aspiration reduces the surgical trauma to the eye; the lens is soft, thus lending itself to such aspiration techniques.

Aphakic birds can be kept in aviaries and used in breeding projects (unless the cataract is thought to be inherited) and they have been used in flying displays, but are not considered suitable for release to the wild.

antibiosis may be required, but the crucial therapeutic technique is nasal flushing with saline and antibiosis (for a 1kg bird use 20ml saline + 1ml antibiotic) (see Chapter 18 for further details). *Chlamydia psittaci* is an uncommon but significant pathogen (in view of zoonosis and infectivity). If doubt exists, birds should be screened for chlamydiosis.

Apart from chronic, intractable or repeated bouts of unilateral or bilateral sinusitis or conjunctivitis, chlamydiosis in raptors will present with some or all of the following signs: markedly green stained urates, air sacculitis, hepatomegaly and/or splenomegaly, exercise intolerance, inappetence or weight loss. Chlamydiosis is common in wild and captive raptors, but it is rarely a clinical problem. Clinical cases typically follow episodes of significant stress or concomitant disease. Diagnosis is made on PCR tests, ELISA carried out on air sac or splenic swabs, or on histopathology. Treatment of an infected and clinically infected collection of birds has been effective using

POSTERIOR CHAMBER OF THE EYE

Retinal lesions may be found in birds with visual defects and as incidental findings where there is no evidence of visual dysfunction. There are many reports of chorioretinitis, particularly in captive owls. The aetiology generally remains uncertain, although toxoplasmosis, nutritional deficiencies, photic damage and blunt trauma have been suggested (Greenwood and Barnett, 1980; Buyukmihci, 1985; Murphy,1987).

NEURO-OPHTHALMOLOGY

The large globe has only limited scope for movement within the orbit. Nystagmus may therefore be evident as movement of the eye or the entire head, and may be associated with trauma, toxic damage to the vestibular apparatus, or abscessation of the infraorbital sinus. Central blindness may be a sequela of trauma and can be diagnosed by the exclusion of the other causes of visual deficit, accompanied by a complete neurological examination and possibly CNS imaging.

CARE OF THE OPHTHALMIC PATIENT

Blind birds are likely to require assistance with feeding and it may be necessary to place food in the claws or mouth. These patients may be more easily startled and the handler should ensure that the bird is aware of his/her approach prior to making physical contact. If the bird is to be kept in an aviary, the nurse must check that the bird can locate a suitable perch in order to reduce the risk of foot or feather damage caused by remaining on the ground.

There appears little risk of self-trauma following ocular surgical procedures: Elizabethan collars are not generally required.

Acknowledgement
The authors are grateful to the Cage and Aviary Research Fund for financial assistance in carrying out extensive examinations nationwide of raptor eyes.

REFERENCES

Buyukmihci INC (1985) Lesions in the ocular posterior segment of raptors. *Journal of the American Veterinary Medical Association* **187**, 1121.

Forbes NA (1995) Epidemic and endemic chlamydiosis in a collection of raptors. In: *Proceedings of the Middle East Falcon Research Group Conference 1995*. National Avian Research Centre, Abu Dhabi.

Fox R, Lehmkuhle SW and Westendorf DH (1976) Falcon visual acuity. *Science* **192**, 263.

Gough RE, Dury SEN, Higgins RJ and Harcourt-Brown NH (1995) Isolation of a herpesvirus from a snowy owl (*Nyctea scandiaca*). *Veterinary Record* **136**, 541.

Greenwood AG and Barnett KC (1980) The investigation of visual defects in raptors. In: *Recent Advances in the Study of Raptor Diseases*. Eds JE Cooper and AG Greenwood. Chiron Publications, Keighley.

Mikaelian I, Paillet I and Williams DL (1994) Comparative uses of various mydriatic drugs in kestrels (*Falco tinnunculus*). *American Journal of Veterinary Research* **52**, 270.

Miller WW, Boosinger TR and Maslin WR (1988) Granulomatous uveitis in an owl. *Journal of the American Veterinary Medical Association* **193**, 365.

Murphy CJ, Kern TJ, McKeever K, McKeever L and MacCoy D (1982) Ocular lesions in free-living raptors. *Journal of the American Veterinary Medical Association* **181**, 1302.

Murphy CJ, Brooks DE, Kern TJ, Quesenberry KE and Riis RC (1983) Enucleation in birds of prey. *Journal of the American Veterinary Medical Association* **183**, 1234.

Murphy CJ (1987) Raptor ophthalmology. *Compendium on Continuing Education for the Practicing Veterinarian* **9**, 241.

Porter SL (1990) Vehicular trauma in owls. In: *Proceedings of the Association of Avian Veterinarians Annual Conference 1990*. AAV, Lake Worth.

Samour JH, Bailey TA and Cooper JE (1995) Trichomoniasis in birds of prey (Order Falconiformes) in Bahrain. *Veterinary Record* **136**, 14.

Shlaer R (1972) An eagle's eye: quality of the retinal image. *Science* **176**, 920.

Simpson VR and Harris EA (1992) *Cyathostoma lavi* (nematode) infection in birds of prey. *Journal of Zoology London* **227**, 655.

Snyder AW and Miller WH (1978) Telephoto lens system of falconiform eyes. *Nature* **275**, 127.

Williams D (1994) Ophthalmology. In: *Avian Medicine: Principles and Application*. Eds BW Ritchie, GJ Harrison and LR Harrison. Wingers, Lake Worth.

CHAPTER SIXTEEN

Foot and Leg Problems

Nigel H Harcourt-Brown

INTRODUCTION

In the United Kingdom the majority of raptors are used for falconry. The main purpose of falconry is to fly a raptor at quarry. Falconry pushes the raptor's body to the limit, and occasionally beyond, in a similar manner to the modern day athlete. Many raptors seen by veterinary practices are suffering from 'sports' injuries caused either by hunting accidents or by excessive activity whilst the birds are restrained by their jesses. The major share of these hunting injuries is seen in the legs and feet of hunting birds; wing injuries are seen less frequently in these birds. In veterinary practice the vast majority of captive raptors seen are presented with injuries or diseases of the pelvic limb.

ANATOMY

The pelvic limb can be considered to start caudal to the last movable thoracic vertebra. Articulating with this vertebra is the synsacrum, which is formed from the fusion of a series of vertebrae homologous to the thoracic, lumbar, sacral and caudal vertebrae of mammals. The pelvis is attached to the synsacrum and together they form a single unit. The acetabulum is not a solid cup, the acetabular foramen being closed by the acetabular membrane. The head of the femur articulates with the acetabulum. The trochanter of the femur articulates with the antitrochanter of the pelvis, and when the leg is in its normal position the femur is prevented from abduction.

The tibiotarsus is formed from a fusion between the tibia and the proximal row of tarsal bones. The tendon of the long digital extensor muscle runs through a bony canal at the distal end of the tibiotarsus. In owls there are long, narrow ossifications within the muscles in the tibial region. The fibula is attached by a tight fibrous union to the tibiotarsus at the fibular crest and is also fused to the distal third of the tibiotarsus. The femoral condyles are attached by ligaments to, and articulate with, the tibiotarsus and the head of the fibula. Various ligaments permit movement between the tibiotarsus and the fibula and allow a good degree of rotation of the femorotibial joint around its long

axis. The femorotibial joint is otherwise similar to that of mammals as it contains two menisci, two cruciate ligaments and a lateral and medial collateral ligament. There are other additional ligaments.

The second, third and fourth metatarsal bones fuse at an early age and also combine with the distal row of tarsal bones to form the tarsometatarsus. The first metatarsal bone is separate and joined by ligaments to the tarsometatarsus. The joint between the tarsometatarsus and the tibiotarsus is known as the intertarsal joint.

The intertarsal joint is similar to the femorotibial joint but has a single meniscus and single 'cruciate' ligament. There is little longitudinal rotation at this joint. The main flexor tendons of the digits arise from the tibiotarsal region and run over the caudal aspect of the intertarsal joint through the tibial cartilage and also in a hypotarsal groove. The flexor tendons run the full length of the caudal aspect of the tarsometatarsus. In Falconidae only, there is a long intratendinous ossification in each of the tendons of *mm. flexor digitorum longus* and *flexor hallucis longus*, and these tendons are partially joined by fibrous tissue. All the flexor tendons pass through the plantar flexor canal at the distal tarsometatarsus, where they branch to each digit. At this point the second digit is supplied by fused branches from the tendons of *mm. flexor digitorum longus* and *flexor hallucis longus* as well as tendons from *mm. flexor perforans et perforatus digiti II* and *flexor perforatus digiti II*; in Falconidae only, these tendons pass within cartilage attached to a sesamoid bone ventral to the metatarsophalangeal joint. Accipitridae have neither ossified tendons nor a sesamoid ventral to digit II.

Lateral and medial views of the muscles etc. of a Harris' Hawk are shown in Figures 16.1 and 16.2.

All the Falconiformes, except the Osprey, are anisodactyl, ie. they have their digits arranged with the first digit facing caudally and the second, third and fourth digits facing cranially. Ospreys and all owls have semizygodactyl feet, with the ability either to position the fourth digit cranially alongside the second and third digits or caudally next to the first digit. The plantar aspect of the foot of a Peregrine Falcon is shown in Figure 16.3.

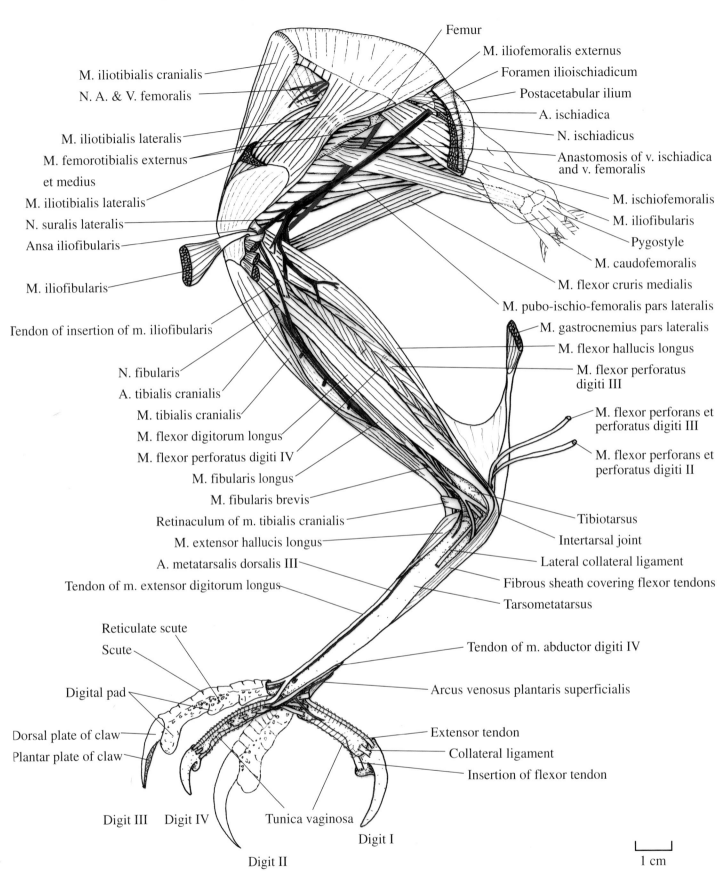

Femur

M. iliotibialis cranialis

N. A. & V. femoralis

M. iliofemoralis externus

Foramen ilioischiadicum

Postacetabular ilium

A. ischiadica

N. ischiadicus

Anastomosis of v. ischiadica and v. femoralis

M. iliotibialis lateralis

M. femorotibialis externus et medius

M. iliotibialis lateralis

N. suralis lateralis

Ansa iliofibularis

M. ischiofemoralis

M. iliofibularis

Pygostyle

M. caudofemoralis

M. flexor cruris medialis

M. pubo-ischio-femoralis pars lateralis

M. iliofibularis

Tendon of insertion of m. iliofibularis

M. gastrocnemius pars lateralis

M. flexor hallucis longus

M. flexor perforatus digiti III

N. fibularis

A. tibialis cranialis

M. tibialis cranialis

M. flexor digitorum longus

M. flexor perforatus digiti IV

M. fibularis longus

M. fibularis brevis

Retinaculum of m. tibialis cranialis

M. extensor hallucis longus

A. metatarsalis dorsalis III

Tendon of m. extensor digitorum longus

M. flexor perforans et perforatus digiti III

M. flexor perforans et perforatus digiti II

Tibiotarsus

Intertarsal joint

Lateral collateral ligament

Fibrous sheath covering flexor tendons

Tarsometatarsus

Reticulate scute

Scute

Digital pad

Dorsal plate of claw

Plantar plate of claw

Tendon of m. abductor digiti IV

Arcus venosus plantaris superficialis

Extensor tendon

Collateral ligament

Insertion of flexor tendon

Digit III   Digit IV

Tunica vaginosa

Digit I

Digit II

1 cm

Figure 16.1: *Lateral view of the pelvic limb of a Harris' Hawk with the integument removed. The body of m. iliofibularis and a portion of m. iliotibialis have been removed; the body of m. tibialis cranialis has been freed and reflected. The bodies of mm. gastrocnemius pars lateralis, flexor perforans et perforatus digiti III and flexor perforans et perforatus digiti IV have also been removed and their tendons of insertion have been reflected. The integument remains on digits II and III. Arteries are red, veins are blue and nerves are green.*

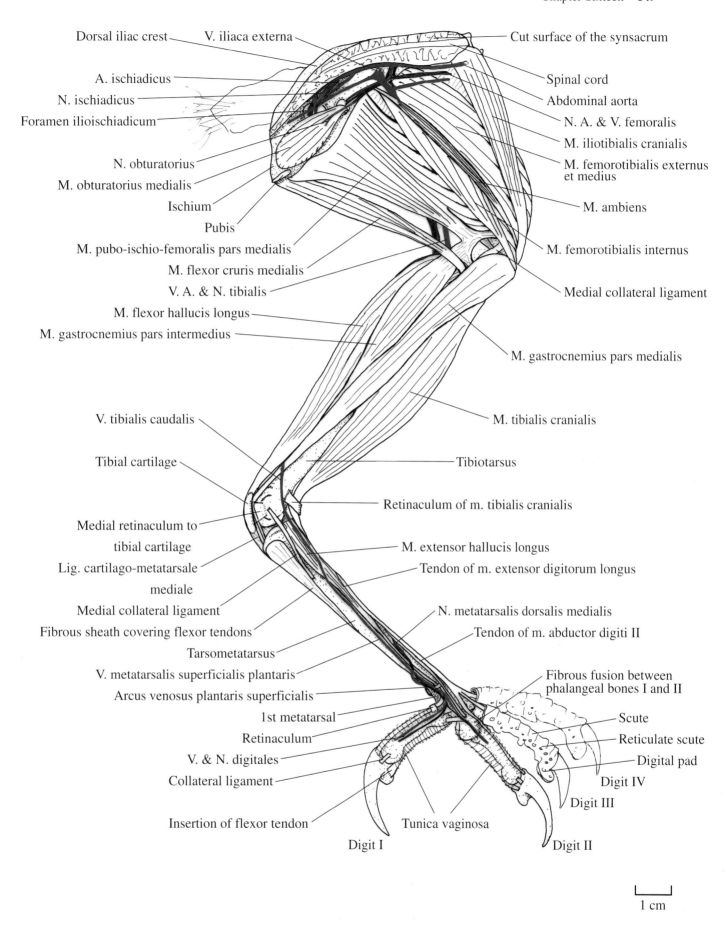

Dorsal iliac crest

V. iliaca externa

Cut surface of the synsacrum

A. ischiadicus

N. ischiadicus

Foramen ilioischiadicum

Spinal cord

Abdominal aorta

N. A. & V. femoralis

M. iliotibialis cranialis

M. femorotibialis externus et medius

N. obturatorius

M. obturatorius medialis

Ischium

Pubis

M. ambiens

M. pubo-ischio-femoralis pars medialis

M. flexor cruris medialis

V. A. & N. tibialis

M. femorotibialis internus

Medial collateral ligament

M. flexor hallucis longus

M. gastrocnemius pars intermedius

M. gastrocnemius pars medialis

M. tibialis cranialis

V. tibialis caudalis

Tibial cartilage

Tibiotarsus

Retinaculum of m. tibialis cranialis

Medial retinaculum to tibial cartilage

Lig. cartilago-metatarsale mediale

Medial collateral ligament

Fibrous sheath covering flexor tendons

Tarsometatarsus

V. metatarsalis superficialis plantaris

Arcus venosus plantaris superficialis

1st metatarsal

Retinaculum

V. & N. digitales

Collateral ligament

Insertion of flexor tendon

Digit I

M. extensor hallucis longus

Tendon of m. extensor digitorum longus

N. metatarsalis dorsalis medialis

Tendon of m. abductor digiti II

Fibrous fusion between phalangeal bones I and II

Scute

Reticulate scute

Digital pad

Digit IV

Digit III

Tunica vaginosa

Digit II

1 cm

Figure 16.2: *Medial view of the pelvic limb of a Harris' Hawk with the integument removed except for digits III and IV. The synsacrum has been sectioned longitudinally along its midline to allow the leg to be shown.*

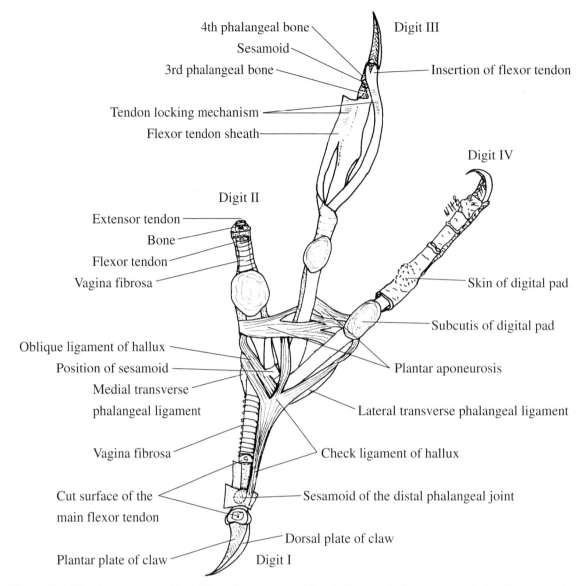

4th phalangeal bone

Sesamoid

3rd phalangeal bone

Digit III

Insertion of flexor tendon

Tendon locking mechanism

Flexor tendon sheath

Digit IV

Digit II

Extensor tendon

Bone

Flexor tendon

Vagina fibrosa

Skin of digital pad

Subcutis of digital pad

Oblique ligament of hallux

Position of sesamoid

Medial transverse
phalangeal ligament

Plantar aponeurosis

Lateral transverse phalangeal ligament

Vagina fibrosa

Check ligament of hallux

Sesamoid of the distal phalangeal joint

Cut surface of the
main flexor tendon

Dorsal plate of claw

Plantar plate of claw

Digit I

Figure 16.3: The plantar aspect of the left foot of a Peregrine Falcon is illustrated after the removal of the integument (except from digit IV) and some subcutaneous fat and the fibrous tissue that forms the metatarsal and digital pads (Harcourt-Brown, 1994). The digital pads are attached to the tendon sheath by fibrous tissue; they allow the bird to have a firm and cushioned grip on its perch or its prey. Roughened areas on the plantar surface of the main flexor tendons and transverse folds on the tendon sheath opposite form the tendon locking mechanism (see digit III). The locking mechanism engages when the toes are flexed and the tendons are held under tension.

In many Falconiformes the pelvic limb is covered with feathered skin to the intertarsal joint; some genera, such as the eagles (*Aquila*), are feathered to their foot. From the intertarsal joint the skin is thickened and is covered by scales (scutes). Each digit ends in a claw, consisting of a phalangeal bone covered with a layer of germinal epithelium which gives rise to a keratinised and calcified downward curved dorsal plate and a softer plantar plate.

The anatomy of the pelvic limb of the Northern Goshawk and the Peregrine Falcon has been described by Harcourt-Brown (1994).

PRINCIPLES OF FRACTURE REPAIR

The bones of the thoracic and pelvic limbs of raptors are very strong and very lightweight. The cortex is thin and brittle and relies on its intact form, as well as internal struts of bone, to give it strength. In the pelvic limb the medullary cavity of the femur is pneumatised by a connection with the abdominal air sac; all the other long bones contain fat or bone marrow in their medullary cavity.

Raptors are frequently presented with fractured bones. The fractures may be simple, greenstick, comminuted or compound; they are usually caused by trauma but may be caused by infection, neoplasia or metabolic disease. Therefore, all fractures must be assessed radiographically as well as by clinical examination.

The aims of fracture repair are to aid healing by promoting the formation of an intact, strong bone, with no involvement with the surrounding structures: muscles, joints, tendons, ligaments, etc. These aims are complicated by a number of factors:

● The rate of healing of avian bone is very rapid, and in wild birds a significant amount of scar tissue and bony callus can form in 7-10 days; possibly before the injured wild bird is presented for treatment.

● Many fractures are comminuted and the bone has broken into a large number of splinters which may be difficult or impossible to reconstruct.

● Greenstick fractures are frequently seen at the distal femur, proximal tibiotarsal, mid to distal tibiotarsus and mid-tarsometatarsus; however, they are often multiple and involve other areas of the body as well. This can cause major complications.

● External immobilisation of the limb above and below the fracture site may immobilise one or two joints. In many cases this would allow scar tissue to form around the joint and permanently reduce the ability of the joint to function. Immobilisation of joints must therefore be avoided if at all possible.

● A large number of fractures are compound, especially in injured wild birds. The protruding bone is usually desiccated and dead. The exposed medullary cavity is a portal of entry for bacteria and, occasionally, fungi or foreign bodies. The bone which is dead or going to die must be removed. The medullary cavity must be picked clean if possible: lavage tends to wash material deeper into the cavity where it is trapped by the internal struts. Lavage is also contraindicated in the pneumatised femur. Dead tissue surrounding the fracture site should also be debrided.

● Purulent material in birds is solid and does not flow; the provision of drainage in these cases is ineffective. Compound fractures that are repaired should be radiographed weekly and purulent material should be removed surgically when it forms.

A raptor that is presented with a fracture of the limb should have the limbs examined grossly. The number and position of the fractures, as well as other injuries, should be ascertained. The whole bird should be fully examined for signs of intercurrent disease. This is especially important in injured wild birds. All injured wild birds have failed the 'fitness test'; they should be assumed to be ill and treated appropriately. Prophylactic treatment is indicated even if the bird appears healthy (see Chapters 2 and 3). When the bird's general condition has been stabilised, it should be anaesthetised, examined physically to assess the extent of the injury and radiographed. If a bird is not to be operated on immediately, it should be restrained by being placed in a small, dark confined space: a cardboard box is usually ideal. Supporting the fractured limb is often impossible and allowing the bird to stand quietly on the uninjured limb is usually the safest course. Splinting the limb is usually counterproductive. It is often sensible to wait 1-3 days before surgery,

especially in wild birds, to allow the bird's general condition to be stabilised.

METHODS OF FRACTURE REPAIR

Splint

This is usually the most inappropriate method of repair; few fractures benefit from the application of a splint. Mid to distal tarsometatarsal fractures are repairable using an L-shaped finger splint (see Figure 16.4). A ball bandage is a useful splint for fractured phalangeal bones if required (see Figure 16.5).

Intramedullary Pin

Intramedullary pinning using trochar pointed 0.8-

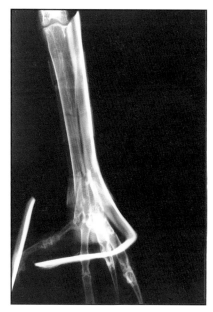

Figure 16.4: *A fracture of the distal tarsometatarsus of a Red-tailed Hawk has been immobilised with a piece of finger splint, the proximal half bent into a gutter and the distal half made into an L-shape to conform to the contour of the bone. It is held in place for 3-4 weeks with zinc oxide tape.*

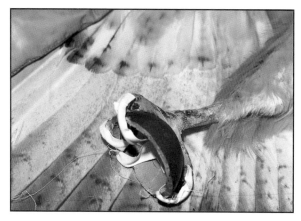

Figure 16.5: *Taping the foot to half a ball and covering with a bandage forms a flexible splint for the toes. A cotton-wool ball may be used instead, but it can become very heavy when waterlogged.*

1.2mm Steinmann pins is a reliable method of repair for many fractures. For this method to be satisfactory the pin must stabilise the bone, therefore stack pinning, which reduces the likelihood of longitudinal rotation, may be necessary. The majority of avian long bones have a large medullary cavity and subtle bends in their length: a single pin will not fill the medullary cavity. A hemicerclage wire technique using 22G orthopaedic cerclage wire can be used to overcome the problem of a small diameter pin in a large medullary cavity in large birds (see Figures 16.6.1, 16.6.2). Pins and a compression wire can be used to repair fractures of extremities of long bones. It is possible to drill holes in the avian cortex using a 21G or 23G 3\4" hypodermic needle on a 2ml syringe, but a 1·1mm drill bit and compressed-air powered orthopaedic drill or a dental drill with a small drill bit is more satisfactory. Hand-cranked drills are usually unsatisfactory and are likely to fracture the fragment being drilled. Cross pinning may also be used to replace the condyles in distal femoral or tibiotarsal fractures (see Figures 16.7.1, 16.7.2).

Very small birds may have long bones pinned with 'old-fashioned' reusable hypodermic needles or the stylets from spinal needles. If possible, all pins should be removed after bony union.

Full-Pin or Half-Pin Fixation

These methods are very useful in a number of potentially difficult fracture repairs: when there is a small piece of bone with little shaft; when there is infection; or where the bone is so comminuted that repair by pins and wire is impossible. Steinmann pins (0.8-1.2mm) are ideal but must penetrate both cortices, whether being used in full-pin or half-pin techniques. The pins are joined by bolting to a cross member or by fixing through silicon or PVC tubing which is filled with methylmethacrylate (Technovit). In small birds and straight bones a 1ml syringe barrel can be used; the pins are drilled through the syringe barrel and held in place with zinc oxide tape, so no methylmethacrylate is needed. There are a number of drawbacks to full-pin and half-pin fixation: it is difficult to align the bone fragments correctly; the bird is encumbered with the external fixation; methylmethacrylate takes a relatively long time to harden and can become hot enough while curing to cause burns; it is possible to injure nerves etc. or entrap tendons with the placement of the pins; and it is possible to cause another fracture by pinning a small bone. However, these techniques often allow the limb to become fully weight-bearing with no joint immobilisation almost immediately postoperatively.

Intramedullary Non-Absorbable Shuttle Pin

Shuttle pinning a simple fracture of a long bone is a useful technique (Coles, 1984). The plastic plunger of a 1ml or 2ml syringe is used to fill the medullary cavity.

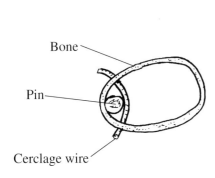

Bone

Pin

Cerclage wire

Figure 16.6.1: *Cross section showing a large medullary cavity with a relatively small intramedullary pin placed down the inner face and trapped against the cortex with a hemicerclage wire.*

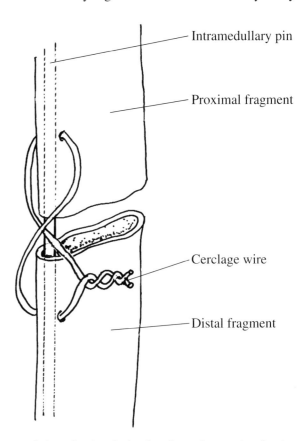

Intramedullary pin

Proximal fragment

Cerclage wire

Distal fragment

Figure 16.6.2: *View of the same technique showing the hemicerclage wire trapping the pin as well as preventing rotation and compressing the fracture when it is finally tightened.*

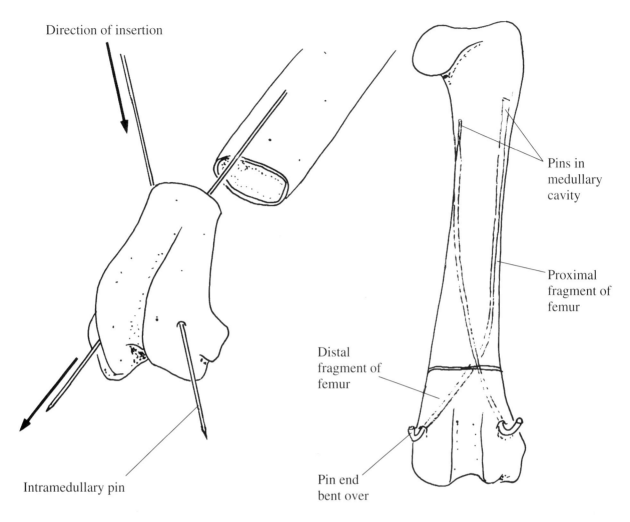

Figure 16.7.1: For fixing fractures involving the condyles of small bones, the pins are introduced into the medullary cavity of the distal fragment to form a cross. The pin ends should be left flush with the fractured bone.

Figure 16.7.2: Reduction of the fracture is then followed by the pins being pushed cranially to occupy the medullary cavity of the proximal fragment. The pins hold the bone as they are bent and in tension.

It is anchored against rotation of the fracture or movement of the prosthesis by two small cross pins. It forms an instantly strong repair and does not need to be removed (see Figures 16.8.1, 16.8.2, 16.8.3). The bird should be confined for 2-3 weeks postoperatively to allow callus to form. This technique must not be used if the bone is infected: removal of the prosthesis is extremely difficult.

Other Methods of Fracture Repair

Intramedullary absorbable pins, bone plates and screws, bone cement and even homologous bone grafts have all been used to repair fractures with varying degrees of success. All these techniques are extremely complicated.

FRACTURES

Pelvis and Synsacrum

This single unit may occasionally be fractured in road accidents and other collisions. Fractures which involve the synsacrum may give irreversible spinal cord damage. Fractures of the pelvis are supported by sufficient muscle mass to heal with no external support if the bird is kept restricted. When pelvic fractures are associated with obvious neurological damage, surgical exploration is necessary and the nerve involved freed from the fracture site.

Femur

The femoral head is usually always fractured when the hip is dislocated (see later). The femur should be approached from the lateral aspect (see Figure 16.1), dissecting between the iliofibularis muscle and the femorotibialis muscle (which is attached to the body of the femur). Care should be taken to avoid the major arteries, nerves and vein found beneath the iliofibularis muscle caudolateral to the femur. Proximal femoral fractures can be repaired with a tension band technique using one or several pins (see Figure 16.9). Mid-shaft femoral fractures can be repaired using one of several

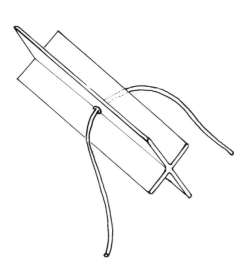

Figure 16.8.1: The shuttle is made from a syringe plunger, a hole is drilled and a piece of nylon is threaded through. Sterility should be preserved.

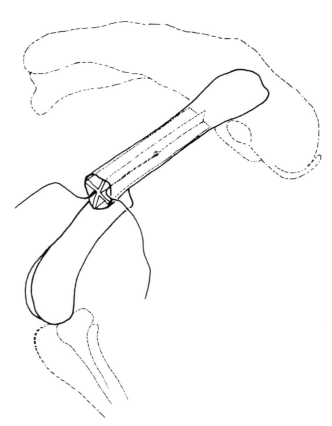

Figure 16.8.2: The shuttle is pushed into the medullary cavity of one fragment. The two ends of the nylon are kept outside the cavity.

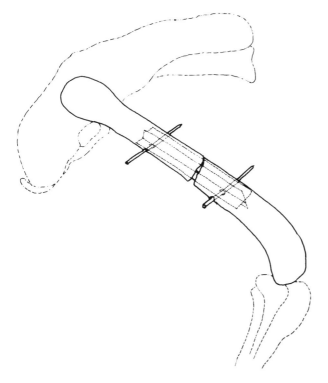

Figure 16.8.3: The fracture is reduced and the two ends of nylon are pulled taut, forcing the shuttle to ride into the distal fragment's medullary cavity. The nylon is then pulled out. The bone may be anchored against rotation by two small pins.

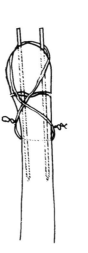
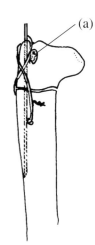

(a)

Figure 16.9: Tension band wiring using two Steinmann pins and orthopaedic wire. Good compression may be achieved. In this repair the trochanteric fossa (a), which allows pneumatisation of the femur, could be closed by callus or prosthesis. This is unlikely to affect the bird.

techniques: pinning with a single pin if the bird is small, eg. a Common Kestrel, or stack pinning with occasionally a cerclage wire in larger birds such as a Harris' Hawk. Shuttle pinning or half-pin fixation are also possible techniques for repairing femoral fractures. The shaft of the femur has a slight craniocaudal curve, which is often lost when pinned; this is of no consequence. Fractures in the condylar region require cross pins, running from the epicondyles and bending up the inner edge of the cortex (see Figure 16.7), or half-pin fixation. Prostheses should be removed from this pneumatised bone; a shuttle pin cannot be removed and long-term complications could occur if it became infected.

Tibiotarsus (and Fibula)

This is the bone most frequently fractured in raptors. The medullary cavity tapers to the distal end. The bone should be approached through a craniomedial incision, between the cranial tibial muscle and the medial gastrocnemius muscle (see Figure 16.2); this approach avoids nerves, arteries and veins. The lateral approach should not be used. It should be noted that two arteries run between the fibula and tibiotarsus, one proximal and one distal to the fibular crest.

The commonest fracture in raptors is seen in newly jessed hawks; the birds are apt to bate violently, pulling and twisting their leg at the same time, and thereby causing the fracture. Falcons are unlikely to do this as they have a calmer temperament and are often hooded when first jessed (see Chapter 13). The tibiotarsus is always fractured within 5mm of the distal end of the fibular crest. The site corresponds to a change in the cross-section of the bone from the almost triangular section formed by the reinforcement of the fibular crest to the round section of the tibiotarsus. Stack pinning using a craniomedial approach and an external splint is a simple method of repair. The initial pin placement is along the cranial surface of the medullary cavity of the proximal fragment; in this manner two pins may be placed without affecting the femorotibial joint. A splint should applied for 10 days to prevent rotation of the fracture around the pins (see Figures 16.10.1, 16.10.2). Half-pin or full-pin fixation in this area may involve the nerves and arteries on the lateral aspect of the tibiotarsus. It is a valuable technique if both legs are broken or if there is a comminuted fracture, as it will allow a rapid return to full function, usually within a day or two. Muscle wastage is common after this technique, but this will resolve providing there is no permanent nerve damage.

Proximal tibiotarsal fractures may be pinned and wired; caudal displacement of the distal fragment can cut the fibular nerve where it passes through the *ansa iliofibularis* (see Figure 16.1), causing motor and sensory deficits.

The repair of fractures of the distal tibiotarsus are complicated by two tendons. The tendon of insertion

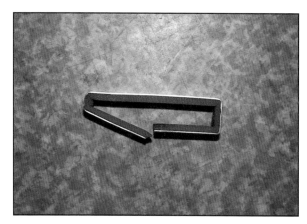

Figure 16.10.1: A splint for preventing the rotation of tibiotarsal fractures around a single pin is made from padded finger splint.

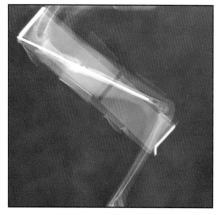

Figure 16.10.2: This radiograph shows the splint taped in place after fracture repair of the tibiotarsus of a Harris' Hawk with a single pin. A cotton wool ball should be placed cranial to the intertarsal joint and caudal to the femorotibial joint, under the tape.

of the cranial tibial muscle runs over the cranial surface of the intertarsal joint through a fibrous retinaculum. The tendon of insertion of the long digital extensor muscle runs under the bony supratendinal bridge, on the cranial aspect of the bone deep to the cranial tibial muscle (see Figure 16.11). Great care should be taken to avoid compromising the free running of these tendons. Any involvement of these tendons in bony callus or fibrous scar will stop the intertarsal joint extending and flexing fully. Care must be taken during surgery; casting or tight bandages in this region often allow scar tissue to compromise the function of this joint. Cross pinning will usually allow adequate fixation of distal tibiotarsal fractures without the need for external support. Placing a pin through the area of the tibial cartilage will trap the flexor tendons and cause permanent disability. Techniques that involve this area should be avoided.

Tarsometatarsus

In owls and falcons there is a medullary cavity running the whole length of this bone. In hawks and eagles

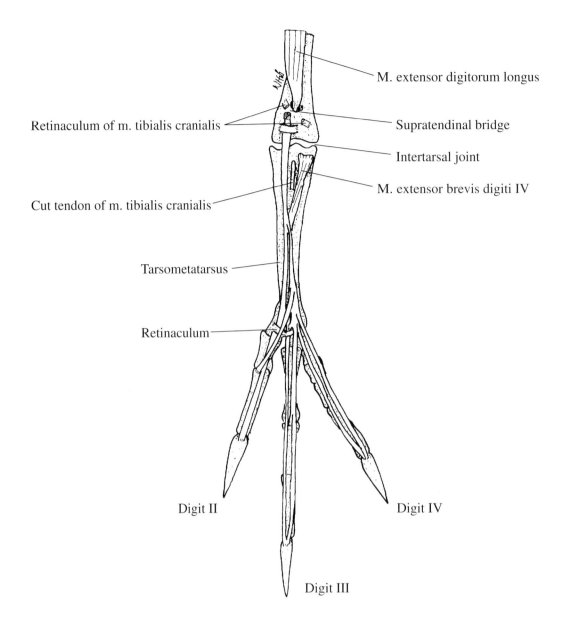

M. extensor digitorum longus

Retinaculum of m. tibialis cranialis

Supratendinal bridge

Intertarsal joint

M. extensor brevis digiti IV

Cut tendon of m. tibialis cranialis

Tarsometatarsus

Retinaculum

Digit II

Digit IV

Digit III

Figure 16.11: The left leg of a Peregrine Falcon showing the path of the long digital extensor tendon over the cranial aspect of the intertarsal joint through the canal formed by the supratendinal bridge (Harcourt-Brown, 1994).

the medullary cavity is absent from the proximal third, and this area is flattened craniocaudally as well. In all these birds the tendons of the extensor and most of the flexor muscles run on either the cranial or caudal aspect of the bone, as do the small intrinsic muscles. The veins are lateral and medial, but the arteries and nerves are mainly cranial. The tarsometatarsus should be approached from the lateral aspect to avoid the medially placed tendon of insertion of *m. flexor hallucis longus* (see Figures 16.1, 16.2). It is impossible to use intramedullary pins to repair the proximal half of this bone in hawks; attempts to use this technique result in the pin being placed in the flexor tendons. Repair of this long bone is possible with an L-shaped splint if the fracture is distal to the tendon of insertion of *m. tibialis cranialis* (see Figure 16.4). Fractures proximal to this insertion are subject

to movement by the muscle and therefore malunion. A combination of half-pin and full-pin fixation can be used to repair this bone in hawks (see Figures 16.12.1, 16.12.2). Care must be taken not to place the pins through the flexor groove on the caudal aspect of the bone and entrap the flexor tendons. Distal tarsometatarsal fractures may be cross pinned.

Casts that hold the tarsometatarsus and the digits rigid result in the flexor tendons being involved in the callus; when the bone has healed the bird is often unable to flex its digits.

Digits

The phalangeal bones are frequently fractured in hunting accidents. The digit has a large flexor tendon surrounded by a thick tendon sheath on the plantar aspect. These structures form a very effective splint.

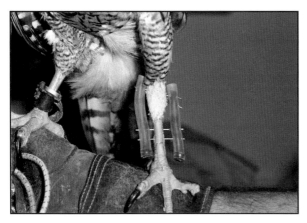

Figure 16.12.1: A combination of full-pin and half-pin fixation three days after surgery. This Northern Goshawk ignored the tubing and methylmethacrylate for four weeks whilst the bone healed. The bird is undergoing its first moult.

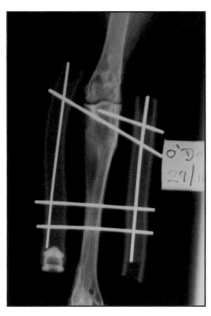

Figure 16.12.2: Radiograph of a fracture of the proximal tarsometatarsus of the same bird. The pins have to be positioned to avoid entrapping the flexor tendons in the flexor groove.

The digit seldom needs support and even fractures involving the joints will heal to give full function if left unsplinted. Splinting the digit usually results in the flexor tendon, and sometimes joints, being trapped in the callus and a stiff or non-functional toe is the result. Large phalangeal bones, eg. as in vultures, can be repaired with laterally placed full-pin fixation. A lateral or medial approach is usual, but the artery, vein and nerve all run in this site. A splint is not necessary.

DISLOCATIONS

Vertebral-Synsacral Joint.

The synsacrum can be dislocated partially or completely from the thoracic vertebrae (see later- Paralysis).

Hip Joint

This joint can be dislocated by avulsing the ligament from the femoral head. When the bird extends its leg the trochanter moves dorsal to the antitrochanter and 'locks', leaving the limb in extension. The bird should be anaesthetised and the diagnosis confirmed on radiographic comparison between both hips. A cranial approach to the joint gives good access as it avoids the antitrochanter. The femoral head should be cut away from the shaft and removed. *M. iliotibialis lateralis* is used to provide a strip of muscle 3cm long and about 5mm wide dissected back to its origin and pushed through the incised joint in the manner of a 'reverse' biceps femoris sling operation. The bird should be kept in a darkened room for one week postoperatively. Postoperative pressure bandages are unnecessary. Birds that have had this operation have made a full recovery, even though the injury may have been several months old.

Femorotibial Joint

This joint is only dislocated as a result of severe trauma. It is possible to make a satisfactory repair by replacing damaged ligaments with Teflon suture material (Gore-Tex). A 21G or 23G hypodermic needle can be used to drill holes through the bone to place the suture material. Meniscal damage is rarely diagnosed. Complete disruption of the joint has been salvaged by using half-pin fixation on the cranial aspect, above and below the joint, holding the joint in reasonable apposition whilst a fibrous union takes place (Rosenthal *et al*, 1992). Although using this technique saves the leg, most falcons and even hawks would soon acquire bumblefoot on the foot of the normal limb. Padding under the foot of the normal limb will help to prevent this occurring.

Intertarsal Joint

This joint in adult birds is usually injured by severe trauma, and dislocation is usually accompanied by damage to tendons, ligaments, integument, etc. It is not usually possible to repair the joint. Amputation is not an option that should be taken as the remaining limb will be quickly affected with bumblefoot.

The tibial cartilage can be damaged on its own: growing birds can easily dislocate many of the structures within or attached to the tibial cartilage. The most frequent dislocation involves the tendon of *m. flexor hallucis longus*. The tendon bursts out of position and lies to the lateral aspect of the tibial cartilage, usually as a sequela to trauma (see Figure 16.13.1). The displacement of the tendon makes the bird unable to use the affected leg; there is an obvious thickening of the joint and, if recently displaced, the tendon can be palpated; the foot is rotated away from the body. If seen within a day or two of the event, the tendon is easily repositioned surgically. The tunnel that the tendon occupied is identifiable and the tendon can be replaced.

4\0 polydioxanone suture (PDS II, Ethicon) is used to repair the tear. No external support is needed for the limb, but the bird should be kept quiet in a darkened room for one week. Less frequently, the insertion of the medial gastrocnemius muscle will pull away from the tibial cartilage and allow the tibial cartilage, flexor tendons and the tarsometatarsus to rotate laterally, or the whole tibial cartilage can displace medially with rotation of the tarsometatarsus (see Figure 16.13.2). Immediate surgical correction is required, but is difficult to achieve as the sutures tend to pull through the tissue used to anchor the muscle insertion. Failure to repair this defect will lead to euthanasia of the patient.

In some cases, whether as a cause or by effect, the intertarsal joint becomes rotated around the long axis of the leg, with a distortion of the tibiotarsus and the tarsometatarsus. When the dislocation of the tibial cartilage is secondary to a growth defect involving the bones, the growth defect should be corrected as well. Osteotomy at the distal third of the tibia, rotation of the bone and full-pin fixation will allow the tibial cartilage to return to its correct position. In some cases this is impossible due to contraction of *m. tibialis cranialis* and permanent flexion of the intertarsal joint.

Phalangeal Joints

These joints can be dislocated without any ligamentous damage. The dislocation is easily replaced under general anaesthetic and usually requires no external support. External support will causes loss of function. If a collateral ligament is broken and there is no additional trauma, the ligament should be sutured using a 3\0 or 4\0 suture of polyglycolic acid (Dexon).

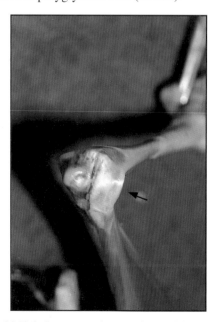

Figure 16.13.1: Dissection showing the caudal aspect of the intertarsal joint of a 34-day-old Harris' Hawk. The dislocation of the whole tibial cartilage (arrow) and related structures was accompanied by contracture of m. tibialis cranialis.

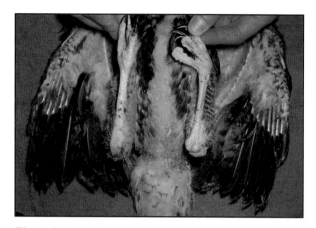

Figure 16.13.2: The clinical appearance showing a flexed and medially rotated left limb and a normal right limb.

COMPLICATIONS SEEN AFTER FRACTURE REPAIR

Malunion

Instability of a repaired fracture, allowing constant movement, causes the bone ends to become reduced in diameter, rounded and smooth, and with no periosteal proliferation: atrophic malunion. Debridement of the bone ends followed by adequate support of the fracture will allow healing. Birds do not have cancellous bone and so this form of bone grafting is not possible.

Osteomyelitis

Many avian fractures, especially in wild birds, are compound (see Chapter 23). Almost invariably, the fracture has become infected prior to the initial examination. If it is possible, the affected bone should be removed at the time of surgery, but often the infection has invaded the medullary cavity and it proves impossible to prevent pus from forming. It is an unfortunate fact that purulent material in avian species collects as a caseous mass that will not clear with drainage. There is rarely formation of a sinus as there is in mammals. In long bones the cortical bone becomes distorted by the continuing growth of the relatively hard purulent mass in the medullary cavity; this may be seen radiographically (see Chapter 10). Because of the caseous nature of the purulent material, drainage is ineffective; flushing the marrow cavity will push the infection further into the cavity, especially in the femur. Single purulent masses may be cured by surgical removal of the lump of purulent material and administration of appropriate antibiotic therapy. Lincomycin (50mg/kg bid) or clindamycin (50mg/kg bid) may be given orally for a minimum of 14 days, and these are usually the drugs of choice. If the bone is known to be infected, the fracture should be repaired using a full-pin or half-pin fixation technique; if some of the cortex has to be removed, there is still support for the weakened bone whilst healing occurs. Multiple caseous masses are usually impossible to remove and the prognosis in these cases is very poor. Unresponsive osteomyelitis should be reappraised for the presence of *Mycobacterium avium*. Acid-fast staining of impression smears of pus are preferable to culture for a quick result.

Occasionally, osteomyelitis develops sufficiently to cause the bone to fracture: surgical repair should be accompanied by culture and impression smears or histopathology which must again include examination for the presence of acid-fast bacteria.

Sometimes, in bones that were fractured and not infected, radiographic evidence of small areas of apparent osteomyelitis frequently occur around the pin during the healing process. Pin removal after the bone has healed will bring a coating of purulent material with it. If antibiotic is administered, the radiographic lesions disappear in a few weeks.

Osteoarthritis

Osteoarthritis is rarely seen in birds in comparison to dogs and cats. It is usually a sequela to fracture involving a joint, or a repair where the pin has been left within the joint.

Septic Arthritis

The commonest joint to be affected with a septic arthritis is the distal interphalangeal joint. Infection usually enters from a scab under the claw or from a bite. Some birds may develop septic arthritis as a sequela to a compound fracture involving a joint; occasionally, from a haematogenous infection of an already bruised joint; and infrequently as a sequela to surgery, unless a compound fracture has involved the joint.

As a general rule, birds where lytic bone changes (see Figure 10.10) can be seen radiographically in the joint rarely recover. If no lytic bone changes can be seen, daily irrigation of the joint with normal saline, followed by 0.25-0.5ml of either lincomycin or tobramycin injected into the joint, is the treatment of choice. Cytology prior to culture will show the presence of Gram-positive or Gram-negative bacteria and will help to make the choice. This technique requires an indwelling catheter and is more difficult in the leg joints than the wing joints; in combination with oral antibiotic it allows some birds to make a full recovery.

Septic arthritis carries a very poor prognosis. Unless amputation is possible, more severe cases should be euthanased. Only the digit can be amputated; whole limb amputation causes bumblefoot on the remaining foot.

Dry Gangrene of the Skin

Occasionally, after surgery, the skin around the surgical site will lose its blood supply and die. This happens very suddenly and produces an area of dry gangrene, which may also include deeper structures. Severe cases involving muscles and ligaments around the joints should be euthanased. Less severe cases can be treated with debridement of the devitalised tissue and application of Granuflex. This topic is covered more fully in Chapters 3 and 14.

Amputation of the Digit

Fractures of the digit which are or have become infected, with or without a septic arthritis, will require amputation; this is the only amputation that is commonly performed on the pelvic limb. Amputation of the digit is usually the last resort for a hunting bird. Loss of function due to irreparable tendon damage, loss of skin or septic arthritis are the usual causes. The digit should be amputated as close to the damaged part as possible; however, the remaining joints have to be functional or the toe is a useless encumbrance. The skin and tendon sheaths are incised and retracted cranially from the phalangeal bone. The phalangeal bone is cut with fine bone cutters so that none of the joint is left behind. The flexor and extensor tendons are sutured together over the end of the cut bone. The skin is then sutured over the top of the amputation. The suture material normally used is 3\0 or 4\0 chromic cat gut and the suture line and toe should be covered with Granuflex. Postoperative antibiotic should be used: lincomycin (50mg/kg p/o bid for five days) is useful.

Digits II, III and IV may be amputated singly with good results; amputation of digit I will stop the bird from gripping its perch, and the results are therefore less satisfactory.

Amputation of the whole limb invariably leads to the formation of an intractable bumblefoot in the remaining limb.

Disturbances of Growth of Bones

The growth plates in birds are different from those in mammals. The process of ossification of the long bones of the pelvic limb of birds has been extensively studied in chickens and turkeys and to a lesser extent in pigeons, quail and passerines. There has been little published work in raptors, but the subject has been studied and the literature in other species reviewed by Fowler (1981).

The main difference between mammals and birds is that birds do not have a calcified epiphysis until the end of their growth period. The proximal and distal ends of the femur and the proximal end of the tibiotarsus therefore appear to be absent on radiographs of growing raptors. The distal end of the tibiotarsus and proximal end of the tarsometatarsus look more like the familiar mammalian growth plates, but this is because the tarsal bones are present and form a centre of ossified bone that resembles the mammalian epiphysis. The growing areas of a 34 day old Harris' Hawk are shown in Figure 16.14.

Young, growing raptors are seen with osteodystrophy; nearly every case is related to incorrect nutrition (see Chapter 22). Some apparently experienced falconers still refuse to supplement the diet of their growing birds with vitamin and mineral supplement; others also use large carcases and give too large a quantity so that the birds do not or cannot eat the bone provided. The clinician should not accept the statement that the owner is 'feeding a good mixed diet and has raised many chicks before with no problems' as proof that the chicks are being fed correctly. Weakened chicks, with folding fractures or complete fractures of the long bones, are seen each breeding season (see Figure 16.15). Falcons grow more quickly and therefore present with more dramatic problems than hawks. Owls are often sold to their new (and inexperienced) owners at five days old with no dietary advice. Affected

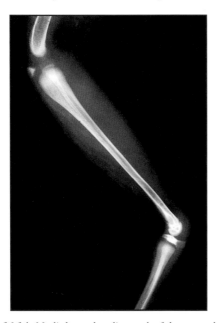

Figure 16.14: Mediolateral radiograph of the normal limb of the 34-day-old Harris' Hawk in 16.13.

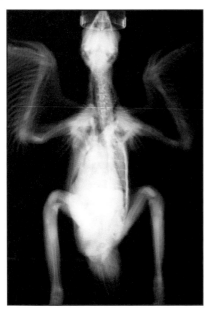

Figure 16.15: Multiple osteodystrophic fractures in a 16-day-old Northern Sparrow Hawk which had been reared for a week on an all meat diet. The ribs are distorted and the cortex of the long bones was irregular in thickness. (See also Figures 22.13, 22.14.)

birds should have a whole body radiograph taken so that all the birds' bones can be assessed for fractures and distortions. Birds with multiple fractures must be euthanased. It should also be remembered that the birds may be suffering from more than a calcium\vitamin D deficiency (see Chapter 13).

Further problems in growing bones are related to the fusion of the second, third and fourth metatarsal bones which takes place in the first few weeks after hatching. The first metatarsal bone remains small and separate from an early embryonic stage; the fifth metatarsal bone disappears; the second, third and fourth metatarsals fuse. Little is recorded about the time of fusion in raptors, but in some species the bones are still fusing as late as five weeks after hatching and so still have separate growing centres. Harris' Hawks have been reported to have damaged one of the growing areas of a single metatarsal bone sufficiently to stop or slow the growth of that side of the limb (Harcourt-Brown, 1994). The result was a considerable deviation of the tarsometatarsus by about five weeks of age (see Figures 16.16.1, 16.16.2). The Harris' Hawk is the only species to be seen by the author to suffer from this deviation, either because of overrepresentation due to the popularity of the Harris' Hawk and the large numbers that are bred annually, or because of their behaviour in the nest. Other species can be affected as well.

The deviation may be corrected by opening up the side of the tarsometatarsus where it has stopped growing and removing a portion of the distorted cartilage from just below the tarsus. The bone is then forcibly straightened, which enlarges the deficit further, and the wound closed with 4\0 chromic catgut. To keep the tarsometatarsus straight it must be held for about

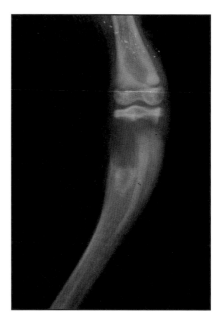

Figure 16.16.1: Craniocaudal radiograph of a five-week-old Harris' Hawk, showing distortion of the proximal metatarsi due to cessation of growth of the second metatarsus.

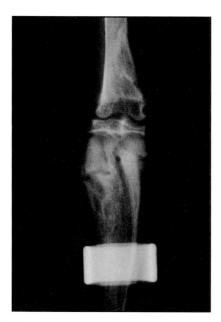

Figure 16.16.2: Two weeks after the limb has been straightened along with removal of some of the cartilage from the area between the tarsus and the second metatarsus. A plaster cast was placed around the intertarsal region for two weeks, while the bird was suspended through a towelling sling with its legs hanging below.

10-14 days in a plaster cast from just above the intertarsal joint to half way down the tarsometatarsus. The bird should be suspended in a towelling sling to allow it to stand on the normal limb. Whilst the leg is plastered the created deficit will fill with bone and the growing centre continues to grow for a further week. The bone should remain straight after cast removal if the bone has stopped growing. Because no other damage has occurred to surrounding structures, the intertarsal joint will function normally. There may be a slight shortening of the affected tarsometatarsus but this does not seem to affect the bird long term.

PARALYSIS OR PARESIS OF THE PELVIC LIMB

Damage to the Vertebral-Synsacral Junction

Subluxation due to trauma is a common cause of paralysis. There is a history of an accident and a lateral radiograph will reveal separation of one or both joints between the notarium and the synsacrum. Occasionally, there is paresis and no obvious subluxation. Stress radiography, by pulling the neck and legs in opposite directions, will show an increased joint space in some of these cases. Birds that are only bruised in this area will make a recovery with steroids and antibiotic treatment; the other cases carry a poor prognosis. Birds with only a paralysed tail may have a dislocation distal to the synsacrum causing a permanent or temporary paralysis of the tail.

Some birds present with a slow developing paresis, extending to paralysis, with a history of trauma some weeks previously. Lateral radiographs will reveal the formation of an intervertebral abscess (see Figure 16.17). The abscess has arisen from haematogenous spread to the joint when it is bruised after trauma. As in other cases of septic arthritis, the prognosis is usually hopeless.

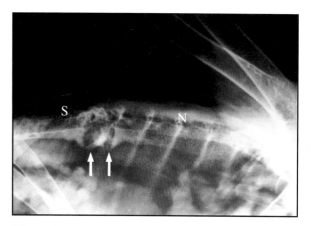

Figure 16.17: Lateral radiograph of a Peregrine Falcon which had slowly become paralysed. Both the joints (arrowed) between the synsacrum (S) and the notarium (N) were involved.

Lead Poisoning

In the early stages of lead poisoning the bird may be presented with paresis of the legs. A pathognomonic sign of lead poisoning in raptors is that they will sit 'holding hands' with themselves. Radiography may reveal lead in the ventriculus; rarely elsewhere. The disease, if left untreated, will progress to convulsions (see Chapter 20). On rare occasions the lead has been cast from the proventriculus, or the cause is not shotgun pellets. The typical signs of lead poisoning should be confirmed in these cases by blood lead levels; treatment before the results are obtained will not cause problems if the bird is unaffected by lead poisoning.

Nephritis

The nerve supply to the pelvic limb is from the femoral, obturator and ischiadic nerves (see Figures 16.1, 16.2). These nerves all arise from the synsacral area and run across the ventral synsacrum and through the pelvis to the limb (see Figure 16.18). The ischiadic nerve supplies the majority of the limb and runs from the synsacrum to the ilioischiadic foramen in close proximity to the middle and caudal divisions of the kidneys. This relationship is sufficient for a nephritis to cause a neuritis. Birds of any species may be presented with paresis and no history of previous trauma; they often appear unwell. Plain radiographs and intravenous pyelography may show increased renal density etc. An intravenous bolus of 175-700mg of iodine in the form of iohexol should be used. The dose is dependent upon the size of the bird. Gentle palpation *per cloacam* will sometimes confirm enlargement of the kidneys if radiography is not available. A barium meal may be useful to outline enlargements that are not renal but can still cause paresis by pressure, eg. renal cysts, neoplasia of the gonad, etc. Birds with renal infection and neuritis may have an increased blood uric acid level and often a leucocytosis. Antibiotic therapy is usually sufficient to effect a rapid improvement and cure. Co-trimazine (30mg/kg s/c or 12-60mg/kg p/o bid for 7-14 days) is usually the drug of choice, in spite of the compromised renal function, as this condition is usually coliform related. Occasionally, the disease will progress and a different antibiotic should be tried; in these cases the paresis may be quite marked and the bird may take some weeks or even months to recover full use of its limbs.

Paramyxovirus

This virus is able to cause a rapid and irreversible paralysis (see Chapter 20).

DISTRACTION OF THE FIRST METATARSAL BONE

This condition is seen mainly in Northern Goshawks.

The first metatarsal bone is connected to the tarsometatarsus by three small ligaments on the caudal aspect of the bones. Affected birds are usually presented with an inflamed, soft, swelling on the medial aspect of the distal tarsometatarsus (see Figure 16.19.1). Radiography reveals the first metatarsal bone displaced proximoplantar, with a slight rotation. There is often a lytic area in the metatarsal fossa indicating an area of purulent material; this area may also be surrounded by bony proliferation (see Figure 16.19.2). Antibiotic therapy in the form of lincomycin (50mg/kg p/o bid for 7-14 days) and sodium fusidate ointment usually stops the active infective process. Once the leg is less swollen it may be necessary to remove the plug of infected material from the metatarsal fossa, or the process will start again. It is very difficult to replace the first metatarsal bone surgically due to the presence of the flexor tendons in the flexor tendon groove and the plantar metatarsal nerve. This condition is due to repetitive concussion on the plantar aspect of the foot while hunting or occasionally while perching (Harcourt-Brown, 1994). It does not occur in falcons because of the check ligament of the hallux (see Figure 16.3).

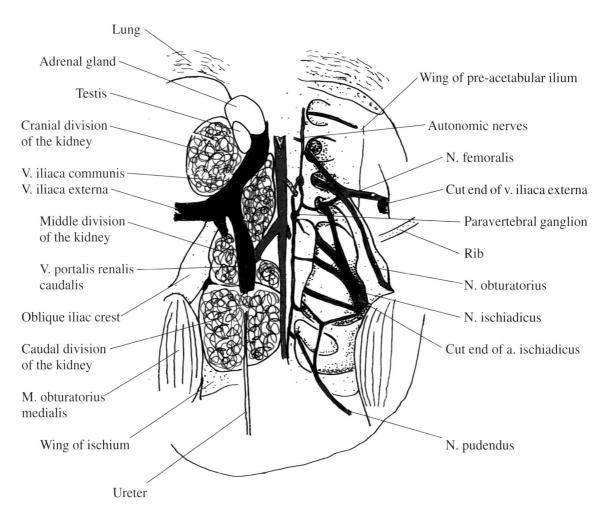

Figure 16.18: Ventral view of the lumbosacral plexus of a Saker Falcon after the removal of the left kidney and its related vasculature, showing the relationship between the nerves and the kidneys.

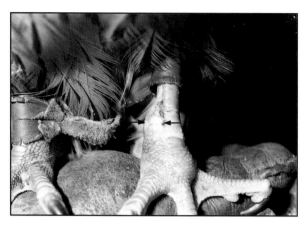

Figure 16.19.1: The clinical appearance of the leg of an immature Northern Goshawk suffering from a distracted first metatarsal bone (arrows).

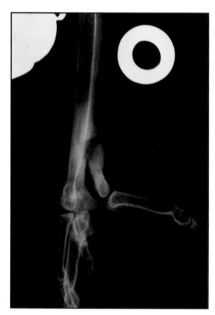

Figure 16.19.2: Mediolateral radiograph of distraction of the first metatarsal bone in the same Northern Goshawk.

SEVERED TENDONS

Birds are often seen with the flexor or extensor tendons to the digits severed. This can happen in several ways:
● Squirrel (*Sciurus carolinensis*) bites can sever the tendon directly or cause the tendon to become infected and the infection separates the tendon by necrosis.
● Infection under a scab around the claw will cause separation of the flexor tendon from the flexor prominence on the distal phalangeal bone.
● The closed ring can sometimes result in compression around the leg and cause tissue necrosis; the tendon of insertion of *m. extensor hallucis longus* runs over the tarsometatarsus at this point and will become separated.
● Brass eyelets in the aylmeri which are not surrounded by sufficient leather, or traditional leather

jesses that are insufficiently greased, can rub a hole in the dorsal aspect of digit I and cause extensor tendon separation.
● As a sequela to bumblefoot infection, at the metatarsophalangeal junction.

The tendons are very long and have no apparent blood supply; nutrition is possibly via the tendon sheath fluid (Harcourt-Brown, 1994). Joining the tendons by end to end anastomosis fails as there is no healing response at the joined tendon ends. A blood supply to the affected site must be obtained from the tendon sheath by either waiting for 3-4 weeks to allow the tendon ends to adhere to the tendon sheath and vascularise, or suturing the tendon to the tendon sheath soon after injury. Once the tendon ends are vascularised, usually 3-4 weeks after the initial injury, they can be joined; providing the new blood supply is preserved, the tendon will heal. A ball bandage applied for 3-4 weeks is useful to allow some degree of movement without allowing the full muscular force to disrupt the repair (see Figures 14.8.1, 14.8.2, 14.8.3, 14.8.4).

TENDON SHEATH INFECTIONS

The flexor and extensor tendon sheaths are contiguous from the distal phalanx to just proximal to the intertarsal joint (see Figures 16.1, 16.2). Infection gaining admission at one point can settle out a relatively great distance from the original injury. It is often necessary to treat these infections by removing the pus and irrigating the tendon sheath with an indwelling catheter for seven days, combined with oral antibiotic. Culture and antibiotic sensitivity is required, but as the organism is invariably S*taphylococcus* spp., lincomycin (50mg/kg p/o bid for 7-14 days) is the initial drug of choice.

BUMBLEFOOT

Pathogenesis
This common condition of captive raptors has been recorded since medieval times. It occurs only on the plantar aspect of the foot. Cooper (1978) suggested a three stage classification of the disease:
● Type I is mild and localised, and either degenerative, giving a thin flattened epithelium, or proliferative, causing hypertrophy of the epithelium to form a corn. Both of these stages degenerate to form a scab. There may or may not be heat and swelling.
● Type II is always more extensive and bacteria play a major role in the disease, causing heat, swelling and pain. This second stage is believed to be caused by either a puncture by the claw or a foreign body, or further degeneration of a type I condition. Bacteriological tests usually disclose *Staphylococcus aureus*, and histology confirms the presence of large numbers of this bacterium. *Escherichia coli, Corynebacterium*

spp., *Pseudomonas* spp. and yeasts are also seen sometimes. Although the clinical impression is that the condition is acute, histologically there seems to be a chronic reaction.

● Type III is characterised by a long-standing, infected and degenerate lesion. The infection is deep enough to involve ligaments, tendons and even the phalangeal tarsometatarsal joints. The feet are intermittently hot and painful.

Remple and Al-Ashbal (1993) carried out bacteriological and histopathological investigations on the feet of 15 raptors with bumblefoot. *Staphylococcus aureus* was found in all cases. The following aetiology was postulated: repeated trauma to the foot, followed by skin devitalisation, followed by colonisation with pathogenic staphylococcal bacteria, followed by phagocyte inhibition, hypersensitivity and chronic granulomatous inflammation. It was also suggested that the reason why bumblefoot is not found in wild raptors is that staphylococci are not found on the feet of wild birds and may be an introduction from the captive environment. The authors commented on the remarkable vascular changes and suggested that these are caused by bacterial hypersensitivity.

Harcourt-Brown (1994) postulated that bumblefoot starts with a condition analogous to a bed sore and its production in humans. He also suggested that only falcons become affected with bumblefoot. Latex casts prepared of the vascular system of the feet of birds with advanced bumblefoot showed a total lack of circulation to the affected area. The lack of circulation is the root cause of the lack of response to infection and the reason that the degenerate areas heal so poorly.

The chain of events that produce a bumblefoot are dynamic. If a falcon with normal feet is taken up, kept restricted in its flying, fed so that it is heavy relative to its flying weight and allowed to perch on hard and unyielding surfaces of wood or concrete, then the following sequence of events invariably occurs: the plantar aspect of the foot, on the metatarsal pad and occasionally the digital pads, loses the rough appearance of the plantar reticulate scales; the skin in this region becomes flattened, smooth and shiny; the epidermis appears to be thinner. If these areas are cleaned and viewed closely, small red streaks are visible having the appearance of 'dead' blood vessels. These changes always correspond to the sites of maximum weight bearing. Occasionally, the skin mounts a proliferative response, but there is always a degenerative smooth area around the proliferation. Histological examination shows thrombosis of the small blood vessels in the pressured and degenerative regions, as well as death of epithelial cells.

Unfortunately, in many cases the condition is allowed to progress as the preceding changes are not noticed. The thin skin at the edge of the bumblefoot lesion separates, allowing access for bacteria to the

subcutis. The bacteria produce the chain of events that form the caseous, inflammatory process, so typical of bumblefoot. The foot becomes hot, swollen and painful. From this point it is no longer possible to cure the foot conservatively. As the condition deteriorates an increasing number of structures are involved: infection of the tendon sheaths with pus tracking towards the intertarsal joint and towards the digits; rupture of the flexor tendons; osteomyelitis of the sesamoid bone ventral to digit II; and septic arthritis of the tarsometatarsal phalangeal joints. Many of these changes can be reversed by treatment, but in some cases recovery is impossible.

Lack of exercise, poor perching surfaces and increased weight are the primary factors in the development of bumblefoot. Infection is secondary.

Captive falcons take less exercise than their wild counterparts. Vascular pooling and venous return must be important factors in the production of bumblefoot. Long-lasting pressure, from having to perch on a hard surface for very long periods, will cause pressure ischaemia and local hypoxia. Excessive weight will also increase the pressure on the foot, as will standing on one leg because of injury or disease to the other. For this reason **NO** falcon should have a limb amputated. The remaining limb will be affected by bumblefoot within a few weeks (see Figure 16.20).

Puncture wounds are not a common cause of bumblefoot. If devitalised skin is punctured it is more likely to develop into a bumblefoot.

Hawks are more active when they are not flying than falcons. Infections of the plantar aspect of the feet of hawks heal very quickly and easily, as does infection of the dorsal surface of the feet of both hawks and falcons. Hawks do not, therefore, suffer from bumblefoot as there are no vascular problems to

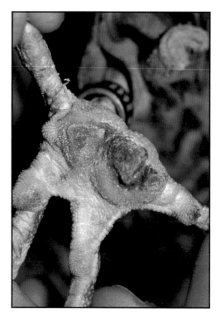

Figure 16.20: *The plantar aspect of the foot of a female Peregrine Falcon two weeks after amputation of the other leg.*

prevent healing. Well-fed wild falcons still fly more in a day than many falconer's birds fly in a week. It is significant that falconers who hunt with their birds on a daily basis seldom have birds with bumblefoot. It is also significant that many birds that have perfect feet through the hunting season are at great risk of developing bumblefoot when 'put down' to moult in an aviary: more food, increased weight, poor perching surfaces, less exercise.

Some birds are presented with bilateral bumblefoot that do not respond as expected to treatment. Many of these birds will be found to have other diseases, especially chronic kidney disease, and fatty liver and kidney syndrome. Ill health causing decreased exercise, and blood pressure problems caused by chronic kidney disease, produce poor perfusion of the distal pelvic limb, encouraging the formation and prevention of healing of bumblefoot.

Pododermatitis has become a term synonymous with bumblefoot. Blood and Studdert (1988) defined pododermatitis as 'inflammation of the skin of the foot'. On this basis, pododermatitis seems an inadequate description of this disease.

Treatment

The aim of bumblefoot treatment is to return the plantar surface of the foot to its normal appearance. This may be a time consuming, laborious task. Birds affected with bumblefoot should be examined fully for sources of other injury to the limbs and also for signs of internal disease. In birds with a poor prognosis, euthanasia should be considered at the outset, rather than later.

All cases of bumblefoot, regardless of their stage of development, should have the following changes in their husbandry:

- A good diet plus vitamin and mineral supplement.
- Cover all perching surfaces with Astroturf (see Figure 16.21): concrete, wood or perches with rope wound around them are all unsatisfactory.
- If the bird is housed indoors, wood shavings should be used to cover the floor, especially if the bird is lying down rather than perching. A dry substrate to put the shavings on and new, dry, *Aspergillus*-free shavings should be used as a layer about 8-10cm deep. If the bird is housed outdoors, new grass is the surface of choice. Move the bird off gravel, concrete, etc.
- Reduce the bird's weight to its flying weight.
- Aviary birds should be jessed and manned as soon as possible. This allows more direct management of the condition. It will also allow the bird to be fed on the fist to avoid the bird eating wood shavings with its food, a possible source of ventricular impaction.
- Increased exercise: even flying three times a day on a 'creance' will help the resolution of bumblefoot; flying free is even better.

For birds with hyperaemia of the foot and a smooth epithelial surface (see Figure 16.22), with or without

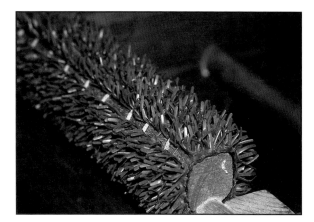

Figure 16.21: A cadge with the perching surfaces covered with Astroturf.

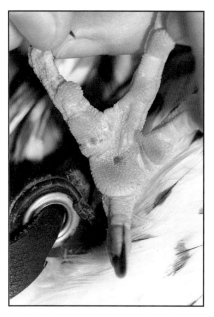

Figure 16.22: Typical early changes of bumblefoot. The papillae are flattened, there is reactive hyperaemia and two scabs are present. Correct perching surfaces and increased exercise allowed a rapid return to normality.

a scab, the above changes are all that is required for the bird to return to normal. Occasionally, there is infection but no pus formation; these cases require antibiotics: lincomycin (50mg/kg p/o bid) or cloxacillin (250mg/kg p/o bid) for 7-10 days. If there is a large scab, sodium fusidate should be applied to the scab and surrounding skin twice daily until the scab lifts and can be removed. Dry feet may need dressing with hand cream.

Birds with epithelial changes, ie. a large scab and a swollen plantar aspect of the foot, require surgical investigation and antibacterial treatment as well as the above changes in management. Five days pre-operative antibiotic is often useful. Bacteriology may be carried out to find the most appropriate antibiotic; the bacteria in these cases are usually *Staphylococcus* spp. The bird should be anaesthetised, placed in dorsal recumbency and the whole foot cleaned, sterilised and draped. The anatomy of the plantar aspect of the foot is illustrated in Figure 16.3. A circular incision should be made between the normal and abnormal tissue. The whole scab plus the underlying purulent material should be removed In many cases the pus is solid and hopefully contained in the fibrous subcutaneous tissues. All abnormal tissue should be removed; the smallest Volkmann's scoop is most useful. Bleeding can be controlled by digital pressure around the mid-tarsometatarsal region. Once the wound has been cleared to healthy vascular tissue, the wound is sutured. First intention healing may be attempted: Remple (1993) and Riddle and Hoolihan (1993) suggested a new treatment for bumblefoot: surgery followed by foot-casting. The plantar surface of the foot is raised from contact with the perch by the application of a rigid cast supporting the base of each digit (see Figures 16.23.1, 16.23.2). It was suggested that foot-casting allowed first intention healing by preventing the normal mechanical forces that are applied to the foot from disturbing the wound. It would seem as likely that the lack of pressure allows better circulation and healing. This is borne out by the fact that without care, 'bumblefoot' will start to occur on the digits where they stand on the foot cast.

Harcourt-Brown (1994) suggested that in cases where a large lesion has been removed, a purse-string suture should be used to reduce the size of the wound. Ketanserin was applied to the wound on a non-adherent dressing, the whole being held in place with zinc oxide tape. Ketanserin is a vasodilator but is no longer available in the ointment form. Oil of proflavine or Dermisol Cream (Pfizer) may be used instead of ketanserin. Foot-casting is helpful in the early stages of treatment in these cases as well. Bacteriology should be performed on the pus; until the results are obtained, lincomycin is the drug of choice. Antibiotic therapy should be continued until the foot wound has granulated or until first intention healing has taken place, ie. a minimum of 14 days. The foot should be dressed daily and once granulation has occurred the wound should be covered with Granuflex to allow epithelialisation. The Granuflex should be changed every five days and left until full thickness normal skin covers the deficit; this may take some months. The majority of these birds will be cured, and if care is taken by the falconer over weight, perches and exercise, there should be no recurrence. If there is recurrence, further surgery and secondary intention healing should be adopted to stop the formation of micro-abscesses; the bird must be checked for intercurrent disease or injury.

Treatment of Difficult or Unresponsive Cases of Bumblefoot

Satterfield and O'Rourke (1981) suggested vaccination and immunomodulation with levamisole as a treatment for bumblefoot. Oaks (1993) could provide

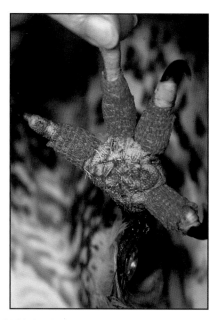

Figure 16.23.1: After removal of the pus and suturing the foot, a conforming bandage is wrapped around the base of each digit to form a cushion. This technique also works well when used in cases where the foot is healing by secondary intention.

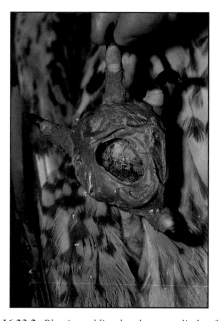

Figure 16.23.2: Plastic padding has been applied to form a foot cast. The suture line is protected whilst casting with a covering of Granuflex. Once set the cast is held in place with zinc oxide tape or glued to the bandaged toes. The cast prevents pressure from affecting the blood supply.

no support for the theory that systemic immunosuppression was an important factor in the pathogenesis of bumblefoot and surgery was judged to be the best method of treatment. Riddle and Hoolihan (1993) recorded the poor success rate in curing more advanced forms of bumblefoot.

Suggestions for treatment of advanced bumblefoot must be modified to suit each case as there is usually a combination of problems.

Some birds have a bilateral, sudden-onset, swelling of the foot (and sometimes the distal tarsometatarsal region) and necrosis of skin, to form a large, moist wound. Bacteriology and sensitivity are mandatory. Many of these cases have *Pseudomonas* spp. present; some are fungal. They have infection invading the joint capsule of the metatarsophalangeal joints, and also the tendon sheaths of the flexor tendons and sometimes the extensor tendons. For treatment, the initial husbandry changes are instituted. Surgical investigation and removal of all necrotic tissue and pus must be combined with irrigation of the tendon sheaths and joint capsule if these are affected. The swollen tendon sheaths should be squeezed. If fluid can be expressed from the bumblefoot wound by squeezing the joint capsule or tendon sheath, this can be considered to demonstrate their involvement. A curved pair of Halstead's artery forceps is introduced through the wound on the plantar aspect of the foot and passed in between the flexor tendons and up the caudal aspect of the tarsometatarsus where the jaws of the forceps are pressed against the skin. A small incision allows the jaws to be pushed through to grasp the end of an intravenous cannula. The cannula should be cut to length so that it will allow irrigation of the infected structures. The cannula should be held in place with zinc oxide tape and irrigation should be carried out at least once daily for five days using an appropriate antibiotic. Irrigation with several millilitres of fluid seems as important as the drug used, but lincomycin, metronidazole, tobramycin, enrofloxacin, ketoconazole or itraconazole may be used, usually diluted, where appropriate. The foot should be placed in a foot cast, or have a non-adherent padded bandage in place which should be changed after flushing (see Figures 16.23.1, 16.23.2). This technique will allow resolution of some of these cases.

Some birds lose the use of a toe due to necrosis of the main flexor tendon in the plantar flexor canal. This is impossible to repair and the toe should be amputated.

Septic arthritis of a single metatarsophalangeal joint may be cured by amputation of that toe and the related trochlea of the tarsometatarsus. A dorsal approach is used and a high speed air drill with a 1.2mm burr is needed. The trochlea of the relevant metatarsal can be removed, totally amputating the digit. This method is only satisfactory for a single digit. Total amputation of more than one digit gives a very small bearing surface and therefore a more likely recurrence of bumblefoot.

Some cases of recurrent bumblefoot have osteomyelitis of the sesamoid bone ventral to digit II. Radiography will confirm this and careful dissection will allow the successful removal of this structure.

Infection of the flexor tendon sheath of the digit should be treated initially with oral antibiotics. The pus should then be removed surgically and the sheath irrigated. It should be borne in mind that the tendon sheath runs to a point about 1cm cranial to the tibial cartilage, and care should be taken not to distribute the infection rather than remove it. In many of these cases, long-term antibiotic therapy is needed. Courses of several months' duration are possible. Often during these long courses the antibiotic has to be changed as different bacteria, resistent to the antibiotic, invade the healing tissue.

The above measures will allow resolution of a further percentage of cases.

BROKEN CLAWS

Some broken claws are trivial and just a few millimetres of claw are broken off, accompanied by a lot of bleeding. Cautery with potassium permanganate crystals will stop the bleeding. More frequently, a large proportion of the claw is torn off leaving the bone and some germinal epithelium. This area must be cleaned with a povidone-iodine solution and covered with Granuflex to prevent the germinal epithelium drying out. A course of antibiotic is usually necessary. Changing the Granuflex every 5-7 days and removing the fibrin clot will allow complete regrowth of the claw. If the exposed bone is allowed to dry out, infection will invade the dead bone and enter the distal phalangeal joint. The end of the digit would have to be amputated.

SUBCUTANEOUS ABSCESSES

Large pea-like subcutaneous abscesses are frequently seen in raptors. Staphylococci are introduced through the skin from a puncture wound and form a caseous abscess, which cannot be drained. The abscess should be removed, including the surrounding capsule (see Figure 16.24). The remaining dead space must be obliterated, usually with mattress sutures through the skin. Leaving the abscess capsule will allow the abscess to regrow in many cases.

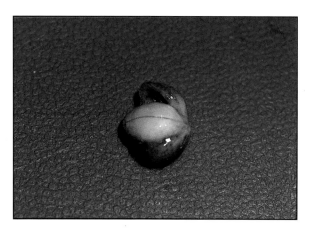

Figure 16.24: *A subcutaneous staphylococcal abscess and its surrounding capsule removed from the toe of a Harris' Hawk.*

Abscesses will also form on the scaly areas of the leg when cracks occur between the scutes. This is very common in Northern Goshawks. The loose scutes should be removed, the abscess debrided and granulation stimulated with oil of Proflavine, applied with a non-adherent bandage. Once the wound is granulating, Granuflex should be used to cover the wound to promote and protect the epithelialisation.

CONGENITAL ABNORMALITIES

Young Merlins may be presented with two or more digits joined by a web of skin. If the birds are young, this may be cut with minimal problem. Adult birds require a more major surgical procedure. This abnormality may be seen in wild and captive birds.

Some immature falcons have feathers in the metatarsal region; usually these are not replaced at the first moult.

GOUT

Gout is uncommon in Falconiformes but can be seen in Strigiformes. Pasty white deposits may be seen subcutaneously over the whole body.

TUMOURS

Tumours are rare. Bone tumours can be seen; fiborosarcomata are the most usual. These cases invariably require euthanasia.

REFERENCES

Coles BH (1985) *Avian Medicine and Surgery*. Blackwell Scientific Publications, London

Cooper JE (1978) *Veterinary Aspects of Captive Birds of Prey*. Standfast Press, Saul.

Fowler ME (1981) Ossification of long bones in raptors. In: *Recent Advances in the Study of Raptor Diseases*. Eds JE Cooper and AG Greenwood. Chiron Publications, Keighley.

Harcourt-Brown NH (1994) *Diseases of the Pelvic Limb of Birds of Prey*. FRCVS Thesis. Royal College of Veterinary Surgeons, London.

Oaks JL (1993) Immune and inflammatory responses in falcon staphylococcal pododermatitis. In: *Raptor Biomedicine*. Eds PT Redig, JE Cooper, JD Remple and DB Hunter. University of Minnesota Press, Minneapolis.

Remple JD (1993) Raptor bumblefoot: a new treatment technique. In: *Raptor Biomedicine*. Eds PT Redig, JE Cooper, JD Remple and DB Hunter. University of Minnesota Press, Minneapolis.

Remple JD and Al-Ashbal AA (1993) Raptor bumblefoot: another look at histopathology and pathogenesis. In: *Raptor Biomedicine*. Eds PT Redig, JE Cooper, JD Remple and DB Hunter. University of Minnesota Press, Minneapolis.

Riddle KE (1981). Surgical treatment of bumblefoot in raptors. In: *Recent Advances in the Study of Raptor Diseases*. Eds JE Cooper and AG Greenwood. Chiron Publications, Keighley.

Riddle KE and Hoolihan J (1993) A form-fitting, composite-casting method for avian appendages. In: *Raptor Biomedicine*. Eds PT Redig, JE Cooper, JD Remple and DB Hunter. University of Minnesota Press, Minneapolis.

Rosenthal K, Hillyer E and Matthiessen D (1994) Stifle luxation repair in a Moluccan Cockatoo and a Barn Owl. *Journal of the Association of Avian Veterinarians* **8(4)**, 173.

Satterfield WC and O'Rourke KI (1981) Immunological considerations in the management of bumblefoot. In: *Recent Advances in the Study of Raptor Diseases*. Eds JE Cooper and AG Greenwood. Chiron Publications, Keighley.

CHAPTER SEVENTEEN

Wing Problems

Greg N Simpson

INTRODUCTION

Raptors are frequently presented with a single droop-ing wing. This chapter discusses the treatment and prognosis of the various conditions associated with this syndrome. The most common cause of abnormal wing carriage is traumatic injury to the musculoskel-etal system of the wing (see Figure 17.1).

EXAMINATION

The resting, unrestrained bird should be viewed to as-sess wing carriage. Injuries to specific regions of the wing result in the wing 'drooping' and being held in a position peculiar to that injury (see Figures 17.2.1, 17.2.2, 17.2.3).

Each wing should be examined, starting at the shoul-der and working distally. The full length of each bone is examined in conjunction with adjacent joints and surrounding soft tissue. Normal and abnormal wings should be compared as this will facilitate the diagno-sis of genuine abnormalities. Initial examination may be carried out with the bird conscious; however, an-aesthesia will often reduce patient stress and simplify the process for the clinician (see Chapter 9). Radio-graphs should be taken with the patient anaesthetised

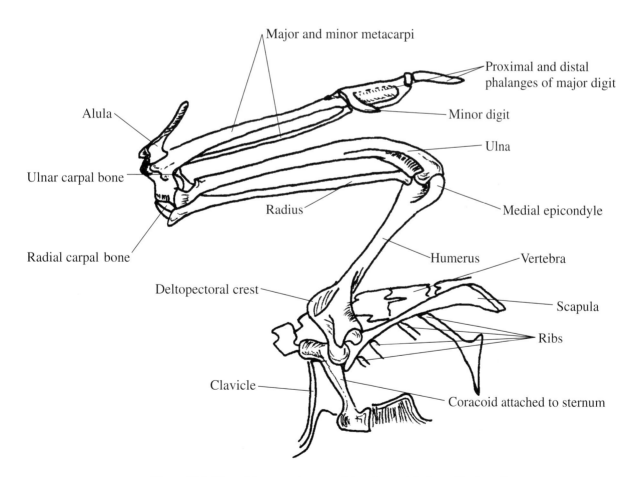

Figure 17.1: *View of the ventral aspect of the wing and the lateral body wall.*

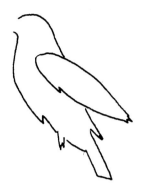

Figures 17.2.1: Shoulder and proximal humerus.

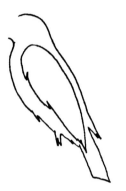

Figure 17.2.2: Mid-humerus to mid-radioulnar region.

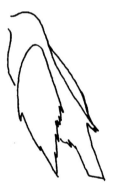

Figure 17.2.3: Distal to the mid-radioulnar region.

(see Chapter 10). It is important that both wings are radiographed for comparison and that two views are taken of the limb at 90° angle. Radiography is essential if an accurate diagnosis is to be made.

FRACTURES

Trauma represents the most frequent cause of wing problems in raptors that are presented at veterinary practices. Howard and Redig (1993) described 542 wild bird fracture cases: 81.5% of the cases had wing fractures. The degree of initial soft tissue damage and the successful management of these tissues during surgical treatment is of significant prognostic importance.

Soft Tissue Wound Management

Swabs for bacterial culture and antibiotic sensitivity should be taken in all cases and before contaminated tissues are irrigated, cleaned and covered with appropriate materials. Until sensitivity results are available, the bird should be treated with a broad-spectrum antibiotic, eg. amoxicillin (150mg/kg i/m or p/o, bid). Three important considerations in wound management are cleaning, closing and covering. These procedures are best carried out with the patient anaesthetised (see Chapter 9). The wound is prepared by plucking or clipping some of the surrounding feathers to expose a 2cm circumference of skin (see Chapter 3). All necrotic material should be removed. The wound should be gently irrigated using warm, sterile saline solution to remove all surface contaminants. In cases where bacterial infections are likely the wound should be lavaged with 1% povidone-iodine in sterile water. In view of the pneumatisation of the humerus, lavage of humeral fractures should be kept to a minimum because of the risk of inhalation or air sacculitis. This procedure may need to be repeated after a few days.

The principles of treating open, severely contaminated wounds where there are large amounts of necrotic material are similar to those employed in mammals (Bojrab, 1981). Wet-to-dry bandaging (warm, saline soaked gauze swabs) are used in the first 3-4 days, with daily changes to encourage debridement and removal of necrotic tissue. Following this, hydroactive dressings, eg. BK Biodress (C-Vet), are applied to encourage epithelialisation and wound contraction whilst at the same time preventing excessive desiccation of the tissues. These dressings may be kept in place by suturing them to the body. Open wounds on the leading edge of the carpus are slow healing and are best treated using this method: in these cases, Granuflex (Squibb) acts additionally as a protective shield against the repetitive trauma experienced as a fractious hawk flies against the sides of its cage.

Paraffin impregnated gauze, although readily available and cheap, may lead to excessive oiling of the plumage and should be avoided.

A variety of topical medicines may be used beneficially. Bacitracin, neomycin and polymyxin may be used in combination and provide a wide spectrum of antibiosis (see Appendix - Formularies). Products containing the basic esters of benzoic acid and para-aminobenzoic acid, eg. benzocaine and lignocaine, are best avoided because of their potentially toxic side effects.

Considerations Prior to Formulating a Surgical Plan for Fracture Repair

Treatment protocols should suit the nature of the injury and facilitate 'normal wing function' postoperatively. Soft tissue injuries and fractures of wild birds which have a good prognosis for complete recovery and a rapid return to the wild should be treated. If this is not possible, injured wild birds should be euthanased. If a wild bird does not recover fully from its injuries, consideration must be given to its rarity and the degree of handicap in order to justify keeping the bird in the hope that it will breed successfully in captivity. It may be humane to consider destroying the more common species unless they can be used for educational purposes (see Flow Chart 3.3 and Chapter 23).

If a falconer's hawk is to continue hunting, the prognosis after surgery must be favourable. However, birds that can be maintained in an aviary for breeding will tolerate substantial loss of wing function. If amputation is considered, it should be noted that male amputees are rarely (if ever) fertile.

Factors Determining Prognosis

There are a number of prognostic factors that should be considered when assessing the likely fracture response to treatment (see Table 17.1).

The fracture site has a bearing on successful healing with normal limb function. Fractures adjacent to joints frequently have concurrent periarticular soft tissue damage; if this is not the case, careful selection of surgical techniques is required to protect these tissues. Similarly, prognosis is influenced by which wing bone or bones are fractured. Table 17.2 highlights the fracture incidence and healing rates of the different wing bones; this helps to predict the likely success and healing rates before attempting fracture repair.

Only 33% of the total number of cases in Howard and Redig's (1993) survey were released back to the wild; significantly fewer (15%) hawks with open contaminated fractures were released compared to the 36% which had closed fractures. From this it would appear that fractures with exposed, devitalised, necrotic or infected bone close to joints, or those with extensive surrounding soft tissue damage, are not likely to heal with functional repair. Birds should only be kept in captivity if they are of value in breeding projects or can be used for educational purposes. In all other cases where injured wild birds cannot be released back to the wild, euthanasia should be recommended.

Applied Physiology and Anatomy

Avian bones are thin and brittle and certain bones are connected to the air sacs (pneumatised bones), eg. humerus, thoracic girdle and certain ribs. Care must be exercised with intraoperative bone handling to prevent iatrogenic fractures. The proximal portions of pneumatised bones should be covered prior to judicious wound irrigation to prevent aspiration, air sacculitis or pneumonia.

Primary and secondary remiges are often attached by fibrous ligaments to the periosteum of the metacarpal and ulnar bones. To prevent periosteal stripping, these feathers should not be removed when preparing the bird's wing for surgery, nor should interremigeal ligaments be damaged.

Table 17.1. Factors affecting fracture treatment prognosis.

Prognosis good	Prognosis guarded	Prognosis poor
Mid-shaft fractures.	Humeral fractures (59% compound). Often associated with fragments of devitalised bone.	'Old', open fractures with devitalised, necrotic or infected bone.
Closed fractures.	Humeral fractures may cause damage to radial or medianoulnar nerve.	Impaired nerve function.
Little soft tissue damage.	Mild infection with good vascularity.	Fractures near to or involving joints. Considerable soft tissue damage.

Table 17.2. Fracture incidence and healing rates of the different wing bones.

Bone	Number of factures	% of cases treated	% of cases healed	% of cases released	Healing time (days)
Humerus	206	39	18	12	34
Ulna	192	66	39	28	37
Radius	133	48	31	14	28
Metacarpal	72	54	33	28	31
Coracoid	28	75	61	53	29

From Howard and Redig (1993).

Fracture Repair Techniques

External Coaptation (Bandages and Splints)

This simple, rapid, inexpensive fracture stabilisation technique should only be considered for primary stabilisation when limited post-recovery range of motion is acceptable, the patient is too small to facilitate surgical correction, there is reasonable stability and good bone alignment, or if the anaesthetic risk is excessive.

Bandages are sometimes used to provide additional support for fractures repaired by other means (see Figure 17.3). These should be removed within three days if at all possible. These birds should then be housed in a dark confined area to reduce wing movement.

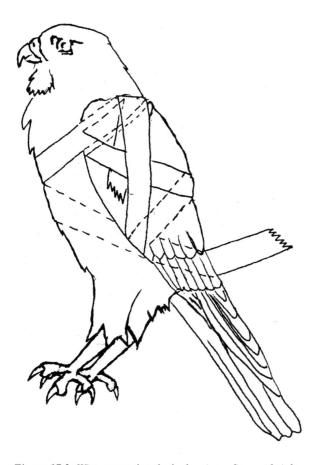

Figure 17.3: Wing secured to the body using a figure-of-eight non-adhesive bandage.

External coaptation is particularly useful for treating mid-shaft radius or ulna fractures where the adjacent bone is intact and acts as a natural splint.

Young chicks under 50g in weight can have wing fractures stabilised by 'glueing' the injured wing in its natural position against the body wall. Albumen is collected from a chicken's egg and used as the 'glue'. After five days the wing is freed by bathing it with warm water and the condition is reassessed. It may be necessary to repeat the procedure for a further five days.

External Fixators

External fixation is regarded as the best stabilisation technique when recovery with a normal range of movement is desired. The equipment is cheap, light, usually well-tolerated, and easily removed. Joints and periarticular structures are preserved postoperatively and immediately function normally. These techniques induce minimal intraoperative soft tissue damage and are particularly suited in corrective osteotomies and comminuted fractures, and to stabilise open fractures while maintaining access for wound management. Birds recover rapidly and have use of the limb within a few days of surgery. Management of the convalescent patient is simple.

Principles of external fixation (see Table 17.3)

● Fixator pins should not be placed through open wounds.

● Avoid large muscle bodies to minimise loosening.

● Avoid nerves and major blood vessels.

● Place three or four pins on either side of the fracture.

● Kirschner pins and hypodermic needles are commonly used as fixator pins. Positive profile threaded pins are useful for larger birds such as eagles as they maintain a stronger bone-pin interface and are more reliable (see Figure 17.4).

● Decrease the risk of fixator slip by placing unthreaded pins at an angle of up to 55° perpendicular to the bone.

● Place connecting bar for fixators as close as possible to skin.

● In addition to Kirschner-Emer clamps, connecting bars can be secured using methylmethacrylate

Table 17.3. External fixator types used to stabilise avian fractures.

Type I fixator.	Half-pin splintage. Pins penetrate one skin surface and both cortices. Weak and loosen rapidly.
Quadrilateral frame type I fixator.	Two half pins placed at 90° to one another. The two connecting bars are secured with a stabilising bar. This technique is particularly useful for correcting humeral fractures (see Figure 17.4).
Type II fixator.	Full-pin splintage. Pins penetrate both skin surfaces and bone cortices.

(Technovit), dental acrylic or araldite. A useful technique is to construct connecting bars with plastic tubes, eg. drinking straw, filled with Technovit. Positioned and aligned fixator pins are passed through the straw. Technovit mixed to the consistency of dough is injected into the straw. Before the material sets the stabilising bar is malleable, so minor malalignments may be corrected. The plastic straw should never be allowed to kink and the diameter of Technovit should equal the diameter of the fractured bone.

Modified type I fixators (see Figure 17.4) offer maximal stability and are particularly useful for treating humeral fractures where a connecting bar (type II fixator) placed on the medial aspect of the wing would cause soft tissue damage. The ends of fixator pins can be bent parallel to the long axis of the bone to increase the strength of and help connect the connecting bar.

Intramedullary Fixation

Although providing adequate alignment and neutralising bending forces, intramedullary fixation on its own does not counteract rotational or shear forces applied to fractures. Even slight malunion can affect the wing's aerofoil and compromise a raptor's hunting ability. Properly placed, normograde or retrograde intramedullary (IM) pins that exit near a joint can injure periarticular tendons and ligaments, significantly reducing joint movement. IM pins and postoperative bandaging should only be considered if the client accepts moderate post-surgical wing function.

Principles of intramedullary fixation.
● IM pins should be large enough to fill one half to two thirds of the medullary cavity.
● Excessively large pins may encourage iatrogenic fractures or damage endosteal blood supply. Stack

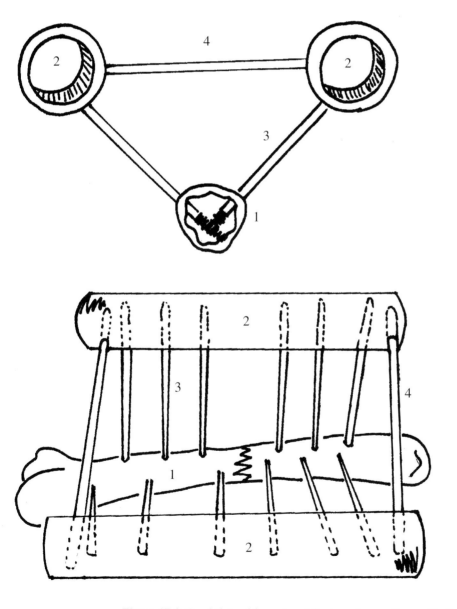

A type I modified biplanar fixator offers maximum stabilisation for humerus or femur fractures. A connecting bar cannot be placed on the medial aspect of either of these bones.

1 Humerus
2 Connecting bars
3 Positive profile
  threaded pin as
  stabilising bars.
4 Cross bar

Figure 17.4: *Quadrilateral frame type I fixator using positive profile threaded pins.*

pinning, cross pinning or Rush-type pinning with several small diameter pins may be considered. This may help prevent postoperative rotation.

● Cerclage wires may be used to counteract shear and rotational forces.

● Intramedullary polymer rods, eg. plastic plunger of a syringe, may be fashioned and used together with external fixators. These are cheap and biologically inert and need not be removed after fracture healing. Birds show rapid post-surgical recovery and are often flying within 14 days. The rods are inserted using a shuttle technique (see Figure 17.5) which may limit the rod length and may not provide adequate stability. External fixation must always be used simultaneously.

● Methylmethacrylate injected into the medullary cavity, together with an implant to aid fracture stabilisation, has been described (Ritchie, 1994). The damage to endosteal blood supply, the loss of endosteal callus and the intramedullary bone necrosis thought to occur does not appear to inhibit bone union. The technique is contraindicated in cases where infectious agents are likely to occur and non-union results if the polymer leaks along the fracture line.

Bone Plates
Bone plates are used infrequently because of the the the thin cortices associated with avian osteology, the relative lack of soft tissues and the degree of technical difficulty.

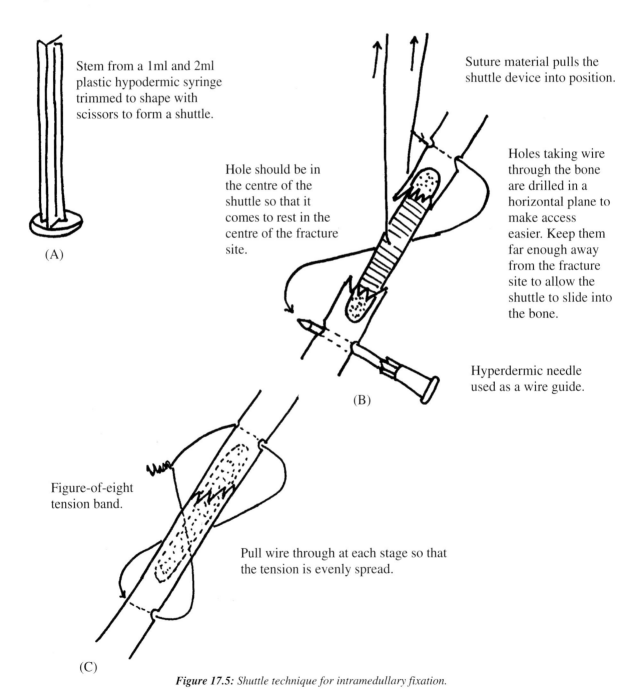

Stem from a 1ml and 2ml plastic hypodermic syringe trimmed to shape with scissors to form a shuttle.

(A)

Hole should be in the centre of the shuttle so that it comes to rest in the centre of the fracture site.

Suture material pulls the shuttle device into position.

Holes taking wire through the bone are drilled in a horizontal plane to make access easier. Keep them far enough away from the fracture site to allow the shuttle to slide into the bone.

Hyperdermic needle used as a wire guide.

(B)

Figure-of-eight tension band.

Pull wire through at each stage so that the tension is evenly spread.

(C)

Figure 17.5: Shuttle technique for intramedullary fixation.

MANAGEMENT OF SPECIFIC INJURIES

Shoulder

Radiography is essential in any investigation of shoulder injuries. Comparative radiographs of both shoulders in the same position simplifies interpretation. Three bones (scapula, clavicle and coracoid) make up the pectoral girdle. The clavicles are fused to form the furcula or 'wish bone'. The tendon of the supracoracoideus muscle passes through the foramen triosseum where these three bones meet. Concussion injuries, caused when raptors fly into solid stationary objects or heavy quarry, frequently result in fractures, rupture of the supracoracoideus tendon and periarticular ligament damage. Fracture of the humeral head and dislocations occasionally occur.

Rupture of the supracoracoideus tendon causes dorsal subluxation of the humeral head and a typical wing carriage. The surgical approach is not challenging; if a bird is presented for treatment within four hours of sustaining injury, surgery should be considered. The tendon is sutured using 2\0 polypropylene, nylon or PDS, with a swaged, round-bodied needle. The wing should be immobilised with a figure-of-eight bandage for two weeks followed by confined cage rest (not loose in an aviary) for eight weeks.

The coracoid is the most frequently fractured bone in the pectoral girdle, where the presence of the supracoracoideus muscle limits surgical access and stabilisation. If significant displacement of bone fragments is evident, referral should be considered (Martin and Ritchie, 1994). In other cases, conservative treatment involving cage rest for 14-21 days is indicated. The cage rest should allow the bird to flex and extend its wings but not flap vigorously. Similar treatment should be applied to other pectoral girdle fractures and periarticular ligament damage management.

Humerus

Fractures normally occur in the mid-shaft or distal third of the humerus. The proximal segment rotates medially due to action of the pectoralis muscle, lacerating the skin and resulting in a compound fracture dorsally (in 59% cases). The distal fragment is frequently sharp and may puncture the skin ventrally. Gross wound contamination encourages osteomyelitis and delays or prevents wound healing. Swabs from the fracture site must be taken for bacteriology and sensitivity. All necrotic tissue and bone should be debrided before stabilising the fractures. Most birds can lose up to 25% of their wing length, yet learn to adapt and fly adequately. Specialist hunters such as the Peregrine Falcon require agility and near perfect recovery to hunt successfully. Buzzards, which soar on thermals, can tolerate greater deformities yet still forage successfully for food. Surgical fixation is required to stabilise humeral fractures if good postoperative recovery is required.

Surgical Approach

The dorsal approach is preferred for most aspects of the humerus, thus avoiding the basilic vein and the brachial artery, as well as the medianoulnar nerve. The bird is anaesthetised and placed in sternal recumbency. The radial nerve can often be identified prior to making a careful incision dorsocaudally from the proximal third of the humerus to the ventral epicondyle. The radial nerve in the mid-humeral section should be retracted. The humerus is covered by the biceps brachii and deltoideus muscles proximally but lies beneath the skin distally (see Figure 17.6).

External fixators (Type I used in combination with shuttle pins, or Modified type I - see Figure 17.4) are preferred for compound fractures and free-ranging birds. Shuttle pins used on their own give poor stability, particularly if fractures are close to joints and the bone fragment is short.

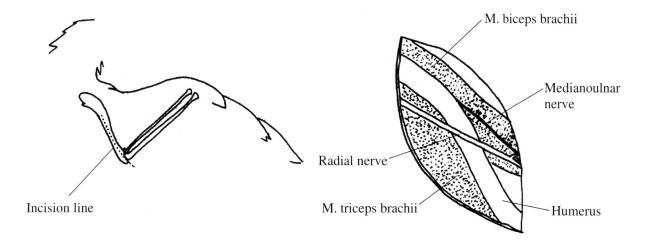

M. biceps brachii

Medianoulnar nerve

Radial nerve

M. triceps brachii

Humerus

Incision line

Figure 17.6: Dorsal approach to the mid-humerus region.

When using intramedullary fixation, the curved humeral shaft and the relatively large diameter of the medullary cavities encountered in avian bones greatly increases the risk of rotation if only one Steinman pin is used. It is better to stack several narrow Steinman pins or Kirschner wires within the medullary cavity. The pins are introduced through the fracture site, advanced proximally out through the humeral crest of the proximal fragment and then retrograded into the distal fragment (Redig, 1993). Full or hemi-cerclage wires may be used in addition to stabilise fractures (see Chapter 16).

Postoperative coaptation should be restricted to five days if combined with intramedullary stabilisation techniques. Coaptation for longer periods frequently compromises wing function. Conservative cage rest management of these cases is similar to that described under shoulder injuries.

Propatagium

The propatagium, lying in the cranial angle of the elbow and running from the lateral thoracic wall to the carpus, is a delicate, vulnerable structure. Damage to the propatagium (feathers or soft tissues) interferes with the wing's ability to produce aerodynamic lift. An understanding of the anatomy of the propatagium is essential when assessing the prognosis and initiating surgical repair.

The dermal, collagenous and elastic ligaments (see Figure 17.7) receive their vascular supply from the radial artery and branches from the subscapular artery and vein running caudal to the *ligamentum propatagiale*. Injuries to the propatagium which present with severe bruising and soft tissue damage, but with no apparent lacerations, may still result in tissue breakdown due to vascular damage and avascular necrosis of the *ligamentum propatagiale*.

Propatagial injuries should be corrected with the wing in an extended, ie. flying, position. There is no 'spare' dermal tissue available to consider incorporating skin grafts in an attempt to correct dermal lacerations. Repairs that reduce the size of the propatagium are likely to fail even after lengthy healing periods. It is important that the supporting collagenous ligament structures are retrieved and individually repaired.

Dissection between the dermal layers of the propatagium must always begin with an incision through the ventral skin surface (hence avoiding the feather tracts of the dorsal surface) and worked cranially.

Radius and Ulna

Elbow joint luxation is a common injury, often compound and with a very poor prognosis. There is very little collateral muscle support and the joint capsule is weak. Ruptured ligaments repair slowly and protracted joint immobilisation after reduction inevitably results in fibrosis and severe loss of joint mobility. The elbow joint is immobilised by strapping it to the body or by using external fixators anchored in the humerus and ulna. These support bars are then stabilised with connecting bars (see Figure 17.8).

Often, fractures of the radius do not involve the ulna. In these cases the affected wing may be strapped to the body using a figure-of-eight bandage (see Figure 17.3). The dressing is left on for 10 days followed by conservative management as described for shoulder injuries. Some cases may be managed without dressing by keeping the bird restrained in a small cage so that it is unable to flap its wings. In some species (especially Northern Sparrow Hawks) the avoidance of strapping is advantageous.

When both the radius and ulna are fractured, stabilisation of the ulna fracture with an external fixator

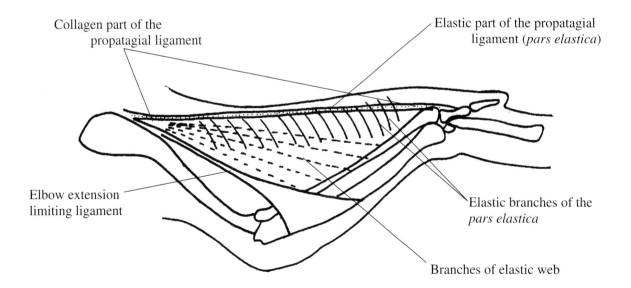

Figure 17.7: Supporting structures of the propatagium.

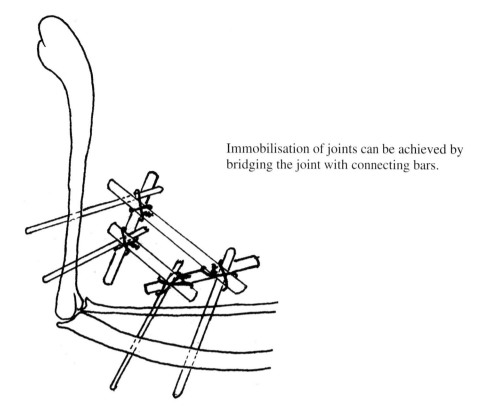

Immobilisation of joints can be achieved by bridging the joint with connecting bars.

Figure 17.8: External fixation used to stabilise luxation of the elbow joint.

(with or without an intramedullary device) is regarded as being adequate. If an intramedullary pin is used, it may be introduced blind from the caudolateral surface of the proximal ulna at the level of the second or third from last secondary feather, just distal to the elbow. The elbow and carpal joints are unaffected by this technique and move freely while healing occurs. Surgical access to the ulna is through a dorsal incision just cranial to the insertion point of the secondary feathers. The deep radial artery and deep radial nerve, which lie in tissue between the radius and ulna, should be preserved. To approach the radius separately, a dorsal incision is made over the radius between the *m. extensor carpi radialis* anteriorly and the *m. extensor digitorum communis* posteriorly. For minimally displaced mid-shaft fractures, external coaptation may be adequate if compromised elbow and carpal range of motion is not an issue.

Carpometacarpus

Carpal wounds are frequently encountered where fractious hawks injure the leading edge of the carpus by flying into the side of their cages or bating whilst tethered on a perch. The wound is open and tendons are often exposed. The wound should be swabbed for bacteriology and antibiotic sensitivity, closed with 3\0 monofilament nylon or catgut, and protected by suturing a pad of Granuflex over the wound.

Carpal wounds should not be confused with **carpal bursitis** (which falconers refer to as 'Blaine') where

tethered hawks, connected by a leash to a perch, inflame the carpal tendon sheaths by knocking the carpus against the ground as they attempt to fly from their perch. Cytology from the carpal bursa reveals a modified transudate. Secondary infection is often confirmed by the presence of heterophils. Treatment includes corrective husbandry, collecting samples for bacteriology and sensitivity, joint irrigation and appropriate antibiotic treatment.

Carpal luxations are best stabilised with external fixators. Postoperative fibrosis and loss of joint mobility means these injuries carry a poor prognosis for free-ranging birds.

Carpometacarpal fractures are best stabilised with small, light external fixators. Surgical correction of metacarpal fractures are largely unrewarding. In this area, damage to the vascular supply frequently occurs and the wing tip is often lost. The fractures are stabilised by introducing an intramedullary pin (blind) or strapping the bird's wing to its body.

OTHER DISEASES

Specific Infectious Diseases

Although uncommon, fungal (*Aspergillus fumigatus*) and yeast (*Candida albicans*) infections of the skin may be associated with wing cases which are persistent and unresponsive to antibiotic therapy. Cutaneous aspergillosis or candidiasis should be treated by daily debridement of the lesion and topical application of enilconazole (1:10 dilution) with or without parental therapy (see Chapter 14).

Infection of the clavicular air sac with aspergillosis, bacterial infection or a foreign body reaction should be considered as a differential diagnosis in a lame bird with no apparent skeletal defect.

Septic arthritis, often caused by *Salmonella typhimurium*, is occasionally encountered. The route of infection is haematogenous. Any number of joints may be involved. They are severely swollen and contain a caseous, purulent, inflammatory exudate. Adult or juvenile birds may be affected; cases often show concurrent hepatomegaly. An attempt should be made to culture pathogens from the joint. An indwelling catheter and daily flushing of the joint with saline followed by tobramycin or linocomycin may be of assistance, but the prognosis is grave.

Carpal and elbow joint synovitis caused by *Mycobacterium avium* may be encountered. The condition carries a poor prognosis and the birds should be euthanased because of the zoonotic implications and the risk of exposing other birds in the collection to infection (see Chapter 19).

Degenerative Diseases

Osteoarthritis is rarely encountered in birds and is usually restricted to those which have sustained earlier injuries. Salicylic acid and other non-steroidal anti-inflammatories, eg. ketoprofen (1mg/kg sid) or flunixin (1-10mg/kg sid), have been used with variable success.

Circulatory Diseases

Wing Tip Oedema and Dry Gangrene Syndrome

This syndrome has been recognised in raptors for many years, but the incidence has increased greatly in the period 1989-1996. The disease is characterised by a sudden, cold, wet pitting oedema of one or both wing tips (see Figure 17.9). The swelling, comprised of a sterile clear transudate, forms around the insertion points of the distal primary feathers and extends proximally. Occasionally, the owner may not recognise the initial oedematous stage, only becoming aware of the condition when one or both wing tips fall off. Some cases have demonstrated concurrent areas of avascular necrosis on the feet.

The swelling gradually subsides. However, the wing tip often darkens, becoming dry and wrinkled before dropping off some six weeks after the initial insult. The portion of wing tip lost often includes the dermal papilla of the distal primaries. Those which regrow are often loosely secured to the wing and usually fall out. Species originating from warmer climates appear more frequently affected, but the condition has been seen in most raptors.

The precise aetiology of the syndrome is not fully understood. The disease has a seasonal distribution with all cases occurring between October and April in association with cold weather. Birds attached to perches at ground level are affected more commonly compared with those loose in aviaries. The peripheral vasculature appears to be compromised with this condition and tissue loss is possibly due to avascular necrosis.

This condition is readily differentiated from all other conditions affecting the distal wing. The condition has been erroneously confused with 'blaine', which affects the carpal joint (see Carpometacarpus).

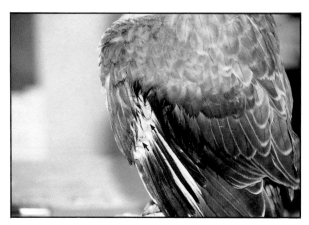

Figure 17.9: *Acute phase of wing tip oedema. Note the swollen oedematous subcutaneous area, showing as blister-like protrusions at the base of each primary feather (arrows).*

Treatment. Treatment in the acute oedematous phase consists of warming the bird and improving peripheral perfusion by massaging the wings. The bird should continue flying throughout the course of therapy. Laser therapy can be used to assist tissue recovery. Medication includes corticosteroids, prophylactic antibiotics to guard against associated bacterial vegetative endocarditis and enteritis, and vascular stimulants, eg. isoxoprine (5-10mg/kg p/o sid for 20-40 days) or propentofylline (5mg/kg p/o bid for 20-40 days). Topical vascular stimulants, eg. Preparation H (Whitehall Laboratories), have been used with apparent success, although it must be applied sparingly to avoid oiling and damage to the bird's plumage. Treatment if initiated during the chronic phase is the same, but the prognosis is poor as loss of the distal portion of the wing is common.

Control. The condition is best prevented by leaving birds loose in sheltered aviaries or housing them inside in a heated mews during the colder months of the year.

Metabolic Diseases

Nutritional hyperparathyroidism (rickets) is now relatively rare in captive-bred raptors. It occurs occasionally in young birds, particularly in the first three weeks of life, when there is a Ca:P:vitamin D_3 imbalance (see Chapters 13 and 16). Affected birds are unable to stand and they have lateral bowing of their legs with numerous folding fractures; however, the wings can be affected, though less commonly. In all cases, whole body radiography must be undertaken so that the full situation can be evaluated (see Chapter 10).

Neoplasia

Neoplasia is uncommon in raptors. However, one of the commonest tumours encountered is **spindle cell tumour** of the distal wing. These appear as firm discrete masses, or diffuse thickenings of the metacarpal area if detected early. The growths can be removed by careful dissection, but more often part of the wing tip requires amputation. Recurrence or metastasis has not been reported.

REFERENCES AND FURTHER READING

Bojrab MJ (1981) *A Handbook on Veterinary Wound Management*. Kendall, Massachusetts.

Bush M (1981) Avian fracture repair using external fixation. In: *Recent Advances in the Study of Raptor Diseases*. Eds JE Cooper and AG Geenwood. Chiron Publications, Keighley.

Cooper JE (1976) *Veterinary Aspects of Captive Birds of Prey*. Standfast Press, Saul.

Coles BH (1985) *Avian Medicine and Surgery*. Blackwell Scientific Publications, Oxford.

Forbes NA (1991) Wing tip oedema and dry gangrene in birds. *Veterinary Record* **129**, 3, 58.

Howard DJ and Redig PT (1993) Analysis of avian fracture repairs: implications for captive and wild birds. In: *Proceedings of the Association of Avian Veterinarians Annual Conference 1993*. AAV, Lake Worth.

MacCoy DM (1983) High density polymer rods as an intramedullary fixation devise in birds. *Journal of the American Animal Hospital Association* **19**, 767.

Martin HD, Ringdahl RPT and Scherpelz J (1993) Physical therapy for specific injuries in raptors. In: *Raptor Biomedicine*. Eds PT Redig, JE Cooper, JD Remple and DB Hunter. University of Minnesota Press, Minneapolis.

Martin HD, Bruecker KA, Herrick DD and Scherpelz J (1993) Elbow luxation in raptors. In: *Raptor Biomedicine*. Eds PT Redig, JE Cooper, JD Remple and DB Hunter. University of Minnesota Press, Minneapolis.

Martin HD and Ritchie BW (1994) Orthopedic surgical techniques. In: *Avian Medicine: Principles and Application*. Eds BW Ritchie, GJ Harrison and LR Harrison. Wingers, Lake Worth.

Redig PT (1981) A clinical review of orthopedic techniques used in the rehabilitation of raptors. In: *Proceedings of the American Federation of Aviculturalists, San Diego, 1981*. WB Saunders, Philadelphia.

Redig PT (1986) Basic orthopedic surgical techniques. In: *Clinical Avian Medicine and Surgery, including Aviculture*. Eds GJ Harrison and LR Harrison. WB Saunders, Philadelphia.

Redig PT, Lind PJ and Degernes L (1990) Of wires, bone cement and hexcelite in the repair of avian fractures. In: *Proceedings of the Association of Avian Veterinarians Annual Conference 1990*. AAV, Lake Worth.

Redig PT (1993) A clinical review of orthopedic techniques used in the rehabilitation of raptors. In: *Zoo and Wild Animal Medicine*. Ed ME Fowler. WB Saunders, Philadelphia.

Redig PT, Howard D and Talbot B (1993) Of pins, wires, bone cement and hexcelite for the repair of avian fractures. In: *Proceedings of the Association of Avian Veterinarians Annual Conference 1993 (Guide to Practical Laboratories)*. AAV, Lake Worth.

Sattersfield W and O'Rourke KI (1981) External fixation in avian orthopedics using a modified through and through Kirschner-Emer splint technique (The Boston Technique). *Journal of the American Animal Hospital Association* **17**, 635.

Scott C (1968) Intramedullary fixation of a fractured humerus in a wild owl. *Canadian Veterinary Journal* **9**, 98.

CHAPTER EIGHTEEN

Respiratory Problems

Neil A Forbes

INTRODUCTION

Successful treatment of respiratory disease in raptors is directly related to the speed at which an owner notices a problem and presents the bird to the clinician, who in turn makes a specific diagnosis and instigates therapy. However, in contrast to many other organ systems a provisional diagnosis can be made before the bird is examined clinically by simple visual and aural observation from a short distance.

At rest, respiratory effort should not be evident and the mouth should remain closed. Respiratory disease commonly causes excessive chest movement, nasal discharge, head or tail bobbing - frequently with mouth breathing rather than nasal breathing - abduction of the wings from the body, neck stretching, coughing, alteration of voice or, on occasions, vomition. Birds must if possible be observed for these signs prior to handling. The resting respiratory rate should be compared with the expected normal rate for birds of that weight (see Table 18.1). The presenting signs are determined by the cause and the site of the pathology.

In raptors it is relatively easy to differentiate between upper respiratory tract (URT) (nares and sinuses) and lower respiratory tract (LRT) (trachea, lung and air sacs) conditions.

UPPER RESPIRATORY TRACT

The upper respiratory tract may be divided into the following functional regions: the naris, the vestibular region, the respiratory region and the olfactory region.

The centre of the naris is occupied by the rostral nasal concha, a hard, fibrous raised structure which should be dry, smooth and shiny. Exudate often builds around the rostral nasal concha thus blocking the nares. The exudate should be removed with a fine blunt instrument (prior to the cause of the exudate being treated).

The vestibular region has a vital function in warming and hydration of inspired air. The most important baffling and warming structure is the rostral nasal concha. The two sides of the nasal passage are separated by the nasal septum. Young Falconiformes have a fontanelle between the two sides; this closes early in life. The main source of moisture is the nasal gland whose duct is situated on the medial aspect of the rostral nasal concha, discharging to form a shallow reservoir. The function of the gland is to produce fluid and hydrate inspired air. The vestibular region is separated from the respiratory region by the nasal crest, which is particularly steep in Falconiformes. Mucus is produced within the respiratory region. This is essential for olfaction, respiration and prevention of infection in the LRT. The mucus is moved by the action of cilia at a rate of 10mm/minute. The middle concha is situated in the respiratory region, as is the nasolacrimal duct and the aperture of the infraorbital sinus, which is of considerable clinical importance.

Birds with URT disease are frequently presented with stained or matted feathers around the nares, sneezing, head flicking, mouth breathing or an audible inspiratory and expiratory noise; the latter noise ceases if the mouth is opened. Frequently, there will be an

Table 18.1. Normal resting respiratory rates in birds.

Weight of bird (g)	Respiratory rate (per minute)
100	40-52
200	35-50
300	30-45
400	25-30
500	20-30
1000	15-20

Harrison and Ritchie (1994).

oculonasal discharge, blockage of the nares, excessive movement of, or abnormal depression of, the skin overlying the infraorbital sinus, or swellings in the periorbital area. The complex nature of the sinus system is demonstrated in the contrast radiographs in Figures 18.1.1, 18.1.2 and 18.1.3. Each part of the respiratory system must be examined methodically.

The external appearance of the nares is often indicative of URT conditions. Rhinoliths are frequently present, and are typically related to bacterial, myco-

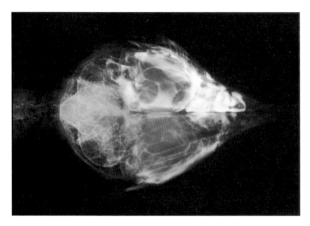

Figure 18.1.1: Contrast radiograph of the sinus structure of a normal Northern Goshawk - dorsoventral view.

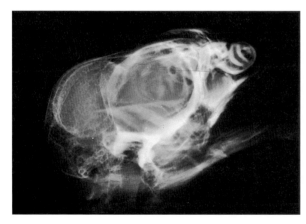

Figure 18.1.2: Lateral view.

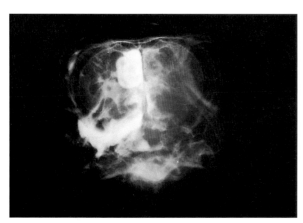

Figure 18.1.3: Craniocaudal view.

plasmal, fungal or viral infection. Severe infections with avipoxvirus or *Cnemidocoptes* spp. (see Chapter 15) can lead to marked proliferation of the cere with resultant occlusion of the nares. Falcon pox (one serotype of avipoxvirus) is not currently present in the UK, although severe disease is encountered in warmer climates, such as the Gulf States. The value of using fowl or pigeon pox vaccines is disputed by workers familiar with the condition. Birds incubating the disease at the time of vaccination will rapidly develop severe clinical signs. In the UK, raptors will occasionally be presented with very minor pox lesions. These are caused by non-falcon serotypes of avipoxvirus and typically resolve in a few days.

The sinuses are entered from the respiratory region, between the middle and caudal concha. Significantly, the entry points into the sinuses are at rostral level. Infection may enter the sinuses, and infection, cellular debris and mucoid secretion from the glands in the sinuses fills the sinuses with fluid. Because of the level of the entry points, the fluid is often unable to drain away. It has been lack of drainage, with the resultant reservoir of infected debris, which has previously rendered sinus infections difficult to treat. As can be seen from Figure 18.1, the interconnection of the nasal chambers and sinuses of either side, together with the multiple ramifications of the infraorbital sinus, mean that if the sinuses become infected, many of the surrounding structures of the head may also be affected. Therefore, sinusitis may present as a persistent unilateral or bilateral ocular discharge. The level of tissue destruction is dependent on the ability or propensity of the pathogen involved to cause lysis. Tissue destruction can also be a consequence of pressure necrosis caused by the production of inspissated caseous material.

Diagnosis

The presence of URT infection is easily recognised. The exact site and nature of the infection may be diagnosed by endoscopy of the choanal slit and the vestibular region (in larger species), by detailed radiography of the nasal chambers and sinuses, and by swabs and aspirates from the nares, choana or sinuses. Culture and sensitivity testing should be carried out. The normal flora of the choana should be predominantly Gram-positive, eg. *Staphylococcus* spp. and *Streptococcus* spp., with less than 10% Gram-negative (Ritchie and Gerlach, 1981) and few fungal hyphae. Fungal infections of the URT are very rarely seen in raptors. The normal cytology of the nasal and infraorbital sinuses reveals occasional non-cornified squamous epithelial cells with low levels of extracellular bacteria and debris (Campbell, 1994). Cytological evidence of sinusitis is denoted by the presence of inflammatory cells in the aspirate. If bacterial infection is present, septic, heterophilic or mixed cell inflammation will be evident. Mycotic infections will typically be demonstrated by mixed cell or macrophagic inflammation together with fungal hyphae or spores. *Mycoplasma* spp. have been frequently implicated in URT infection, although authenticated cases are rare. This may be due to difficulty in culturing these organisms. *Mycoplasma* spp. respond well to tetracyclines, tylosin, spectinomycin or enrofloxacin. *Chlamydia psittaci*, although not common in raptors, should always be eliminated as a cause of conjunctivitis or URT.

Treatment

Parenteral therapy may be required for organisms such as *Pseudomonas* spp. However, sinus flushing or intrasinus injections of antibiotics are invariably essential. In the absence of microbiological testing the author favours the use of enrofloxacin in saline (0.75ml of 5% Injection in 20ml of saline for a 1kg bird). Birds should be held upside down (to enable the more distant diverticulae of the sinus to be penetrated), the syringe nozzle (without a needle) held tight against the nares (the mouth should not be held closed) and the total contents of the syringe evacuated forcibly through the nasal chambers. Treatment is continued daily for ten days. The technique is simple and may be easily demonstrated to the owner to carry out at home.

White caseous or necrotic lesions may be found in the nasal chambers, in the area of the choana or in the oropharynx. These may be caused by *Trichomonas* spp. (usually contracted by eating fresh pigeon), certain bacteria, *Candida* spp. or *Capillaria* spp. Swabs must be taken, a definitive diagnosis made and appropriate therapy instigated. Trichomoniasis is treated with carnidazole or metronidazole; candidiasis with flucytosine, itraconazole or nystatin. Capillariasis is treated with fenbendazole (25mg/kg p/o daily for five days) (ivermectin and single doses of fenbendazole are ineffective against *Capillaria* spp.). When debriding oral or nasal abscesses, care should be taken to avoid causing severe haemorrhage. Chemical cautery (silver nitrate or ferric sulphate) and/or electrosurgical equipment should be available. In raptors, opening or trephination of sinuses is rarely necessary. Very occasionally, nasal aspergillomata occur. In these cases the author favours identification of the site, removal of the lesion and placement of an indwelling catheter. Therapy is continued with parenteral and topical medication (see later).

LOWER RESPIRATORY TRACT

Most species of birds have four paired and two non-paired air sacs. Inspired air passes down the trachea, through the lung field via the intrapulmonary primary bronchi and through the neopulmonic parabronchi to the caudal air sacs (see Figures 18.2.1, 18.2.2). The neopulmonic part of the lung possesses a highly efficient and active scavenging system. Any inspired particulate matter is usually removed at this point. The caudal air sacs comprise the abdominal and caudal thoracic air sacs. No gaseous absorption occurs in the air sacs; they act as a bellows system. (See Chapter 9 for more detailed respiratory physiology).

Trachea and Primary Bronchi

The trachea commences at the glottis, which is the slit-like opening in the posterior segment of the tongue. The glottis is not protected by a soft palate, but closes when the bird swallows. The vocal apparatus is located at the bifurcation of the primary bronchi (syrinx) and not at the larynx as in mammals, although the larynx will modify sounds in birds. The avian (raptor)

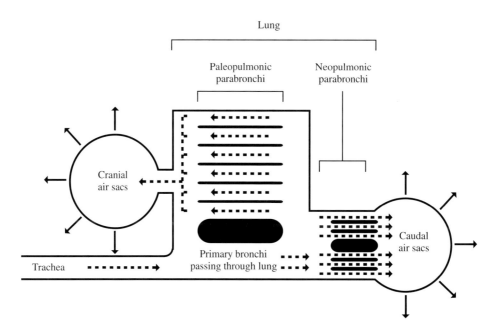

Figure 18.2.1: Schematic diagram of the LRT during inspiration (after Fedde, 1993).

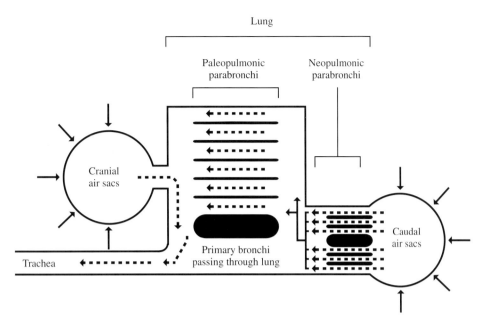

Figure 18.2.2: Schematic diagram of the LRT during expiration (after Fedde, 1993).

trachea differs in two main respects from mammals: firstly, the tracheal rings are complete; and secondly, the tracheal length and diameter are comparatively greater and often longer.

Diseases of the trachea and primary bronchi are varied and differential diagnosis provides one of the most important and potentially rewarding challenges of avian practice. Clinical signs will include loss or change of voice, coughing, rasping or rattling inspiration and/or expiration, and dyspnoea. The significant clinical diseases affecting the trachea are parasitic, bacterial and fungal diseases.

Parasitic Diseases of the Trachea

Syngamus trachea is a common parasite, particularly in members of the buzzard group. A retrospective study of 18 cases by the author showed that 14 involved members of the buzzard group. The life cycle of the parasite is either direct or the parasite may utilise a paratenic ('transfer') host, eg. earthworms, snails, slugs, flies and other arthropods. The staple winter diet of the Eurasian Buzzard is predominantly earthworms, slugs, snails and other invertebrates (Kenward, personal communication). Other buzzard species are thought to utilise similar diets, hence the increased incidence in these species. The parasite may live in the paratenic hosts for months or years. Passage via earthworms renders the parasite more infective to the main host (Morgan and Clapham, 1934). After ingestion, the larvae pass via the bloodstream into the lungs within six hours and from there they pass into the trachea. Faecal ova may be present 17-21 days after ingestion of ova.

Bacterial Diseases of the Trachea

The commonest respiratory bacterial pathogens isolated from raptors are *Klebsiella pneumonia*, *Pseudomonas aeruginosa* and *Pasteurella multocida*. Other organisms, such as *Yersinia pseudotuberculosis*, *Escherichia coli*, *Streptococcus* spp. and *Staphylococcus* spp., have also been implicated on occasions. *Mycoplasma* spp. have frequently been incriminated, but due to the difficulty in recovering these pathogens, there are few authenticated cases. Although the clinical signs are similar to those seen with parasitic infestation, a mucopurulent exudate may be seen in the trachea or the trachea may be excessively erythematous with copious mucoid discharge. If bacterial infection is suspected, aspirates or tracheal swabs should be taken, impressions smears examined and isolation and sensitivity testing performed.

Fungal Diseases of the Trachea

Aspergillus fumigatus infection may occur after a bird has been kept in a spore-rich environment, eg. birds kept close to rotting or decaying vegetable material (Forbes, 1991). However, because of the ubiquitous nature of the organism, it is possible for birds to inspire *A. fumigatus* spores in most environments. Clinical disease is precipitated under conditions of immune supression or incompetence.

A number of species, eg. Golden Eagle, Great Sparrow Hawk, Gyr Falcon, Snowy Owl and Northern Goshawk, appear to be very much more susceptible to aspergillosis. If any of these species are kept in a potentially contaminated or stressful situation, prophylactic therapy is justifiable (Forbes, 1992). Furthermore, every effort should be made to ensure that the environmental *A. fumigatus* loading is minimised. Aspergillosis is not transmissable between birds. Birds should be kept distant from all forms of rotting or decaying vegetable matter, eg. shredded bark, compost, hay, etc.; poorly stored, mouldy travelling boxes can be a significant source of *Aspergillus* spp.

Clinical disease is most commonly seen following an episode of stress, eg. transport, mixing of groups, isolation of gregarious birds, etc. In birds being trained (often a stressful process), owners often state that the bird is not reacting as quickly as expected. Despite a good appetite, affected birds show a marked weight loss. In the chronic form the bird's condition will sometimes decline, due to extensive granulomata formation in the air sacs (see Figures 18.3.1, 18.3.2), but in fact the bodyweight remains constant. In the tracheal/syringeal form, where an aspergilloma obliterates one or both primary bronchi at the level of the syrinx, there is often a change in voice. Other forms will present with vomiting, lethargy, a drooping wing or, occasionally, respiratory signs. In some cases, polydipsia and polyuria are also present. Clinical signs are dictated by the part of the respiratory system in which the lesion is situated. A good resumé of clinical findings and diagnostic techniques is given by Redig (1980).

Diagnosis of Tracheal Diseases

Faecal examination should be carried out for the ova of *S. trachea* or *Cyathostoma* spp. (gapeworms);

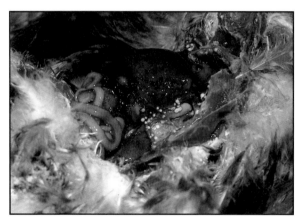

Figure 18.3.1: Acute multifocal aspergillosis in a Red-tailed Hawk.

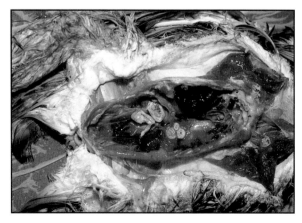

Figure 18.3.2: Five more chronic air sac lesions in a Northern Goshawk.

a positive diagnosis is significant, although a negative result is not definitive. If the result is negative, but the clinical signs are suggestive of tracheal disease, it is imperative that the trachea is swabbed for bacteriology prior to endoscopic examination.

Tracheal swabs can be taken in a conscious raptor by using a fine swab, eg. an ear, nose and throat (ENT) or clittoral swab, which may be passed through the glottis and need not enter further than the proximal 2cm of the trachea. Tracheal washes may be carried out by one of two methods. If the bird is severely dyspnoeic, it should be anaesthetised and an air sac breathing tube placed in the caudal abdominal air sac (see Chapter 9). In the first method a sterile endotracheal tube is placed in the trachea and a plastic respiratory (or male dog) catheter is passed through the tube to the level of the syrinx (just caudal to the thoracic inlet). Sterile saline (0.5-1ml/kg bodyweight) is introduced and then withdrawn. In the second method an 18-22G plastic catheter is introduced through the skin and into the trachea in the caudal cervical area and advanced to the level of the syrinx. This method may occasionally be carried out in a conscious bird. The bird is held horizontally and the sample aspirated. The author favours the first method as tracheal endoscopy, which requires general anaesthesia, can be carried out at the same time. The tracheal wash sample in a normal bird should have a low cellular content with minimal or no macrophages or inflammatory cells. An increase in heterophils, macrophages or other inflammatory cells is clinically significant. In bacterial conditions, bacterial phagocytosis will be evident. In fungal infections, characteristic thick septate hyphae that branch at 45° will be seen (Campbell, 1994).

Radiography may help diagnosis and may reveal the presence of aspergillomata at the syrinx. However, careful, experienced interpretation of the radiographs is required in view of the interspecies variation in normal shape and size of the syrinx (from Pygmy Falcon to Andean Condor).

Endoscopy is the most useful aid to diagnosis. The trachea should be examined for *S. trachea*, the degree of inflammation, hyperaemia and the presence of excessive mucoid secretion. Collection of aspirates and, most importantly, full visualisation of the trachea and syrinx is easily and confidently achieved with endoscopy.

Treatment of Tracheal Diseases

An accurate and specific diagnosis is important when assessing the therapy and progress of a respiratory case. Treatment of *S. trachea* involves the use of an anthelmintic (fenbendazole or ivermectin); the initial dose is usually repeated after 7-10 days. Following anthelmintic therapy, a quantity of dead worms (the females being up to 2cm in length) may be found in the trachea and primary bronchi. These may cause a foreign body pneumonia, so clinical signs will not disappear (for up to six weeks) despite the fact that the primary pathogen has been effectively treated. Birds should be maintained on parenteral or droplet antibiotic therapy, eg. gentamicin, for the duration of clinical signs. Therapeutic protocols for parasitic, bacterial and fungal diseases of the trachea are shown in Table 18.2.

Nebulisation

Nebulisation has been thought of as being complicated and requiring expensive equipment. It is now within the financial reach of any avian practice, most bird breeders and many general veterinary practices. Human nebulisers as used by asthmatics are suitable for birds; they are stocked and are usually available for sale from general human hospitals or from hospital suppliers (cost approximately £100). Nebulisers are run off mains electricity or a car battery. Nebulisation is typically used for 15-20 minutes 4-5 times daily. If particle size as low as 0.3 microns can be achieved, medication can reach the lungs and parts of the air sac system. Drugs such as amphotericin B, gentamicin, polymixin B and tylosin have been shown to be poorly absorbed from the respiratory system. However, they are highly effective at a local level. It is possible to use potentially toxic drugs, eg. gentamicin, which are highly effective, in confidence and safety. Suitable drugs and dose rates are shown in Table 18.3.

The bird is confined in a cage or night quarter and the door is covered with a towel or sheet of perspex. The medication is placed in the administration chamber, which is placed in an upright position within the cage. Nebulisation can be easily carried out without any stress or handling of the patient, and can be of benefit in sick dyspnoeic birds.

Intratracheal medication

All the drugs listed in Table 18.3 can also be used by the intratracheal route. Intratracheal medication can be easily accomplished in conscious raptors. Medication is given with a 1ml syringe with a blunt needle attached; the drug is administered into the trachea via the glottis. A volume of 0.5ml can be administered to a 1kg bird without causing respiratory embarrassment.

Surgical Conditions of the Trachea

Traumatic injuries to the trachea occur occasionally. Often, these injuries are because of 'crabbing' (claw attack) by other raptors. Punctures, lacerations or avulsions of the trachea may occur. The primary action is to maintain a respiratory airway; this is often best achieved by placing an abdominal air sac breathing tube (see Chapter 9). Reconstructive surgery can then be attempted.

Devoicing

The commonest form of tracheal surgery which is requested is devoicing of imprinted birds (screamers). In the UK this procedure is considered by the Royal College of Veterinary Surgeons (RCVS) to be an unnecessary mutilation and as such is an unethical procedure which may not be carried out under any circumstances by an MRCVS. The latter fact is not listed in the 1993 RCVS Guide to Professional Conduct, although it appeared in the 1986 Mutilations Report, under category c, which was fully endorsed by RCVS Council in 1986. Some clinicians may be ignorant of these details, although they are relevant and should be adhered to. (Devoicing is accomplished by exposing the distal trachea cranial to the thoracic inlet, applying moderate traction, transecting the trachea and causing chemical or physical damage to the syringeal membranes. The procedure carries a degree of risk; the effects may not be permanent.)

Syringeal Aspergilloma

Acute obstruction of the airway of raptors is usually caused by the formation of a syringeal aspergilloma (see Figure 18.4). The condition is common and is initially characterised by an alteration in the voice of the bird. From the onset of signs, complete respiratory obstruction will occur in 10-15 days.

Table 18.2. Therapy for parasitic, bacterial and fungal tracheal diseases.

Organism	Medication	Route and duration
Syngamus trachea, Cyathostoma spp.	Fenbendazole, ivermectin + antibiosis.	Anthelmintic: p/o. Repeat in 10 days. Antibiosis: p/o, s/c or topical, i/t, nebulisation. Up to six weeks.
Bacterial	Antibiosis.	Parenteral +/- i/t or nebulisation.
Fungal	Amphotericin plus flucytosine	1.5mg/kg i/v tid for five days (+ fluids) and/or i/t or nebulisation. 7.5mg/kg p/o bid.
	Itraconazole plus enilconazole	10-15mg/kg i/v or p/o. I/t (1:10 dilution - 0.5ml/kg bid) or nebulisation (1:10 dilution - 20 minutes qid) .

Table 18.3. Suitable drugs and dosages for nebulisation.

Drug	Dosage
Amphotericin B *	100mg in 15ml saline
Chloramphenicol succinate **	200mg in 15ml saline
Erythromycin	200mg in 10ml saline
Gentamicin *	50mg in 10ml saline
Polymixin B *	333,000 iu in 5ml of saline
Spectinomycin	200mg in 15ml saline
Sulphadimethoxine	200mg in 15ml saline
Tylosin *	100mg in10ml saline/1g in 50ml dimethyl sulphoxide
Amikacin *	50mg in 10ml saline
Enrofloxacin	100mg in 10ml saline

* Poorly absorbed from the respiratory epithelium.
** Not permitted in 'food producing animals'.

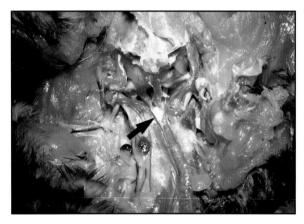

Figure 18.4: Syringeal aspergilloma (arrowed).

Placement of an Abdominal Air Sac Breathing Tube
Birds with acute lower respiratory dyspnoea must be examined endoscopically as an emergency procedure. An abdominal air sac breathing tube may need to be placed prior to endoscopy or surgery, depending on the severity of dyspnoea. A number of different sites have been recommended; each varies in ease of placement and effectiveness. The author favours the placing of the tube into the caudal abdominal air sac, gaining access caudal to the thigh and ventral to the caudofemoralis muscle. The leg is pulled forward and an incision made in the skin. A path is taken between muscle masses in a craniomedial direction and as large a tube as possible (5mm for a 750-1000g bird) is in-

troduced at least 2cm into the caudal abdominal air sac. The exact muscle positioning varies between species. Once introduced the tube is sutured to both the muscle wall and the skin. The tube may be left in place for several weeks if necessary. If the breathing tubes are intended for temporary retention *in situ*, some form of Elizabethan or neck collar may be required to prevent removal. The tube may be used for topical treatment of the air sacs as well as maintenance of respiration. Anaesthesia may be induced and maintained via an air sac breathing tube using a volatile agent. The minute volume of gaseous anaesthetic must be increased by a factor of x2-3 in order to maintain anaesthesia. In all cases involving birds with dyspnoea, isoflurane is the recommended anaesthetic agent.

Surgical Treatment of a Syringeal Aspergilloma
With the breathing tube in place, the trachea may be operated on safely. Although retraction and transection of the trachea to gain access to the syringeal region has been described, in raptor species it is usually impossible to gain direct access to the lesion and it is still necessary to operate down a length of distal trachea. The author favours the per-glottis approach. A 2.7mm rigid endoscope and a 'cut off' male dog catheter are passed simultaneously through the glottis. The lesion is seen easily on one or both sides of the syrinx. By careful positioning of the bird, the bulk or all of the lesion can be removed by a rotational cutting

motion with the catheter, whilst at the same time applying suction to the catheter (using a 60ml syringe). Segments of the aspergilloma are sucked up or impaled on the end of the catheter and recovered. If the segments cannot be recovered, they may be pushed down the primary bronchi, from where they will emerge on the ventral aspect of the lung in the thoracic air sac. These segments may be either recovered from the thoracic air sac or treated *in situ*. The latter is not an ideal solution, but at least the life threatening obstruction has been removed. Following surgical removal or debulking of the aspergilloma, long-term medical treatment is essential to prevent recrudescence (see later).

Medical Treatment of Fungal Conditions of the Trachea (see also Chapter 3)

If an antifungal drug is to be effective, the organism must be susceptible to the drug at concentrations achievable at the site of infection. The drug must be able to penetrate to the centre of the infection and must not be toxic to the patient at the levels and durations of treatment that are required to control the infection. It has been reported that the azole compounds do not reach adequate minimum inhibitory concentration (MIC) levels for the first 3-5 days of therapy (Flammer, 1993), although this point is refuted by Janssen Animal Health who manufacture itraconazole and other members of this group of compounds. In view of this, amphotericin B (1.5mg/kg i/v tid for 3-5 days) is recommended. However, because of the potential for renal toxicity if the bird is dehydrated, 15ml/kg of fluids should also be given intravenously each time amphotericin B is administered. There are several medical treatment regimens that are recommended by different workers. The method preferred by the author is a combination of surgical removal or debulking of the lesion, followed by topical (intratracheal) enilconazole (diluted 1:10) concurrently with amphotericin B for the first 3-5 days as well as either itraconazole or flucytosine orally. Topical treatment is maintained for two weeks and parenteral treatment for two months after disappearance of the lesion.

AIR SACS

Bacterial Air Sacculitis

Air sacculitis can occur in raptors. It is often a sequela to *Serratospiculum* spp. (air sac nematode) infestation, although this is only likely to be seen in the UK in birds imported from warm climates, eg. Saker Falcons from the Gulf States (75% of all wild-caught Saker Falcons are likely to be carrying this organism). If, subsequently, the birds are ill with some other disease, or if treated with an anthelmintic, bacterial air sacculitis will often ensue. In cases of air sac parasitism, daily therapy with mebendazole (20mg/kg for 14 days) followed by surgical or endoscopic removal of the worms is recommended.

Chlamydiosis

Chlamydia psittaci infection may present with air sacculitis, hepatosplenomegaly, green faecal staining of the urates or intractible conjunctivitis. The condition is seen most often in stressed birds which may have *Serratospiculum* spp. infection and air sacculitis concurrently (Forbes, 1995)

Aspergillosis

Fungal infection is the commonest condition of the air sacs. Aspergillosis of the air sacs typically affects the caudal air sacs. As the air sacs surround the digestive system, cases of air sac asperillosis typically show lethargy, inappetence or vomiting, with dramatic loss of condition. They do not usually show any respiratory signs.

Diagnosis

Diagnosis of air sac aspergillosis is made on high quality lateral and dorsoventral radiographs (see Figure 18.5), followed by endoscopy. The value of endoscopy cannot be overemphasised (see Chapter 23). Not only can the lesions be visualised, but samples can be aspirated for culture and biopsies (of air sac tissue and lung) taken for pathology.

Treatment

Unless detected very early, drug therapy alone is unlikely to be effective because of the thick leathery caseous encapsulation which develops (see Figure 18.3.2). In these cases, surgical removal should be attempted. Surgery is difficult and risky, but is often the only possible chance of survival. Surgery will usually involve midline and paracostal incisions on one or both sides of the bird.

Clavicular Air Sac Disease

Although this condition is rare, the presenting signs may be misleading. The bird shows unilateral wing lameness in the absence of any evident wing pathology. Radiographs will often reveal a loss of air space and an increased radiodensity of the clavicular air sac

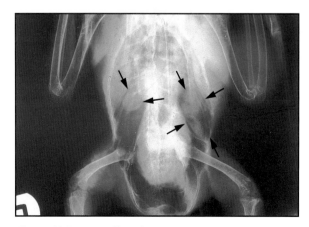

Figure 18.5: Aspergillosis lesions (arrowed) in the caudal thoracic air sac of a Gyr Falcon.

on that side. This condition may be caused by foreign body penetration, eg. a blackthorn whilst flying into thick cover, or aspergillosis.

REFERENCES

Campbell TW (1994) Cytology. In: *Avian Medicine: Principles and Application*. Eds BW Ritchie, GJ Harrison and LR Harrison. Wingers, Lake Worth.

Fedde, MR (1993) Structure and function of the avian respiratory system. In: *Avian Medicine and Surgery: Core Topics*. Association of Avian Veterinarians, Lake Worth

Flammer K (1993) An overview of antifungal therapy in birds. In: *Proceedings of the Association of Avian Veterinarians Annual Conference 1993*. AAV, Lake Worth.

Forbes NA (1991) Aspergillosis. *Veterinary Record* **128**, 263.

Forbes NA (1992) Diagnosis of avian aspergillosis and treatment with itraconazole. *Veterinary Record* **130**, 519.

Forbes NA (1995) Chlamydiosis in Falconiformes: clinical signs, diagnosis and treatment in a collection. In: *Proceedings of the Middle East Falcon Research Conference 1995*. National Avian Research Centre, Abu Dhabi.

Harrison GJ and Ritchie BW (1994) Making distinctions in physical examination. In: *Avian Medicine: Principles and Application*. Eds BW Ritchie, GJ Harrison and LR Harrison. Wingers, Lake Worth.

Morgan DO and Clapham PA (1934) Some observations on gapeworm in poultry and game birds. *Journal of Helminthology* **12**, 267.

Redig PT (1980) Aspergillosis in raptors. In: *Recent Advances in the Study of Raptor Diseases*. Eds JE Cooper and AG Greenwood. Chiron Publications, Keighley.

Richter T and Gerlach H (1981) The bacterial flora of the nasal mucosa of birds of prey. In: *Recent Advances in the Study of Raptor Diseases*. Eds JE Cooper and AG Greenwood. Chiron Publications, Keighley.

CHAPTER NINETEEN

Chronic Weight Loss, Vomiting and Dysphagia

Neil A Forbes

INTRODUCTION

Birds have a great ability to hide illness. The majority of avian clinical cases presented to the clinician show a rapid deterioration. The duration of the illness is generally short and results in early death or rapid recovery. This chapter deals with a number of clinical situations which have a lengthy pathogenesis. The clinician has more time to make a specific diagnosis, although the treatment may not be any easier. Affected birds may be presented with any of the following signs or histories:

- Exercise intolerance or reluctance to exercise.
- Weight loss.
- Insufficient weight gain with respect to food consumed.
- Failure to respond as expected to training.
- Alteration in appearance of faeces (mutes) or casting (pellet).
- Inappetence, head flicking, vomition or regurgitation.

Most of these signs are non-specific and may be ignored by the inexperienced owner or veterinary surgeon. However, any one of them may be of great significance and therefore necessitate a full clinical examination. Familiarity with falconry terminology, training methods, feeding and husbandry is essential (see Chapter 13).

A full history should be taken, including age, sex, previous exercise or training, ie. falconry as opposed to breeding bird, expected 'flying' and 'fat or top' weights, recent weight trends, diet fed, eg. have any quarry or wild caught birds been fed in previous two year period, has fresh pigeon been fed at all, and appetite. A falconer will generally have a much better idea of the individual bird's well being, state of training, expected response to training, etc. than other bird keepers. A falconer's relationship to a trained bird is similar to that of an experienced race horse trainer. Keepers should always be requested to obtain a faecal (mute) sample from the bird. The sample should be examined by direct microscopic wet preparation for parasites prior to examination and handling of the bird. As most falconers' birds are fed partially or entirely on avian derived food (fresh or frozen), there is always

a potential for the passage of subclinical or non-pathogenic infection from quarry/food species to the raptor. These infections may be parasitic, bacterial, protozoan or viral. Having examined the faecal sample (even if positive for parasites), the bird should be 'cast' and examined clinically (see Chapter 2). Even if the bird appears to the clinician to be healthy, a full haematology and full or limited biochemistry should be performed (see Chapters 7 and 8). Table 19.1 shows key clinical signs, investigative procedures, differential diagnosis, therapy and prognosis for these conditions.

Table 19.2 lists clinical signs, investigative procedures, differential diagnosis, therapy and prognosis for systemic conditions causing similar signs to those considered in Table 19.1.

MANAGEMENT OF THE UNDERWEIGHT BIRD WITH NON-SPECIFIC SIGNS

In many cases, irrespective of the cause of anorexia, weight loss, etc., birds fail to gain or maintain weight. This may be as a result of underlying illness or simply a management problem.

Some raptor keepers believe it is necessary to give flying birds one enormous meal daily (as much as the bird will eat). An excessive meal on its own is occasionally enough to cause an upset to the bird. Ill, inappetent or underweight birds should be fed several times a day with smaller meals, during which time 'casting', ie. roughage in the diet (fur and feather), should be withheld. Falconers in some countries, especially the Middle East, never feed 'casting'. Wild birds often pluck their quarry, ingesting very little 'casting'. Feeding 'casting' is not essential, particularly in the short term. Small meals of finely cut nutritious meat (including fat as a source of energy) should be given, together with additional fluid, by crop tube. As soon as one meal has been 'put over', ie. the crop has emptied into the proventriculus, a further meal should be offered.

SOUR CROP

Sour crop is an acute toxaemia which arises if food is

consumed by a bird but does not pass from the crop into the proventriculus. The food is held at body temperature in the absence of any digestive action. The consequence is a rapid putrefaction of the meat, toxaemia and rapid death of the bird. Birds which have taken over four hours to empty their crop should receive treatment as a matter of urgency. The first aim is to encourage the crop to empty, either by regurgitation,

manual emptying or digestion. Initially, the bird should be given oral fluids by crop tube (7ml/kg bodyweight). This will often aid onward passage of food. If no improvement is seen within one hour, the bird should be encouraged to regurgitate. Some birds will regurgitate when travelling or when lightly sprayed with warm water. If this fails to produce crop emptying the bird should be anaesthetised, intubated and the crop

Table 19.1. Clinical signs, diagnosis, therapy and prognosis of chronic diseases in raptors.

Clinical signs	Investigative procedure	Differential diagnosis	Therapy and prognosis
Inappetence, head flicking whilst eating, regurgitation, crop slow to empty into proventriculus, slow to cast (bring back undigestible fur or feather).	1. Examine mouth fully. 2. If white lesions, microscopic examination of impression smear, wet prep (saline), hanging drop or Diff Quik. Find source of infection and prevent re-exposure. (Fresh pigeons should not be fed to raptors. Freeze first, as trichonomads are temperature sensitive.)	*Capillaria* spp. (bi-operculate nematode eggs).	Fenbendazole (100mg/kg p/o once or 25mg/kg p/o daily for five days). Resistant to ivermectin. Prognosis good. Secondary bacterial stomatitis can occur, therefore use concurrent antibiosis. Reinfection may occur from the environment via direct life cycle.
		Trichomonas spp. (known by falconers as 'frounce') (motile protozoa seen in saline wet prep or hanging drop).	Metronidazole (50mg/kg p/o daily for five days) or carnidazole (25mg/kg p/o once). Prognosis good.
		Candida spp. (budding yeast) readily visible on Diff Quik. *Candida* spp. infection often occurs secondary to antibiotic therapy.	Nystatin (300,000 units [3ml]/kg p/o bid for seven days). Prevent by routine use of probiotics at times of stress or following antibiotics.
		Bacterial stomatitis; seen on Diff Quik. Gram staining and sensitivity testing required (infection may be primary or secondary).	Effective antibiosis. Prognosis good. Tube feeding may be required initially as bird is often inappetent.
	If no white lesions present: 3. Microscopic examination of impression smear; wet prep (saline), hanging drop, Diff Quik of crop smears or aspirates.	Trichomoniasis, candidiasis, bacterial infection, abdominal conditions.	Give therapy specific to diagnosis. If tests uninformative, progress to stage 4 (see below).
	If no white oral lesions and no organisms in crop aspirate or wet prep, continue with: 4. Endoscopy (intubate and place saline in crop to aid visualisation). Collect samples, examine lining of crop.	As earlier. If all tests negative, progress to procedures 5-8 (see next page).	The crop lining may be haemorrhagic, have a pseudomembrane, show avipoxvirus or other lesions. Until a diagnosis is made, symptomatic therapy should be given.

Table 19.1. Continued.

Clinical signs	Investigative procedure	Differential diagnosis	Therapy and prognosis
Regurgitation, vomition.	Procedures **1**, **2**, **3**, **4** and also: 5. Bacterial testing of crop, casting and faeces (mutes). 6. Parasitological examination of faeces. 7. All vomiting birds should have a full haematology and biochemistry profile. 8. Lateral and dorsoventral radiographs should be taken in order to check abdominal organ size, placement, abdominal masses and air sac conditions. If any abdominal abnormalities are observed on radiography: 9. Abdominal endoscopy is indicated. In the case of air sacculitis, this may be hampered practically in view of thickened, tough air sac walls.	Bacterial enteritis, *Candida* spp., parasitic enteritis; septicaemia; toxaemia; or any air sac condition, eg. aspergillosis, air sacculitis (see Chapter 18).	Any vomiting bird should receive i/v or i/o fluid therapy via a catheter (1% of bodyweight in 10 minutes); metoclopramide (2mg/kg i/m or i/v tid), antibiosis, eg. amoxycillin (200mg/kg p/o tid for 5-7 days or 200mg/kg i/m sid for 5-7 days), and any other relevant therapy. After an initial period of 3-4 hours, fluid should be given orally via a crop tube (1% of bodyweight every two hours). If this is well tolerated, after 2-3 doses give diluted liquidised convalescent-type food instead, eg. Hills A/d diet, Critical Care Formula (Vetark). Do not give solid food for 36-48 hours or until the bird is willing to take food voluntarily (see Chapter 3).
Inappetence, vomition, weight loss, abdominal straining, cloacal prolapse, fresh or digested blood in faeces. Occurence of these signs is rare.	**1-9.** Also barium contrast abdominal radiographs.	As listed earlier; gut impaction with casting, foreign bodies or endoparasites; gut torsion; or intussusception.	Nursing and supportive care; specific therapy for any pathogens or parasites; surgery if required. Prognosis guarded to grave if intestinal surgery required.

Table 19.2. Systemic diseases causing chronic debilitation.

Clinical signs	Investigative procedures	Differential diagnosis	Therapy and prognosis
Exercise intolerance or reluctance to exercise. Weight loss. Insufficient weight gain with respect to food consumed. Failure to respond as expected to training.	History, clinical examination, haematology, biochemistry, radiology, endoscopy (biopsy if relevant).	Aspergillosis. Avian tuberculosis. Parasitism. Enteritis. Liver disease. Others.	See Chapter 18. See later. See later. See later. See later.

contents milked manually back to the mouth and removed with forceps. Such birds should receive metoclopramide (or cissapride), fluid therapy (i/v and oral) and antibiosis (see Flow Chart 3.4).

ASPERGILLOSIS

Aspergillus fumigatus is an extremely common

pathogen in raptors. Infection may arise as a consequence of a bird being kept in a spore-rich environment, eg. when birds are kept close to rotting or decaying vegetable material (Forbes, 1991). However, because of the ubiquitous nature of *A. fumigatus* many birds will be exposed to spores, which will enter their lungs and air sac systems. If individual affected birds have concurrent immune system suppression or immuno-incompetence, clinical disease will occur (see Chapter 18).

Diagnosis

Diagnosis of aspergillosis may often be complex and misleading due to the variety of clinical signs encountered. As stated earlier, an alteration or loss of voice is almost pathognomonic for the aspergillosis-syringeal form. This occurs where a single lesion forms at the bifurcation of the trachea in the area of the syrinx. Tracheoscopy will confirm the diagnosis. Aspergillous rhinitis is rarely encountered in raptors, although it is not uncommon in psittacines (Bauck *et al*, 1992). Diagnosis of these cases is made on aspiration, radiology, endoscopy and culture. Serological diagnosis of avian aspergillosis is currently unreliable in the UK. The commonest forms of the disease, where single or multiple aspergillomata form in the abdominal or thoracic air sacs, are the most difficult to diagnose and treat. (Very occasionally, aspergillomata may be seen in the clavicular air sac, leading to paresis of a wing.) The commonest clinical signs are rapid weight loss, loss of appetite, vomition and diarrhoea; respiratory signs are usually only seen in the terminal stages.

Haematology, although not diagnostic, is extremely useful in narrowing the differential diagnosis. As with avian tuberculosis, a dramatic rise in white blood cells (WBC) is noted. The acute onset early cases, ie. rhinitis and tracheal forms, do not show this increase initially. The WBC count is expected to be in excess of $15 \times 10^9/l$ and is often $25\text{-}40 \times 10^9/l$. High definition, well-positioned radiographs and endoscopy of each air sac on each side is helpful. A useful comparative study of diagnostic techniques has been reported by Redig (1980). Endoscopic examination is difficult if concurrent air sacculitis is present.

There is a particularly unusual form of aspergillosis which may well be confused with viral hepatitis. This is the septicaemic form, where numerous *Aspergillus* filaments are found in the liver sinusoids on histopathology *ante* or *post mortem*. Discrete lesions are not seen at any sites; diagnosis can only be made on serology or liver biopsy.

Treatment (see Chapter 18)

AVIAN TUBERCULOSIS

Avian tuberculosis is rare in raptors, although common in ground-living birds. The disease usually presents as a chronic wasting disease characterised by weight loss, despite a well-maintained food intake. Pallor or jaundice of the mucous membranes may be apparent. Frequently, diarrhoea is present, indicated by a soiling of the feathers around the vent. The disease leads terminally to extreme weakness and dyspnoea. Vomition is an occasional sequela. The rate of pathogenesis and onset of clinical signs is most rapid at or following times of stress. Infection can affect any part of the body. If the bones of the limbs are affected (see Chapter 16), body condition usually remains good.

Diagnosis

A number of different diagnostic techniques have been used for the diagnosis of avian tuberculosis in non-poultry species. It has been reported recently in a comparative study that infected birds showed heterophilia, monocytosis and hyperfibrinogenaemia as well as a tendency to develop hypochromic, microcytic anaemia (Hawkey *et al*, 1990). Monitoring of these changes has proved to be the most accurate method of diagnosis. This method proved useful in setting up a control for an endemic infection in raptors (Forbes, 1990).

Haematology shows a raised WBC count in excess of $18 \times 10^9/l$: this is made up predominantly of monocytes. Heterophilia, hyperfibrinogenaemia and anaemia will often be noted. In suspect cases, endoscopy of the liver will usually reveal the typical white tuberculous lesions (see Figure 19.1). Although *Mycobacterium avium* has a predilection for the intestinal tract and associated organs, it can be found in almost any site in the body.

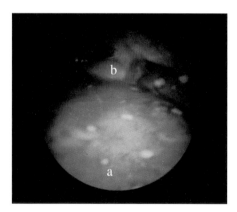

Figure 19.1: *Tuberculous lesions in the liver: a. liver; b. lung. (Compare with Figure 23.10.)*

Treatment

It is now generally accepted that when avian tuberculosis occurs in a collection of raptors all positive cases should be eliminated. This is particularly important because of the resistant nature of the organism, which can remain viable for up to four years in the ground. By the time a clinical case is diagnosed, there is likely to be considerable contamination of any areas of soil to which the birds have had access. Screening of the whole collection and elimination of all positive cases is advisable whenever a member bird is found to be positive. Birds are blood tested every three months (for one year), and suspect birds are examined endoscopically. This protocol results in a high level of accuracy. Positive cases are removed either for euthanasia or for solitary confinement during therapy. Successful medication for avian tuberculosis has been described by Rosskopf *et al* (1991). However, medical treatment of avian tuberculosis is difficult, carries a zoonotic risk and is both expensive and time consuming. Most importantly, at least during the initial part of the treatment course, the bird will continue to contaminate the environment, thereby running a risk of infecting the other birds in the collection and the aviculturalist. Since the increased incidence of AIDS in humans, *M. avium* has become a much more important zoonosis. The risk of human infection, particularly in immune suppressed individuals, must be stressed to owners who wish to treat their bird(s). The treatment regime recommended by Rosskopf *et al* (1991) is as follows:

- Enrofloxacin injectable (15mg/kg i/m bid for 7-10 days).
- Clofazimine 50mg capsules (1.5mg/kg once daily).
- Cycloserine 250mg pulvules (5mg/kg bid).
- Ethambutol 100mg tablets (20mg/kg bid).

Enrofloxacin is given for 7-10 days only, whilst the oral drugs are all given for three months to one year depending on the severity of the infection and its granulomatous nature. The treatment protocol involves considerable handling of the birds and, therefore, increases the zoonotic risk. Taking into consideration the zoonotic potential and the physical and psychological welfare aspects of treating birds affected with tuberculosis, the author advises euthanasia in all cases.

PARASITISM

Ectoparasites
Ectoparasites are common in raptors (see Chapter 14). Large numbers may cause weakness and lethargy through anaemia. However, high levels of ectoparasite infestation are usually indicative of birds which were ill prior to parasitism, rather than as a consequence of parasitism.

Endoparasites
Endoparasites will commonly cause loss of condition and other clinical signs. Veterinarians are frequently approached by clients requesting a dose of the best all-round wormer for their birds. As with all species, an antiparasitic drug must be specific to the parasite type. This is particularly true for birds as there are few dual purpose anthelmintics available. Wild raptors have a high incidence (60% nematodes) of subclinical parasitism. However, if wild birds enter captivity the stress incurred may well precipitate clinical parasitism. All ex-wild birds should either receive prophylactic therapy and/or have faecal examinations performed. Parasitism is commoner in wild raptors compared with captive raptors. Table 19.3 shows the main parasitic problems which may arise.

ENTERITIS

Raptor chicks are born with little or no gut flora; as a consequence, bacterial overgrowths and enteritis are common. The use of a probiotic, eg. Avipro Paediatric (Vetark), in hand-reared chicks in the first 14 days of life will greatly reduce such infections. As the staple diet of many captive raptors is avian derived, there is always the potential for the spread of avian pathogens between food species and raptor. Enteric infections may be parasitic (see earlier), bacterial or viral. Common bacterial infections include *Salmonella enteriditis* and *S. typhimurium, Escherichia coli, Pseudomonas* spp.

Table 19.3. Common parasitic infestations of raptors.

Species and host susceptibility	Clinical signs	Treatment
Capillaria spp. (thread worm). Commonest nematode. Lemon shaped, bi-operculate egg. Frequently responsible for clinical disease. Direct infection or by ingestion of molluscs, earthworms, etc.	White necrotic oral lesions or enteric lesions. Head flicking, weight loss, diarrhoea.	Ivermectin often ineffective. Use benzimidazoles at the highest levels, eg. fenbendazole (100mg/kg p/o once or 25mg/kg p/o daily for five days). Repeat after 10 days. Beware source of infection and possible reinfestation. The bird's environment should be cleaned or replaced. Levamisole (40mg/kg i/m or p/o) has a narrow safety margin.
Ascaridia spp. Typical ascarid-type egg (thick shelled); some show discrete bi-operculum, eg. *Porrocaecum* spp. Individual worms are large; found in small intestine, ventriculus and large intestine. Relatively uncommon (more common in young birds); rarely found in high numbers.	Rare, unless high numbers. Can cause weight loss and gut impaction or rupture, especially in young birds.	Ivermectin (200mcg/kg of 1:11 dilution). Benzimidazole at the standard dose (25mg/kg p/o daily for five days or 100mg/kg once). Levamisole has narrow safety margin; rarely justifiable in individual raptors.

Table 19.3. Continued.

Species and host susceptibility	Clinical signs	Treatment
Spirurid spp. (stomach worm). Rarely pathogenic. Thin-walled, larvated egg.	Found in lumen and mucosa of ventriculus and proventriculus. Cause inappetence and weight loss.	Ivermectin (200mcg/kg), benzimidazole (25mg/kg p/o daily for 3-5 days or 100mg/kg once). Benzimidazole does not appear to be toxic or cause feather abnormalities in raptors.
Syngamus spp. (gapeworm). Commonest in buzzards and other scavengers. Faecal ova.	See Chapter 18. Cause dyspnoea, neck stretching, coughing.	Ivermectin (200mcg/kg), benzimidazole (100mg/kg p/o, repeat after 10 days) plus antibiosis. Beware reinfestation from environment. Concrete aviary floors prevent mollusc and arthropod intermediate hosts.
Serratospiculum spp. (air sac worm). Common in warm climates; not found in UK, unless imported birds. Faecal ova.	Pathogenicity low in healthy birds. May cause air sacculitis if birds concurrently ill. Dead worms in air sacs may lead to potentially fatal air sacculitis.	Mebendazole (20mg/kg daily for 14 days), antibiosis; if still present, remove dead worms by endoscopy.
Trematodes Rare in UK; 30% incidence in warmer countries. Usually large singe operculate egg.	Non-pathogenic unless in very large numbers (rare). Enteric or hepatic signs with respect to species of fluke.	Treat with chlorsulon (20mg/kg p/o on three occasions at two week intervals) or praziquantel (5-10mg/kg s/c or p/o daily for 14 days); not effective against all species.
Cestodes Rare. Faecal ova.	Rarely of significance.	Treat with praziquantel (5-10mg/kg p/o or s/c, repeat after 14 days). Also chlorsulon.
Caryospora spp. (rare).	Sudden death in juvenile birds 25-45 days of age. Inappetence, abdominal pain in adult birds.	Clazuril (5-10mg/kg p/o daily three times on alternate days.
Eimeria spp. (rare) and *Isospora* spp.	Weight loss, enteritis. Usually juvenile or weak birds affected.	Sulphonamide (75mg/kg daily 3:2:3) or clazuril (as above).
Sarcocystis spp. (rare).	Weakness, inappetence, lethargy, death.	Pyrimethamine (0.25-0.5mg/kg p/o bid for 30 days).
Toxoplasma spp. (raptors, with the exception of owls, appear relatively resistant).	Conjunctivitis, blindness (retinal damage), circling, anorexia, diarrhoea.	Pyrimethamine (as above).
Trichomonas spp. (frounce).	Inappetence, dysphagia, white lesions in mouth/oesophagus/crop.	Metronidazole (50mg/kg p/o daily for five days). Carnidazole (25mg/kg p/o once). Always freeze pigeon carcases prior to feeding to raptors. *Trichomonas* spp. are temperature sensitive.

and *Proteus mirabilis*. Birds with enteritis should have Gram stains, microbiology and sensitivity testing carried out on their faeces.

METABOLIC DISEASE - HEPATOPATHY

As stated earlier, infection may be easily passed from food to raptor. There are a number of bacterial and viral infections which can give rise to significant debilitating disease. The commonest chronic disease has been described by Forbes (1996) as 'hepatopathy'. The term 'hepatopathy' was chosen because cases demonstrated significant pathological changes in the liver tissue, although by the time of presentation and diagnosis, there was often no active inflamation present. All cases present with poor exercise tolerance. Birds kept and fed in aviaries will not appear ill; only when exercised will it be appreciated that they are unwell. In severe cases a short period of exertion will lead to a hypoglycaemic fit. To date the condition has only been recognised in falcons (not hawks). The bird generally recovers from the fit, more rapidly if glucose is administered orally. Blood samples taken at the time of the fit confirm hypoglycaemia. Other signs which may be seen are somnolence, lethargy, anorexia and diarrhoea. Secondary infections may be common. In severe 'hepatopathy' cases, tremors and other central nervous system signs occur, even at rest.

Aetiology

The full aetiology of 'hepatopathy' has not been ascertained. Epidemiological evidence indicates an infectious agent. The condition will suddenly occur in a collection, clinical signs arising in 30-40% of falcons over a period of one month.

Hepatopathy is a non-specific disease condition which may be caused by a multitude of different agents or factors. Hepatopathies may be divided into acute or chronic forms, although some agents can lead to either. Many different aetiologies have been implicated in birds - for example, drugs or chemicals, eg. mebendazole and chemical poisons; infections, eg. *Campylobacter jejuni, reovirus, Yersinia pseudotuberculosis, S. typhimurium*, although these pathogens present acute clinical signs, frequently leading to the birds rapid demise; or metabolic inbalances, eg. diabetes mellitus, hypothyroidism. Cavill (1982) described both an acute and a chronic form of viral hepatitis. The chronic form presented with similar signs of lethargy and anorexia as seen in the cases described by Forbes (1996). Greenwood and Cooper (1982) described an inclusion body hepatitis in raptors in the UK which they attributed to herpesvirus infection, whilst Gough *et al* (1993) isolated a herpesvirus from a case involving a falcon in the UK. However, both the latter cases resulted in acute clinical signs and death. In the cases described here the signs have all been chronic in nature.

Diagnosis

Hepatopathy was suspected in most cases after taking a full history. Blood profiles revealed the following abnormalities:
- Haematology showed a lowered WBC count (1.5-2.5x10⁹/l; normal range 4.0-8.75x10⁹/l).
- Raised blood cholesterol (x = 11.2: 9.1-13.2mmol/l; normal ranges 5.2-6.8mmol/l.
- Raised alkaline phosphatase (x = 957: 743-1172iu/l; normal range 213-407iu/l at 37°C.
- Raised LDH levels (x = 2210, 1855-2675iu/l at 37°C; normal range 740-1270iu/l).
- Normal CK levels (380-590iu/l at 37°C).

- Raised bile acid levels (fasting) (x = 280, 264-310µmol/l; normal range 12-99µmol/l).
- Fibrinogen levels ranged from 4.5-6.5g/l (normal range 1.6-3.5g/l).
- Fasting uric acid levels were raised (745-1100µmol/l; normal range 236-578µmol/l).
- Glucose levels were also raised in the non-exercised birds, although once exercised, levels were below normal.
- All figures are from Forbes (1996); the normal ranges refer to falcons).

Lateral radiographs showed enlarged liver, spleen and kidneys. At *post mortem* the liver was 1.5 times normal size and pale and friable. Histopathology of the liver showed chronic active or non-active hepatitis, with both granulocyte and mononuclear cell infiltrate, particularly in the portal areas. Multiple fatty cysts or granulomata were present throughout the parenchyma. Normal lobular architecture was present and bile duct hyperplasia was not a feature. These changes are non-specific and indicated a marked chronic hepatitis of unknown aetiology. It was not possible to determine the cause of the initial insult. No pathogenic organism could be demonstrated. Serology for falcon herpesvirus was negative, as was serology and ELISA for chlamydiosis.

Treatment

Birds were treated initially by reducing dietary fat intake, encouraging exercise and increasing metabolic rate by the use of thyroid hormone. This produced no improvement. Subsequent cases have been rested, with a low fat diet, for a period of 3-6 months. Blood profiles have been repeated and exercise has only been recommended once fibrinogen levels have returned to normal (<4g/l). These birds have made a full recovery, although some have taken six months for this to happen.

MISCELLANEOUS

A number of other causes of chronic ill thrift do present, particularly in older birds.

Neoplasia has been rarely reported in raptors, despite a relatively large captive population. Various abdominal tumours are occasionally found, eg. terratomata and adrenal, gonadal or renal tumours. Malignant lymphoma is also occasionally encountered and these birds are characteristically presented with suspected swellings in the crop. The swellings are usually situated in lymphatic tissue in the cervical region dorsal to the crop. The lesion should be readily diagnosed on radiography (with contrast media if necessary) by the time it has been recognised and the bird presented to the veterinarian.

Other metabolic disorders such as **renal failure** and **diabetes** do occur. **Chronic air sacculitis** and **egg**

peritonitis often lead to similar signs of lethargy, inappetence and exercise intolerance (see Chapters 18, 21 and 22).

REFERENCES

Bauck L, Hillyer E and Hoeffer H (1992) Rhinitis case reports. In: *Proceedings of the Association of Avian Veterinarians Annual Conference 1992*. AAV, Lake Worth.

Cavill JP (1982) Viral diseases. In: *Diseases of Cage and Aviary Birds*. 2nd Edn. Ed ML Petrak. Lea and Febiger, Philadelphia.

Flammer K (1993) An overview of antifungal therapy in birds. In: *Proceedings of the Association of Avian Veterinarians Annual Conference 1993*. AAV, Lake Worth.

Forbes NA (1990) Diagnosis and control of avian tuberculosis in a collection of raptors, using haematology and endoscopy. In: *Proceedings of the British Veterinary Zoological Society Autumn Meeting 1990*. BVZS, London.

Forbes NA (1991) Aspergillosis. *Veterinary Record* **128**, 263.

Forbes NA (1992) Diagnosis of avian aspergillosis and treatment with itraconazole. *Veterinary Record* **130**, 519.

Forbes NA (1996) Diagnosis and treatment of the chronically ill raptor. *Journal of the British Veterinary Zoological Society* (in press).

Forbes NA and Cooper JE (1991) Diseases and pathology of the European Merlin (*Falco columbarius*). In: *Biology and Conservation of Small Falcons*. Eds MK Nicholls and R Clarke. Hawk and Owl Trust, London.

Forbes NA, Cromie RL, Brown MJ, Montali RJ, Bush M and Stanford JL (1993) The development of an ELISA test for the early detection of *M. avium* infection in wildfowl. In: *Proceedings of the Association of Avian Veterinarians Annual Conference 1993*. AAV, Lake Worth.

Gough RE, Drury SEN, George AD and Randall CJ (1993) Isolation and identification of a falcon herpesvirus. *Veterinary Record* **132**, 220.

Greenwod AG and Cooper JE (1982) Herpesvirus infections in falcons. *Veterinary Record* **111**, 514.

Hawkey C, Kock RA, Henderson GM and Cindery RN (1990) Haematological changes in domestic fowl (*Gallus gallus*) and cranes (*Gruiformes*) with *Mycobacterium avium* infection. *Avian Pathology* **19**, 223.

Redig PT (1980) Aspergillosis in raptors. In: *Recent Advances in the Study of Raptor Diseases*. Eds JE Cooper and AG Greenwood. Chiron Publications, Keighley.

Rosskpof WJ, Woerpel RW and Asterino R (1991) Successful treatment of avian tuberculosis in pet psittacines. In: *Proceedings of the Association of Avian Veterinarians Annual Conference 1991*. AAV, Lake Worth.

CHAPTER TWENTY

Fits, Incoordination and Coma

John E Cooper

INTRODUCTION

This chapter is concerned with diseases that produce clinical signs that might be broadly classified as 'neurological', but where the underlying aetiology and pathogenesis can involve a number of different organs and tissues. As the title of the chapter suggests, affected birds show such clinical features as fits (convulsions), locomotor incoordination, muscle fasciculations, stupor and coma. Diseases that fall into these categories have long been recognised in raptors kept for falconry (Cooper, 1978). Terms sometimes used by falconers include 'fits', 'cramp', 'convulsions', 'epilepsy', 'apoplexy', 'seizures' and 'stroke'.

Investigation and treatment of many of the disorders covered in this chapter need to be carried out promptly and proficiently. Failure to do so can result in the bird's death or irreversible deterioration: secondary problems, eg. trauma, asphyxia or inhalation of ingesta, can also occur.

A recommended approach to birds with signs of 'fits, incoordination and coma' is shown in Figure 20.1. The speed with which each stage must be carried out will depend upon the type and severity of the clinical signs.

Figure 20.1: Recommended approach to birds with signs of 'fits, incoordination and coma'.

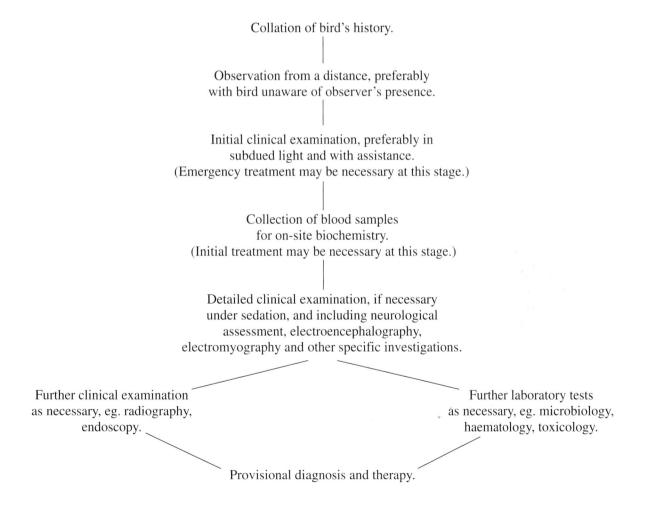

Collation of bird's history.

Observation from a distance, preferably with bird unaware of observer's presence.

Initial clinical examination, preferably in subdued light and with assistance.
(Emergency treatment may be necessary at this stage.)

Collection of blood samples for on-site biochemistry.
(Initial treatment may be necessary at this stage.)

Detailed clinical examination, if necessary under sedation, and including neurological assessment, electroencephalography, electromyography and other specific investigations.

Further clinical examination as necessary, eg. radiography, endoscopy.

Further laboratory tests as necessary, eg. microbiology, haematology, toxicology.

Provisional diagnosis and therapy.

AETIOLOGY

The causes of 'fits, incoordination and coma' (and similar signs) are many and varied, and sometimes more than one is involved. However, the main headings are:

- Poisons.
- Nutritional/metabolic.
- Traumatic.
- Infectious.

In domestic fowl a number of conditions are recognised that produce neurological or locomotor signs (Calnek *et al*, 1991) and some of these may have parallels in raptors. Much research is still needed.

Poisons

Both exogenous and endogenous toxins can produce a range of clinical signs in raptors (see Figures 20.2, 20.3). Table 20.1 lists some of the more important poisons, their effects and a recommended approach to treatment and/or control.

Raptors that die following nervous signs frequently show intraosseous haemorrhage *post mortem*. This is agonal change due to pooling of blood in the bones of the skull (see Figure 20.4) and is not significant in terms of diagnosis.

A range of other substances is known to be toxic to poultry and other birds and could possibly be associated with 'neurological' or other signs, especially terminal depression resembling stupor or coma. In raptors, various compounds, including certain drugs, can prove toxic, eg. procaine or metronidazole, and may cause marked clinical signs (Cooper, 1978). These should be considered in any differential diagnosis.

Endogenous poisons can produce a range of clinical signs, some of which simulate neurological disease. For example, bacterial endotoxins, such as from *Escherichia coli*, can cause pathological changes in the liver, blood vessels, etc., resulting in 'Gramnegative shock' with associated clinical signs. Another

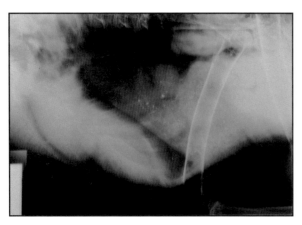

Figure 20.2: *Dilated proventriculus as a result of chronic lead poisoning in a Golden Eagle. (Photo courtesy N A Forbes)*

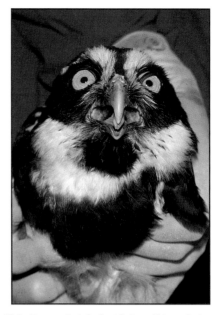

Figure 20.3: *Spectacled Owl with fits. Although the convulsions could be controlled with diazepam, the bird did not respond to treatment and died. The diagnosis was organochlorine poisoning.*

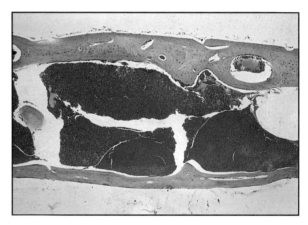

Figure 20.4: *Intraosseous haemorrhage in the skull.*

example of endogenous intoxication occurs in renal or hepatic disease when toxic metabolites, eg. uric acid or metabolic by-products, accumulate and can cause clinical disease characterised by depression, lethargy, unresponsiveness and (occasionally) muscle fasciculations or fits.

Nutritional/Metabolic

Table 20.2 lists some of the nutritional/metabolic disorders that can cause fits, incoordination and coma in raptors. Much remains to be learned about the aetiology and pathogenesis of these conditions, and the practitioner can help his colleagues, as well as his clients, by collecting and disseminating data on such cases, even when therapy has proved unsuccessful.

Other metabolic disorders that may cause clinical signs of relevance to this chapter include uricaemia (and associated gout) - mentioned earlier - and electrolyte imbalance. These and others should be considered in any differential diagnosis.

Table 20.1. Exogenous poisoning associated with signs of 'fits, incoordination or coma'.

Poison	Clinical signs	Diagnosis	Control	Comments
Lead.	Nervous signs. Lethargy, weakness, anorexia, ataxia, blindness, convulsions. Sometimes weight loss. Green faeces. First sign is often leg weakness. Birds rest on their hocks, frequently with medial rotation of the feet, one foot grasping the other.	Radiography (presence of lead, proventricular dilatation) (see Figure 20.2). Blood lead analysis. Detection of lead in the gastrointestinal (GI) tract by endoscopy. Haematology (hypochromic anaemia). Elevated liver enzymes.	Prevent access to lead shot or other sources. Treat with sodium calciumedetate (10-40mg/kg i/m bid for 5-10 days) or other chelation therapy. Remove lead from the GI tract by endoscopy and/or gavage. Can be removed by midline laporatomy and opening of the gizzard (quick and easy). Give additional castings to encourage oral recovery or give magnesium sulphate to hasten passage of lead through the GI tract. Supportive measures.	Associated with ingestion of shot or other materials containing lead, usually in prey or carrion. Shot in own muscles generally not a danger. See Reiser and Temple (1981). Occasionally, lead poisoning can occur due to lead in other situations, eg. bone marrow or coelomic cavity.
Other heavy metals, eg. cadmium, mercury, zinc.	Range from non-specific to weakness, lethargy, weight loss, convulsions, recumbency and death.	Blood analysis. *Post-mortem* toxicology. Endoscopy. Radiography.	Varies. Sodium calciumedetate. D-penicillamine (55mg/kg p/o bid) for copper poisoning. Remove metal from GI tract.	Relatively little published information on raptors. See poultry (Calnek *et al*, 1991) and pet bird (Dumonceaux and Harrison, 1994) literature.
Strychnine.	Convulsions, muscle fasciculations. Rapidly fatal (usually less than 30 minutes).	Analysis of contents of GI tract, or *post-mortem* toxicology. History.	Supportive measures. Sedation or anaesthesia. Remove ingesta from GI tract.	Raptors can ingest strychnine when the latter is used (sometimes illegally) to kill pest species or is put in bait. See Redig and Arendt (1982).
Alphachloralose.	Lethargy, stupor, hypothermia. Frequently occurs as a secondary poisoning when a raptor ingests poisoned pigeons etc.	As above.	Maintain body temperature, fluids, hand feeding. Remove ingesta. Prevent access to poisoned birds.	Associated with ingestion of bird pests for which alphachloralose is used as a control measure. See Cooper (1978).

Table 20.1. Continued.

Poison	Clinical signs	Diagnosis	Control	Comments
Barbiturates, eg. phenobarbitone.	Lethargy, stupor, anaesthesia, hypothermia, respiratory depression, cardiac abnormalities.	As above.	Maintain body temperature. Supportive measures. Respiratory stimulants. Remove ingesta (empty crop). Ensure that carcases of animals killed with barbiturates are properly discarded and are not available to raptors.	See Cooper (1978) and Langelier (1993).
Pesticides.	See below.	Diagnose on clinical signs and history. Seen after plant spraying inside (accidental exposure) or crop spraying outside (drift of toxic agent). See below.	See below.	See below for differentiation between toxin groups.
Organochlorines (chlorinated hydrocarbons), eg. aldrin, dieldrin (see Figure 20.3).	Acute effects - convulsions, apparent blindness, torticollis, ataxia. Chronic effects - reduction in eggshell thickness, embryonic mortality. Possibly minor clinical signs in adult birds.	Blood analysis or biopsy. *Post-mortem* toxicology.	Supportive measures. Increase bird's condition (fat reserves). No specific treatment. Avoid contact between raptors and organochlorines.	Organochlorines are stored in fat and may be liberated when a bird loses condition. Raptors may ingest organochlorines or suffer toxicity from contact with insecticides.
Organophosphates and acetylcholinesterase inhibitors, eg. carbamates.	Ataxia, convulsions, paralysis, altered pupillary reflexes, bradycardia. Organophosphates can take 1-3 weeks before effect, whereas acetylcholinesterase inhibitors are usually acute in onset.	Blood analysis, biopsy or food analysis. *Post-mortem* toxicology.	Atropine (0.1mg/kg i/v or i/m every 3-4 hours) or pralidoxime chloride (2-PAM) (10-40mg/kg). **NB**. 2-PAM is non-proprietary: contact National Poisons Bureau for availability. Treatment can prove effective in cases of acetylcholinesterase inhibitors (where inhibition slowly reverses), but usually not with organophosphates (where irreversible inhibition occurs). Supportive measures. Use insecticidal preparations sparingly on raptors.	See Cooper (1978) and Porter (1993).

Table 20.1. Continued.

Poison	Clinical signs	Diagnosis	Control	Comments
Clostridium botulinum toxin ('botulism') and other clostridial toxins ('enterotoxaemia').	Botulism - flaccid paralysis, lethargy, sometimes diarrhoea, oedema and haemorrhage. Enterotoxaemia - incoordination, diarrhoea and haemorrhage.	History. Demonstration of toxins in GI tract and food.	Antitoxin if available. Supportive measures including respiratory stimulants. Avoid food contaminated with *Clostridium* spp. or preformed toxin, including maggots and other invertebrates. Remove carcases. Make sure excess food is not left in the aviary. Beware caching of food by birds.	See Cooper (1978). Vultures and certain other carrion-eating raptors may be relatively resistant to botulinum toxicity.

Table 20.2. Nutritional/metabolic disorders associated with signs of 'fits, incoordination or coma'.

Aetiology	Clinical signs	Diagnosis	Control	Comments
Thiamine deficiency.	Nervous signs, including fits and 'star gazing'.	Circumstances, including history and response to therapy. Analysis of food for thiamine or thiaminase.	Treat with thiamine orally and by injection. Prevent by encouraging a mixed diet and being wary of fish. (Thiaminase may also be produced by non-pathogenic enteric organisms.)	Probably common in fish-eating birds, eg. Ospreys, but also Harris' Hawks. See Cooper (1978). Thiamine deficiency seen in Harris' Hawks in the UK is not a dietary deficiency but an inability to metabolise and utilise thiamine. Can be prevented by supple-menting the diet with 100-150mg/kg thiamine daily. Condition is seen in certain breed lines only (Forbes, 1987). Other B vitamin deficiencies may also play a part.
Hypocalcaemia, nutritional osteodystrophy and hyperpara-thyroidism.	Muscle fasciculations and tremors; often associated with soft bones and/or 'spontaneous' fractures. Seen most commonly in neonates fed meat diets, or in egg laying females. Hypocalcaemia may be seen following multivitamin injection (too much D_3 given to a potentially calcium deficient bird).	Blood chemistry (calcium). Clinical examination and whole body radiography may reveal skeletal disease. Response to therapy.	Immediate injection of 10% calcium (1-5ml/kg i/v) followed by correct Ca:P:D_3 ratio in diet. Prevent by feeding an adequately balanced diet.	Vitamin D_3 may also be involved: this should be administered **with caution** in clinical cases.

Table 20.2. Continued.

Aetiology	Clinical signs	Diagnosis	Control	Comments
Hypoglycaemia.	Nervous signs, including convulsions. Early signs often subtle - birds easily alarmed, abnormal behaviour, including unusual vocalisation.	Blood chemistry (glucose). Response to therapy. Normal blood glucose level is 12-17mmol/l.	Immediate injection of glucose, followed by high energy diet (handfed if necessary). Prevent by monitoring weight and condition of birds, especially when used for falconry.	Particularly common in small birds with a high metabolic rate, eg. Northern Sparrow Hawk, when flown too light in weight or on a cold or windy day. Advise falconers who fly these birds to carry glucose and a crop tube for use in an emergency. See Cooper (1978). Can also be seen in birds with impaired liver function, especially when exercised.
Hyperglycaemia.	As above. Occurs inevitably during the initial stages of training or retraining, particularly in sensitive species such as Northern Goshawks.	As above.	Treat birds with slightly elevated blood glucose levels (22-27mmol/l) with a benzodiazepine; higher levels (27-32mmol/l) with 0.1 units of protamine zinc insulin; treat until blood glucose level normal. Prevent by minimising stressors when training birds, eg. accustom to humans, reduce diet slowly.	Probably particularly in Northern Goshawks (Forbes, 1995). See Hochleithner (1994).
Hepatic encephalopathy (see Chapter 19).	Hepatic disease causes: (1) Inability to mobilise glucose when required, therefore hypoglycaemic fits when exercised. (2) Inability to clear metabolic by-products, therefore fits/tremors 3-4 hours after digestion of food.	Biochemistry, haematology, radiography, endoscopy and liver biopsy.	Rest, symptomatic treatment.	Increasingly diagnosed in the UK (Forbes, personal communication).

Traumatic

Physical damage to the central nervous system can cause clinical signs ranging from abnormal stance and ataxia to 'concussion' in which the bird shows reduced responses to stimuli, slow pupillary reflexes (sometimes unilateral) and depression that may manifest itself as docility or unconciousness. Diagnosis is based on clinical findings coupled with radiography and other imaging techniques. Shotgun pellets and other foreign bodies can also cause nervous signs. Treatment is discussed elsewhere in this manual (see Chapter 4).

Hyperthermia can cause clinical signs suggestive of nervous disease, especially if coupled with dehydration. This occurs occasionally in the tropics if birds are denied access to shade, and elsewhere when birds are confined in an excessively hot environment, eg. next to a radiator or fire - especially young neonates that are being hand reared. The treatment consists of cooling, including fluids intravenously.

Infectious

Many infectious agents can cause relevant clinical signs. Some examples are given in Table 20.3.

It seems likely that other organisms, including protozoa, may be associated with relevant clinical signs in raptors. They should be considered in any differential diagnosis.

TREATMENT

In the Tables the word 'immediate' is used frequently. Many of the conditions that cause 'fits, incoordination and coma' in raptors are emergencies. They demand prompt diagnosis and prompt treatment. Treatment of emergencies can be considered under three headings:
● Immediate care by the owner.
● Initial therapy by the veterinary surgeon.
● Long-term therapy by the veterinary surgeon in consultation with the owner.

The author prefers midazolam (0.5-1mg/kg i/v or i/m, bid or tid) to diazepam (0.5-1mg/kg i/v or i/m, bid or tid) for birds. Because midazolam is water-soluble it is (a) more rapidly absorbed by the intramuscular route than is diazepam, (b) less irritant to muscles or other tissues, and (c) miscible with other agents, eg. ketamine hydrochloride.

Sometimes there is merit in sedating or lightly anaesthetising a 'fitting' bird, especially if it fails to respond adequately to a benzodiazepine and is damaging itself. A low dose of ketamine (5-10mg/kg i/m or i/v) can be used for this purpose.

Both sedated birds and those that are in a stupor or coma need careful monitoring. Important considerations are respiration, colour of the mucous membrane and response to stimuli. If respiratory depression or distress is a problem, the following actions should be considered:
● Check that the airways are clear.
● If respiration does not start/improve following build-up of CO_2, administer doxapram by injection.
● Consider use of O_2.
● Improve ventilation by air sac cannulation (see Chapter 9).

PERIPHERAL NERVE PROBLEMS

Under the general heading of 'incoordination' can be considered peripheral nerve injuries. These may cause paralysis or locomotor disturbances.

Cooper (1978) discussed peripheral nerve lesions in captive raptors and described a number of syndromes, some of unknown aetiology and pathogenesis, that occur. These and other conditions are listed and described in Table 20.4.

POST-MORTEM EXAMINATION

Research on nervous diseases of raptors has been hampered by a dearth of both pathological and normal material of good quality. The central nervous system autolyses rapidly *post mortem*, and histopathological and electronmicroscopical examination and interpretation are often extremely difficult. Peripheral nerves are more resistant to *post-mortem* changes but, even so, artefacts can complicate investigation.

Post-mortem examination is covered in detail elsewhere in this manual (see Chapter 11). However, it should be noted that good quality nervous material for examination can be obtained if (1) (preferably) the carcase is perfused with buffered formol saline or

Immediate care by owner.	**Reduce stimuli by:** ● Placing bird in a padded box in the dark in a warm place. ● Applying the bird's hood (check regularly in case the bird vomits). ● Avoiding unnecessary noises and interference.
Initial therapy by the veterinary surgeon.	**Control clinical signs by:** ● Injecting a benzodiazepine (diazepam or midazolam). ● Minimising handling or other contact other than essential blood sampling.
Long-term therapy by veterinary surgeon (and owner).	**Treat specifically by:** ● Administering appropriate agent - antidote to poison, thiamine, calcium borogluconate, protamine zinc insulin, antibiotics. ● Giving supportive therapy as necessary, eg. fluids, hand feeding, corticosteroids. ● Commencing long-term measures to prevent recurrence, eg. adequately balanced diet, improved training programme.

Table 20.3. Infectious diseases associated with signs of 'fits, incoordination or coma'.

Aetiology	Clinical signs	Diagnosis	Control	Comments
Bacteria producing bacteraemia (including septic thrombi), septicaemia or toxaemia. Bacterial sinusitis.	Nervous signs or depression/coma. Head tilt, incoordination.	Blood culture. Haematology. Detection of local lesions elsewhere on body. Sinography, aspiration.	Immediate administration of antibiotics. Fluids. Corticosteroids. Attention to local lesions. Prevent by prompt treatment of bacterial diseases. Include antibiotic cover during surgery of infected lesions.	Bacterial infections may arise within the central nervous system or spread to it from ear, eye, sinuses or elsewhere. Abscess formation in pre-auditory diverticulum of infraorbital sinus, causing pressure on the vestibular apparatus or the brain. See Cooper (1978).
Newcastle disease (paramyxovirus infection).	Sometimes nervous signs, including torticollis. Sometimes generalised weakness, diarrhoea, etc.	Serology (rise in titre). Virus isolation from affected bird or its prey, eg. pigeons.	No specific treatment - supportive measures plus isolation. Prevent by avoiding contact between raptors and sources of infection. Vaccinate twice yearly (Columbovac PMV, Solvay Duphar).	Raptors are described as of 'low' or 'moderate' susceptibility. See Gerlach (1994).
Trichomonas gallinae ('frounce').	Usually stomatitis. Occasional cases (especially in owls) involve ears, nasal cavity and brain.	Clinical signs. Detection of flagellate organisms in fresh, wet preparations or stained smears.	Metronidazole (50mg/kg p/o once daily for five days) and appropriate topical treatment, including debridement. Prevent by avoiding pigeons as food and treat early lesions promptly.	See Pokras *et al* (1993) and Samour *et al* (1995).
Sarcocystis sp.	Head tilt, depression, apparent blindness.	Difficult in live bird (immuno-histochemistry).	Not known.	A case has been reported in a Golden Eagle.

Table 20.4. Peripheral nerve problems.

Condition	Aetiology/ pathogenesis	Clinical signs	Diagnosis	Control	Comments
Brachial plexus avulsion.	Damage to the roots of the brachial plexus.	Paralysis of affected wing, sometimes together with other paralysis and analgesia. Atrophy of muscles.	Electrodiagnosis (EMG) (live bird). Histopathology (dead bird) - atrophy of plexus and ganglia, skeletal muscle atrophy.	No specific treatment at present. Amputation of affected wing can be considered in captive birds.	See Smith (1993).

Table 20.4. Continued.

Condition	Aetiology/ pathogenesis	Clinical signs	Diagnosis	Control	Comments
Vertebral column injuries: (1) Cervical. (2) Between notarium (fused thoracic vertebrae) and synsacrum. (3) Caudal to synsacrum.	Trauma.	(1) Usually dead before seen. (2) Flaccid paralysis of legs, cloaca, etc. Incontinence, loss of sensation. (3) Usually legs only temporarily impaired; no total loss of function. Tail shows flaccid paralysis. (**NB**. Full tail function is required by raptors for braking and turning.)	Clinical signs. Radiography (will detect skeletal damage). Magnetic resonance imaging (MRI) may detect nerve tissue damage.	(1) Usually hopeless prognosis. (2) Nursing, corticosteroids. Surgery occasionally possible. Euthanasia if no improvement after three weeks. Full recovery after 2-3 months. Beware cloacal calculi. (3) Normally full leg function regained after 7-10 days; full tail function in 6-8 weeks. Prognosis good.	Careful and systematic investigation is necessary to distinguish between cases with a reasonable as opposed to a poor prognosis.
Aspergilloma of the lumbar vertebrae or bacterial abscessation.	Usually *Aspergillus fumigatus* infection or bacterial infection secondary to trauma.	Paralysis (sometimes bilateral), weakness, occasional vertebral collapse.	Radiography. Serology. Laparoscopic or other diagnosis of concomitant aspergillosis.	Attempt therapy with antifungal agents (usually unsuccessful) or antibiotics (see Chapter 18).	Often missed in diagnosis.
Marek's disease.	Herpesvirus infection.	Paralysis, sometimes cutaneous and visceral lesions.	Clinical signs and characteristic histopathological findings.	None at present.	Predominantly a disease of galiform birds. Rare in raptors (Cooper, 1978).
Posterior paresis due to pressure.	Space occupying lesions in abdomen, eg. renal or gonadal diseases/tumours, tuberculosis or other infections, eggs.	Unilateral or bilateral, flaccid or spastic paralysis of leg(s). Sometimes other signs associated with lesion.	Detection of underlying lesion by radiography, ultrasonography, laparoscopy or cloacal examination. Biopsy. Haematology and biochemistry can be useful.	Surgery. Removal of egg. Chemotherapy where appropriate.	See Cooper (1978).

Table 20.4. Continued.

Condition	Aetiology/ pathogenesis	Clinical signs	Diagnosis	Control	Comments
Paralysis due to nerve damage.	Laceration of brachial or sciatic nerve following fracture, surgery, eg. on bumblefoot, or injections.	As brachial plexus avulsion plus signs associated with fracture or other underlying lesion. Haematology and biochemistry can also be useful.	As brachial plexus avulsion, but single nerve usually involved.	Regeneration or repair sometimes occurs if nerve not completely severed. Nerve damage following injection usually resolves after 5-7 days. Otherwise amputation required.	See Cooper (1978).
Curled toe paralysis.	Riboflavin deficiency.	Rotation of plantar digits at up to 15 days of age.	Clinical signs and history of inadequate diet. Clinical signs can be confused with straddle leg component of vitamin E deficiency - treat for both.	B vitamin supplementation, plus vitamin E.	See Chapter 22.
Paralysis of legs.	Unknown - sometimes possibly a B vitamin deficiency. (See Chapter 16 re kidney infection causing paresis/ paralysis of the lumbosacral plexus.)	Complete or partial paralysis. Digits tightly clenched, marked tone in leg muscles. Sensation present, but possibly impaired.	Clinical signs.	Some cases appear to respond to B vitamin complex.	See Cooper (1978). Birds with debilitating disorders, eg. chronic diarrhoea, may 'go off their legs'.
Vitamin E/ selenium deficiency.	Acute nutritional deficiency in neonates (see Figure 20.5).	Opisthotonus, 'star gazing', ataxia, weakness, straddle legs, tremors.	Clinical signs. Age. Rapid response to therapy.	Improve diet of parents. Prevent excessive storage of food. Inject selenium (0.05mg) and vitamin E (3.4iu) subcutaneously and repeat after 72 hours, eg. 0.05ml/ chick of Dystosel (Intervet). Follow with oral supplementation, eg. ACE High (Vetark).	

alternative fixative (some are suitable for both light microscopy and transmission electron microscopy) by intravenous injection immediately following euthanasia, or (2) small pieces of appropriate tissues are fixed in buffered formol saline, by immersion, within a few minutes of death.

Advice on these techniques can be obtained from a veterinary pathologist, preferably the one who is going to examine the tissues.

'Normal' samples are also required for comparison with pathological material, and the veterinary surgeon who has to kill a raptor - for example, one that has been injured - should consider fixing tissues as described earlier as reference specimens. The only disadvantage of the perfusion technique, other than the need to perform it proficiently, is that all tissues are fixed and microbiological investigations are not then possible.

CONCLUSIONS

This chapter has dealt with a range of conditions that can produce clinical signs suggestive of a neurological disorder. These cases can be difficult to diagnose and difficult to treat. Often they need to be considered as emergencies and the veterinary surgeon must be prepared to act quickly.

Some cases will not respond to treatment or will die before it can be given. These birds should be examined *post mortem*, preferably by an experienced avian pathologist. Despite the antiquity of 'fits' and allied conditions in raptors, many questions remain unanswered: the practitioner can contribute substantially to unravelling the solutions.

REFERENCES

Calnek BW, Barnes HJ, Beard CW, Reid WM and Yoder HW (1991) Eds *Diseases of Poultry*. 9th Edn. Wolfe, London.

Cooper JE (1978) *Veterinary Aspects of Captive Birds of Prey*. Standfast Press, Gloucester.

Dumonceaux G and Harrison GJ (1994) Toxins. In: *Avian Medicine: Principles and Application*. Eds BW Ritchie, GJ Harrison and LR Harrison. Wingers, Lake Worth.

Forbes NA (1987) Fits in the Harris' Hawk. *Veterinary Record* **120(11)**, 264.

Forbes NA (1995) Differential diagnosis and treatment of fitting in raptors with particular attention to the previously unreported condition of stress induced hyperglycaemia in Northern Goshawks (*Accipter gentilis*). In: *Proceedings of the European Association of Avian Veterinarians Conference, Jerusalem, 1995*. AAV, Lake Worth.

Gerlach H (1994) Viruses. In: *Avian Medicine: Principles and Application*. Eds BW Ritchie, GJ Harrison and LR Harrison. Wingers, Lake Worth.

Hochleithner M (1994) Biochemistries. In: *Avian Medicine: Principles and Application*. Eds BW Ritchie, GJ Harrison and LR Harrison. Wingers, Lake Worth.

Langelier KM (1993) Barbiturate poisoning in twenty nine bald eagles. In: *Raptor Biomedicine*. Eds PT Redig, JE Cooper, JD Remple and DB Hunter. University of Minnesota Press, Minneapolis.

Lumeij JT, Westerhof I, Smit T and Spierenburg TJ (1993) Diagnosis and treatment of poisoning in raptors from the Netherlands. In: *Raptor Biomedicine*. Eds PT Redig, JE Cooper, JD Remple and DB Hunter. University of Minnesota Press, Minneapolis.

Pokras MA, Wheeldon EB and Sedgwick CJ (1993) Trichomoniasis in owls. In: *Raptor Biomedicine*. Eds PT Redig, JE Cooper, JD Remple and DB Hunter. University of Minnesota Press, Minneapolis.

Porter SL (1993) Pesticide poisoning in birds of prey. In: *Raptor Biomedicine*. Eds PT Redig, JE Cooper, JD Remple and DB Hunter. University of Minnesota Press, Minneapolis.

Redig PT and Arendt TD (1982) Relay toxicity of strychnine in raptors in relation to a pigeon eradication programme. *Veterinary and Human Toxicology* **24**, 335.

Reiser MH and Temple SA (1981) Effects of chronic lead ingestion in birds of prey. In: *Recent Advances in the Study of Raptor Diseases*. Eds JE Cooper and AG Greenwood. Chiron Publications, Keighley.

Samour JH, Bailey TA and Cooper JE (1995) Trichomoniasis in birds of prey (Order Falconiformes) in Bahrain. *Veterinary Record* **136**, 358.

Smith SA (1983) Diagnosis of brachial plexus avulsion in three free-living owls. In: *Raptor Biomedicine*. Eds PT Redig, JE Cooper, JD Remple and DB Hunter. University of Minnesota Press, Minneapolis.

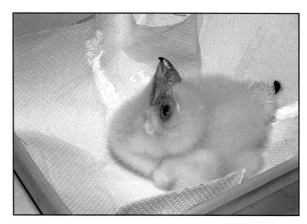

Figure 20.5: *Vitamin E/selenium deficiency in a neonate. (Photo courtesy N A Forbes)*

CHAPTER TWENTY ONE

Breeding Problems

Richard Best

INTRODUCTION

Captive breeding of raptors is now widely used to produce birds for falconry and exhibition, and also to produce offspring of endangered species for multiplication in captivity and release to the wild. The productivity of breeding birds can be increased by removing fertile eggs before or early in incubation and hatching them under foster birds or in incubators. Artificial insemination is used in some centres to produce pure-bred species and hybrids.

NORMAL BREEDING

Breeding activity is mainly stimulated, in temperate regions, by a decreasing day length prior to an increasing day length. Mature ova are released from the ovary and enter the oviduct at the infundibulum, where fertilisation occurs. As the ovum passes through the oviduct, albumen and shell membranes are laid down. Albumen is added in the magnum (3-4 hours) and the shell membranes in the isthmus (one hour). The shell is laid down in the uterus (shell gland) (20-22 hours) which is a discernible pouch-like structure. This complete process usually takes 24-26 hours. It has been shown that after insemination the spermatozoa of an American Kestrel will reach the infundibulum within at least 12-24 hours. After copulation or insemination the spermatozoa can remain viable in storage tubules in the anterior vagina and storage grooves in the infundibulum for periods as long as 12 days (Pendleton *et al*, 1987): in spite of this, most falcon breeders inseminate before each egg is laid. The reproductive tract of a female bird with an egg in the uterus is shown in Figure 21.1

CLINICAL EXAMINATION

The abdomen of breeding birds should be examined for signs of general enlargement or palpable masses. The lumen of the cloaca should also be examined either digitally or endoscopically for evidence of inflammation, calculi or other space-occupying lesions. Before the breeding season a routine clinical examination will ascertain that the birds are healthy and that any potential problems are identified. This is also an ideal time for routine parasite control. Owners should be encouraged to keep breeding birds under regular observation and to maintain accurate records.

LEGISLATION

Following amendments to the Wildlife and Countryside Act 1981, which took effect in May 1994, all indigenous diurnal raptors (with the exception of Eurasian Buzzards, Northern Sparrow Hawks and Common Kestrels) and certain non-indigenous species must be registered and ringed when kept in captivity. Metal alloy closed rings are used for captive-bred birds and plastic cable ties for others. Registration and ringing are controlled by the Department of the Environment.

Closed rings are placed around the tarsometatarsal region of a fledgling at 7-12 days of age, when the foot is just small enough to slip through the ring. Usually, both a male bird (smaller) and a female bird ring are applied at this time. The male bird ring is placed on last as this helps to hold the female bird ring on the leg. Once the sex of the bird has been established, the inappropriate ring should be removed.

HUSBANDRY PROBLEMS

Sex Determination

In many species of raptor there are few reliable plumage characteristics to determine sex. However, there is a marked, and generally reliable, difference in size in most species. Where the female is approximately 30% larger than the male, this is known as reverse sexual dimorphism. Some species show a weight range overlap between the sexes, which makes this method of sex determination unreliable.

Determination of sex in monomorphic species can be made by laparoscopic examination (see Chapter 23). This has the advantage of enabling the gonads and other organs to be examined as the same time. In some avian species, sex determination is possible by demonstration of deoxyribonucleic acid (DNA) associated with the sex chromosomes. However, at present, this procedure is not available for raptors other than owls. Chromosome examination (karyotyping) has also been used for sex determination.

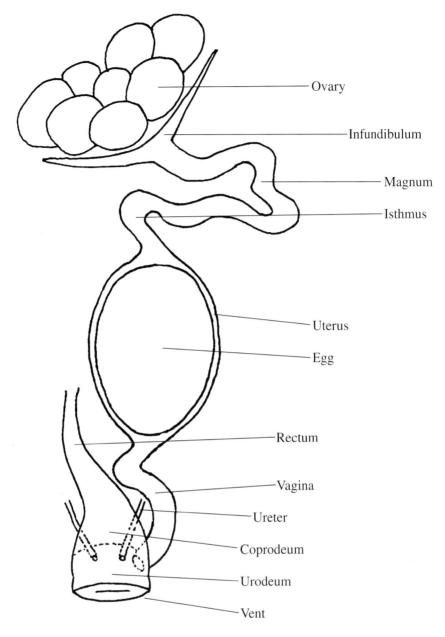

Figure 21.1: Reproductive tract of a female bird with an egg in the uterus.

Behavioural Problems

When a male and a female of the same species are placed together they may not necessarily form a pair bond. This incompatibility may show itself simply as absent or partial courtship and breeding behaviour, or it may lead to aggression, commonly from the female, often leading to injury or death of the male. Such aggression is a particular problem with Northern Goshawks and Merlin's, and is so common in captive Northern Goshawks that it must be viewed as normal. The male must be provided with an escape route and refuge as he would in 'the wild'. Many compatible pairs go through a female dominated aggressive phase. Problems of incompatiblity may be prevented by placing the male in the breeding aviary several weeks before introducing the female, and providing him with a screened refuge. Alternatively, the birds may be kept in adjoining aviaries and the smaller male only allowed with the female when she is truly receptive; at this time her aggression towards the male will be in temporary abeyance. Human imprinted birds, ie. those who think they are human, may fail to pair bond with a member of their own species.

Disturbance

Most pairs of breeding raptors are sensitive to disturbance. This may lead to problems with courtship, incubation or the rearing of young. Siting and design of breeding aviaries must be aimed at protecting the birds from unnecessary close disturbance. Many experienced breeders favour an aviary designed with solid walls and an open mesh roof, the so-called 'skylight seclusion' aviary. Others prefer to allow the birds some visibilty to the outside through partially netted or slatted walls. Observation ports should allow views, without disturbance, into every part of the aviary, especially the nest ledge. Feeding hatches should be similarly designed (see Chapter 22).

Nutrition

Breeding imposes a strain on the metabolic reserves of a bird, especially on the egg laying female. Deficiencies in calcium and vitamin D_3 may predispose to poor eggshell quality and eggbinding. Other deficiencies cause poor hatchability and problems in newly hatched chicks. The development of the embryo depends on nutrients stored within the egg and these, in turn, depend on the nutritional status of the female.

Overfeeding, lack of exercise and obesity in breeding birds is detrimental. However, care should be taken in advising restricted feeding as food items play an important part in courtship with most species. Food should be restricted prior to courtship and the male fed *ad libitum* (if kept separately) to encourage the concept of the male as the provider for the female.

MALE BREEDING PROBLEMS

Testicular Inactivity and Disease

Breeding failure due to testicular inactivity should be suspected if there is a lack of courtship behaviour and copulation and the production of unfertilised eggs. Unfertilised eggs are identified by the lack of any embryonic development, which can only be detected by candling (see later - Infertile Eggs and Hatching Problems) or opening the egg after a minimum period of 3-4 days incubation. Testicular inactivity will occur in sexually immature birds. In mature birds the gonads may be underactive for physiological or pathological reasons (including old age). Testicular activity can be partly assessed by laparoscopy. The testes may be small and obviously inactive with no visible vasculature, or larger and more active with a well-developed blood supply. Semen samples can be obtained by massage techniques. Sexually imprinted males can be trained to 'copulate' with their handlers. Semen can be examined to assess sperm density, motility and morphology employing similar techniques to those used to examine mammalian semen (Pendleton *et al*, 1987).

Synchronisation of Breeding Activity

Pairs may be compatible, yet not be in full breeding condition at the same time. Male birds are generally sexually mature 1-2 years before female birds. The age of maturity is variable from species to species (see Table 21.1). Members of the same species may not synchronise breeding activity if they originate from different global regions.

Behavioural Problems (see also Husbandry Problems)

Males who have previously been exposed to an aggressive female may lose their confidence and not breed even when provided with a different mate.

Table 21.1. Biological data of some common raptor species (CJ Griffiths, personal communication).

Species	Minimum age for breeding (years)	Clutch size	Incubation period (days)	Interval between eggs (days)	Start of incubation
Northern Goshawk	2-3	3-5	35-38	2-3	1st-2nd egg
Northern Sparrow Hawk	1-2	4-6	35-35	2-3	3rd-4th egg
Eurasian Buzzard	(2)-3	2-4	36-38	3	1st-2nd egg
Harris' Hawk	2-3	2-5	32	2-3	last egg or penultimate
Common Kestrel	1	3-6	27-29	1-2	2nd-3rd egg
Peregrine Falcon	2	3-4	29-32	2-3	last egg or penultimate
Barn Owl	1	4-7	30-31	2-3	1st egg
Northern Eagle Owl	2-3	2-4	34-36	2-3	1st-2nd egg
Snowy Owl	2	3-9	30-33	2-3	1st egg

Skeletal Problems

Successful copulation requires both birds to bring their cloacae into contact. To perform this acrobatic act each bird must be physically fit. Birds with permanent skeletal abnormalities may be unable to copulate successfully. In male raptors, loss of a wing can be a major obstacle as the male uses his wings to maintain his position on the female. Generally, male birds require all four limbs to be fully functional, though one-legged hawks may have normal conception rates.

Cloacal Disease

Any cloacal lesion in a male may lead to infertility by affecting his ability to copulate. Severe obstructive cloacal conditions will be life threatening.

Cloacal calculi, caused by accumulation of urates, will lead to partial or complete impaction of the cloaca. They are usually associated with cloacitis, seen as soiling of the vent region with urate deposits. There is often urate nephrosis. Cloacal calculi can be detected radiographically, by palpation of the cloaca externally through the abdominal wall, or internally with an auriscope, lubricated probe or finger. Affected birds may suffer intestinal and urinary blockages and require supportive fluid therapy. The calculus may be expressed through the vent by manual pressure either directly or following a single ventral midline cloacotomy incision.

Cloacitis, without associated calculus formation, will cause discomfort on defecation and be associated with soreness and cracking of the skin around the vent and soiling of the area with urates. Bacterial infection, commonly *Escherichia coli* or occasionally *Pseudomonas* spp., is associated with cloacitis and can be treated with antibiotics given systemically, eg. piperacillin (150mg/kg i/m bid), and/or locally. Inflammatory conditions of the cloaca may lead to granulation tissue developing on the cloacal mucosa and treatment must continue until this resolves.

An **oviduct prolapse** must be differentiated from a prolapsed cloacal tumour (see Figure 21.2) or an intestinal intussusception (see Figure 21.3) by careful examination of the presented tissues, radiography and, in an acute case, by laparotomy. Only a cloacal prolapse can be retained either by a purse-string suture placed in the skin immediately around the vent or by transverse stay sutures placed at the lateral aspects of the vent. Cloacopexy can be performed by suturing the ventral cloacal wall to the abdominal musculature via a midline laparotomy.

FEMALE INFERTILITY

Ovarian Inactivity and Disease

Breeding failure due to ovarian inactivity will occur in young sexually immature birds and in mature birds where activation of the gonads has failed for physiological or pathological reasons (including old age).

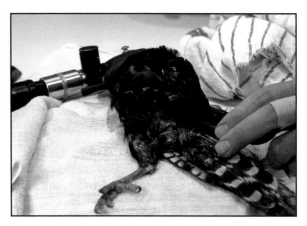

Figure 21.2: Oviduct prolapsed per cloacum. (Photo courtesy N A Forbes)

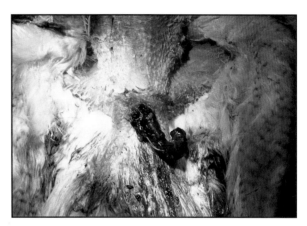

Figure 21.3: Intestinal intussusception prolapsed per cloacum. (Photo courtesy N A Forbes)

Ovarian activity can be assessed by laparoscopy.

Behavioural Problems

(see Husbandry Problems)

Oviduct Disease and Associated Problems
Eggbinding

Eggbinding is the inability of a bird to expel an egg from the reproductive tract and is an emergency requiring accurate diagnosis and appropriate treatment.

Eggbinding most commonly occurs in the lower part of the oviduct, but it can also occur from the upper oviduct to the cloaca. The severity of the condition depends largely on the position of the egg. When in the lower oviduct the egg can cause pressure, firstly, on the nerves and blood vessels, causing leg weakness, and secondly, on the kidneys, ureters and lower intestine, causing potential urinary and intestinal obstructions. Leg weakness may also be associated with hypocalcaemia.

Eggbinding is more common towards the end of a clutch and may be associated with low levels of dietary calcium or vitamin D_3 causing hypocalcaemia, physical or psychological trauma, inclement weather, or other factors, eg. oviduct or cloacal tumours. The obstructing egg often has a roughened, thin shell which may indicate a nutritional deficiency, oviductitis or a dysfunction of the shell secreting tissues of the shell gland.

Affected birds will often be found by the owner on the floor of the aviary. They will appear lethargic, often unable to perch, and may be seen to strain. They must be caught and handled with care so that the egg is not damaged. Palpation of a hard lump in the caudal abdomen is suspicious of eggbinding. Diagnosis should be confirmed on radiography; this will also assist in differentiating an egg from other abdominal masses. Laminated, unshelled eggs are found rarely and are not easy to diagnose radiographically. The main diagnostic confusion is between a bird exhibiting egg laying lethargy and one that is eggbound (see later).

Some eggbound birds will be suffering from shock and should be given fluid therapy (see Chapter 3). However, all eggbound birds should be treated initially with oxytocin (3-5 IU/kg i/m) and calcium gluconate 10% or calcium borogluconate 10% (1-5ml/kg i/v or s/c). Alternatively, a single dose of a prostaglandin may be given: dinoprost (0.02-0.1mg/kg i/m or directly into the cloacal mucosa) is thought to relax the vagina and increase the tone of the uterus, thus facilitating expulsion of the egg. Joyner (1994) suggested that dinoprost may be superior to oxytocin for expelling the egg. The cloaca should be lubricated and the bird placed in a warm environment (20-25°C). If the egg is not passed within 2-3 hours, or if the condition of the bird deteriorates, further intervention is indicated. Eggs that are bound in the cloacal region may be expressed through a well-lubricated vent by gentle pressure with finger and thumb on the abdominal wall in a caudal and ventral direction.

Eggs bound in the lower oviduct can be pressed gently towards the vent until the opening of the oviduct is identified as an open ring surrounded by a raised 'rosette' of tissue. This opening is explored with a blunt probe, eg. the plastic nozzle of a suitable oily medication which also acts as a lubricant. The shell is identified and, in many cases, may be delivered through the vent by steady, gentle pressure. If no progress is made, the shell may be breached with a metal instrument, the egg collapsed and the contents expelled. The shell can be removed carefully with forceps or left to be passed out on its own, which should occur naturally within two days.

These manipulations should be carried out under general anaesthesia, which must be administered with care in weak and distressed birds (see Chapter 9). If the anaesthetic risk is assessed to be great, the egg contents can be aspirated by abdominal paracentesis using a large bore needle directly through the ventral abdominal wall (see Figure 21.4) (Rosskopf and Woerpel, 1993). The egg may then collapse spontaneously if the shell is thin or absent, or be gently collapsed manually and the shell left to be passed within a few days.

Routine treatment with antibiotics for at least five days must be given to all cases. Recovery of cases that have been identified and treated in the early stages is usually good. Eggbinding of one egg will often cause retrograde peristalsis within the oviduct; if the subsequent egg has already entered the oviduct, egg peritonitis may ensue.

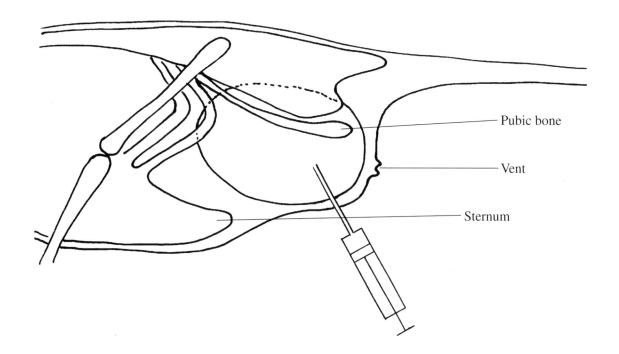

Figure 21.4: Site for needle aspiration of a retained, soft-shelled egg. (After Rosskopf and Woerpel, 1993)

Egg Peritonitis
Yolk material within the peritoneal cavity, usually associated with bacterial infection, will cause severe, acute and often fatal disease. This yolk material can originate directly from the ovary or from an ovum expelled from the oviduct. Evidence exists that yolk material on its own will only initiate a mild reaction. Peritonitis only follows a secondary bacterial infection, commonly with *Escherichia coli*. Bruising following eggbinding and retrograde peristalsis predisposes to egg peritonitis.

Egg peritonitis and eggbinding need to be differentiated as they produce similar symptoms in females in breeding condition. Radiography may exclude the presence of an egg and may show the distinctive ground glass appearance and loss of abdominal differentiation that occur in peritonitis. Raised white blood cell counts (>20 x 10^9/l) and serum fibrinogen levels (>4g/l) will indicate the presence of an inflammatory process which, together with cytology and bacteriology on fluid obtained by abdominal paracentesis, will help establish a diagnosis of egg peritonitis.

General supportive treatment by placing the bird in a warm environment (20-25°C), oral or intravenous fluids (via an indwelling catheter - see Chapter 3), together with antibiotic therapy, eg. piperacillin (150mg/kg i/m bid), should be effective in cases where diagnosis and treatment are instigated early.

Salpingitis
Bacterial infection of the oviduct may follow eggbinding. Large accumulations of inspissated material may be found in an infected oviduct.

Consideration should be made of a bird's future breeding career following repeated eggbinding, egg peritonitis or salpingitis. These conditions carry a high risk of fatality and, in many cases, future breeding should be prevented. Ovidectomy may be the treatment of choice.

Prolapse of the Oviduct
Prolapse of the oviduct tissue through the cloaca must be differentiated from a cloacal prolapse, a tumour or intestinal intussusception. The prolapse may follow egg laying or accompany the passage of an egg. It may even precede egg laying, especially if remnants of eggs from the previous year are fibrosed in the oviduct. The prolapse may also involve the cloaca, the ureters and the rectum. Affected birds will require immediate surgical attention and supportive fluid therapy. A midline laparotomy should be performed and the prolapsed part of the organ returned to the abdomen by gentle traction on the retained segment of the oviduct. The oviduct can then be secured within the abdomen by suturing to the abdominal wall. In a long-standing case the damage may be irreversible and surgical removal of the whole oviduct would be indicated.

An ovidectomy can be performed by sectioning the oviduct at the level of the vagina and dissecting the infundibulum from the ovary. Ovariectomy is not normally performed as adequate surgical access to the ovary is difficult and the risk of uncontrollable haemorrhage is high due to the short, inaccessible ovarian blood vessels. (Ovulation appears to cease in an ovidectomised bird.)

Cloacal Disease
A recurrent or persistent cloacal prolapse can occur following egg laying. This must be differentiated from a cloacal tumour, prolapsed oviduct or intestinal intussusception by careful examination of the presented tissues, contrast radiography and, in an acute case, laparotomy. The diagnosis and treatment of cloacal prolapse, cloacal calculus and cloacitis has been described earlier (see Male Breeding Problems).

Egg Laying Lethargy
Some females in breeding condition will show an apparent malaise for some days prior to the start of egg laying. Such birds become very lethargic and may have ruffled body plumage and partially closed eyes. The abdomen may look enlarged and the droppings become voluminous. This condition is normal and must be differentiated from eggbinding and egg peritonitis.

INFERTILE EGGS AND HATCHING PROBLEMS

The development of the embryo and the successful hatching of the chick are dependent partly on external environmental factors, ie. temperature and humidity, and partly on internal factors such as shell quality, nutritional content, genetic make-up and infections. Microorganisms can reach the egg from an infected ovary or oviduct before the shell is deposited, or gain entry through the porous shell. The egg is especially vulnerable to infection immediately after laying when, on cooling, the contents contract and the inner shell membranes separate and draw in air which forms an air cell.

Eggs may be left with the parents to hatch naturally, or they may be removed either immediately they are laid or after a period of natural incubation. Eggs left under the parents for the first 7-10 days will 'set' better and show a higher hatchability. Such eggs can be incubated artificially in an incubator or naturally under other broody females, including poultry. Only young poultry should be used in view of the risk of older hens excreting *Mycobacterium avium* and infecting the chicks.

The development of the embryo can be followed by 'candling'. Unhatched eggs are classified as 'clear' if no obvious embryonic development is apparent on candling, or 'dead-in-shell' if embryonic development is advanced. The investigation of unhatched eggs requires laboratory examination (Bird, 1980; Cooper,

1993) (see Chapter 11): the common causes are summarised in Table 21.2.

A normal egg (see Figure 21.5) should lose approximately 15-16% of its weight during incubation due to water loss through the shell. Hatching failure may occur if this loss is either too little or too great, and may be due to factors such as incorrect humidity or abnormal shell porosity. Incubators are usually kept at between 36.75-37.75°C with a relative humidity of 40-45%. Eggs may be weighed every 3-5 days to ensure correct weight loss. Regular weighings of an incubated egg can be compared with a projected optimal weight loss to indicate any possible incubator humidity problems (see Figure 21.6) (Weaver and Cade, 1987). Eggs may be moved to a second incubator kept at a slightly lower temperature and a higher

relative humidity at the first sign of 'pipping', ie. chicks breaking out of the eggs. Most incubated eggs will 'pip' at about 30 days and hatch after a further 48 hours.

PERINATAL DISEASE

Illness in the immediate post-hatching period may be a result of faulty incubation. Chicks may hatch in an exhausted state, weakened by prolonged effort. They may also be dehydrated or oedematous due to abnormal fluid loss during incubation, or have deformities, usually of the limbs, due to malposition within the egg. Hypothermia will occur rapidly if newly hatched chicks are not dried and kept warm. In aviaries, neonatal chicks may be injured or killed by the parents. Chicks may be weak and sickly due to infections

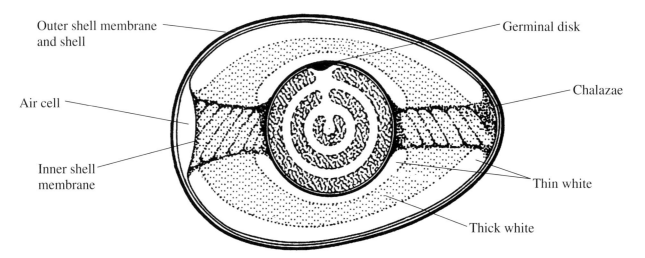

Figure 21.5: Structure of a normal egg. (From Anderson-Brown, 1979)

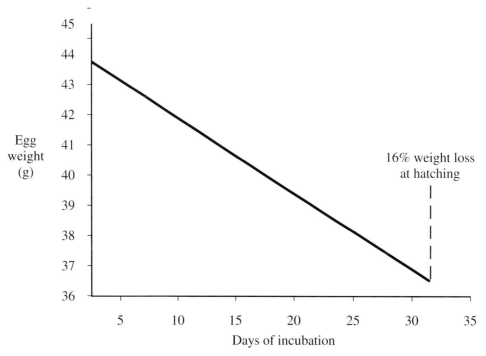

Figure 21.6: Typical weight loss during incubation of a normal raptor egg. (After Weaver and Cade, 1987)

Table 21.2. Causes of hatching failure in raptor eggs.

Appearance on candling	Stage of embryonic failure	Possible causes of failure	Additional causes associated with artificial incubation
Clear egg - no embryonic development.	No fertilisation apparent. Eggs may be fertilised but not developed.	Both birds female. No copulation. Infertile male. Disturbance, so no incubation. Non-synchronous breeding activity.	Incorrect temperature. Rough handling or excessive storage of egg.
Clear egg - early embryonic development.	Fertilisation - early death.	Chilling/disturbed incubation. Infection. Genetic make-up.	Incorrect temperature. Rough handling of egg.
Dead-in-shell: embryo not entered air cell.	Death in mid to late incubation.	Chilling/disturbed incubation. Nutritional deficiency. Infection. Excessive or impaired fluid loss.	Incorrect temperature. Incorrect turning. Incorrect humidity. Poor ventilation. Dirty eggs.
Dead-in-shell: embryo entered air cell; shell may be 'pipped'.	Death in last few days of incubation.	Chilling/disturbed incubation. Nutritional deficiency. Infection. Excessive or impaired fluid loss. Malposition of chick.	Incorrect temperature. Incorrect turning. Incorrect humidity. Dirty eggs.

contracted whilst in the egg. These chicks usually fade in the period up to 10 days of age (see Chapter 22).

HYGIENE OF AVIARIES AND INCUBATORS

Breeding Aviaries

Breeding aviaries cannot be cleaned regularly due to the problems associated with disturbance. However, the design of the aviary and the positioning of the perches should limit the soiling of the walls and food ledges, and the provision of a well-drained concrete or gravel floor will minimise contamination.

The whole aviary, and especially the nest ledges, should be thoroughly cleaned and disinfected prior to the breeding season.

Incubators

Control of hygiene in incubators is essential to reduce bacterial contamination of the eggs. If eggs are to be washed prior to setting, which is rarely recommended, a proprietary disinfectant must be used and the manufacturer's instructions regarding temperature and time followed exactly. As most raptor eggs will already have started to be incubated naturally, washing and disinfection at this stage might be dangerous for the developing embryo. Incubators should be cleaned and disinfected before use and then every two weeks. A variety of disinfectants can be used, eg. bleach, Virkon (Animalcare) or Chicgard (Antec), applied either directly to the incubator surfaces or using aerosol/fogging equipment. Fumigation with formaldehyde is effective and widely used. In contrast to the techniques

adopted in poultry hatcheries, routine disinfection is best performed with the eggs removed to a spare incubator.

REFERENCES

Anderson-Brown AF (1979) *The Incubator Book.* World Pheasant Association, Reading.

Bird DM (1980) Some microbiological aspects of egg hatchability in captive American Kestrels. In: *Recent Advances in the Study of Raptor Diseases.* Eds JE Cooper and AG Greenwood. Chiron Publications, Keighley.

Coles BH (1985) *Avian Medicine and Surgery.* Blackwell Scientific Publications, Oxford.

Cooper JE (1993) Pathological studies on egg embryos. In: *Raptor Biomedicine.* Eds PT Redig, JE Cooper, JD Remple and DB Hunter. University of Minnesota Press, Minneapolis.

Joyner KL (1994) Theriogenology. In: *Avian Medicine: Principles and Application.* Eds BW Ritchie, GJ Harrison and LR Harrison. Wingers, Lake Worth.

Pendleton BAG, Millsap BA, Cline KW and Bird DM (1987) Eds *Raptor Management Techniques Manual.* Institute for Wildlife Research, National Wildlife Federation, Washington DC.

Rosskopf WJ and Woerpel RM (1993) Avian obstetrical medicine. In: *Proceedings of the Association of Avian Veterinarians Annual Conference 1993.* AAV, Lake Worth.

Weaver JD and Cade TJ (1987) *Falcon Propagation.* The Peregrine Fund, New York.

CHAPTER TWENTY TWO

Neonate Husbandry and Related Diseases

Graham Butterworth and Nigel H Harcourt-Brown

INTRODUCTION

Until about twenty years ago, falconers were able to take birds from the wild in the UK, or import them from abroad, with little or no restriction. Nowadays, it is almost impossible to obtain a wild caught raptor unless the bird is too badly injured to return to the wild. This has required falconers to breed birds for either sporting purposes, as breeding birds, a combination of both roles, or for release back into the wild. Baby birds and even eggs are potentially valuable, especially if they are from the rarer species. Rearing raptors in captivity can be undertaken completely by the parent birds, or at the other extreme the falconer can undertake the entire process from the time the egg is laid. The various methods are an attempt to produce as many perfectly nourished and psychologically normal offspring as is reasonable.

IMPRINTING

Raptors have, like most other birds, a very poor ability to think and their behaviour is primarily controlled by reflex actions. These reflex actions are modified during the development of the chick by external stimuli. In the wild, most external stimuli related to social behaviour are provided by the parent, especially the mother; in captivity the stimuli may be modified to a greater or lesser extent by contact with the handler. This process is known as imprinting. Imprinting has four aspects:
● The learning process is confined to a brief well-defined period in the bird's development.
● Once the imprinted lesson is learnt, the memory is very stable and in some cases is irreversible
● The imprinting process is often completed long before what is learnt is relevant in the bird's behaviour, eg. some of what is imprinted in a chick may not be relevant until the chick is mature and starts to breed some years later.
● The imprinted lesson is generalised and the bird will respond to any member of the species relevant to the lesson that is imprinted, not just the individual that has caused the imprinting. In the case of adversely imprinted captive raptors, this can be any human.

In the natural environment the most effective stimuli are provided by the mother, approaches to the mother being rewarded by body contact and warmth or by food. The imprinting process attaches the baby bird to the parent and therefore to birds of the same species as the mother; imprinting also attaches the chick to its siblings.

Newly hatched chicks show no fear of a new object or event. As the chick's ocular and auditory senses develop, so do the fear responses, eg. avoidance, alarm calls, 'freezing', etc. As these fear responses develop, the ability to become imprinted decreases. In species of a nervous disposition, such as Northern Sparrow Hawks, the period of sensitivity to imprinting decreases rapidly at around 18 days of age. In other species of calmer disposition, such as the Harris' Hawk, this period of sensitivity lasts for longer and declines more gradually up to 16 weeks of age. Birds reared in isolation retain the ability to imprint for longer than those reared in groups, especially if the group has external stimuli.

When baby birds are reared with no contact with their parents, it is very likely that they will become imprinted on their keeper; this causes many undesirable behavioural characteristics. Adversely imprinted birds will regard humans as another bird and scream for food, attack or behave in a number of undesirable ways; they also fail to recognise other birds of the same species as mates etc. The methods of rearing birds discussed below are centred around minimising adverse imprinting and, in some instances, specifically imprinting 'desirable' behaviour.

METHODS OF REARING RAPTORS

Wild Birds
Adults birds select their nest site in a secure place with a good view. The young birds see and hear everything, recognise parents and siblings in adult and immature plumage respectively, and finally are taught to hunt by their parents. Wild birds seldom rear the maximum number of young; the main reason for this is the amount of food available. A survival of the fittest rule applies and the strongest and most dominant youngsters survive. These birds are psychologically normal as wild

birds, which includes being fearful of any new objects or events. To be trained successfully for falconry, these birds need lots of manning, initially and throughout their life, coupled with drastic weight control. These birds are imprinted on their own species. It is no longer legal to use these wild birds for falconry.

Captive-Bred Birds: Parent-Reared in Skylight and Seclusion Aviary

Skylight and seclusion aviaries have solid sides and an open roof; they shelter the adult birds completely and give maximum opportunity for nervous birds to breed. The young birds have contact with adult birds and siblings but see no humans or other external stimuli. Their only contact with the outside world is auditory. Small numbers of birds are produced by this method. Close inspection of the young is not possible and disease problems will therefore go unnoticed. Birds bred by this method are often given food *ad libitum*. This can result in nutritional deficiencies as the parents will take only the meat from the carcases instead of feeding the whole carcase. The young birds are not taught to hunt by their parents and are nervous and fearful of humans and their surroundings outside the aviary. Training for falconry is similar to that for wild birds, with lots of manning and strict weight control. The young birds do not have any flying or hunting experience prior to training and they are imprinted on their own species.

Peregrine Falcons reared by this method are more nervous than wild birds. Northern Goshawks will be similar to wild caught birds, whilst birds with placid temperaments, eg. Harris' Hawks, are unaffected by this method of rearing.

Using the above method, but adding slatted windows or having partially meshed open-fronted aviaries to allow the birds to become accustomed to humans and outside life, produces better adjusted birds from a behavioural point of view: they need less manning and can often be flown at a higher weight than the 'secluded' youngster. These birds can become partially imprinted on humans, dependent upon the degree of contact.

Some falconers modify this procedure to produce a large number of parent-reared youngsters. The female does not usually start to incubate until the third egg has been laid; she is allowed to incubate the eggs for 7-10 days and the eggs are then removed for artificial incubation. In a short time she will recycle and lay another clutch of eggs: in about 14 days for Peregrine Falcons, 11 days for Merlins, 18-21 days for Northern Goshawks and 17-18 days for Harris' Hawks. The young birds from the first clutch hatch and are hand reared. They are usually about seven days old by the time the second clutch has been laid and incubated for 7-10 days, so these chicks are placed in the nest at the time that the second clutch of eggs is removed. By the time the second clutch has been hatched and hand

reared to seven days old, the first clutch is big enough to place on the floor of the aviary when the second clutch is placed in the nest. The parents are willing to feed both groups of chicks. By the time the first chicks can fly up to the nest the second clutch chicks are strong enough to survive the competition.

This method allows almost 100% hatching and rearing to seven days; however, it puts a great deal of strain upon the laying female's reserves. If the diet is inadequately supplemented the second clutch of eggs can be inadequately nourished. Some breeders will produce a third clutch of eggs by this method, but the chicks from this clutch are even more likely to be nutritionally compromised.

Captive-Bred Birds: Behavioural Imprints

The young birds are reared solely by a human handler who takes the place of the parent bird completely: no attempt is made to disguise the handler. The birds are carried about from an early age and placed into maximum contact with people, other animals, different places and traffic. When the birds begin to fly they are not restricted: they can follow the handler outside and fly around. There is no need for a creance etc. Also, the birds start to fly when fat and still on several meals a day. When the birds are flying strongly the amount of food is decreased to gain some measure of control and to stop the birds becoming too independent and straying. At this point the birds generally start to scream for food as young wild birds do when their parents are weaning them. If the birds are encouraged to hunt and are successful, the screaming will decrease, as it does with wild birds. If the birds are not successful at hunting, the screaming will persist. These birds are usually aggressive to birds of their own species and will not usually breed naturally when sexually mature. Owls are an exception to this; many will still breed naturally when reared as behavioural imprints.

Shutting a screaming bird away from human contact in a large aviary for about a year will often allow the bird to become apparently normal.

Theoretically, behavioural imprints are the best birds for falconry as they do not require their weight to be reduced drastically to be flown. They can be flown at weights approximating to the weight that they would be in the wild. This is the only way that Northern Sparrow Hawks should be reared for hunting. The birds can be closely monitored throughout their development, and in the right hands these birds will attain their full potential.

Other Methods of Rearing

Production of social imprints or the skylight and seclusion bred birds are at opposite ends of a spectrum of methods for breeding and rearing raptors in captivity. Between these two methods there are many variations.

Crèche Rearing

Crèche rearing involves groups of young of similar ages being reared together with human contact. This method produces birds that accept humans and can also react socially to other birds of the same species; when sexually mature they are able to breed naturally, or by artificial means, dependent upon their degree of exposure to either humans or birds.

Isolated Crèche Rearing

Isolated crèche rearing is similar to standard crèche rearing but with the birds having minimal contact with humans. The young birds are fed by sending the food down a chute. This method of rearing produces birds that are more nervous than the preceding method, but they are still tamer than parent-reared birds. Young birds reared in this manner are still able to be bred by natural or artificial methods.

Hand Rearing

It is also possible to hand rear young birds and place them with their parents or foster-parents at 10 days old. This allows the production of two clutches of eggs/young from one pair of birds. Another method is to allow the parents to rear the young to about 35 days and then fly them at hack, with or without close contact with humans.

In general, rearing methods that involve human contact should produce maximum numbers of good quality young birds. Any problems that arise can be detected early and appropriate remedial action taken. Young birds that are being parent reared are difficult to monitor as closely, and in many cases the young birds will have died and/or disappeared before any problem is noticed.

FEEDING AND GROWTH

Feeding - General Considerations

Growth can occur only if the organs and tissues receive the nutrients needed for their synthesis; it is therefore dependent on an adequate diet. Insufficiency of energy and available protein are the commonest causes of raptors failing to grow or showing disproportional growth. However, in theory, a dietary deficiency of any one of the 35 or more nutrients known to be essential for raptors could be responsible for impairment of growth. Growth is also impaired when disease of the alimentary tract prevents adequate absorption of nutrients, eg. repeated occurrences of gastroenteritis, sour crop, etc. Many disorders of metabolism prevent normal utilisation of nutrients and so retard growth or development. Chronic infectious diseases severely retard growth; they can do this by reducing appetite or by preventing normal absorption or utilisation of nutrients.

The adage 'We are what we eat', as well as applying to human nutrition, also applies to all animal nutrition, including that of raptor chicks. A chick needs to be fed a type of food that (a) can be digested, absorbed and utilised with maximum efficiency, and (b) provides all the required nutrients that it needs for energy, maintenance and growth in the correct amounts for the current stage of growth. For example, it is inefficient for a one-day-old raptor chick to be fed a type of food that provides the ideal nutrient combination that would enable the feather growth that it would require if it was about four weeks old. Put simply, a one-day-old chick needs food that will make it into a two-day-old chick in the most efficient way, and when the chick is two days old it needs food that will make it into a three-day-old chick, and so on; the chick's nutritional requirements are constantly changing during its period of growth. Details of the sources and types of food that should be fed to raptor chicks are given in the captions to Figures 22.1 to 22.9.

A secondary effect of feeding a diet that does not have an ideal nutrient combination for a particular type of raptor chick is that the chick, to achieve normal growth, may have to eat a larger amount of food to obtain sufficient limiting nutrients. This large volume of food places a greater load upon the digestive system, not only because of the amount of food that needs to be processed, but by the amount of time that the food is present in the gut. Food that spends too long in the gut can upset the balance of bacteria, and the young chick will not yet have maximum resistance to infection. The same problem is caused by feeding a diet that is not easily digestible; tough food also spends too much time in the gut.

Young chicks up to one week old, with their still developing digestive systems, need to be fed easily digestible foods such as skinned day-old poultry chicks or baby mice. These foods should be as fresh as possible. If frozen, they should have been rapidly frozen when fresh, and fed newly thawed. Both of these foods will pass through the gut very quickly and are easily digestible; this is vital to avoid bacterial infections in young chicks. Feeding probiotics at this stage may be helpful. Older chicks need a diet that contains adequate minerals during periods of maximum skeletal growth and high levels of relevant amino acids during periods of maximum feather growth (see Figures 22.7-22.9). All raptor chicks should be supplemented with a suitable avian vitamin and mineral supplement from two to three days old.

Immediately after hatching the chick is only able to lie upon its side with its head bowed over, pointing towards its feet. This position is partly due to the prominent 'hatching muscle' (*m. complexus*) that is located on the dorsal aspect of the neck. However, the prominence of this muscle is transitory and it starts to regress; by about 4-6 hours after hatching it has reduced considerably. The chick is then able to lie upon its stomach and raise its head to beg for food.

First attempts at begging for food are usually quite feeble and the chick soon tires and needs to rest. However, with adequate feeding the chick can usually beg for food quite strongly by the end of the first day.

At one day old the chick has usually mastered the food begging and food taking actions. Its range of movements also starts to become more extensive: it will roll up when too cold, stretch out when too warm, and if there is a concentrated heat source it will attempt to move away from or approach it to regulate its temperature (see Figure 22.1).

By three days old the chick is growing fast. Its digestive system starts to become more efficient and the throughput of food it can handle starts to increase dramatically (see Figure 22.2). During this period the chick's visual capabilities increase. Diurnal raptors usually have their eyes open directly after hatching and by seven days old they can distinguish individual objects as distinct from their earlier perception of just light and dark. Nocturnal raptors (owls) have their eyes closed after hatching and their eyes usually start opening between 4-6 days old.

At seven days old most chicks are starting to grow their second, much thicker coat of down (see Figures 22.3, 22.4). Their vision continues to improve until at about 14 days old most chicks have normal adult vision.

At 14 days old the chicks are still sitting upon their haunches, but most chicks are starting to pull at pieces of food held in their feet. They have also acquired a voluminous coat of secondary down and therefore require less brooding than before (see Figures 22.5, 22.6).

Between two and four weeks old the chick's previously slowly developing nervous system, along with its now fully functioning vision and auditory systems, have developed sufficiently for it to absorb much more information and to react accordingly. Imprinting can now occur, as can fear responses, and the chick can show significant ability to react to its own experiences. Feather growth is now considerable and by four weeks old most chicks are starting to lose their down as feather growth continues. They are also starting to stand upright on their feet as opposed to sitting on their haunches. As a result of this they stand and can therefore feed upon whole carcases more readily (see Figure 22.7). The wings develop at a similar rate to the legs, and by four weeks old the wing feathers are three quarters grown, allowing the birds to flap and flutter on the nest. Their feathers continue to grow: by five weeks old the birds are able to fly onto the floor, where they will feed on food dropped to them (see Figure 22.8); by six weeks old they are strong enough to fly back to the nest ledge and their feathers are full grown. Peregrine Falcons develop at the above rate; smaller birds develop faster; hawks grow more slowly; and eagles and vultures slower still.

NEONATE DISEASES

Many diseases that are seen in young birds are due to inadequate nutrition of the parents in the months leading up to laying and during the laying period. Some females are expected to lay up to 16 eggs in a season, and unless the diet is correctly supplemented many of these eggs will fail to hatch or, less noticeably, the chicks fail to thrive. A chick from a nutritionally deprived egg will fail to grow at the correct rate and will also have a greater incidence of abnormalities and disease than a chick from a normal egg. In the opinion of the authors, all birds should be supplemented with a good quality avian vitamin and mineral supplement, such as A1 Raptor (G Butterworth), Avimix (Vetark) or Vitahawk (distributed in UK by Ben Long), the quantity of which varies with the birds' requirements; supplementation should start from day two. Many raptor keepers think that it is adequate to feed what they describe as a good varied diet and no supplement because this is what the birds eat in the wild; wild birds seldom rear more than half their clutch and skeletal abnormalities such as deviation of the keel can be seen in wild birds.

Many diseases are seen as a result of incorrect incubation temperature and/or humidity levels. Gross variations from the norm will stop all the chicks from hatching, but mild abnormalities may result in failure of retraction of the yolk sac, torticollis, curled or crooked toes, ataxia or stargazing, as well as the chicks being weak, stunted or poor growers. These conditions may have other causes, but if they are seen in young birds where there has been a poor hatch rate, then incubation technique as well as the nutritional status of the parents must be assessed. Further information on causes of incubation faults at different stages can be found in Chapter 40.

Failure of Retraction of the Yolk Sac

The yolk sac should retract into the chick prior to hatching, and then the umbilicus closes (see Figure 22.10). Some birds hatch with a yolk sac the size of a pea or smaller protruding from the body. Keeping the bird in a brooder on clean paper towels will allow the yolk to be absorbed and the sac to dry up and drop off over a period of 4-5 days. Heck and Konkel (1983) recommended povidone-iodine as a navel antiseptic; this is often not necessary. Sometimes, the yolk sac is larger than this and may burst; the stump should be tied off with nylon. The yolk sac is a source of nutrition to the young bird for the first few days of life and so the bird is deprived of a large amount of vital nutrient if the stump is tied off. The chick must be heavily supplemented with double the normal quantity of vitamins, otherwise nutrition-related abnormalities such as poor or abnormal growth will occur.

Heck and Konkel (1983) recommended that a large unretracted yolk sac should be pushed into the

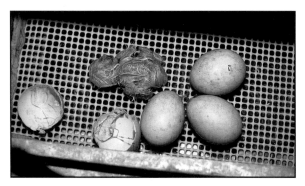

Figure 22.1: A clutch of four Northern Goshawk eggs in the hatcher at a temperature of 37.5°C. One has just hatched, the others have pipped. The chick will take 5-10 minutes to dry, but will need to be rubbed 'fluffy' with cotton wool. Although the yolk sac will be absorbed over two days and will provide nourishment, the chick will beg for food by 8-12 hours after hatching, when it may be fed on day-old chick muscle meat, either fresh or newly thawed.

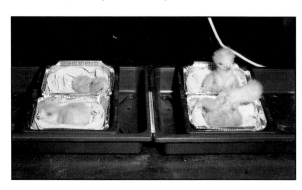

Figure 22.2: Harris' Hawks at 2-3 days old. A dull-emitting heat lamp is suspended above them to provide a temperature of approximately 32.2 °C. The young birds are fed on pieces of day-old chicks (not skin or yolk sac) or pieces of baby rats or mice (pinkies), plus an avian vitamin and mineral supplement. Probiotics may also be useful. The birds are fed using forceps every 4-6 hours as soon as their crops are empty and they beg for food. They are kept on paper towels which are changed after each feed.

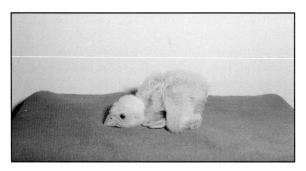

Figure 22.3: Seven days after hatching, this Peregrine Falcon is in its typical lying position. It can raise its head to beg for food and is able to sit for short periods on its intertarsal joints. It is still covered with the first coat of down feathers. It is now eating cut up day-old chicks, unskinned but with their yolk sac removed, and with some vitamin and mineral supplement. It is still too young to receive fur or feathers. It is just starting to feed from a saucer four times per day. At this age it is still important to feed the chicks only when their crops are empty, and to feed until full. Carpenter et al (1987) stated that an eaglet should eat 8% of its bodyweight per feed and increase its weight by 10% daily.

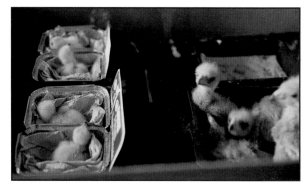

Figure 22.4: A group of 10-day-old Harris' Hawks and three-day-old Northern Goshawks. The beer mats are to retain the mutes which are sliced (squirted) over the side of the trays, and also to protect the Northern Goshawks from the squabbles and fights between the Harris' Hawks.

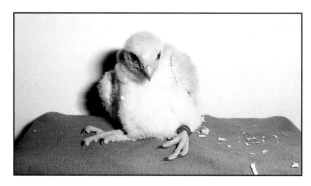

Figure 22.5: By 14 days old a Peregrine Falcon is able to stand for brief periods and is eating 3-4 meals per day off a saucer. This bird was ringed at 11 days using both male and female rings obtained from the Department of the Environment. Both rings may be placed on the same leg with the female ring proximal to the male. When grown, the male ring must be cut off if the bird is female. The bird is covered with a second coat of down and no longer needs brooding. It has fully developed its senses of hearing and vision. The bird is kept on wood shavings, the mutes are picked out after each meal, and the shavings are changed daily. Care must be taken to avoid the bird eating food covered with shavings as the bird cannot 'cast' and will become impacted.

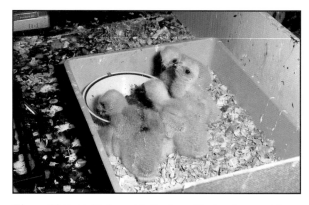

Figure 22.6: At 14 days old, Northern Goshawks are at the same stage of development as a Peregrine Falcon. A brood can be together in the same tray. They are kept at approximately 17°C, and will huddle together if they are too cold. They are fed from a saucer and eat chopped day-old chicks, with a vitamin and mineral supplement on each meal. At this age and stage of development, Northern Sparrow Hawks are sold to be reared as social imprints.

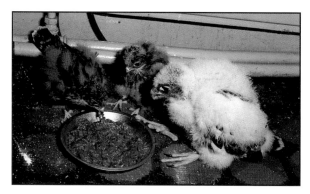

Figure 22.7: A male Peregrine Falcon and two male Merlin chicks at 28 days old. These birds are being reared as social imprints. The Merlins have developed and are feathered; their primaries and tail feathers are half the full-grown length. The Peregrine Falcon has quarter-grown wing and tail feathers. They are eating whole four-week-old, chopped-up quail or chickens, still with vitamins and minerals added. Buzzards, Harris' Hawks and eagles are developing more slowly by this stage.

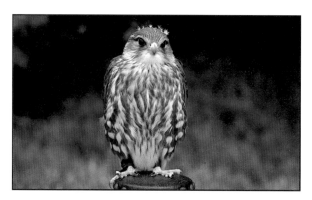

Figure 22.8: At five weeks old this Merlin is almost fully fledged, is eating a whole small quail or small chicken carcase, is still having three meals a day, and will go to a new home at seven weeks old; Northern Goshawks and Peregrine Falcons take 10 days longer to reach the same stage. These birds are unlikely to become adversely imprinted after 7-8 weeks of age.

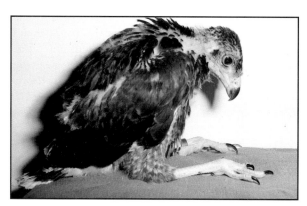

Figure 22.9: A Harris' Hawk at five weeks old has grown all its contour feathers, its wing and tail feathers are only a quarter grown, and it is eating chopped whole carcases three times a day. It is able to stand but still spends a lot of time on its intertarsal joints, in this typical pose. Harris' Hawks are very boisterous and fight frequently. They are fully grown at 12-14 weeks old but are still able to become adversely imprinted until 16 weeks old; this seems to be linked with their unique social behaviour.

coelomic cavity and sutured into place; intestine that has prolapsed through the umbilicus should also be replaced and the umbilicus surgically closed. These procedures carry a high risk of omphalitis and peritonitis, even with care, sterility and postoperative antibiotics.

Nutritional Osteodystrophy

This is also dealt with in Chapters 13 and 16; however, it is seen in some very young birds. The chicks are presented gasping and apparently unable to swallow or feed. Owners complain that the chicks' throats are obstructed. These birds are usually from nutritionally deficient parents and, in addition, the chicks have

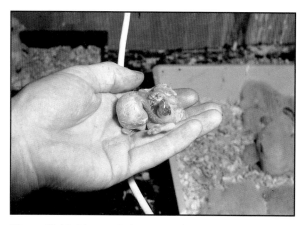

Figure 22.10: This newly hatched Peregrine Falcon has not retracted its yolk sac. With care this had dried up by day four when the shrivelled remnant dropped off.

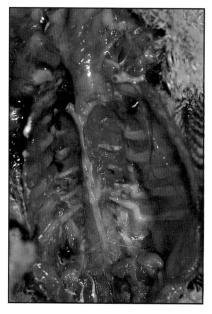

Figure 22.11: Post-mortem examination of a five-day-old Eurasian Buzzard. The chick had come from unsupplemented parents. Many of their eggs had failed to hatch. The diet of the adults and the youngsters was unsupplemented day-old chicks. The distorted ribs can be seen after removal of the lungs and kidneys. All the long bones were more pliable than usual.

usually had no supplement. The birds have become weakened, the ribs are deformed (see Figure 22.11) and the lungs distorted, the food has caused an inhalation pneumonia and the birds invariably die. Parent birds that are allowed too much food will overfeed their young with muscle meat with the same result.

Splay Legs

Splay legs is the name given to a condition that can be caused by lack of support for a well-nourished growing chick. The bird attempts to stand but its leg muscles are not strong enough and the legs splay out. If the chick is left like this a permanent deformity can result. Placing with several other chicks and reducing the temperature to encourage huddling can prevent this condition occurring. If the chick is on its own or is badly affected, it should be placed in a suitably sized, high-sided bowl lined with padding. Unsupplemented birds will have splay legs but with concomitant folding fractures of legs and wings (see Figures 22.12, 22.13). If badly affected, these birds should be euthanased as they rarely develop into normal adult birds.

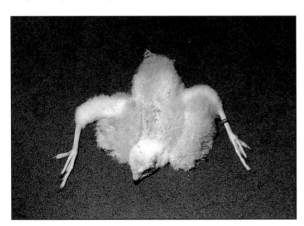

Figure 22.12: A 16-day-old Northern Sparrow Hawk presented with splay legs. The bird had been fed on day-old chicks with no vitamin supplement since being sold some six days previously. It had been kept with other chicks of the same age which were similarly affected. Radiography showed folding fractures of all the major wing bones and the tibiotarsi, as well as the femurs.

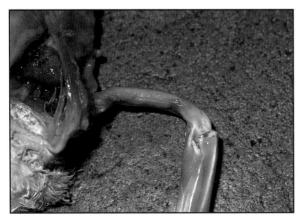

Figure 22.13: Post mortem. The left femur from the same chick. The bone is bent at the distal and proximal thirds.

Starvation: Hypoglycaemia

A seven day-old Merlin that has had no food for 12 hours will become incoordinate, its feet will bunch up and it will start to have fits. The administration of glucose by crop tube or injection will reverse the condition immediately. Larger birds take longer for these symptoms to show: 18 hours for a Peregrine Falcon. Older birds with these symptoms and no starvation may be suffering from lead poisoning, especially if fed with minced rabbit, pigeon or pheasant (see Chapter 20).

Starvation caused by lack of food or illness in older birds will frequently produce an interval of poor growth across the growing feathers: fret marks. All the growing feathers are affected at the same time and so the fret mark appears as a line across the tail and wing feathers. These feathers will break very easily when the bird is flown (see Chapter 14.2). Individually marked feathers can often be caused by mites.

Star Gazing

In poultry this is generally attributed to incorrect incubation or nutritional failure. If the birds are fed on an incorrect diet then it must be supplemented. Vitamin E and selenium deficiencies are common causes of this condition (see Chapter 20; Figure 20.5). Harris' Hawks can exhibit this trait at about seven days old even when well supplemented with vitamin E and selenium. Their star gazing will be made worse if the bird is fed by forceps from directly above; the bird should be fed from in front and its head stopped from going up by the gentle use of a finger.

Bacterial Hepatitis and/or Septicaemia

Parental passive immunity is transferred through the egg in birds. The parents have produced antibodies to the antigens in the aviary environment. Artificial incubation and rearing will subject young and immunoincompetent chicks to a different range of infections compared with those to which their parents may have been exposed. Infections may pass through the eggshell or may enter via the umbilicus; infections can also occur orally, usually with the food, when the new gut is immunoincompetent and before it has its normal gut flora. The chicks will look tired and lethargic (see Figure 22.14), fail to be as willing to eat, and will die very quickly. The urates are often green rather than white. The skin of the bird may appear crinkley and the bird's face wizened: these are signs of dehydration. Dehydration due to hyperthermia must not be confused with this condition. Oral fluid therapy and antibiotics will save the early cases. The bacteria are often Gram-negative. Drugs that are useful include enrofloxacin, co-trimazine, or a combination of tobramycin and lincomycin (see Appendix - Formulary [Raptors]). A 5-7 day course is necessary to prevent recurrence. It is often useful to use probiotics in the first few weeks of life in breeding facilities where this condition is common.

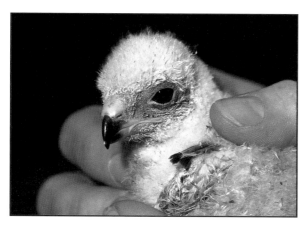

Figure 22.14: A 14-day-old Northern Sparrow Hawk which had become unwell with a bacterial hepatitis. Even when stimulated the bird looked sleepy, and it had stopped eating. The egg tooth is still clearly visible.

Coccidiosis

Coccidiosis, due usually to *Caryospora falconis*, is seen in young birds, especially Merlins and some owls, at 4-6 weeks of age. The birds have usually been stressed by moving them into different surroundings. The birds appear lethargic and unsteady, and they die within six hours of these symptoms. Some cases are less acute and develop diarrhoea containing coccidial oocysts. All raptors with coccidial oocysts in their faeces should be medicated with clazuril (5-10mg/kg p/o once daily three times on alternate days). Breeders who have had cases should be advised to give a single prophylactic dose at between 17-20 days of age and again at six weeks of age.

Haemoproteus

These protozoa will cause acute weight loss and collapse due to anaemia in many species of birds. Recent warm summer weather in the UK has increased the incidence of this disease. Cases have been seen most frequently in Snowy Owls and Harris' Hawk. These birds have been bred in the UK and were not in the vicinity of imported birds. Diagnosis is made on examination of a blood smear. Treatment is with a single dose of primaquine (Primaquine Phosphate, Winthrop) (0.75-1mg/kg p/o) and three doses of chloroquine (Aralen, Winthrop) (15mg/kg p/o at twelve hour intervals) (Redig *et al*, 1993), together with supportive therapy.

REFERENCES

Carpenter JW, Gabel RR and Wiemeyer SN (1987) Captive breeding: eagles. In: *Raptor Management Techniques Manual*. Eds BAG Pendleton, BA Millsap, KW Cline and DM Bird. Institute for Wildlife Research, National Wildlife Federation, Washington DC.

Heck WR and Konkel D (1983) Incubation and rearing. In: *Falcon Propagation*. Eds JD Weaver and TJ Cade. The Peregrine Fund, New York.

Redig PT, Talbot B and Guarnera T (1993) Avian malaria. In: *Proceedings of the Association of vain Veterinaries Annual Conference 1993*. AAV, Lake Worth.

Thorpe WH (1964) Imprinting. In: *A New Dictionary of Birds*. Ed A Landsborough Thomson. T Nelson, London.

CHAPTER TWENTY THREE

Miscellaneous (Raptors, Pigeons and Waterfowl)

Neil A Forbes and Nigel H Harcourt-Brown

INTRODUCTION

There are a number of conditions that do not fall readily into the format of the other chapter headings within this manual. This may be due to their multifactorial nature or simply that it is not possible to place them elsewhere. The result is a miscellany of conditions and topics which are unrelated but could not be left out of this manual. This chapter is placed at the end of the raptor section but it should be noted that it does include information relating to raptors, pigeons and waterfowl.

INDIVIDUAL IDENTIFICATION

Raptors, pigeons and waterfowl may all have identifying closed rings (leg bands) placed around the tarsometatarsal region soon after hatching. This is essential for pigeons which are to be used for racing and which therefore require a specific ring, and for those raptor species listed in Schedule 4 of the Wildlife and Countryside Act 1981 (this includes Peregrine Falcons, Gyr Falcons, Merlins, Northern Goshawks, Golden Eagles, any hybrid of the above, as well as a number of very rare species) which require a ring from the Department of the Environment. If captive-bred raptors of other species are to be sold, they require an individually numbered closed metal ring, eg. British Bird Council or AC Hughes. All breeders of birds should be encouraged to carry out permanent identification of all their progeny. In this way accurate breed records and stud lines can be maintained.

Some form of identification is recommended in raptors, especially those species no longer on Schedule 4 and which are not therefore legally required to be ringed. Rings are easily removed after a bird has been stolen. Therefore, other forms of permanent identification should be maintained, preferably either DNA 'fingerprinting' or electronic identification chips. DNA fingerprinting is very expensive; electronic chips are relatively cheap and have been used safely in many thousands of raptors without problems. The British Veterinary Zoological Society (BVZS) recommend that the microchip is injected into the pectoral muscle at the caudal margin of the sternum. In this site the chip is not visible or palpable and it may be read whilst the bird is on the fist or perch. No sedation or anaesthesia is required for implantation. If the implant leaves a large hole in the bird's skin, a catgut suture should be placed to stop the chip being extruded. Birds should not be flown for 72 hours after a microchip is implanted. Even birds that are ringed should have an identichip to allow permanent proof of identity should the ring be removed or become illegible.

Waterfowl may have British Trust for Ornithology (BTO) or Darvid rings placed at any time.

SEDATING LOST BIRDS

Clinicians are frequently approached regarding the sedation of lost or injured raptors or waterfowl. Under the Wildlife and Countryside Act 1981, many raptors may only be recaptured in the first two weeks after their escape or loss. If the bird will not come close enough to catch when hungry and tempted with food, trapping in a humane trap, eg. Larsen trap, purse net or mist net, can be recommended. It is possible to sedate birds with oral diazepam (2-5mg/kg; proportionally less for larger birds). All sedatives take some time to work and the bird has usually flown away before the sedative has taken effect. However, it does make it easier to chase the bird and occasionally makes it easier to catch, especially if one is climbing a tree at night!

Ketamine (100mg/kg in a 30g piece of meat) has been used to immobilise a captive Harris' Hawk which had flown off and was avoiding recapture (Garner, 1988). This method may also be used for catching ducks on a pond.

SEX DIFFERENTIATION

Raptors

Captive breeding of raptors is extremely important to many bird keepers. Some species of raptors demonstrate reverse sexual dimorphism, ie. the females are generally 30% larger than the males. However, some species have more than one race, each of different size, eg. *Buteo* spp. Therefore, there may be an overlap in the weights of the sexes and it is difficult to be sure if the bird is a large male or a small female. Some species are sexually monomorphic, eg. owls. DNA chromosomal sex differentiation is not currently possible in raptors. Standard endoscopic techniques may be safely employed (see Laparoscopy).

Waterfowl

Most waterfowl can be differentiated by plumage colouration or by size, weight or long bone measurement. DNA differentiation is possible in an increasing range of waterfowl species. The laboratory (Vetgen Europe, Winchester, UK) should be contacted for details. Occasionally, endoscopic examination is required (see Laparoscopy).

SUDDEN DEATH IN RAPTORS

Causes of sudden death in raptors are listed in Table 23.1.

REHABILITATION OF INJURED WILD BIRDS

The rescue, care and re-release of injured wild birds is a highly emotive subject amongst well-meaning members of the public. The clinician has a duty to help, assist and advise rescue organisations. The advice may sometimes be hard to accept and unwelcome; many

Table 23.1. Causes of sudden death in raptors.

Cause of death	*Post-mortem* signs	Prevention	Species susceptibility
Respiratory obstruction, most frequently when a bird attempts to cast whilst in transit or whilst hooded.	Tracheal or choanal and oral obstruction.	Do not give casting the day before travelling. Do not hood a bird when it is due to cast.	Any.
Hypocalcaemia.	Extensor rigidity, post-fitting.	Susceptible species should be 'manned' before transport or other stressful events.	Northern Goshawks in particular.
Hyperglycaemia.	Extensor rigidity, post-fitting.	Slower, more gentle 'manning' or the use of socially imprinted birds, so that training is less stressful to the bird.	Northern Goshawks in particular.
Hypoglycaemia	No significant signs.	Beware flying small susceptible species at too light a weight or in inclement weather.	Northern Sparrow Hawks.
Trauma (in particular intersex aggression in breeding pairs).	Traumatic injuries.	Great care should be exercised regarding the timing of the mixing of sexes in breeding birds.	Northern Goshawks and Merlins.
Caryospora spp. Acute death in young birds 28-45 days of age. Clinical disease is often preceded by a minor episode of stress, eg. moving birds from one aviary to another. Chicks are found dead or are lethargic for 24 hours prior to death.	Haemorrhage in small intestine.	Faecal oocyst counts on adults prior to breeding, in an attempt to reduce nest ledge contamination. Treatment of 'at risk' chicks before clinical disease, eg. with clazuril (see Chapter 19) .	Merlins are most commonly affected, but any species may be affected.
Poisoning, eg. strychnine, carbon monoxide, severe lead poisoning.	Variable with respect to agent.	Avoidance of toxic agents.	Any species.
Arteriosclerosis. Commonest in middle to old aged breeding birds, especially females.	Thickening of great vessel walls.	Prevent obesity, feed low fat diet, encourage exercise.	Any species. Commoner in falcons, especially Gyr Falcons.

Table 23.1. Continued.

Cause of death	*Post-mortem* signs	Prevention	Species susceptibility
Acute bacterial infection.	Air sacculitis, visceral gout affecting serosal surface of liver and pericardium, many other possible variable signs.	Good husbandry, feeding pathogen-free food.	Any species.
Acute viral infections, eg. Newcastle disease, Falcon herpesvirus, adenovirus, etc.	Variable depending on pathogen.	Good husbandry, correct quarantine procedure.	Any species. Mauritius Kestrel is particularly susceptible to a variety of virus infections.
Tick toxicity reaction due to *Ixodes* spp. infestation.	The tick is likely to be found on the corpse, with significant oedema and vasculitis in the surrounding tissue.	Prevent or reduce risk of contact with ticks.	Any species.
Urogenital tract, eg. egg peritonitis, eggbinding, orchitis, prolapsed oviduct.	Variable, characteristic signs.	Minimise stress during breeding season.	Any species.
Gut obstruction or prolapse.	Characteristic *post-mortem* signs.	Careful observation.	Any species. Red-tailed Hawk most commonly affected.

injured wild birds should be euthanased as soon as they are presented for examination. **It is the authors' firm opinion that only those birds which have a realistic opportunity of release to the wild should receive treatment.** The maintenance of handicapped or crippled wild birds in captivity can very rarely be justified. If handicapped birds are kept they fill the rescue centre, acting as a drain on precious time and resources. They can prevent sufficient time and care being given to those birds which have a good chance of return to the wild.

Raptors

The single largest cause for admission of raptors to rescue centres (apart from 'orphans') is traumatic injuries with fractured bones. The bone which is fractured, the type of fracture, the proximity of the fracture to a joint, and the condition of the fracture and the surrounding tissue all have a bearing on the potential outcome. The following figures (Howard and Redig, 1993) give respective recovery rates and are of great value in assessing the likely outcome in different situations:

Total admissions	802
Birds with fractures	542

Number of fractured long bones		733
Incidents with:	1 fracture	398
	2 fractures	21
	3 fractures	27
	4 fractures	3

Eighty eight percent of all cases had one or more fractures as a consequence of a single point trauma incident. The condition of the fracture and the surrounding soft tissue at the time of admission were the most significant factors in the decision as to whether the bird received treatment or was euthanased. Twenty four percent of all fractures were deemed to be beyond realistic repair at the time of admission, and were euthanased.

Fifty percent of all fracture cases were finally euthanased. The majority of birds which were not going to make a good recovery had become apparent 14 days after initial admission. The fracture type was also of great significance; closed fractures not only had a better chance of healing, but also healed seven days sooner.

The percentage of birds finally released was greater for closed fractures (36%) than for open fractures (15%). However, if the open fracture did heal, the bird

Days after admission	Euthanased due to fracture	Euthanased for other reasons	Died spontaneously
0	24%	4%	2%
3	29%	5%	9%
7	31%	6%	11%
14	32%	7%	12%
Totals	**40%**	**10%**	**15%**

Fracture type	Closed			Open		
	Number fractured	% Healed	Days	Number fractured	% Healed	Days
Comminuted	73	51	30	125	27	36
Oblique	46	70	32	22	27	36
Segmental	29	45	28	20	25	69
Transverse	155	46	33	82	27	33
Unknown	18	28	28	84	0	-

Bone fractured	Number of fractures	% of cases treated	% of cases healed	% of cases released	Days to release
Humerus	206	39	18	12	34
Ulna	192	66	39	28	37
Radius	133	48	31	14	28
Metacarpal	72	54	33	28	31
Coracoid	28	75	61	53	29
Femur	27	55	33	22	31
Tibiotarsus	51	51	33	21	30
Tarsometatarsus	22	45	14	9	25

had a similar chance of release. The bone which was fractured also had a major effect on the final outcome. The reasons for this were associated with:

● The degree of soft tissue damage which must have occurred in order for that bone to have become fractured.

● Whether that bone was affected by necrosis, displacement of fractures, or proximity to vulnerable nerve tissue.

● The likelihood for fragment protrusion through the skin causing osteomyelitis.

Waterfowl

Full, normal flight is not crucial for the release of waterfowl, so long as they go to a sheltered lake, with an island (to give protection from predation), which is not overpopulated.

Disease Control in Rescue Birds

Figures varying from 35-65% are given for the rates of parasitic infection in wild birds. The parasite infection can make the birds ill enough to be the cause of their entry to the rescue centre. Even if this is not the case, in birds which are injured, subclinical infestations are likely to become clinically significant. All birds entering a rescue centre must be treated for endoparasites using either fenbendazole, ivermectin or praziquantel. If necessary, they should be treated for ectoparasites, using ivermectin, carbaryl, or permethrin (see Appendix - Formularies).

By the time a wild bird is sufficiently weak to be caught by a member of the public, it is likely to be suffering from shock and may well have secondary bacterial or viral infections. Great care must be taken by any rescue centre in order to prevent cross-infection between one bird and the next. Some infections may be rapidly apparent; others, eg. *Mycobacterium avium*, might not cause clinical disease for months or years after infection, but can contaminate the environment. Cage design for rehabilitation birds is as described in Chapter 4. Alternatively, disposable cardboard boxes may be used. Aviaries are not so easily cleaned and are not disposable; careful design is important. Although more expensive than an earth floor, the authors recommend the use of a concrete floor sloping to a drainage system, covered with ten centimetres of soil or pea gravel. Plants or shrubs are advantageous in aviaries but should be planted in pots, not in the ground. If infection should become apparent, the aviary can be cleared back to concrete and solid walls, cleaned, disinfected and then repainted and refurnished.

Human Contact

Rehabilitation birds should have minimum contact with people prior to release; this is especially important for young birds (see Chapter 22). There is an exception to this: some raptors have to be trained using traditional falconry techniques prior to release in order that their fitness may be increased and their ability to hunt and kill their own food proven.

Monitoring of Released Birds

It is important that the success rate of any rescue centre should be monitored as closely as possible. For this reason, birds should be identified, by the application of a British Trust for Ornithology (BTO) ring, prior to release. Only an individual trained to ring birds under the auspices of the BTO is able to do this. In time, the post-release survival times can be assessed as the rings are sent to the British Museum by people who find the birds dead. Although the rings state British Museum London, they should in fact be returned to the BTO at Tring, Hertfordshire, UK.

Release of Birds

Birds should not be released to the wild if they are unable to hunt, kill and feed effectively, or unable to integrate safely with their own species. Birds should not be released if they suffer from:
● Loss of an eye or eyesight, which may be difficult to assess.
● Loss of the claw of digits I or IV, which prevents perching and killing.
● Permanent loss of any part of the beak, usually due to damage to the bone and beak forming tissues.
● Inability to waterproof their plumage.

Release Techniques

The longer a bird is kept in captivity, the more problematic its release is likely to be. If a bird is fit for release within 14 days of the initial injury, then it should go back to its original territory. If, however, release has been delayed, it is usually better if the bird is released in another suitable area.

Birds must only be released in a suitable location which is known to be able to support their species. There must be suitable terrain, vegetation and prey, and only a small number of the same species of bird. The weather should not be extreme. Timing of release should not be close to migration time (where relevant). Time of day is also important: diurnal birds should be released early in the day whilst owls should be released shortly before sunset.

To return the bird to the wild effectively, a range of differing methods exist, each having its own advantages and disadvantages. The simplest method involves the release of a fit bird from a mobile or permanent aviary into an area which the bird has been able to see for several days. Following release, food is supplied at the aviary for as long as the bird comes back for it. More complex techniques involve the training of a bird using traditional falconry techniques, so that the bird becomes truly fit and proves its ability to kill prior to release.

EUTHANASIA

On occasions, captive or wild injured birds will require euthanasia. This is often a hard decision, particularly for an inexperienced clinician when presented with a mainly healthy but handicapped bird. Experienced clinicians should use pentobarbitone injection intravenously via the ulnar vein (see Figures 3.1, 3.2). If an intravenous injection would be technically or psychologically difficult, an intramuscular injection of ketamine (40mg/kg) is recommended prior to intravenous barbiturate. It is also possible to administer the barbiturate into the pectoral muscles or the liver. It is inadvisable to give the dose into the abdominal cavity as it will enter the air sacs where it will be very irritant and painful prior to death.

Rescue centres may seek advice from clinicians on euthanasia of hopeless cases, often presented to them moribund. Clinicians could advise on physical methods of euthanasia, eg. decapitation or a single hard blow to the head. However, many people find this advice hard to accept. Alternatively, if the clinician has a good rapport with his/her client and believes the client to be capable and reliable, he may train him/her in the proper storage, recording and use of barbiturates, which could be administered by the intraperitoneal route. The clinician may then dispense a small volume of barbiturate, which would be replaced on a named patient basis.

ENDOSCOPIC EXAMINATION

Endoscopy Equipment

Endoscopy is a very useful diagnostic tool in avian practice. It is a sensible always to use the largest endoscope possible for the procedure. The most useful general purpose endoscope is a rigid 4.0mm 0° cystoscope with a sheath. This is a robust endoscope with a good field of view and good illumination; it is also the cheapest. A rigid 2.7mm 0° endoscope can be used in smaller orifices and is surgically less invasive; as such it is invaluable, but it is shorter, much more easily damaged and more expensive than the cystoscope. It is possible to buy even smaller diameter rigid endoscopes, but these are not recommended for avian work. For an initial purchase, the 4.0mm 0° cystoscope is the most satisfactory.

Auriscopes and the Focuscope are not very useful in comparison to an endoscope and, although cheaper, they are, in the authors' opinion, a false economy.

Endoscopy in the Clinical Examination

Many of the raptors that are presented for examination are regurgitating or flicking their food. It is very useful in these cases to examine thoroughly the upper alimentary tract (see Figure 23.1). This can be accomplished using a 4.0mm 0° endoscope (cystoscope) with a sheath fitted. The bird should be restrained by a handler holding the wings against the body; this also prevents the legs being raised to grab the endoscopist. The endoscopist should hold the bird's head with the left hand and place the thumb in the commisure of the jaw as a gag. The endoscope can be introduced from the left side of the bird (from the endoscopist's right) and passed gently down the oesophagus and into the crop if this is present. A sheath should be fitted to the endoscope; this will allow mild insufflation of the oesophagus and crop with air so that the endosocopist can look down the endoscope as it is advanced into the bird. The authors use a length of tubing attached to the irrigation port, and blow down the tube whilst examining the bird. If the bird has been starved, the endoscope can be passed from the crop into the proventriculus, and even into the gizzard, with little difficulty.

This technique is invaluable for visualising foreign bodies, abscesses or tumours. It can also visualise and obtain diagnostic samples in generalised bacterial or yeast infections or parasitic infestations of the upper alimentray tract. This is usually possible in the conscious bird.

It is also possible to examine the cloaca in the conscious bird, using either an endoscope or an auriscope. It is easier to make this examination with the bird unconscious as this allows a thorough cleansing by irrigation of the whole cloaca.

Under anaesthesia, it is possible to enter the oviduct of a bird that has recently laid an egg and examine a significant amount of the oviduct.

When a clinician is presented with a dyspnoeic bird it is important to examine the upper respiratory tract endoscopically from the glottis to the syrinx (see Figures 23.2, 23.3); this requires a general anaesthetic. Larger birds the size of a female Harris' Hawk upwards require a 4.0mm endoscope; smaller birds a 2.7mm endoscope; and birds the size of a male Northern Sparrow Hawk or smaller an endoscope of less than 1.0mm. Only endoscopic examination can reveal the presence of parasites, eg. *Syngamus trachea.*, or a growth of *Aspergillus* spp. infection on the tracheal wall, as well as foreign bodies etc.

Laparoscopy

Birds are well suited for laparoscopy as they have air-filled spaces throughout their body in the form of air sacs. This allows easy visualisation of all their internal organs. General anaesthesia is mandatory.

Some species are so rare in captivity or in the wild, and so little is known about them, that laparoscopy is the only method to allow accurate gender determination. An incision on the left side of the bird, between the last two ribs (see Figure 23.4), allows the endoscope to enter the caudal thoracic air sac. The endoscope must be pushed through the oblique septum to see into the

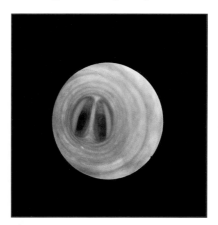

Figure 23.2: Normal trachea and syrinx of a normal Saker Falcon.

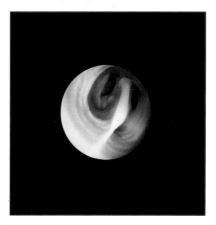

Figure 23.3: Syringeal bulla of a normal male Blue-winged Teal.

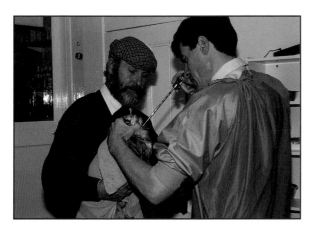

Figure 23.1: Endoscopic examination of the upper alimentary tract of a conscious female Northern Eagle Owl who had become inappetent. The bird is wrapped in a towel and the body and legs are held by the owner.

abdominal air sac; there may be an audible 'pop' when this happens. The gonad is seen in combination with the cranial division of the kidney and the adrenal gland (see Figures 23.5, 23.6). In the female bird the dorsal oviductal ligament is usually seen running over the cranial lobe of the kidney (see Figure 23.7); the presence of this ligament is very useful as a guide to the gender in immature birds where the ovary may be small, underdeveloped and difficult to see. Laparoscopy gives a guide to the age and state of maturity of the bird as well as the disease status of the gonad. In competent hands it is a safe and reliable procedure.

The same site of entry will also allow examination of the caudal border of the lung (see Figures 23.8, 23.9), the pericardial sac, and the liver (see Figure 23.10), spleen, proventriculus, gizzard, intestines and kidney. It is also possible to biopsy the liver or kidney using an endoscope to guide the forceps or by introduction down a specifically designed sheath. This is an ideal method of diagnosis for many diseases, eg. avian tuberculosis, herpesvirus hepatitis.

NB. All the endoscopy illustrations were obtained using a 4.0mm 0° endoscope.

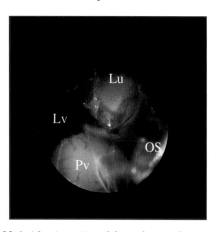

Figure 23.4: After insertion of the endoscope between the last two ribs, the lung (Lu), liver (Lv) and proventriculus (Pv), and the oblique septum (OS), can be seen.

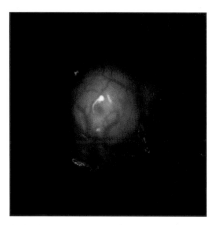

Figure 23.5: The testis of a male Red-tailed Hawk in breeding condition. The testis is considerably larger than the adrenal gland.

HERPESVIRUS INFECTIONS

Herpesvirus infections occur in many avian Families. A typical characteristic is their ability to produce individuals that are symptom-free carriers of the disease for weeks, months or even a lifetime after recovery from the disease. Intercurrent disease or stress has been associated as the cause of shedding of virus from these individuals. Three serologically related herpesvirus infections can be seen in Falconiformes, Strigiformes and Columbiformes. Pigeon herpesvirus infection is discussed in Chapters 28 and 31.

Falcon Herpesvirus or Inclusion Body Hepatitis

This infection is seen in the USA and has been rarely recorded in the UK (Gough *et al*, 1993). The disease is typified by sudden death or a short period of weakness and anorexia; there are no external signs. *Postmortem* examination typically reveals signs of viraemia with enlargement of the liver, spleen and kidneys, and pale coloured necrotic foci in the liver, spleen and the

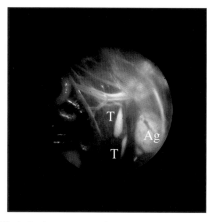

Figure 23.6: Both testes (T) of a 6-month-old Lanner Falcon. The adrenal gland (Ag) is larger than the testes.

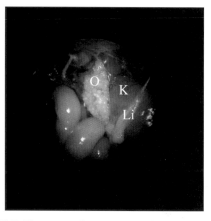

Figure 23.7: The ovary of a mature Northern Eagle Owl outside the breeding season. The dorsal oviductal ligament (Li) is visible running over the kidney (K). When in breeding condition the ovary (O) is more vascular and single ova become much larger. When immature the ovary has an amorphous appearance as the ova are undeveloped

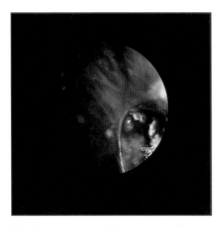

Figure 23.8: *Cases of aspergillosis are usually easy to diagnose endoscopically. In this view in the caudal thoracic air sac, fungal plaques can be seen on the inflamed air sac. The ostium to the lung can be seen to contain active fungus and the fruiting bodies are protruding into the air sac. (Photo courtesy Wolfe Publishing Limited)*

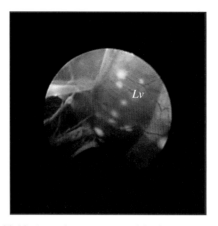

Figure 23.10: *An endoscopic view of the liver (Lv) of a terminally ill Snowy Owl. The bird also had necrotic plaques on the roof of its mouth, and caseous lesions similar to those on the liver on its spleen and caeca. Liver biopsy confirmed a case of owl herpesvirus. (Compare with Figure 19.1)*

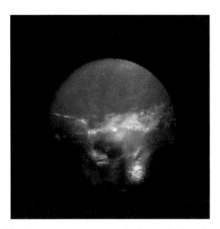

Figure 23.9: *The appearance of the lung of a Northern Goshawk with an inhalation pneumonia caused by glucose solution administered to an ill bird using a syringe and no crop tube.*

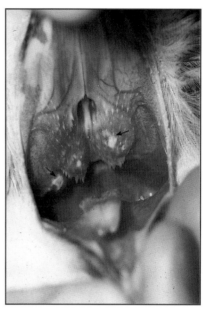

Figure 23.11: *The oral cavity of a Northern Eagle Owl showing the necrotic foci (arrows) typical of owl herpesvirus in the posterior palate. (Compare with Figure 15.8.)*

intestines. Histopathology demonstrates predominantly eosinophilic intranuclear inclusion bodies in the cells surrounding necrotic areas in the liver and other organs.

Owl Herpesvirus

Owl herpesvirus infection is seen in captive and wild Strigiformes in the UK and elsewhere. There are no recorded cases in Barn Owls, although they have been infected experimentally with falcon herpesvirus, as have some Strigiformes. A typical case of owl herpesvirus has been described by Gough *et al* (1995). The course of the disease is usually slower than in falcons, with the owls being unwell for up to a week before dying. Typical clinical signs are depression, anorexia and weight loss. Affected owls are seen to have multiple 1-2mm caseous necrotic foci in the lining to the posterior palate (see Figure 23.11); these foci resemble trichomoniasis and misdiagnosis is common at this stage of the disease, especially as these foci can be invaded by both *Trichomonas* spp. and

fungi (Gerlach, 1994). Ill birds invariably die; at *postmortem* examination they are found to have dramatic white necrotic foci in their liver, spleen and intestines (see Figure 23.12). These foci could be mistaken for avian tuberculosis. However, cytological examination of slides stained for acid-fast bacteria will be negative and histopathology will reveal multifocal areas of coagulative necrosis and large numbers of predominantly eosinophilic inclusion bodies. In living birds the disease may be confirmed endoscopically (see Figure 23.10).

Gough *et al* (1995) suggested that because of the close antigenic relationship between the herpesvirus of pigeons, falcons and owls, pigeons should not be used as a food source for falcons or owls. Prevention of the disease in falcons can also be helped by

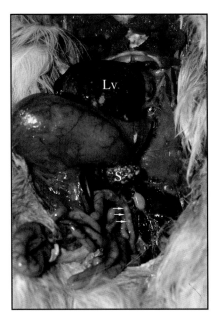

Figure 23.12: *The typical white, necrotic foci (arrows) caused by owl herpesvirus can be seen post mortem in the liver (Lv), spleen (S) and intestines of this Northern Eagle Owl.*

quarantine of newly acquired birds, especially if imported from the USA. Captive owls should be kept out of contact with wild owls, especially ill wild owls. Indirect contact with captive owls via a keeper must be borne in mind when injured wild birds are being nursed (see Chapter 4).

REFERENCE

Garner MM (1988) Use of an oral immoblising agent to catch a Harris' Hawk (*Parabuteo unicinctus*). *Journal of Raptor Research* **22(2)**, 70.

Gerlach H (1994). Viruses. In: *Avian Medicine: Principles and Application.* Eds BW Ritchie, GJ Harrison and LR Harrison. Wingers, Lake Worth.

Gough RE, Drury SEN, George AD and Randall CJ (1993) Isolation and identification of falcon herpesvirus. *Veterinary Record* **132**, 220.

Gough RE, Drury SEN, Higgins RJ and Harcourt-Brown NH (1995) Isolation of a herpesvirus from a Snowy Owl (*Nyctea scandiaca*). *Veterinary Record* **136**, 541.

Howard DJ and Redig PT (1993) Analysis of avian fracture repairs: implications for captive and wild birds. *Proceedings of the Association of Avian Veterinarians Annual Conference 1993.* AAV, Lake Worth.

CHAPTER TWENTY FOUR

Husbandry and Nutrition

Frank D W Harper

INTRODUCTION

Domestic pigeons are believed to be derived from varieties of the native Rock Dove; other species of the Family Columbidae may be kept in mixed avicultural collections. The terms 'dove' and 'pigeon' are interchangeable, but dove is usually applied to the smaller species.

Pigeons were amongst the earliest of domesticated livestock and the association of pigeons with man and human religion predates written history (Levi, 1974). The ability of pigeons to carry messages reliably has been exploited in warfare, trade and political administration. Pigeons have also been a valuable food source. The manorial dovecot has been replaced by commercial plants which produce juvenile birds for human consumption. These are common in the United States of America and in continental Europe; in the UK, however, most pigeon keeping is recreational. The keeping of pigeons for pleasure has a fascination for all social classes, in part attributable to the intelligence of the pigeon and its ability to recognise and interact with people without constraints on the liberty of the bird.

Selective breeding has produced many varieties (or breeds) with marked differences in size, conformation and plumage. Table varieties can weigh up to 2kg, more than four times the weight and size of the ornamental Fantail Dove. The exhibition varieties show the greatest diversity of shape and plumage and, pre-Darwin, many were thought to be different species. The sporting varieties are less changed from the ancestral form. Tumblers and rollers are small-bodied breeds (300-400g) bred to perform 'aerobatics'; tipplers, of similar size, are entered in competitions for duration of home flights (up to 20 hours). Racing pigeons (450-550g) are the most commonly kept sporting breed.

The sport of pigeon racing exploits the ability of what is by nature a sedentary, non-migratory species to orientate and navigate reliably over considerable distances. There are some 60,000 active participants in the sport in the UK who rear some two million young birds annually. Commercial breeding 'studs' also exist. There is a multi-million pound supporting industry with medicine and 'tonics' comprising a large proportion of the budget. Racing is at local, regional, national and international level. Birds fly from a common release point (up to 1,000km distant) to the home loft. The result is determined by 'velocity' - total distance/time, expressed as yards per minute(average 1,250ypm/75kph). Racing speed, altitude and line of flight are all influenced by wind conditions. Racing is on a weekly basis over progressively increasing distances; for old birds from April to July and for young birds from July to September. Large convoys may carry many thousands of birds. Transportation is by road, in crates holding 15-30 birds of mixed ownership, and there is an obvious risk of contact with, and spread of, potential pathogens. Crates are usually cleaned between races, but are seldom disinfected.

Some biological data and reproductive and developmental data are given in Tables 24.1 and 24.2.

HOUSING AND MANAGEMENT

Ornamental varieties are usually kept (at full liberty) in a garden dovecot, wall boxes or in the upper storey of an outbuilding; functioning medieval dovecots still exist. Exhibition varieties are usually housed in closed bird rooms, often as individually penned pairs; conformation, feathering and display behaviour are the priorities. Performing varieties are housed in a facility that allows entry and exit for periods of controlled exercise. Stray birds (strappers) may be a source of infection if they join the flock and gain entry.

Racing pigeons are kept in 'lofts' or 'cots'. Designs vary, but the effective headroom is usually about 2m, allowing control of the birds. A minimum of 0.25sqm floor space per bird should be provided. This minimum would apply to young birds; stocking rates should be lower for adults. Floors may be scraped daily, deep littered or slatted, but each system has defects. Scraping does not remove coccidial oocysts; deep litter can allow accumulation of nematode eggs; and slatted floors, with spilt food, can attract mice.

Perches and boxes are designed to minimise feather soiling or damage, but a sufficient number should be provided: an easily established and stable 'pecking order' puts less stress on the immune system. The arrangement of perches is of particular importance where

Table 24.1. Biological data (domestic pigeon).

Parameter	Comment
Bodyweight	350-500g (breed extremes 200-2000g).
Body temperature (cloacal)	40-41°C (limited diagnostic value).
Respiratory rate	25-30 per minute (remains constant in a fit bird).
Heart rate (resting)	240 per minute (rises with exertion or stress).
Life span	Up to 30 years. Females seldom fertile after 10 years. Racing life up to seven years.
Food consumption	Approximately 30g per bird per day.
Water consumption	30-60ml per bird daily (one litre to 20 birds); drinking is by beak immersion and suction.

Table 24.2. Reproductive and developmental data.

Parameter	Comment
Sexes	Monomorphic, but with experience the male can be identified by a bolder appearance to the head. During courtship display the male adopts a more upright stance, performs a full circle and 'tap dances'. The display is accompanied by loud cooing with inflation of the cervical air sacs and tail sweeping. Ritual feeding by the male (beak wringing) precedes copulation.
Courtship	A bonding period, 7-10 days of 'driving' (chasing) to nest, and nest building precedes laying. Pigeons are monogamous and pair-bond for life, but this can be manipulated.
Definitive layer	Two eggs in the clutch. The first egg is laid in the early evening; the second some 44 hours later.
Incubation	18-20 days; shared; the male sits by day. Light incubation of the first egg allows synchronised hatching. The average hatch produces one of each sex.
Crop milk	A protein and fat rich, non-carbohydrate secretion which accumulates in the hypertrophied crop epithelium from day 14 of incubation.
Feathering	Commences at seven days of age (coinciding with the change to feeding with regurgitated grain and onset of independent thermoregulation). There is no difference between the sexes.
Fledging	Nestlings (squabs) are weaned from about 24 days of age. They are referred to as 'squeakers' until voice change (about eight weeks of age).
Moulting	From six weeks of age in juveniles; from April to December in adults (see Chapter 26) . There is progressive replacement of remiges and retrices (wing and tail flights). Moult of body contour feathers is heaviest during August and September.

young birds are housed. Dominant birds seek the highest perches and arrangement in a few horizontal rows is preferable to vertical stacking. There should be 10-20% more perches than the number of birds housed. Experience suggests that losses from an overcrowded loft can be high, both in fledglings ('fly-aways') and from training flights, until wastage has established an optimum number of birds for the loft.

A sunny loft is desirable: a well ventilated and dry loft is essential. Construction material, orientation (southeast is optimal) and location (away from frost hollows, surrounding trees and buildings) can influence the health of the inmates.

The terminology applied to sections (or partings) in the loft reflects function and has significance in a clinical work-up.

Stock Loft
Houses the breeding pairs; these are often imports and may not fly out ('prisoners'), but often have access to an attached open aviary. The interior is fitted with large nesting boxes, each provided with one or more nesting bowls (traditionally terracotta but often synthetic or disposable papier mâché). Stock birds may be handled less often than racers and can be subject to less critical observation. Insidious deterioration or subclinical conditions may escape notice and be the source of loft problems.

Natural (Racing) Loft
Houses pairs, racing on a nesting cycle. Loft fittings comprise both boxes and perches for each pair (see Figure 24.1). Birds raced 'on natural' may be subject to the additional stress of rearing whilst racing.

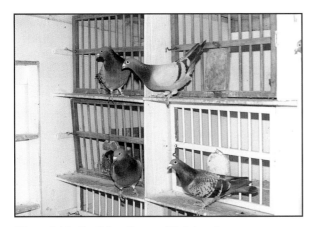

Figure 24.1: Traditional 'natural' loft interior.

Widowhood (Racing) Loft
Houses males only, racing to a sight of the hen on return. There is a low stocking rate and often individual feeding. A 3m x 3m section may house as few as eight racing males. The loft is usually enclosed and often heated; the 2m ceiling may be false, allowing adjustable roof ventilation, with or without extractor fans or humidity control. Double boxes with a divider are provided for each bird, but no perches; the intention is to increase territorial attachment to the nesting box. The racing males rear a single youngster pre-season, after which the hens are removed to a separate section or aviary. Parasitism is usually low, but in the enclosed loft, respiratory conditions may be a problem. As with stock birds, the separated hens may be subject to less observation during the racing season.

Young Bird Loft
Houses current-year banded birds. These juveniles are often of mixed age groups with a proportion of imported birds from a variety of sources. There may be some short-term overcrowding and contact with strays is likely. These are factors of clinical significance.

FEEDING
Feeding methods vary. Birds may be offered a measured amount of food once or twice daily, either individually (widowhood males) or communally on trays. Alternatively, they may be given free access to hoppers. The feed should be a mixture of legumes (field beans, peas, tares) and cereals (wheat, barley, maize) with some smaller seeds; the proportions may vary with personal preference and perceived priority (maintenance, rearing, moulting, etc.). The current practice during racing is to feed cereals early in the week ('depurative', 'breakdown') increasing the protein as the race day (usually Saturday) approaches. Pelleted feeds are marketed and these may be fed either as a supplement or as an alternative to traditional grain mixtures. Water is usually provided in communal fountains (most are three litre capacity): various 'tonics' and vitamins are often added. Grit is offered together with mineral salts and soil/clay minerals: these seem to be a nutritional requirement, especially in prisoner birds. Green food and animal protein should be offered regularly, but the amount eaten will vary. Pigeons show some selectivity with seasonal requirements. Absolute deficiencies are unlikely to be encountered, but considerations of balanced nutrition and calorific and biological values may arise.

GENERAL MANAGEMENT
Racing success is dependent upon a regular routine that encompasses feeding, exercise, basket training and flock discipline. Good stockmanship can be acquired, but the genetic quality of the birds is paramount. The success of the fortunate few is sometimes seen as a result of 'tonics', and so the use of herbs, chemical foods, vitamins and , unfortunately, antibiotics is widespread. An increasing problem, particularly in Belgium, is the use of steroids (ophthalmic preparations administered orally, intranasally or via the conjunctiva) to retard the moult of young birds during racing; 'burn out' and reproduction disorders in later life are the recognised sequelae. An annual pre-season treatment with anthelmintics and antiprotozoals is traditional but may not be necessary, whereas treatment in season is not usual yet may be needed. Vaccination against paramyxovirus infection is a legal requirement for all racing and exhibition birds (see Chapters 28 and 29). A vaccine against pigeon pox is available but its use is optional (see Chapters 26 and 28).

HANDLING
Clinical examination can be approached with safety and confidence. Pigeons are docile birds: they neither bite nor use claws and are not unduly stressed by handling. To catch up a bird, two hands should be used to close the wings and cup the body. If catching up from

a basket, one hand will suffice. Once taken up, the grip should be adjusted and the extended legs forked with the first and second fingers of one hand (palm up) and the thumb closed over the tail and wing tips (see Figures 2.9, 24.2). Most examination procedures are now possible (features of the normal bird are listed in Table 24.3). Generally, the owner can be relied upon to hold the bird in the required position when the clinician needs two hands free for sample collection, eg. skin and feather specimens; oropharyngeal, crop and cloacal swabs; crop aspirates; and blood collection from ulnar or tarsal veins (see Chapter 7).

DOSING

Oral administration of tablets and capsules presents no difficulty, but liquids are best given by crop tube. Drugs can be delivered on food using a binding agent to mix the medication with half the rations. Drinking water medication is convenient. However, pigeons sip before drinking and may reject strong tasting solutions. Baths and other sources of water must be removed. Water medication must be approached with caution in birds that are rearing; water consumption rises, particularly in hot weather, and there is a risk of toxic overdose (to the adults, eg. dimetridazole). Furthermore, some anthelmintic and antibiotic preparations can damage the developing feathers of nestlings (see Chapter 27).

Parenteral administration is more reliable but intramuscular injection via the pectoral muscles is best

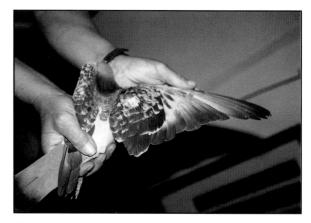

Figure 24.2: Method of holding a pigeon. Note the wing is held so as to demonstrate the Salmonella spp. lesion of the elbow.

avoided in the racing bird; injection into the leg muscles or subcutaneously is preferable. Subcutaneous injection in the dorsal midline of the lower neck is the recommended site for the administration of paramyxovirus vaccine. The clinician should be aware that there is an extensive venous plexus (*plexus venosus intracutaneous collaris*) laterally which extends dorsally in the upper neck. The extensive crop and air sacs, especially in the 'blower' varieties (those with exaggerated air sac development, eg. pouters and croppers), must also be considered when using this route. Intravenous administration can be via the superficial ulnar vein or the tarsal veins.

Pigeon pox vaccine is applied by brush to freshly

Table 24.3. Signs of health.

Examination	Observation
Demeanour	Alert with no nervous symptoms. **NB**. Some fancy varieties show congenital postural and behavioural peculiarities.
Plumage	Soft with no soiling (from faeces) or damage (from ectoparasites).
Body	Full, but with a buoyant and 'corky' feel.
Feet and legs	Red and clean with distinct annular scales.
Skin	Clean with 'reptilian lustre'.
Eyes	Bright with no swelling or discharge; strongly pigmented iris and brisk pupillary response.
Eye ceres and nasal wattles	'Chalky' appearance; free from staining (except when rearing).
Oropharynx	Clean and dry.
Respiration	Inaudible.
Faeces	'Droppings' of normal appearance, ie. semi-solid, coiled pellets with a white cap of solid urates.

plucked feather follicles (see Appendix - Formulary [Pigeons]). The percutaneous route may be used for some parasiticides and some anti-inflammatory preparations.

CLINICAL BIOCHEMISTRY AND HAEMATOLOGY

Information on avian clinical biochemistry and haematology can be found in Chapters 7 and 8 and in relevant references in this manual. Published data indicate a wide range in many reference values for pigeons. Variations arise from differences between sexes, ages and sampling techniques. Significant changes in the blood film can often be identified subjectively, eg. heterophilia in acute salmonellosis and erythrocyte sickling in some liver conditions.

REFERENCES AND FURTHER READING

Keymer IF (1991) Pigeons. In: *Manual of Exotic Pets.* New Edn. Eds PH Beynon and JE Cooper. BSAVA, Cheltenham.

Levi WM (1974) *The Pigeon.* 2nd Edn. Levi Publishing Company, Sumter.

Stam JWE (1987) *Pigeon Racing Today and Tomorrow.* Mardis, Oaklahoma. (English edition available from The Racing Pigeon, 21, Wren Street, London. Subtitled *35 Years in the Practice: Knowledge, Experience, Realisations and Opinions of a Veterinary Pigeon Enthusiast.*)

CHAPTER TWENTY FIVE

Head and Neck Problems

Alan S Wallis

ANATOMY

The external features of importance in terms of disease include the eyes, ceres, wattles and nares. The ears open caudally to the eyes and are covered with feathers. The mouth is large and the tongue relatively immobile. Numerous glandular ducts open on the palate laterally and caudal to the choanal cleft. The existence of a very extensive *plexus venosus subcutaneus collaris* is a special feature.

The crop lies subcutaneously at the opening of the thorax. Its importance lies not only as a part of the digestive system, but as a secretory organ in the nutrition of the young. The thyroid glands, and the parathyroid glands which are separate from the thyroid glands, lie laterally at the entrance to the thorax.

CLINICAL EXAMINATION

Birds should be observed undisturbed in the pannier or loft and any postural or behavioural abnormalities noted. The head and neck are best examined with the bird held on either side by an assistant. A small light source, eg. a pen torch, is useful for examining the eyes and reflexes, the oropharynx and, by transillumination, the interior of the trachea. The eye should be bright and free from discharges. Pupillary reflexes are not reliable but should be noted (see Chapter 15). Owners should be asked if there has been a recent change in iris colour.

The ceres and wattles should be clean and, in mature birds, almost snowy white (see Figure 25.1). In males the structure of the wattles may be complex (physical dimorphism is unreliable in determining the gender of pigeons). The structures may be obviously stained by ocular or nasal discharge.

The mucous membrane within the oropharynx should appear healthy. Encrustations of the commissures of the beak and around the glottis or oropharynx must be investigated. Cytology on fresh material is best. Diphtheritic membranes are often present, and should be considered abnormal. They may extend into the oesophagus.

The presence of almost any noticeable secretion within the oropharynx is an indication of abnormality

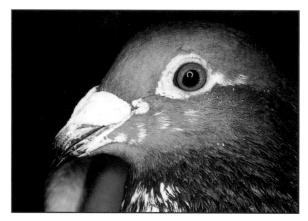

Figure 25.1: Ceres and wattles.

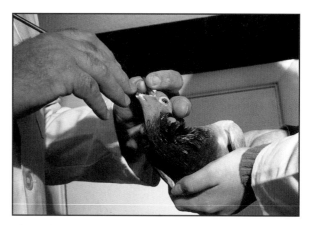

Figure 25.2: Collecting pharyngeal mucus.

and should be investigated (see Figure 25.2). Pustular lesions may be noted on the hard palate. Mucus samples can be easily removed for microscopic examination using a bacteriological loop (small amounts tend to get lost on a swab). Samples of mucus and discharges for cultural examination are best collected on a swab.

The crop should be palpated. It is normally a thin-walled, very elastic organ in which food can readily be palpated. Thickening, sponginess and fetid odours are indications of abnormality.

Pigeon fanciers tend to describe particular signs as if they were specific conditions, eg. one-eyed cold or greasy wattle. The evidence is that such signs are commonly responses to local infections rather than specific conditions and, as such, they often fail to respond to purely symptomatic treatment. Therefore, it is important that samples should be collected for further examination as a matter of routine so that a specific diagnosis can be made whenever possible.

Because pigeons live in colonies and the mixing of populations is an inherent part of the sport of pigeon racing and showing, infectious diseases are widespread and readily transmitted. Investigation of possible predisposing causes is a necessary part of the understanding and successful treatment of loft problems.

ABNORMAL HEAD POSTURE

Abnormal head posture may be an indication of paramyxovirus type 1 (PMV-1) infection, systemic paratyphoid (*Salmonella typhimurium*), polyneuritis, otitis or meningitis.

Paramyxovirus Type 1

PMV-1 infection is a notifiable disease. The abnormalities associated with PMV-1 characteristically involve the central nervous system (see Chapter 29). Any of the following signs may be observed singly or variously amongst a group of birds, or all of the signs may be exhibited by one specimen, though not necessarily simultaneously. The bird may be unable to hold its head normally. It may rotate upon the neck. The bird may look backwards more or less continuously either via a 180° twist of the neck or by looking between its legs. Tremor of the head and neck is often noticeable when the bird is held; this is an early sign of PMV-1 infection. Characteristically, the bird may be unable to pick up grain, apparently the result of a lack of co-ordination between eye and beak, the bird pecking in the wrong place consistently perhaps a few centimetres to the right or left of the target.

A history of vaccination against PMV-1 does not necessarily preclude the occurrence of this condition. Some birds seem unresponsive to vaccination and, under conditions of mass vaccination within the loft, missed vaccinations, eg. due to a faulty gun, deposition of vaccine in the feathers, etc., must occur from time to time. The incubation period for this infection may be unexpectedly long; nervous signs associated with PMV-1 infection have been observed to develop in young birds as late as nine weeks post vaccination.

Birds showing nervous involvement resulting from PMV-1 infection will typically show a strong serological reaction to PMV-1 in a haemagglutination inhibition (HAI) test. The HAI test will not distinguish completely between the serological response due to vaccination and that due to clinical infection.

Virus investigation of birds showing clinical signs involving the central nervous system is often unrewarding. Such signs usually occur in the late post-acute phase of the infection when viraemia has subsided. Whilst recovery of PMV-1 from the brain of such a bird is diagnostic, virus investigation may prove negative despite clinical, serological, epidemiological and immunological evidence which is very strongly indicative of the existence of PMV-1. The histological examination may also provide useful supportive evidence.

Treatment

There is no effective specific treatment for this condition, but if the bird can take food and water, a period of up to 12 weeks of quiet, rest and nursing may result in a remarkable degree of recovery, sufficient at least to enable the bird to remain as a useful breeder. Recovered birds are not considered to be infectious carriers of this condition.

Salmonellosis (Paratyphoid)

All isolations of *Salmonella* spp. from pigeons must be reported to the State Veterinary Service. Paratyphoid is also described in Chapter 29.

Invasion of the body tissues by *Salmonella* spp., classically *S. typhimurium* phage type 99, leads to the formation of small abscesses in various locations. The brain is one such site. The posture of the head and neck in these birds is often consistently abnormal, eg. the head is held to one side, the posture being not greatly exacerbated by excitement.

Abscesses due to *Salmonella* spp. have been recorded in the fundus. There may be swelling (in chronic cases not very marked) and noticeable opacity. Birds showing clinical signs of chronic abscess formation due to *S. typhimurium* infection will invariably show strong serological reaction to killed suspensions of this organism. A rapid plate test is easily carried out and a very strong agglutination reaction occurs in positive cases. Abscesses of the brain are inaccessible to culture other than at *post mortem*. However, the use of the rapid plate test on a loft basis may well indicate which birds should be selected for euthanasia and *post-mortem* examination, including culture. The culture of the droppings of birds with chronic abscess formation due to this cause is unlikely to reveal *S. typhimurium*.

Isolation of the causative organism from a loft outbreak is of great potential value. Sensitivity tests should be carried out and a suitable antibiotic chosen. There are occasions when the preparation of a specific, emergency licensed vaccine is necessary for the control of this condition, in which case isolation of the causative agent is a licensing requirement.

There is no commercially available vaccine for the control of paratyphoid in pigeons in the UK.

Treatment

Individual cases showing nervous signs of this nature are generally untreatable. However, loft treatment is generally extremely effective. Following sensitivity testing, an appropriate antibiotic should be given, eg.

amoxycillin (1.5g/litre drinking water for 5-7 days) or enrofloxacin (150-300mg/litre drinking water for up to 10 days). Experience suggests very strongly that clinical outbreaks of paratyhpoid are usually complicated (very commonly by coccidiosis, trichomoniasis and/or hexamitiasis). Appropriate antibiotic therapy of paratyphoid is only likely to prove satisfactory when intercurrent infections are simultaneously and effectively treated. **NB.** A history of recent routine antiparasitic treatment does not rule out reliably the existence of intercurrent infection.

Paratyphoid is a persistent, slowly spreading infection and as such is liable to recur in an affected loft. Intensive loft hygiene involving the frequent removal of droppings and their safe disposal, together with the application of an appropriate Ministry of Agriculture, Fisheries and Food (MAFF) approved disinfectant, eg. C.S. Fluid (Ciba Geigy), is a necessary adjunct to therapy. Antibiotic therapy may be repeated monthly over three months or so in association with intensive loft hygiene; recurrence is then unlikely. The use of deep litter systems in paratyphoid infected lofts is inappropriate. Where paratyphoid is a persistent recurring problem, despite all of the above considerations, vaccination is generally very helpful and well worth consideration despite its high cost.

POLYNEURITIS

Polyneuritis is a condition of uncertain aetiology often manifesting itself as fits. Generally, individual specimens only are affected. Birds appear normal at rest, but excitement, eg. feeding, will precipitate a fit, the bird spinning round on the loft or pannier floor. Clinical signs may be similar to those described for PMV-1 infection.

The condition may be induced experimentally in pigeons by feeding a vitamin B_1 deficient diet such as polished rice, but it is unlikely that this deficiency could occur on a diet of mixed seeds. However, the possibility of a thiaminase in the food should be considered.

The diagnosis of polyneuritis due to vitamin B_1 deficiency is easily confirmed by the administration of vitamin B_1 either in the form of yeast tablets or as a water soluble preparation. A rapid clinical response follows if a deficiency is present. (See Chapter 29.)

OTITIS

Inflammation of the ears has not been commonly reported. Bacterial infections, including tuberculosis, have occasionally been recorded.

A condition loosely described as 'vertigo' has been reported quite commonly and, whilst this is a non-specific term which may be applied to a variety of pathologies, eg. PMV-1, paratyphoid or polyneuritis, the possibility of otitis should not be overlooked nor should the ears be forgotten during *post-mortem* examination.

MENINGITIS

Menginitis can be caused by infection other than PMV-1 or paratyphoid. Routine culture and histological examination of the cranial contents should be carried out in any significant outbreak of postural abnormality of the head.

INFLAMMATION OF THE MUCOUS MEMBRANES

Many clinical signs result directly from inflammation of the mucous membranes, eg. one-eyed cold, but the mucous membranes of the head and neck are closely related and it is unusual for problems of this nature to be limited to a single area.

The signs vary in intensity from very slight to severe. Single birds may be affected or the signs may appear epizootic. In milder cases, birds may show little or no clinical indisposition, though race performance is usually adversely affected. In more severely affected cases, exercise tolerance may be impaired; birds may alight after only a few minutes flight showing distressed beak breathing or they may be unwilling to fly at all. There may well be mucoid or mucopurulent discharges from the eyes and nares.

Trichomoniasis

Microscopic examination of oropharyngeal mucus is essential. The parasites are easily identified under carefully adjusted light and x200 magnification. Chronic trichomoniasis is one of the commonest pigeon diseases, often referred to as 'canker'.

In its most commonly reported form, extensive caseous deposits are found in the pharynx and oesophagus (see Figure 25.3). These can be moved fairly easily with a swab, exposing inflamed areas. However, subacute trichomoniasis, in which no plaques are visible, is a much more common clinical problem. The parasites may well be present in vast numbers and, whilst the presence of the odd parasite is unlikely to precipitate clinical signs, their presence may be no less significant if only as a source of infection. Following treatment, the number of parasites may be very small and difficult to detect microscopically over a period of 7-10 days. However, culture of trichomonads is a very sensitive diagnostic technique. The presence or absence of pus cells in pharyngeal mucus should also be noted under the microscope. The presence of pus cells is important as it suggests a significant primary or secondary bacterial infection. Routine bacterial culture and sensitivity testing of discharges is worthwhile. Commonly, organisms such as *Pasteurella* spp., *Haemophilus* spp., *Streptococcus* spp. and *Staphylococcus* spp. are encountered. *Mycoplasma* spp. are

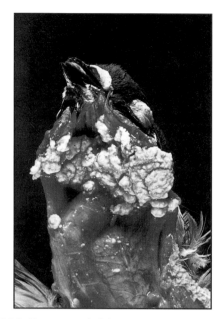

Figure 25.3: Very severe diphtheritic trichomoniasis.

widely distributed in the upper respiratory tract but their isolation and culture is difficult and slow. Their presence as a complicating factor in the aetiology of upper respiratory tract infection is generally assumed.

Treatment

The number of medicines effective against trichomoniasis is relatively small and most of these are readily available to the fancier in pet shops etc., eg. dimetridazole, carnidazole, aminonitrothiazole. Resistance to these drugs is widespread (abuse is common) and their effectiveness may not be safely assumed. A useful strategy is to provide a medicine different from that used prophylactically in the loft (if any).

In cases of unresponsive trichomoniasis a combination of tetracycline (400mg/l) plus furaltadone (440mg/l) given in the drinking water over seven days has been found to be very effective (also for the primary treatment of coccidiosis), but this combination should not be given to birds feeding young less than 10 days of age.

Bacterial infections should be treated with antibiotics indicated by bacterial sensitivity tests, but it is usual to chose an antibiotic which, in addition, has good antimycoplasmal activity as well as specific activity against the bacteria isolated.

Individual birds may be treated parenterally. For sensitive infections, parenteral tetracycline is the treatment of choice. Whilst individual cases obviously occur, this generally suggests the presence of widespread infection in the loft. Therefore, parenteral treatment is usually accompanied and supported by medication of the whole loft (or section) with a comparable antibiotic given via the drinking water (see Appendix - Formulary [Pigeons]).

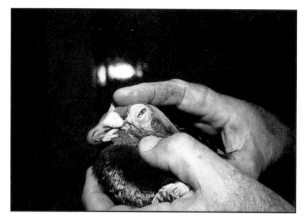

Figure 25.4: Chlamydiosis.

The clinical appearance of bacterial or mycoplasmal infection of mucous membranes is usually secondary to parasitic infection which is often subclinical or chronic in nature. Where this is the case, effective treatment of the secondary problem will only be achieved when the primary problem has been successfully addressed.

Chlamydiosis

Infection with *Chlamydia psittaci* is common in pigeons (see Chapter 31) and most frequently seems to be subclinical. Unresponsive and fairly widespread respiratory or ophthalmic conditions should be investigated specifically with this in mind (see Figure 25.4). Referral of appropriate swabs in transport medium to a specialist laboratory is probably the most sensitive diagnostic means, or a polymerase chain reaction (PCR) test can be carried out by MAFF. However, examination of impression smears of corneal conjunctiva for typical chlamydial inclusion bodies is both quick, positive and inexpensive.

Pustules may well be observed on the palate. They have been associated with trichomoniasis, but they are very common in otherwise normal healthy pigeons, and histologically have the appearance of blocked salivary glands.

Treatment

Chlamydiosis is one of the more important zoonoses so far as pigeon fanciers are concerned. Treatment, though tedious, is usually very effective not only in dealing with clinical disease but in elimination of the carrier state as well. Tetracycline (400mg/l of drinking water continuously for three weeks supported by parenteral tetracycline administered on alternate days) is the treatment of choice. Doxycylcine (500mg/l for 45 days) has also been recommended. During the course of treatment of the birds, the loft should be thoroughly cleansed using an MAFF approved disinfectant at least twice. Droppings must be burnt or deep buried.

Where the existence of chlamydiosis is suspected, the pigeon fancier should be advised to take specific hygienic precautions whilst working in the loft. These should include the use of a particle mask, boots, overalls and gloves. The fancier should be advised to seek medical advice promptly in the case of personal ill health. The medical advisor may not be aware of his patient's activity as a pigeon fancier.

Pigeon Pox

The classical pustules of pigeon pox may well be observed within the oropharynx. They may also occur on the wattles and ceres, but less commonly in the feathered areas of the skin. Usually, pox lesions are multiple and their appearance is largely diagnostic, but where such lesions are noted only within the oropharynx, the possibility of herpesvirus infection should be considered. More information on pigeon pox can be found in Chapter 26.

CROP

Sour Crop

The most common problem associated with the crop is so-called 'sour crop'. The crop becomes thickened, and distended with fermenting impacted food. There is a fetid odour. Affected birds lose condition and their droppings may be loose. Diagnosis presents no problems, but the condition itself may be complicated by trichomoniasis, candidiasis, capillariasis or bacterial infection. Stained smears from crop samples should be examined microscopically for pathogens.

The contents of the crop should be gently massaged out or, if this is impossible, removed surgically. The bird should be maintained on a minimum quantity of a light diet whilst recovery occurs. Fluid therapy, including electrolytes, and also antibiotics may be helpful. The traditional use of bicarbonate of soda solution to wash out the crop is contraindicated due to potential renal damage.

Capillariasis

Acute capillariasis of the crop may be associated with intense vomiting and a high mortality. The intense vomiting associated with this condition precludes effective oral administration of anthelmintics. Levamisole (0.1ml i/m) and ivermectin (dilute 1% Injection 1:9 immediately before use - give 0.2ml/kg i/m) are effective anthelmintics which can be given parenterally or percutaneously.

THYROID GLANDS

Goitre has been reported, with the thyroid glands enlarged. Sluggishness, overweight, poor feathering and poor reproduction have been reported. The condition is rare in the UK since most fanciers give vitamins and mineral supplements to their pigeons. Some fanciers, however, have extreme nutritional ideas and careful enquiry as to management practices may give evidence of nutritional deficiency in apparently 'well fed' birds.

INJURIES

Skull and neck injuries as a result of collision do occur. Fighting amongst males is frequent in the breeding season and superficial injuries, particularly to the eyes, ceres and wattles, can occur.

Vaccination against pigeon pox during the breeding season is contraindicated since such injuries often become extensively infected with vaccine virus, leading to severe exacerbation of otherwise comparatively minor injuries. (**NB**. Pox vaccination should be given at least five weeks before pairing up.) Secondary lesions, whether due to field infection or live vaccine virus, are not necessarily limited to unfeathered portions of the skin.

Injury as a result of PMV-1 vaccination has been recorded. Occasionally, severe local granulomata appear subcutaneously at the site of vaccination, but they may also occur when a vaccine is misdirected subcutaneously over the skull. Oil based vaccines may track subcutaneously and the lesions are not necessarily precisely at the reported vaccination site. The *plexus venosus subcutaneous collaris* is extensive in pigeons, particularly in the male, and vaccine misdirected into this region may lead to sudden death. *Post-mortem* examination reveals a massive congestion of this complex. Vaccination may also be accompanied by a low incidence of collapse and death for no obvious reason - possibly an acute anaphylactic type of reaction. Where mass vaccination of several lofts is carried out at a session, deaths, when they occur, are sometimes limited to birds in only one of the lofts involved.

Table 25.1. Summary of conditions of the head and neck associated with nervous signs.

Condition	Clinical signs	Diagnosis	Differential diagnosis	Treatment	Prognosis
PMV-1 (notifiable disease).	Bizarre head posture, torticollis, incoordination of eye and beak movement. Tremors, fits, death.	Signs. History. Vaccination status. Serology, histology, virology.	Paratyphoid, polyneuritis, otitis, meningitis.	None specific. Rest and nursing. Vaccination.	Guarded. Vaccination provides good loft protection.
Salmonellosis, usually *S. typhimurium* (paratyphoid).	Constant abnormal head posture, paralysis, death, opacity in fundus of the eye, wasting. Affects predominantly first year birds.	Signs, history, *post-mortem* examination, microabscesses in brain or eye. Serology, bacteriology. Check parasite status. (Other localised lesions.)	PMV-1, polyneuritis, otitis, meningitis.	Treat concurrent parasitisms. Appropriate antibacterials, eg. amoxycillin or enrofloxacillin, on a loft basis. Vaccination.	Usually only individuals affected. On a loft basis - excellent. On individual cases - very poor.
Otitis, meningitis.	Paralysis, fits, head tilt, death.	Usually only individuals affected. *Post-mortem* examination, bacteriology.	PMV-1, paratyphoid, polyneuritis.	Appropriate antibiotics in suspected cases.	Satisfactory if treatment initiated early enough.
Polyneuritis (aetiology uncertain).	Fits, bizarre behaviour.	Clinical signs, lack of positive serology etc., history of nutritional abnormality. Response to diet change. Usually only individuals affected.	PMV-1, paratyphoid, otitis, meningitis.	Dietary change. Thiamine supplementation.	Fair.

Table 25.2. Summary of conditions of the head and neck associated with upper respiratory tract and ocular signs.

Condition	Clinical signs	Diagnosis	Differential diagnosis	Treatment	Prognosis
Pox.	Pustules, diphtheritic membranes of oropharynx, eyelids, ceres, wattles. Birds often not severely ill, but performance affected.	Epizootic condition. Appearance not limited to single locus in all birds. Vaccination history. Racing season. Virology, histology.	Trichomoniasis, herpesvirus, trauma, candidiasis, capillariasis, (oral lesions).	Unless complicated, isolate and leave alone. Cautery. Antibiotics if appropriate.	Excellent. Vaccination provides good loft protection.
'One-eyed cold', mycoplasmosis, bacterial ophthalmitis.	Conjuctivitis, not necessarily unilateral. Ocular discharge. Possible wattle staining. Tends to spread through loft.	Clinical signs. Mild condition. Often responds spontaneously. Contagious.	Ornithosis, upper respiratory infections, trichomoniasis, trauma, coccidiosis.	Range of anti-inflammatory ointments (**NB**. grease can damage feathers). Appropriate antibacterials, including antimycoplasmal agents. Ventilation. Drinker hygiene.	Excellent.
'Greasy wattle', infectious rhinitis, mycoplasmosis.	Rhinitis; a mild clinical condition. Sneezing, mucus on surface.	Clinical signs. Usually mild, often contagious. Bacteriology.	Ornithosis, trichomoniasis, coccidiosis.	Appropriate antibiotics, including antimycoplasmal agents. Ventilation. Drinker hygiene.	Excellent.
Trichomoniasis ('canker').	Pharyngitis, diphtheritic membranes, catarrh, upper respiratory signs. Poor exercise tolerance.	Diphtheritic membranes often not deeply adherent. Microscopic examination of mucus for trichomonads or pus cells. Bacteriology.	Pox, herpesvirus, mycoplasmosis, bacterial infection, coccidiosis. Capillariasis. Candidiasis.	Appropriate primary and secondary medication. Beware resistant strains of *Trichomonas* spp.	Excellent.
Herpesvirus.	Pharyngitis with or without diphtheritic membranes/ ulceration.	Lesions may be deeply adherent. Virology. Often complicated by trichomoniasis or other secondary infections and coccidiosis. Chronic epizootic condition.	Pox, mycoplasmosis, trichomoniasis.	Treat intercurrent infections, nutritional support. Vitamins. Acyclovir (0.5mg pipetted into the crop tid for seven days).	Guarded.

Table 25.2. Continued.

Condition	Clinical signs	Diagnosis	Differential diagnosis	Treatment	Prognosis
Ornithosis (chlamydiosis). Important zoonosis.	Very variable in intensity. Intractable conjunctivitis/ rhinitis. Sneezing. Discoloured ceres and wattles.	History of unresponsive signs. Microscopy. Specific examination for *Chlamydia psittaci*. Presence of *C. psittaci* does not eliminate other concurrent infections.	Other respiratory conditions, trichomoniasis, coccidiosis.	Tetracyclines at high dosage over long period of time. Treat intercurrent infections.	Excellent.

Table 25.3. Summary of conditions of the head and neck associated with digestive signs.

Condition	Clinical signs	Diagnosis	Differential diagnosis	Treatment	Prognosis
Sour crop (impaction).	Morbid bird. Distended, thickened crop. Fetid odour.	Clinical signs.	Candidiasis, capillariasis, trichomoniasis.	Empty crop. Light diet. Surgery if required.	Excellent.
Candidiasis.	Morbid bird. Diphtheritic membranes. Diarrhoea. Fetid odour.	Clinical signs, microscopy, culture.	Sour crop, trichomoniasis, herpesvirus, capillariasis.	Nystatin suspension (20,000 units suspended in 1ml of water pipetted into the crop once daily for seven days). Diet.	Good.
Crop capillariasis.	Vomiting. Acute. High mortality, particularly in young birds.	Microscopy.	Acute poisoning, hexamitiasis, candidiasis, trichomoniasis.	Levamisole parenterally. Ivermectin.	Fair.

FURTHER READING

Coles BH (1985) *Avian Medicine and Surgery*. Blackwell Scientific Publications, Oxford.

Keymer IF (1991) Pigeons. In: *Manual of Exotic Pets*. New Edn. Eds PH Beynon and JE Cooper. BSAVA, Cheltenham.

Levi WM (1974) *The Pigeon*. Levi Publishing Company, Sumter.

CHAPTER TWENTY SIX

Skin Conditions

Alan S Wallis

INTRODUCTION

The skin of pigeons is divided into four well-contrasted and circumscribed areas:

- The feathered areas.
- The scaly areas of the feet and legs.
- The ceres and wattles.
- The horny claws and beak.

Examination should consist initially of a thorough inspection of the feathered areas. The underlying skin should be clean and the plumage itself bright and appropriate to the age and stage of moult of the bird. **NB**. Young birds lose their juvenile plumage between about six and 29 weeks of age and subsequently moult annually in the autumn (see Figure 26.1).

Plumage may well be affected by intercurrent disease and feathers growing during such a period may be 'fretted' and lack normal colour, strength and elasticity. The tail and wings should be extended against the light to reveal the existence of ectoparasites and their eggs between the barbs and along the shafts of feathers. The presence of broken feathers requires further investigation.

The ceres and wattles are usually snowy white. They may be discoloured if the bird is in poor health or if any discharges are present (which merit further investigation). Inflammatory and traumatic changes are frequently seen in these areas. These may be the result of insect bites, with or without infection, trauma due to fighting, or infectious disease.

The scales of the legs should be clean and bright and the feet free from swelling and inflammation. Any abnormalities in the claws and beak should be noted.

The aetiology of skin conditions can be listed under eight headings: parasitic, bacterial, viral, fungal, nutritional, toxic, traumatic and neoplastic.

Congenital defects are rare but have been reported, eg. featherless birds and porcupine quills. These conditions are usually incompatible with flight and/or natural breeding.

Despite the above observations, the diagnosis of pigeon skin conditions is often frustrating. Extensive medication of the bird will usually have been tried by the fancier prior to presentation. The absence of ectoparasites can be very difficult to prove. A systematic approach is therefore essential. Careful history taking and observation are crucial. For example, pigeon pox is usually epizootic in nature and frequently coincides with the racing season. Where lesions suspicious of pox are seen, careful examination of other birds is likely to reveal the consequence of the infectious nature of this condition. The appearance of the lesions is fairly characteristic, but vaccination is usually very effective and the disease only appears in unvaccinated birds. The presence of the larger ectoparasites is generally obvious to the naked eye, but confusion can be caused by the appearance of typical feather damage following previous eradication of the parasites. Diagnosis of infestations with parasitic mites or dermatophyte infection without microscopic confirmation is likely to lead only to frustration.

Table 26.1 at the end of this chapter gives a summary of some of the skin conditions found in pigeons.

ECTOPARASITES

Fleas

Two species of fleas are of particular significance, the European chick flea (*Ceratophyllus gallinae*) and the stickfast flea (*Echidnophaga gallinacae*). Other species have been recorded. The diagnosis of fleas does not present any difficulty. Since most pigeon fanciers take a rigorous attitude towards cleansing and the removal of droppings, they are not particularly common.

Lice

Two species of lice are commonly found on pigeons in the UK, the slender louse (*Columbicola columbae*) and the large body louse (*Menapon latum*). The slender louse may be seen particularly between the barbules of the feathers when held against the light. The eggs are laid in the groove between the feather shafts and the barbs. The body louse lays its eggs in a similar situation and causes damage (appearing as pin pricks) to the barbs of the feathers.

Parasitic Mites

Several species of mites live on the outside of the feather. They can be observed resting like beads along

Figure 26.1: *The sequence of moulting in three young birds (Levi, 1974).*
(Reproduced with kind permission of the Levi Publishing Company, Sumter, South Carolina.)

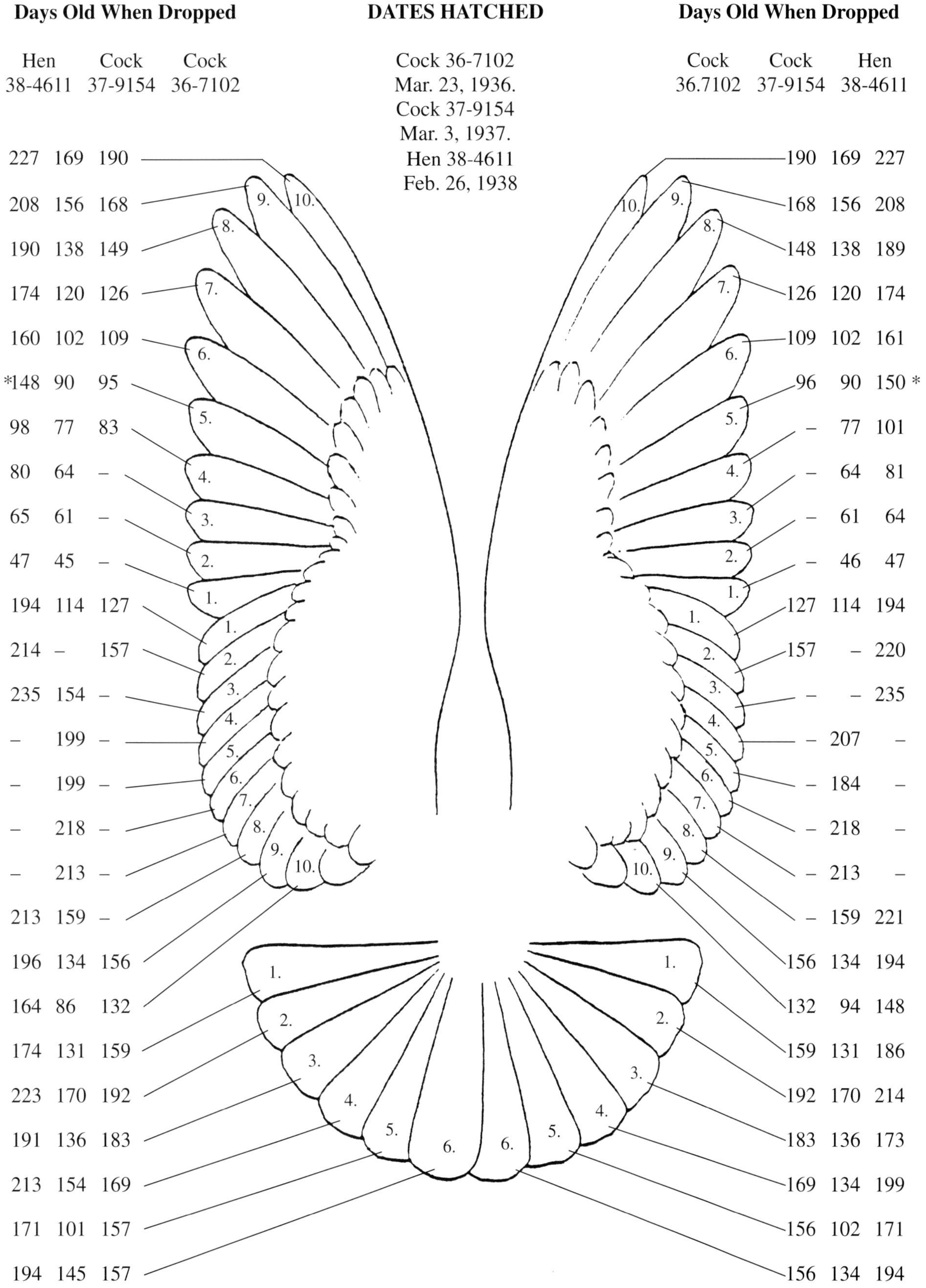

Days Old When Dropped

Hen 38-4611	Cock 37-9154	Cock 36-7102
227	169	190
208	156	168
190	138	149
174	120	126
160	102	109
*148	90	95
98	77	83
80	64	–
65	61	–
47	45	–
194	114	127
214	–	157
235	154	–
–	199	–
–	199	–
–	218	–
–	213	–
213	159	–
196	134	156
164	86	132
174	131	159
223	170	192
191	136	183
213	154	169
171	101	157
194	145	157

DATES HATCHED

Cock 36-7102
Mar. 23, 1936.
Cock 37-9154
Mar. 3, 1937.
Hen 38-4611
Feb. 26, 1938

Days Old When Dropped

Cock 36.7102	Cock 37-9154	Hen 38-4611
190	169	227
168	156	208
148	138	189
126	120	174
109	102	161
96	90	150 *
–	77	101
–	64	81
–	61	64
–	46	47
127	114	194
157	–	220
–	–	235
–	207	–
–	184	–
–	218	–
–	213	–
–	159	221
156	134	194
132	94	148
159	131	186
192	170	214
183	136	173
169	134	199
156	102	171
156	134	194

*   Hen 38-4611 - leg accidently broken, age about 14 weeks.

the shafts of feathers and they can give rise to a good deal of irritation and feather damage.

The depluming mite *(Cnemidocoptes laevis laevis)* is the cause of feather rot. It inhabits the skin at the base of the quill. The feather follicle and the feathers frequently break off leaving a shortened stub, perhaps 2-3mm in length, projecting from the skin. Bald areas occur and, whilst the appearance is characteristic, it can be misleading.

The pigeon quill mite *(Syringophilus columbae)* is less common but causes similar damage. It inhabits the inside of the feather shaft and is therefore difficult to see. However, under a microscope, particularly at x50 magnification under a stereo microscope, they can present a spectactular sight (dodgem cars in three dimensions!). Their habitat makes them inaccessible to routine treatment.

The scaly leg mite *(Cnemidocoptes mutans)* is not primarily a pigeon parasite, but it can cause severe crusty lesions of the legs and feet as a result of burrowing in the scales. It must be differentiated from pox, bumblefoot and gout.

The red mite *(Dermanyssus gallinae)* is a very destructive ectoparasite with a broad avian host range. Much of the life cycle is spent away from the host, but populations may build up explosively, particularly in the summer months, and blood sucking can lead to severe anaemia and even death of the host. Parasites may not be present on the bird when presented for examination as they only feed at night, but the anaemic state of the bird and the unclean appearance of the skin is suggestive. On *post-mortem* examination, ingested, engorged mites may be found within the oesophagus and crop. The mites roost underneath furniture within the loft, eg. nest bowls, or in crevices in the structure.

The Northern fowl mite *(Ornithonyssus sylviarum)* is a rather similar parasite, though a larger proportion of its life cycle is spent on the body of the bird. These are relatively large mites which can be seen, certainly in their adult form, with the naked eye and which, when engorged, are bright red.

Diagnosis

Ectoparasites are numerous and common. It is satisfying to observe these with the naked eye but identification is complex. Ectoparasites may be cleared on a microscope slide in 1% sodium hydroxide. Several specimens may be needed (mounted on one slide) to observe all of the diagnostic characteristics. The presence of an ectoparasite alone does not establish the existence of skin disease.

Birds presented with a deplumed area, probably littered with broken feather stubs, are a particular problem. Detailed examination frequently fails to demonstrate ectoparasites or any other specific causes. Diagnostic techniques which have proved of assistance are the digestion of feather stubs and feathers immediately surrounding the stubs overnight in 1% sodium hydroxide at 37°C (a V-bottomed container such as a 30ml universal or a centrifuge tube is suitable for this purpose). Microscopic examination of the deposit should reveal ectoparasites or their parts clearly against a background of amorphous material.

Sealing of feathers and stubs under suspicion in a small closed plastic envelope for at least 24 hours is often useful. Parasites tend to migrate from such material and become caught in the folds of the envelope. With a microscope they may be found readily under low power magnification by direct examination through the plastic.

Examination of the undersides of furniture in the loft must be carried out carefully if dermacid mites are to be incriminated.

The microscopic examination of suspicious encrustations cleared with 1% sodium hydroxide is potentially useful, but in many cases such examinations prove negative, particularly when extensive earlier treatments have been attempted.

Treatment

Mites and lice may be treated by routine use of dusting powders, eg. Ridmite Powder, Johnson and Johnson. (**NB**. The use of chlorinated hydrocarbon compounds is contraindicated in the treatment of birds.) In general, mite infestations can be treated with cypermethrin 0.5% as a spray or dip (Barricade, Lever).

Burrowing mites in particular may be treated with ivermectin (1% solution diluted 1:9 with sterile water immediately prior to use - give 0.2ml/kg i/m) (Coles, 1985). Application of the same dose directly onto the skin over the back may also be effective. (**NB**. Solutions of ivermectin in water are unstable and must be prepared immediately before use. Stock solutions may be prepared in propylene glycol [beware of wet bottles]).

BACTERIAL INFECTIONS

Specific bacterial infections of the skin appear to be relatively uncommon. Superficial injuries may become infected with *Erysipelothrix* spp., whilst bumblefoot is essentially a chronic secondary infection due to *Staphylococcus* spp. The lesions caused by ectoparasites, pox or fungi may all commonly become secondarily infected. Tuberculosis gives rise to secondary lesions of the skin. These are multiple tubercles which appear as hard nodules with yellow caseous centres, or which may be ulcerated and are seen particularly on the under surface of the wings.

Diagnosis

Diagnosis is confirmed by examination of Ziehl-Neelsen stained smears. Skin tuberculosis is usually secondary to a more generalised condition; caseous polyarthritis is likely to be a concurrent finding. Skin tuberculosis, which is well recognised in pigeons in some parts of the World, but is not common in the UK, must be differentiated from fowl pox and ectoparasitism. Culture and sensitivity testing should be carried out prior to treatment of infected superficial injuries etc.

Chronic skin irritation with patchy feather loss may be associated with bacterial infections, mainly due to *Staphylococcus* spp. In such cases, careful examination fails to identify any other agent.

Differential diagnosis - infection with parasitic mites, nutritional factors, mechanical factors and drug toxicity.

Treatment

Treatment of tuberculosis in pigeons is not a practical proposition. Other bacterial infections usually respond well to antibiotic therapy. Following culture and sensitivity testing, individual birds are best treated with amoxycillin tablets (20mg/bird p/o, sid or bid for five days), or amoxycillin LA injection (15mg/bird i/m) followed by oral treatment (20mg tablets for individuals; 20mg/kg in the drinking water for loft treatment) (see Table 26.1). Chronic conditions such as bumblefoot are generally unresponsive.

VIRAL INFECTIONS

Pigeon Pox

This is a fairly common infection, caused by the virus *Avipoxvirus columbae*. Pigeon pox can be spread by mosquitoes as well as by contact. Contact spread is facilitated by the presence of abrasions. The incubation period is 7-9 days.

Outbreaks usually start in the early weeks of the flying season, ie. May, and may continue throughout the rest of the year. Any part of the skin may be involved, but lesions are most commonly seen on the ceres, wattles, eyelids and the commissures of the mouth (oropharynx), and less commonly on the legs and feet. The appearance of lesions is associated with the simultaneous presence of infectious virus and trauma, thus the vaccination process involves the infection of a few traumatised feather follicles with vaccine virus and results in the appearance of typical lesions at the vaccination site.

The clinical picture is characteristic. Initially, a papule appears with some swelling and oedema. The papule breaks down to become a pustule which is yellowish brown in colour and firmly adherent. If the pustule is removed, a raw bleeding point remains. Lesions may be single or multiple (see Figure 26.2). The course of the disease is normally 3-4 weeks, after which the lesions resolve and the remaining scabs fall away leaving healthy tissue underneath. Recovered birds are strongly immune to further infection, perhaps

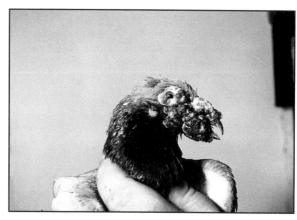

Figure 26.2: *Multiple lesions of pigeon pox.*

for the duration of their life. The incrustations are rich in virus and highly infectious. Secondary bacterial infection of the pustules may occur.

An exotic form of the disease, **epithelioma contagiosa**, is also seen, usually in the feathered areas of the skin. It appears as a tumour-like lesion which grows rapidly and eventually resolves naturally. Epithelioma contagiosa is normally seen in association with the appearance of typical pigeon pox in other birds in the loft.

Diagnosis

Diagnosis of pigeon pox is established by the appearance of typical lesions and the epizootiology of the condition. It may be confirmed by histological or virological examination of lesions.

Differential diagnosis. Trauma, eg. due to insect bites with secondary bacterial infection, capillary haemangio-endothelioma and cutaneous lipoma, bumblefoot, scaly leg and articular gout.

Treatment

Pigeon pox lesions are generally best left alone to resolve spontaneously unless they are in potentially threatening locations, eg. the eyelids, when cautery and antiseptic dressing may be required. The majority of cases recover completely in 3-4 weeks. Vaccination of all the birds in a loft as soon as the diagnosis has been made usually brings outbreaks of the disease under control within 7-10 days. Vaccinated birds should not be flown competitively before the vaccination lesions have resolved.

Capillary Haemangio-Endothelioma

This conditions manifests itself as a vigorously growing tumorous lesion which appears on the feathered areas of the skin, frequently on the neck and the upper side of the wing. It first appears as a disturbance of the feather coat, but grows rapidly and projects through the plumage and is highly vascular. Within a matter of 2-3 weeks the lesion reaches about the size of a hazel nut (1-2cm in diameter) and, if damaged, bleeds very freely. However, it resolves without treatment within a further period of 3-4 weeks. The precise aetiology of this condition is not known but, since it usually appears in more than one bird in a loft, it is assumed to be infectious. The histological appearance is suggestive of a viral infection.

FUNGAL INFECTIONS

Typically, the non-feathered areas of the skin are affected by fungal infections. Young birds are particularly susceptible. The lesions consist of scaly, greyish white patches which may become very much thickened with time. The usual cause is the dermatophyte fungus, *Trichophyton megnini.*

Diagnosis

Diagnosis is based on the appearance of suspicious lesions confirmed by microscopic examination of scrapings cleared in 1% sodioum hydroxide or culture on suitable media.

Differential diagnosis - ectoparasitism, pigeon pox, infected insect bites, trauma, drug toxicity.

Treatment

Fungal infections are difficult to treat and specific treatment should only be administered following a confirmed diagnosis. The use of griseofulvin (10mg/kg daily for 21 days given as a crushed tablet suspension in water pipetted directly into the crop) has been found to be effective. Alternatively, ketoconazole (3mg/kg tid for 7-21 days pipetted into the crop) can also be used without adverse effects (see Chapter 14): this is only indicated in particularly valuable specimens. Topical treatment of lesions with tincture of iodine and glycerine (1part iodine:6 parts glycerine) has been reported. Dermatophyte infections are persistent in the environment and a thorough disinfection of the loft and its furniture with an iodine based disinfectant is indicated.

NUTRITIONAL

Pigeons are naturally omnivorous. For preference they tend to take green foods and seeds and primary nutritional deficiencies are unlikely. However, certain birds are idiosyncratic in their selection of food, as may be observed when birds are caged individually, and pigeon fanciers sometimes develop extreme theories with respect to nutrition. Therefore, nutritional problems cannot be excluded without a very careful consideration of the full history. Particularly during periods of rapid growth of the feathers, the requirement for sulphur-bearing amino acids is high, and any shortfall is likely to lead to weak, poorly coloured or brittle feathers.

Diagnosis

Diagnosis presents great difficulty, but the suspicion may to some extent be confirmed by history. However, since the effect of correction of a deficiency on the feathers will not be apparent until the next moult, the situation is an unsatisfactory one.

Differential diagnosis - concurrent ill health, toxicity, trauma.

Treatment

It is essential that the diet offered is a fully balanced one. The use of commercially available pelleted diets discourages selective feeding, though pigeons reared on natural grains may be slow to recognise pellets as food. The use of nutritional supplements containing trace elements, vitamins and amino acids has a real value. Dried brewer's yeast is a valuable source of amino acids, calcium, phosphorus, trace elements including zinc, and the B vitamins excluding B_{12}. Dried yeast may be included in the diet at up to 4% of the feed. If grains and seeds are mixed with a small volume of light cooking oil prior to the addition of dried yeast, the yeast will adhere satisfactorily to the grains. The addition of a soluble multivitamin, eg. Dupharsol 13/60 (Solvay Duphar Veterinary), to the drinking water is also logical under the circumstances.

TOXIC

The highly selective nature of pigeons as feeders leads to rejection of 'off' grains, so that mycotoxicoses are only rarely seen. The most common toxicity problems associated with the skin appear to be drug associated. The use of benzimidazole anthelmintics has been associated with abnormal feather development: the use of these compounds in parents feeding young is contraindicated. The failure of quills to burst into full feathers seems to be a feature of this condition. The use of pyrimethamine potentiated sulphonamides in the treatment of coccidiosis has been associated with the appearance of brittle and poorly coloured feathers. The injection of betamethasone and possibly other corticosteroids may well result in the appearance of a fret mark in any growing feather. As a general rule, medication of any sort should be avoided during feather growth. Any damage sustained during feather growth can only be made good at the following moult.

Diagnosis

Diagnosis is based upon the appearance of abnormal plumage together with a consistent history. Confirmation is usually impracticable.

Treatment

Treatment of toxic effects of this nature is obviously impracticable. Avoidance is based upon therapeutic caution and good husbandry.

TRAUMATIC

Pigeons are subject to trauma as a result of collisions and fighting. Collisions with wires can lead to extensive skin injuries. Pigeons respond very well to suturing, rest and appropriate antibiotic therapy.

Wire injuries generally involve the lower cervical area, including the crop. Where the injury penetrates the crop, care must be taken to ensure the integrity of the crop wall prior to closure of the skin. A torn crop represents a serious trauma and careful attention should be given to its repair according to sound surgical principles.

Injuries caused by fighting are generally apparent on the head and are seen most frequently, though not exclusively, in males. These injuries normally only present a problem when they become infected. The use of pigeon pox vaccine is contraindicated in the early part of the breeding season when there is considerable competitive activity between cocks (see Chapter 25). Otherwise, insignificant superficial wounds may become infected with vaccine virus and acquire the typical appearance of pigeon pox and take several weeks to resolve.

Extensive crusty lesions about the head are commonly thought to be associated with infected insect bites.

Diagnosis

Because home medication by the pigeon fancier with antibiotics, particularly tetracyclines, is very common, culture and sensitivity testing of extensive superficial wounds is indicated prior to antibiotic medication. Individual pigeons are often presented with lesions of the skin overlying the crop suggestive of parasitic mite infestation. These are naked areas scattered with feather stubs 2-3mm in length, often without obvious inflammation, though the skin may appear superficially scabby. Detailed examination of these lesions microscopically and by digestion frequently reveals no specific cause. It is the author's view that such lesions result from friction with the sharp edge of a feeder or drinker, possibly associated with a nutritional or toxic, brittle feather factor. Usually, in such cases, there is a long history of ineffective treatment with assorted antiparasitic dressings.

NEOPLASTIC

Capillary haemangio-endothelioma and epithelioma contagiosa have been referred to earlier (see Viral Infections). The rapid development of these lesions is more suggestive of infection than a classical neoplasm. Lipomata are often seen on the skin of older pigeons. They are benign tumours, usually slow growing and pedunculated. Normally, they do not give rise to health problems.

Diagnosis

Diagnosis is based on history, appearance and histology.

Treatment

Capillary haemangio-endothelioma and epithelioma contagiosa will resolve naturally. However, the engorged appearance of the former indicates the isolation of affected birds. Where haemorrhage occurs this may be controlled by ligation or cautery. Where necessary, lipomata may be removed by ligation.

Table 26.1. Summary of some skin conditions of pigeons.

Condition	Clinical signs	Diagnosis	Differential diagnosis	Treatment	Prognosis
Ectoparasites					
Fleas	Dirty skin, anaemia.	Direct examination.	Other ectoparasites.	Coumaphos, cypermethrin.	Excellent.
Lice	Dirty skin, feather damage, presence of eggs.	Direct examination.	Other ectoparasites.	Coumaphos, cypermethrin, permethrin.	Excellent.
Mange mites (various)	Broken feathers, irritation, encrustation of legs and feet.	Direct examination. Microscopy.	Other ectoparasites, fungal infections, bumblefoot, nutritional, gout, toxic, mechanical.	Cypermethrin, ivermectin, hygiene.	Fair.

Table 26.1. Continued.

Condition	Clinical signs	Diagnosis	Differential diagnosis	Treatment	Prognosis
Red mite and Northern fowl mite	Dirty skin, anaemic, death. Blood engorged mites may be visible, especially at night.	Direct examination of environment. Examination of birds at night.	Other ectoparasites.	Cypermethrin, ivermectin, hygiene.	Good.
Fungal infections (favus) (zoonosis)	Greyish white scaly lesions.	Microscopy, culture.	Mange mites, pox.	Griseofulvin, iodine and glycerine.	Poor unless treated early.
Pox	Typical pustules on mainly featherless areas and oropharynx. Epithelioma contagiosa appears as a growing tumour, usually of feathered areas.	Direct examination, season, history, epizootiology, histology.	Trauma (fighting and insects) (trichomoniasis etc.). Capilliary haemangio-endothelioma.	Local if indicated. Vaccination on a loft basis.	Excellent.
Bacterial					
Superficial	Irritation, loss of feathers.	Absence of other factors.	Ectoparasites, fungal infection, nutritional.	Hexetidine (Hexocil Solution, Upjohn) shampoo (no longer licensed).	Excellent.
Traumatic	Infected wounds, eg. *Erysipelothrix* spp.	Bacteriology.	None.	Appropriate antibacterials.	Excellent.
Tuberculosis (zoonosis)	Caseous nodules, often under the wings.	Wasting bird. Direct examination. Examination of Ziehl-Neelsen stained smear. *Post-mortem* lesions.	Severe mite infestation, pox.	None directly. Hygiene. Possible eradication by intradermal test.	Individually very poor. Consider colony and loft destruction.
Bumblefoot	Chronic sepsis of foot/feet.	Direct examination. Pain. Usually only odd birds affected.	Scaly leg mite, gout.	Appropriate antibiotics.	Poor unless treated very early.
Neoplastic					
Lipoma	Local swelling, usually slow growing. Old birds.	Appearance, age. Only odd birds affected.	Capillary haemangio-endothelioma, epithelioma contagiosa.	Surgery.	Excellent.

Table 26.1. Continued.

Condition	Clinical signs	Diagnosis	Differential diagnosis	Treatment	Prognosis
Capillary haemangio-endothelioma	Rapid growth and recession. Very vascular.	Appearance. Usually more than one bird affected.	Lipoma, epithelioma contagiosa.	Isolation.	Excellent.
Nutritional	Usually broken feathers, leaving stubs on frictional areas. Loss of colour.	Appearance, absence of other conditions, history, mechanical factors.	Mange mites, drug toxicity.	Soluble multivitamins, dried yeast.	Good, though slow.
Toxic	Brittle feathers as above. Poorly formed feathers. Poorly coloured feathers. Fret marks.	Appearance, history of medication during feather growth.	Nutritional/mechanical factors. Chronic ill health.	Avoid treatment during feather growth unless essential.	Favourable but slow.

REFERENCES

Coles BH (1985) *Avian Medicine and Surgery*. Blackwell Scientific Publications, Oxford.

Levi, WM (1974) *The Pigeon*. Levi Publishing Company, Sumter.

CHAPTER TWENTY SEVEN

Wing and Leg Problems

Frank D W Harper

INTRODUCTION

The limbs of the domestic pigeon are little changed in form from those of the ancestral Rock Dove. Pigeons are a strong flying species, possessing an elliptical wing of low aspect ratio (span divided by width) and moderate wing loading (bodyweight divided by wing area) (King and McLelland, 1984). Such a wing enables rapid take-off, sustained flapping flight and high manoeuvrability, but limited gliding and soaring capability. The common name reflects the nesting and roosting sites on cliff and rock ledges. Feeding behaviour is one of inland foraging to open ground: the legs, therefore, are strongly developed. Little use is made of trees as perches and the relatively small feet (anisodactyl foot - three toes forward, one digit back) have small claws and a weak flexor grip. Pigeons are poor swimmers but on occasion they use both wings and legs for forward propulsion on the water. The skeletal and muscular anatomy of both pectoral and pelvic limbs of pigeons resembles that of the domestic fowl as described in standard texts. Some publications use the Rock Dove as a type species (George and Berger, 1966).

When approaching clinical problems of the limbs, the overlap of function must be considered. Birds presented as unable to fly may have leg problems preventing take-off: this may not be obvious in a bird removed from a box. Similarly, abnormal leg carriage following injury can compromise flying efficiency in the racing bird.

CONGENITAL AND DEVELOPMENTAL ABNORMALITIES

Monstrosities

Monstrosities seldom survive hatching. Wingless or other limb deformed specimens may be presented as curiosities. Correction of webbed feet (syndactylism) (see Figure 27.1) may be requested. Simple incision along a forcipressure line can be performed in juveniles. Affected adult birds are seldom presented. The bird is not inconvenienced and the owner has come to accept the curiosity.

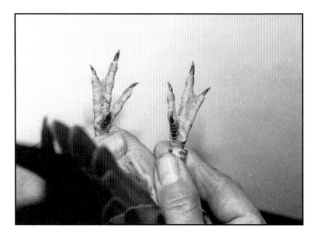

Figure 27.1: *Pigeon with webbed feet (outer toes).*

Abnormal Wing Feathers

Abnormal wing feather development in nestlings frequently gives cause for concern. 'Porcupine' pigeons with no expanded vane to the feathers have been recorded (Levi, 1974). Regarded as of genetic origin, the condition has been reproduced by administration of ivermectin to one-week-old nestlings. 'Pipey' feathers, ie. feathers with delayed expansion of the vane, may reflect a genetic trait or management fault, eg. nutritional, or dry and dusty conditions with low humidity and failure to provide baths. Where the problem is widespread in a loft and associated with blood quills (an extreme form, with failure to resorb the pulp in the growing shaft), an underlying infection is likely to be present. Interference with vane expansion and damage to the feather can be a sequela to administration of ivermectin, benzimidazole anthelmintics and some antibiotics, eg. lincomycin and potentiated sulphonamides. Missed feeding in the parents can result in fret marks or hunger lines on the feathers of the 'youngsters'.

Skeletal Abnormalities

Skeletal abnormalities of pigeons, rachitic or chondrodystrophic, caused by mineral deficiencies are poorly documented and are probably rare (Levi, 1974). Stunting of the second squab can occur for a variety of reasons, eg. poor parenting, intercurrent disease or poorly synchronised fostering, and skeletal development may be poor. Crooked keels (common) and spontaneous fractures (particularly of the proximal tibiotarsus) may reflect a deficiency, but in those cases investigated a heavy burden of *Trichomonas gallinae* and/or *Hexamita* spp. has been found. Perosis, enlargement of the intertarsal joint, with or without displacement of the Achilles tendon ('slipped hock'), is recognised in poultry and other species as a consequence of manganese, zinc or choline deficiency. However, cases have been seen in squabs fed by parent birds which had gained access to 'Growmore' garden fertiliser. A temporary and self-correcting outward rotation of the carpus may be seen in single reared, rapidly growing squabs. Associated with or independent from this phenomenon, such squabs may show the condition known as 'pinwheel'.

PINWHEEL

Pinwheel (splay leg) is a unilateral or, less frequently, a bilateral extension of the knee (femorotibial) joint which develops in the second or third week after hatching (see Figure 27.2). Levi (1974) reported the condition as developing between 14-30 days of age. Squabs seen to be normal when ringed (7-8 days of age) are subsequently found to be thrusting their leg(s) laterally. Affected birds cannot adduct their limb(s) and/or flex the femorotibial joint(s): they spend much of the time 'scrabbling' and circling (pinwheeling) in an apparent attempt to compensate. In established cases there is secondary trauma to the soft tissues over the keel bone. Attempts at treatment by strapping the legs or by surgery have been unsuccessful: when affected limbs are dissected there has been no obvious abnormality. Keymer (1991) gave a comprehensive description of the condition, discussed aetiology and described Walsh's method of prevention by the use of a nest divider when single chicks are hatched. The problem is most often encountered in mid or late season in single reared, usually forward, well grown squabs. Flat bottomed nest bowls and shortage of nesting material are contributory factors, as is a nesting site with little headroom, eg. under a box - it is in such circumstances that a nest pair is likely to be affected. Amongst breeders there is a perception that single chicks are brooded more intensively, and frequently a potato is placed in the nest for 'balance'.

ACQUIRED PROBLEMS

Acquired abnormalities are not common in nestlings, but digits can be damaged or the distal tibiotarsus fractured when attempting to ring over-age or over-large youngsters. Newly weaned squeakers huddle and are at risk of limb injury from sliding doors. Acquired abnormalities constitute the majority of limb problems in the older pigeon.

Abnormalities of feathers and skin are considered

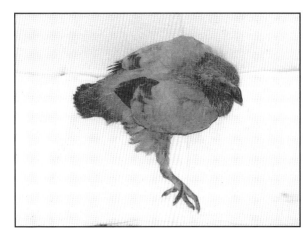

Figure 27.2: Pigeon squab displaying pinwheel (splay leg).

elsewhere (see Chapter 26). The ten primary flight feathers are, however, a major feature of the wing. Interruption or cessation of the normal moulting sequence once it has commenced is an important, but non-specific, diagnostic indicator requiring further investigation. As in nestlings, feather damage can be a result of medication or past infection, eg. paramyxovirus.

The development of blood quills may be the reason for an initial consultation. Blood quills usually arise in one or more of the three distal primaries on one or both wings and may indicate a past or current systemic condition. Affected birds show pain and are reluctant to fly. Popularly attributed to a 'knock', incidence is high in flocks that have shown signs of the adenovirus/*Escherichia coli* complex earlier in the season. Bacterial cultures yield coliforms and *Staphylococcus* spp. and there is a good response to amoxycillin injections (see Table 27.1).

STAPHYLOCOCCAL INFECTIONS

Staphylococcal infections may become established by extension of local lesions or localisation of septicaemic conditions, and may be encountered as a tenosynovitis or septic arthritis, usually of the hocks and feet (see Figure 27.3).

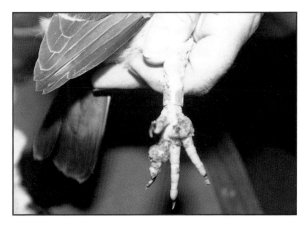

Figure 27.3: Staphylococcal lesions on the toes of a pigeon.

SALMONELLOSIS

Salmonellosis is fully described in the chapter on nervous conditions (see Chapter 29), but in the context of wing and leg problems, infection with *Salmonella typhimuriam* var. *copenhagen* is the pre-eminent cause of septic arthritis of the limbs of pigeons. Wing boil, wing lump or dropped wing are descriptive lay terms for the condition. The elbow joint is most commonly affected and most cases occur in females. In early cases, usually presented because the birds are reluctant or unable to fly, the joint is acutely swollen or suppurating and fluid can be collected for culture or slide agglutination. When other joints of the wing or leg are involved, fluid accumulation is less evident and radiography may be necessary to identify the lesion. Chronically affected joints may ankylose and early treatment is important if this is to be avoided. Suggested treatment is with enrofloxacin (20mg/kg for 10 days). Treatment can be initiated parenterally and maintained orally (repeated injections are irritant). In acutely swollen joints, aspiration and intra-articular dexamethasone (after initiation of antibiotic therapy) may help.

When diagnosed, septic arthritis due to *Salmonella* spp. implies a flock problem and all birds in the loft should be treated. Any suspect individuals should be culled where possible and, during treatment, thorough cleansing, litter disposal and repeated disinfection should be carried out. Septic arthritis due to *Staphylococcus* spp. is usually a problem of the individual bird. A rare infection of the limbs in the individual is by *Mycobacterium avium*. Lesions found in tuberculosis are illustrated in Levi (1974).

STREPTOCOCCAL INFECTIONS

Streptococcal infections are probably underdiagnosed. Devriese *et al* (1989) and De Herdt *et al* (1994) described symptoms which mimic those of salmonellosis, including arthritis. Lesions described were 'areas of necrosis in the pectoral muscles, tenosynovitis of the tendon of the deep pectoral, and arthritis of the stifle, hock or shoulder joints'. An unconfirmed but clinically similar condition, ie. inability to fly, predominantly in hens and with no evidence of *Salmonella* spp. infection, has responded to treatment with amoxycillin. The condition known as 'wing lock', seen in birds after prolonged confinement in baskets and traditionally attributed to 'cramp' in the pectoral muscles, also shows some similarities.

NON-INFECTIOUS ARTHRITIS

Non-infectious arthritis, age related, is common in males from about seven years of age. Affected birds become progressively lame, adopt an increasingly 'pigeon toed' stance and develop obvious enlargement of the knee joints, particularly the distal femur. These birds are usually breeders and they may become infertile due to an inability to copulate successfully. Strategic use of a non-steroidal anti-inflammatory, eg. ketoprofen (0.1ml i/m or s/c repeated once or twice on consecutive days during the driving period), can prolong the reproductive life. Other products, eg. diclophenac, have been used empirically and at various dose rates by fanciers. Artificial insemination can also prolong the reproductive life of valuable males. Differentials to be considered with respect to arthritic conditions are the articular form of gout and neoplasia of the skeletal structures, neither of which are common in pigeons.

BUMBLEFOOT

Bumblefoot (see Chapter 16) is seen occasionally in pigeons. Infection by *Staphylococcus* spp. or *E. coli* causes swelling of the pad overlying the tarsometatarsophalangeal joint with accumulation of caseous pus. More common is infection of, or loss of, the claw on the posterior digit (the inability to hook this claw up to the tail in flight is seen as a handicap). Keratinised excrescences may develop on the toes of older birds and can become infected. The condition is non-parasitic: scaly leg does not seem to occur in pigeons. Type 1 bumblefoot ('corns') can resemble lesions of pigeon pox.

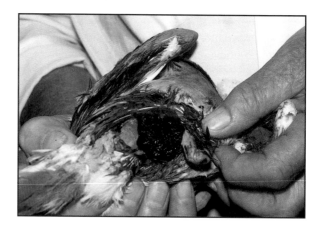

Figure 27.4: Haemangioma on the leg of a pigeon.

MISCELLANEOUS CONDITIONS OF THE WING

Haemangiomata (popularly called 'protein lumps') are pox-related lesions which may occur on the feathered parts of the leg (see Figure 27.4) but are more common on the wings, as are **lipomata** and other **neoplasms**. Ligation or cryosurgery are the recommended procedures for the removal of masses from the wing. Apposition of friable, inelastic skin is difficult and surgical incisions can lead to scar formation and xanthomatosis. **Lacerations** of the wing caused by predators present similar problems of repair.

Self-mutilation and **feather picking** are rare, but can occur in association with liver disease. Usually, the right axillary region and/or the posterior edge of the wing are affected. A condition similar to lovebird dermatitis (an intractable ulcerative condition, probably of viral origin) may also be encountered in this region, but on either wing.

MISCELLANEOUS CONDITIONS OF THE LEGS

The identity band may cause direct injury; sometimes the accumulation of skin debris under the ring can restrict circulation. Plastic secondary markers may crack and the sharp edge may section the common digital extensor tendon. The resulting apparent extensor paralysis, with curling of the toes, is a common sequela to many leg injuries, but it may be the first and only symptom in some cases of paramyxovirus infection and precede the more typical symptoms (polydipsia, polyuria) in loft mates by several days.

Hens sometimes lose the use of both legs after laying. This seems to be pressure related. Recovery occurs within about 72 hours with or without calcium therapy.

Amputation of the digits due to accidental ligature is common, but experience and observation of ferals suggests that pigeons can walk on any (healthy) limb remnant distal to the knee. However, they do not adapt well to the loss of a wing.

TRAUMA AND FRACTURES

Racing pigeons may incur collision injuries in flight or when escaping from predators. The techniques of fracture repair are mentioned elsewhere in this manual (Chapter 16). However, some special considerations apply to pigeons. Pigeons attempt to use a limb early in the healing process and rotational stability is important. Furthermore, leg fractures are frequently bilateral and consideration should be given to suspending the bird in a netting sling during convalescence. If conservative treatment of a wing fracture is adopted, it should be remembered that it can take some days for birds to adapt to a strapped wing: they may fall and suffocate when a strapping is first applied. Rupture of the supracoracoideus muscle and tendon, rare in other species, is a frequent injury in the pigeon (Coles, 1985). There is a characteristic upward subluxation of the head of the humerus. Coles (1985) stated that repair of the tendon is almost impossible.

THERAPEUTICS

Table 24.1 lists some of the drugs used in the treatment of the conditions mentioned in this chapter.

REFERENCES

Coles BH (1985) *Avian Medicine and Surgery.* Blackwell Scientific Publications, Oxford.
De Herdt P, Ducatelle R, Haesebrouck F, Devriese LA, De Groote B and Roels S (1994) An unusual outbreak of *Streptococcus bovis* septicaemia in racing pigeons (*Columba livia*). *Veterinary Record* **134**, 42.
Devriese LA, Ceyssens K, Uyttebroek E and Gevaert D (1989) Streptococcal infections in pigeons. *Proceedings of the 2nd European Conference of the Dutch Association of Avian Veterinarians, Utrecht, 1989.* NVDV, Utrecht.

Table 24.1. Therapeutics for wing and leg problems.

Drug	Indication	Dosage	Authority
Amoxycillin	*Salmonella* spp., *Streptococcus* spp., *Staphylococcus* spp.	150mg/kg i/m, s/c or p/o qid, or 1500mg/l water, for six days.	Gylstorff and Grimm (1987).
Enrofloxacin	*Salmonella* spp.	200mg/l water (20mg/kg) for 10 days.	Uyttebroek *et al* (1989).
Ketoprofen	Arthritis.	0.1ml of 1% solution once daily on one, two or three occasions.	Data sheet (cat dose).
Diclophenac	Arthritis.	12.5mg orally, single dose.	Used empirically by some breeders.
Calcium borogluconate	Post-laying paralysis.	1-2ml of 10% solution by slow i/v or s/c injection.	Coles (1985).
Dimethyl sulphoxide	Reduce swelling of lower limb (trauma); carrier for steroids.	Topically.	Unpublished.

George JC and Berger AJ (1966) *Avian Mycology*. Academic Press, London.

Gylstorff I and Grimm F (1987) *Vogelkrankheiten*. Verlag Eugen Ulmer, Stuttgart.

Keymer IF (1991). Pigeons. In: *Manual of Exotic Pets*. New Edn. Eds PH Beynon and JE Cooper. BSAVA, Cheltenham.

King AS and McLelland J (1984) *Birds: Their Structure and Function*. Baillière Tindall, London.

Levi WM (1974) *The Pigeon*. 2nd Edn. Levi Publishing Company, Sumter.

Uyttebroek E, Gevaert D and Devriese LA (1989) Effects of antibiotics on experimental salmonellosis in pigeons. *Proceedings of the 2nd European Conference of the Dutch Association of Avian Veterinarians, Utrecht, 1989*. NVDV, Utrecht.

CHAPTER TWENTY EIGHT

Respiratory Diseases

David G Parsons

INTRODUCTION

Respiratory problems are a major concern of the pigeon fancier. Clinical examination of affected birds and taking of an accurate history is required. Previous medications administered, dosage and treatment course are particularly important. Seeking veterinary assistance is often the last resort following failure of earlier remedies.

The significance of a respiratory infection depends on the time of year and what is expected of the birds. Mild respiratory problems in the racing season are far more significant than at the end of the season.

Respiratory distress need not simply be the result of a respiratory infection. Any deviation from the normal could indicate a systemic infection with a respiratory manifestation. It is important, therefore, to assess the respiratory problem in conjunction with general bird health, management and nutrition (see Chapters 24 and 30). Loft management is particularly important in predisposing to infection and subsequent recovery from infection.

CLINICAL SIGNS

The following clinical signs could be indicative of a respiratory infection: abdominal breathing/tail bobbing; blocked nares; changes in vocalisation; congestion of mucous membranes; conjunctivitis; coughing; diphtheritic membrane formation; discoloured cere; mucus in the mouth; nasal discharge; ocular discharge; open mouth breathing; panting after a short training toss; pus in the choanal cleft; pus on the loft wall; rattling breathing; scratching the head; sinus swelling; sneezing; sneezing after sinus or tracheal compression; staining of feathers around the eye; staining of feathers on the wing butt.

VIRAL INFECTIONS

Pigeon Herpesvirus (PHV)

Hosts
Pigeons are the natural hosts and reservoir of this disease. Pigeon herpesvirus is serologically related to falcon and owl herpesvirus.

Transmission
Spread is by direct contact with infected pigeons. In Europe, over 50% of pigeons have antibodies to PHV. Many pigeons recover from the disease and become life-long asymptomatic carriers. These carriers will shed the virus from time to time. The majority will excrete virus from the throat during the breeding season, particularly whilst feeding youngsters. Squabs infected at this early age are protected by passive immunity of parental origin; they tend to become asymptomatic carriers. Susceptible birds may be infected at any age, but usually under six months. There is no evidence for egg transmission. Infected birds will excrete virus within 24 hours of initial infection, prior to the appearance of symptoms, with high antibody titres persisting for 7-10 days. Recrudescence can occur without clinical signs, ie. the stress of feeding youngsters. As with many herpesviruses, latency, the period (of virus replication) between absorption and release from the cell, is a feature of this disease.

Clinical Signs
PHV is a common disease, particularly of young pigeons under six months of age.

Acute infection. The following signs may be seen: sneezing; protruding membrana nictitans; conjunctivitis; clear discharges from the nares with subsequent rhinitis; cere turning brown; congestion of the mucous membranes of the mouth; diphtheritic membrane formation; occasionally ulcers. Other signs are more indicative of a systemic infection. These include vomiting, diarrhoea, lethargy, the inability to fly and occasionally death.

Chronic infection. The following signs may be seen: sinusitis; white spots on the soft palate; dyspnoea and secondary complications due to bacterial infections (*Escherichia coli*, *Pasteurella* spp., *Staphylococcus* spp. and *Streptococcus* spp.); trichomoniasis; and *Mycoplasma* spp. infection.

Post-Mortem Findings

Congestion of the mucous membranes of the mouth, pharynx and larynx can be seen on *post mortem* examination. Small white foci of necrosis and small ulcers may also be seen. Diphtheritic membrane formation can occur. If the infection has become generalised, necrotic foci may be seen in the liver. In some birds there may be a caseous obstruction of the trachea, air sacculitis and pericarditis.

Diagnosis

This is usually based on the clinical history and signs. Confirmation can be obtained by virus isolation, serology and histopathological demonstration of intranuclear inclusion bodies in pharyngeal cells, liver or kidney. It is important to ascertain whether trichonomads are a complicating factor. Pharyngeal swabs can also be taken for bacteriological examination.

Differential Diagnosis

Acute PHV must be differentiated from Newcastle disease or pigeon paramyxovirus infection. Chronic infection could be confused with pigeon pox, trichomoniasis, vitamin A deficiency or chlamydiosis.

Treatment

Nursing and supportive therapy are very important. This should include the provision of extra heat, antibiotic therapy and treatment for trichomoniasis if necessary. Chemotherapy has been tried using trisodium phosphonoformate and acycloguanosine, but it failed to prevent infection.

Control

No effective vaccines are currently available. Attenuated and inactivated vaccines have been tried experimentally. Both reduced virus excretion and clinical signs but neither could prevent the development of carrier status. Routine disinfection is essential.

Pigeon Pox (see also Chapter 26)

Host

Pigeons are the natural host. Serological cross reactions can be demonstrated between pigeon pox virus and fowl pox and falcon pox viruses.

Transmission

This is primarily by direct contact via cuts and abrasions, eg. fighting in race baskets or insect bites. Respiratory infection could occur from aerosols in a contaminated environment when the virus has been shed from infected feather follicles and dried scabs. Infected parents feeding squabs will also transmit infection. The incubation period is between 4-14 days. The virus is shed from infected pocks and feather follicles. In chickens a latent infection has been demonstrated for 13 months.

Clinical Signs

Pigeon pox is a common disease of young pigeons. The disease is often reported at the end of the racing season (end of September) when it will not have an adverse affect on the loft's ability to race. However, it can occur at any time, particularly March through to September.

The earliest signs are slight closing of one eye, excessive lacrimation and development of a firm white swelling on the eyelid. This rapidly enlarges, becoming more yellow to brown and crusty. Lesions may also be found around the nares, the commissures of the beak, the pharynx and the larynx. Occasionally, lesions may also be seen on the legs. An internal form can also occur.

An atypical form of pigeon pox is also seen. Isolated cases or a sporadic outbreak of 'warts', 'blood blisters' or 'protein bumps' may be presented. These can be found on the leading edge of the wings, breast and rump. They can vary in size from 5-25mm diameter. If damaged, they will bleed profusely.

The course of infection in both typical and atypical pigeon pox is approximately three weeks. Scars may be left at the site of the pox lesion. In some cases, beak deformities may occur.

Post-Mortem Findings

Post-mortem examination confirms the extent of the lesions and whether or not there has been any involvement of the oesophagus or trachea which has prevented feeding or breathing.

Diagnosis

The owner may report that the pigeons showed poor performance in a race two weeks earlier. This, in conjunction with the clinical signs, is virtually pathognomonic for pigeon pox. Isolation of the pox virus from pox lesions or direct electron microscopy will confirm the diagnosis. Additional tests include histopathology - demonstrating the presence of Bollinger bodies - and the agar gel precipitin test on pox lesions.

Differential Diagnosis

Differential diagnosis should include trichomoniasis, herpesvirus infection, vitamin A deficiency, candidiasis, aspergillosis and ringworm.

Treatment

There is no specific treatment. Surgical removal may be necessary if the lesion(s) interferes with vital functions. Painting the lesions with aqueous iodine may be beneficial. Antibiotics to control secondary infection may also be necessary to ensure that the bird can feed and breathe. Concurrent trichomoniasis must be treated if present, as this will exacerbate the condition.

In large lofts, where stock birds are kept separate from the race teams, it may be decided to vaccinate the remainder of the birds. Under no circumstances should vaccinated birds be allowed to race for at least six weeks. Extreme caution must be exercised, especially if the stock birds are rearing youngsters (this is best avoided).

In uncomplicated cases the lesions of both typical and atypical pox will resolve naturally.

Control
A pigeon pox vaccine is available (Pigeon Pox Vaccine (Living) Nobilis, Vetrepharm). The vaccine is rubbed into plucked feather follicles on the leg (see Appendix - Formulary (Pigeons)). Vaccine must not be allowed to get onto the hands as it might inadvertently be transferred to the pigeon's eye or mouth. Under no circumstances should vaccine be applied to a bleeding feather follicle. All the birds in the loft should be vaccinated at the same time. Annual boosters are recommended. Breeding stock should be vaccinated at least six weeks before pairing up and all race birds should be vaccinated six weeks before the first race. Only healthy birds should be vaccinated. Do not allow recently vaccinated birds to mix with unvaccinated birds.

Following an outbreak, thorough disinfection of the loft is required. Steam cleaning is particularly effective.

Newcastle Disease and Pigeon Paramyxovirus (PMV-1) Infection
Newcastle disease and PMV-1 infection of pigeons are both notifiable to the Divisional Veterinary Officer (DVO) of the Ministry of Agriculture, Fisheries and Food (MAFF). Nervous signs are usually seen first with PMV-1 infection of pigeons. Mortality may be the presenting sign with virulent Newcastle disease infection (see Chapter 29). The two strains of virus can be distinguished using monoclonal antibodies.

Hosts
PMV-1 can infect many species of birds. These include chickens, turkeys, pheasants, ducks and geese (the latter two do not usually show marked clinical signs).

Transmission
Infection can occur by ingestion or inhalation of virus. The commonest method of spread is likely to be by mechanical transmission of infected faeces. The incubation period varies from 2-15 days. Virus can be shed from the respiratory and intestinal tracts.

Clinical Signs
Signs can be seen in unvaccinated birds of any age. Virulent PMV-1 infection is associated with a high mortality, listlessness, rapid breathing and weakness. The degree of respiratory involvement is variable. Oedema around the eyes and head can also occur. Pigeon paramyxovirus infection usually presents as a nervous condition (see Chapter 29).

Post-Mortem Findings
There are no specific lesions in pigeons apart from generalised congestion of the viscera which indicates a septicaemia.

Diagnosis
History and clinical signs. Confirmation requires serology (haemagglutination inhibition test) and virus isolation. Serological diagnosis is more difficult in birds that have been vaccinated against pigeon paramyxovirus infection.

Differential Diagnosis
Should include chlamydiosis, poisoning and other systemic infections.

Treatment (see also Chapter 29)
Treatment will depend on the virulence of the virus isolated. Slaughter of all stock may be necessary. Where strains of low virulence are isolated, slaughter may not be necessary. In this case, nursing and supportive therapy, as for herpesvirus infection, will help.

Control (see also Chapter 29)
Vaccination of all birds in the loft with pigeon paramyxovirus vaccine will protect against clinical pigeon paramyxovirus disease and cross protect against Newcastle disease.

The Diseases of Poultry Order 1994 (SI 1994/3141) states that:
● The show or race organiser must ensure that all racing pigeons entering have been vaccinated with a suitable vaccine against PMV-1 in pigeons.
● A racing pigeon is defined as any pigeon transported or intended for transport from its home loft to be released so that it may freely fly back to the loft or any other destination.

The author recommends annual vaccination of all birds in the loft. This should be done three weeks before pairing up for adults or three weeks before the first race. Pigeons can be vaccinated from three weeks of age. The precise programme will depend on the loft's policy for showing or racing and the current disease situation. Vaccinating all the birds in the loft will help avoid the possibility of the virus becoming endemic in the loft. Vaccination prevents clinical signs of disease. It does not prevent the bird from becoming infected. A vaccinated racing pigeon could therefore become an asymptomatic carrier of virulent virus.

It is important to minimise the risk of buying in infection by purchasing stock from areas where virulent

Newcastle disease does not exist. Virulent Newcastle disease is endemic on the Continent. The local DVO should be able to advise or obtain up to date information on the problem areas.

BACTERIAL INFECTIONS

Chlamydia psittaci

Hosts
Pigeons, chickens, turkeys, pheasants, ducks, geese and many species of wild birds, as well as psittacines, can be infected by *C. psittaci*. Subspecies differentiation of *Chlamydia* spp. has been attempted but currently no one specific system has been adopted. Differentiation has been attempted on the basis of inclusion morphology, plaque neutralisation tests, immunofluorescence and DNA anlaysis. *Chlamydia* spp. strains can be broadly grouped as highly virulent or of low virulence. The latter group has been isolated from pigeons and ducks.

Transmission
Infection is endemic in pigeons. In a survey in England and Wales in 1983, 83% of lofts, retrospectively monitored, had serological evidence for the presence of infection. It is believed that the primary spread of infection is from parent to squab whilst crop feeding. In addition, infection can occur by inhalation of respiratory exudates or contaminated faecal dust. Direct transmission can occur when crop milk is being fed to youngsters. The incubation period is not known for pigeons but it is known to be very variable (42 days to one and half years) for psittacines. The organism is shed in respiratory exudates and faeces. Latent infections are a common occurrence.

Clinical Signs
Fortunately, the pigeon strain of *C. psittaci* seems generally to be of low virulence. However, pigeons can be infected with highly virulent strains. The clinical signs may be variable. Acute disease is accompanied by weight loss, anorexia and green diarrhoea. The respiratory manifestations include swollen eyelids, runny eyes, discolouration of the cere, conjunctivitis progressing to keratoconjunctivitis, and respiratory sounds. These birds can become carriers. Poor performance when racing may be the only indication of subclinincal infection. The severity of the clinical signs will be altered by concurrent infection with inclusion body hepatitis, PMV-1, salmonellosis and trichomoniasis, the latter combinations giving signs of acute infection.

Post-Mortem Findings
The classic *post-mortem* findings of chlamydiosis in pigeons are serofibrinous air sacculitis, peritonitis and occasionally pericarditis. There may also be hepatomegaly, splenomegaly and pneumonia. A recent survey of pigeon diseases at *post mortem* showed that 11 out of 126 were positive on polymerase chain reaction (PCR) test for *Chlamydia* spp. antigen. In eight of these, *Chlamydia* spp. was considered to be the primary cause of the diarrhoea and weight loss (Pennycott, 1994).

Diagnosis
Neither clinical signs or *post-mortem* findings are pathognomonic except in acute cases. Additional confirmatory testing should be undertaken. This includes impression smears, culture, PCR, ELISA, fluorescent antibody, serology and histopathology. The PCR test is the test of choice on faeces. A pooled sample which has been collected over 3-5 days is preferred because of intermittent shedding. Tissues can be examined by direct smear using a modified Ziehl-Neelsen stain to look for inclusion bodies. The ELISA test and culture can be used to confirm these findings.

Differential Diagnosis
Differential diagnosis should include herpesvirus, Newcastle disease and ocular trichomoniasis.

Treatment
All the birds in the loft should be treated. This will probably necessitate administration of medication in the drinking water. Tetracycline (60mg/kg for six weeks) has resulted in a clinical cure. Enrofloxacin (10mg/kg for up to 10 days) is an alternative. There is no specific recommendation by the manufacturer for this latter treatment.

Control
Ensuring that a good routine of general hygiene is employed will help. The owner must be informed that chlamydiosis is a zoonosis and be advised of the signs of human clinical infection.

Mycoplasmal Infections
This infection is believed, by pigeon fanciers, to play an important role in respiratory disease. In their view, it is a significant cause of respiratory disease and mucus at the back of the throat. However, Howse and Jordan (1983) stated that the role of *Mycoplasma* spp. in pigeon respiratory disease was not known.

Host
Three species of *Mycoplasma* have been isolated from both normal and sick pigeons: *M. columborale, M. columbinum* and *M. columbinasale*.

Transmission
Infection is spread by inhalation and ingestion of contaminated respiratory or faecal material. The incubation period is 7-14 days. The organism is shed in respiratory exudates and faeces. As with other mycoplasmal infections, latency is common.

Clinical Signs; *Post-Mortem* **Findings; Diagnosis; Treatment; Control (see 'One-eyed Cold')**
The treatment of naturally occurring mycoplasmal infection with tiamulin (1ml of a 12.5% solution in 560ml drinking water for 35 days) has been shown by Howse and Jordan (1983) to be only temporarily effective, with a rapid recrudescence of infection.

Staphylococcal and Streptococcal Infections

Transmission
Transmission is by inhalation of infectious aerosols and ingestion of infectious exudates. Mechanical damage to the beak and nostrils as a result of fighting in the loft or in the race baskets also permits infection to occur.

Clinical Signs
Staphylococcal and streptococcal infections often cause respiratory problems in young birds. Signs include a purulent discharge from the nostrils, pus in the choanal cleft, head shaking and scratching at the nostrils with brown discolouration of the cere. Sneezing can result in yellow pus on the loft wall. This is often described as the 'snots'.

Diagnosis
Bacteriological culture from the choanal cleft will confirm the bacterial species involved.

Treatment
It is important to determine whether individual or flock treatment is required. It is often convenient for the fancier to treat all the birds in the loft at once. However, this can result in recrudescence a few weeks later when more susceptible birds become infected. Amoxycillin (890mg of 100% amoxycillin trihydrate powder per litre of drinking water for five days) or tetracycline (1g of tetracycline hydrochloride 80% per 1.5 litres of drinking water for five days - equivalent to 60mg/kg) will aid in the control of infection.

Control
General loft management is particularly important. Attention must be given to ventilation, routine hygiene and overcrowding. The latter often occurs in the breeding season. Another source of infection comes from taking in strays (strappers).

Pasteurella Multocida

Transmission
Infection is spread by inhalation or ingestion of nasal discharges and faeces from infected birds.

Clinical Signs
P. multocida infection is an uncommon disease that can affect any age of bird. Experimental infection failed to produce disease but did induce a carrier state. Disease can occur following other predisposing stresses. Acute infection is characterised by respiratory distress, watery discharges which may be seen from the mouth, and mortality. Chronic disease is characterised by respiratory sounds, purulent nasal discharges and conjunctivitis with or without swollen sinuses. In addition there may be nervous signs, arthritis and subcutaneous abscesses.

Post-Mortem Findings
The lesions seen in the acute disease are those associated with a generalised septicaemia with or without petechial haemorrhages. Chronic infection is characterised by rhinitis, sinusitis, conjunctivitis, tracheitis and pneumonia.

Diagnosis
Rapid confirmation of the diagnosis can be obtained by making a Gram stain of an impression smear from heart blood or the liver of the dead bird. Cytological examination of smears from the nares and pharynx of birds with an upper respiratory infection may reveal the typical bipolar staining *Pasteurella*-like organisms. Caution must be exercised in interpretation because these organisms can be found in normal birds. Additional routine bacteriological culture will also detect infection. It may be necessary to incubate plates for 48 hours if negative after 24 hours.

Treatment
Treatment of all the birds in the loft is advisable. Water soluble medication with amoxycillin or tetracycline is preferable (see earlier and Appendix - Formulary ([Pigeons]).

Control
It is important to try to determine the source of infection, paying particular attention to rodent infestation. Cats can be a problem, but they are usually actively discouraged from the loft. Infection may indicate a recent stress such as overcrowding, poor ventilation, change in management or vaccination.

Other Bacteria
Any pathogenic bacteria that cause a systemic illness can give rise to respiratory signs. This includes *Salmonella* spp. and *Erysipelothrix* spp. infection, colisepticaemia, yersiniosis and tuberculosis. Avian tuberculosis can cause disease in pigeons. It is uncommon in racing pigeons but common in feral pigeons.

FUNGAL INFECTIONS

Aspergillosis
Aspergillosis is caused by fungi of the genus *Aspergil-*

lus, most commonly *A. fumigatus*, but *A. flavus* or *A. glaucus* may also be involved.

Transmission
Inhalation or ingestion of fungal spores, usually from environmental contamination, bedding or feed.

Incubation, Shedding and Latency
This depends on the age of the bird, its immuno-competence and the infective dose.

Clinical Signs
There are no specific signs. However, infection is usually chronic and there will be loss of body condition. The respiratory signs will depend on the site of the infection, but will include dyspnoea, rattling sounds, rapid breathing, a fully open larynx, loss of condition and dehydration. Sometimes, infection occurs in the eye with swelling and the formation of a yellow caseous plaque.

Post-Mortem Findings
Diagnosis is most likely to be made on *post-mortem* examination. Miliary white nodules in the lungs, syrinx, bronchioles and air sacs are typical of a mycotic infection. Compression of the lung expresses white strands of pus from the cut surface. White plaques of mature fungal growth with dark green to black centres may be found on the air sacs. In cases of acute *Aspergillus* spp. pneumonia there may be no plaques.

Diagnosis
The combination of clinical signs, *post-mortem* lesions and microscopical examination of smears for fungal hyphae or spores will confirm the diagnosis.

Differential Diagnosis
Acute salmonellosis, trichomoniasis, pigeon pox, 'one-eyed cold'.

Treatment
There is no satisfactory treatment.

Control
Control relies on identification of the potential sources of infection and their removal, eg. mouldy food, straw and damp litter.

PROTOZOAL INFECTIONS

Trichomoniasis (see also Chapter 25)

Clinical Signs
Clinical signs include a failure to fly well and exercise intolerance. On landing, affected birds will pant heavily as though they have been flying very hard. They will also be seen to gape and gasp. Excess mucus can be seen at the back of the throat. The occasional

sneeze may be heard. Lacrimation may be a feature in some birds.

Diagnosis
It is best to assume that every pigeon is infected. Throat swabs should be taken for microscopical examination for the presence of *Trichomonas gallinae*. A freshly warmed slide and normal saline should be used. The use of cold tap water will result in cold shock to the trichomads and loss of motility.

Differential Diagnosis
Mycoplasma spp. infection, pigeon herpesvirus, pox virus.

Haemoproteus spp.
There are two species of *Haemoproteus* spp. that are known to infect pigeons and doves: *H. columbae* and *H. saccharovi*. The former is spread by the pigeon louse fly (*Pseudolynchis canariensis*). The incubation period is not known.

Clinical Signs
This is generally a subclinical infection with any respiratory signs being secondary to anaemia, emaciation and depression.

Diagnosis
Confirmation is by identification of the parasite in the erythrocytes on a blood smear.

Treatment
Treatment is not usually necessary.

Control
Control will involve controlling the vector.

PARASITIC DISEASES

Mites
Both nasal mites (*Neonyssus columbae*, *N. melloi* and *Sternostoma striatus*) and air sac mites (*Cytodites nudus*) are found in pigeons, although the significance of infection is debatable. *N. columbae*, *N. melloi* and *S. striatus* (members of the Family Rhinonyssidae) are regarded as non-pathogenic, but their presence would be expected to reduce a racing bird's potential. *C. nudus* can cause granulomatous pneumonia if a heavy infection is present.

Transmission
The mode of transmission is not known, but is possibly via exudates from the repiratory system.

Clinical Signs
Infection can be subclinical or be involved in secondary damage to the respiratory tract, resulting in emaciation, obstruction of the bronchioles and pneumonia.

Post-Mortem Findings

Small white oval mites, about 0.5mm long, can be found.

Diagnosis

Diagnosis can be made by endoscopy and on *post-mortem* examination. The clinician must beware the presence of other mite eggs and mites, eg. feed mites, in faeces.

Treatment

Ivermectin (200mcg/kg s/c or p/o once) could be tried. The dose can be repeated in 7-10 days.

Control

Control is by good disinfection procedures.

Syngamus trachea (gapeworm)

Transmission

Transmission can be either direct by ingesting embryonated eggs or infective larvae, or indirect by eating earthworms. The minimum time for an infective larvae to develop in the egg is 8-14 days. Infective larvae can remain encysted in earthworms for at least four years. Once infective larvae have been swallowed, they migrates via the blood stream to the lungs and then to the trachea. Maturity is attained about 17-20 days after infection has occurred.

Clinical Signs

Experimental infection has not produced the typical signs of gaping and sneezing. Natural infection, though rare, has been recorded.

Post-Mortem Findings

Typical 'Y' shaped, paired worms are found in the trachea.

Diagnosis

In live birds, infection can be confirmed by the presence of *S. trachea* eggs in the faeces or the demonstration of worms in the trachea by transillumination or endoscopy. At *post-mortem* examination the presence of the worms in the trachea, air sacs or lungs would confirm the diagnosis. Although the life cycle can be direct, the likelihood of infestation occurring with current loft management procedures is minimal. Free flying pigeons will sometimes feed on the ground and can therefore be infected by contact with *S. trachea* shed by game birds, magpies, jays and poultry.

Treatment

Treatment is with fenbendazole (Panacur Capsules for Pigeons, Hoechst) (one 8mg capsule/pigeon over eight weeks of age). Antibiotics may be indicated to control possible foreign body pneumonia caused by dead worms in the lung, as can occur in other species.

Control

Control is by preventing access to infected ground, regular faecal screening and treatment when necessary.

MISCELLANEOUS CAUSES OF INFECTION

'One-Eyed Cold'

This syndrome can be a result of one or more of the following infections: pigeon herpesvirus, chlamydiosis, mycoplasmal infection, trichomoniasis and bacterial infections.

Clinical Signs

'One-eyed cold' is a common infection found primarily in younger birds. It tends to affect individuals over an extended period of time. Usually, only one eye is affected. Initially, there may be swelling of the eyelids with closure of the eye, excessive lacrimation, staining of the feathers about the eye and discolouration of the cere. This can progress to keratoconjunctivitis and permanent blindness if treatment is not instituted quickly.

Diagnosis

Diagnosis is on clinical signs alone. The bird should be screened for trichomonads.

Differential Diagnosis

Pigeon herpesvirus and pigeon pox.

Treatment

An antibiotic ophthalmic ointment should be applied to the eye for at least seven days (chlortetracycline ointment should be used to control possible *Chlamydia* spp. infection). Affected birds should be treated with doxycycline (one 20mg tablet per bird for five days). The slow spread of this infection makes individual bird treatment preferable to flock medication. If trichomoniasis is suspected, all the birds in the appropriate section of the loft should be treated.

TUMOURS

Any space occupying lesion within the air sacs, including tumours, can be expected to result in respiratory signs. Tumours affecting the lungs or heart may also cause respiratory signs.

FOREIGN BODIES

Pieces of straw, shavings or grass can become lodged in the nose, larynx and trachea.

VENTILATION

Poor ventilation of the loft will allow the build up of large quantities of dust, ammonia and bloom.

Overcrowding will only exacerbate this problem. Poor loft placement, eg. in the lee of trees, will restrict ventilation.

TOXINS

Exhaust fumes from engines, sulphur fumigating candles and formalin will all cause respiratory problems.

REFERENCES AND FURTHER READING

Calnek BW (1991) Ed *Diseases of Poultry*. 9th Edn. Wolfe, London.

Harrison GJ and Harrison LR (1986) Eds *Clinical Avian Medicine and Surgery, including Aviculture*. WB Saunders, Philadelphia.

Howse and Jordan (1983) Treatment of racing pigeons naturally infected with *Mycoplasma columborale* and *M. columbinum*. *Veterinary Record* **112**, 324.

Pennycott TW (1994) Pigeon diseases: results from a Scottish diagnostic laboratory. In: *Proceedings of the Association of Avian Veterinarians Annual Conference 1994*. AAV, Lake Worth.

Soulsby EJL (1968) *Helminths, Arthropods and Protozoa of Domesticated Animals*. 6th Edn. Baillière Tindall & Cassell, London.

CHAPTER TWENTY NINE

Nervous Conditions

Tom W Pennycott

INTRODUCTION

Several conditions can cause nervous signs in pigeons, the commonest two conditions being infections with paramyxovirus 1 (PMV-1) and with *Salmonella typhimurium*. Nervous signs resulting from dimetridazole toxicity, following excessive medication for trichomoniasis, and hypocalcaemia in female pigeons around the time of egg laying are fairly common. Less frequently encountered are nervous signs arising from other chemical poisons. Trauma should also be considered (see Chapter 3). Nervous signs may be secondary to another disorder which has reduced appetite and resulted in hypoglycaemia and/or thiamine deficiency.

It is imperative that a full clinical examination (see Chapter 2) is carried out when investigating nervous conditions of pigeons.

PARAMYXOVIRUS 1 INFECTION

PMV-1 infection in pigeons is a notifiable disease, and the local Divisional Veterinary Officer (DVO) of the State Veterinary Service must be informed if PMV-1 is suspected. When investigating nervous conditions of pigeons, the differential diagnosis must, therefore, always include PMV-1. Where infection is suspected, the local DVO must be informed and the birds must be prevented from flying out.

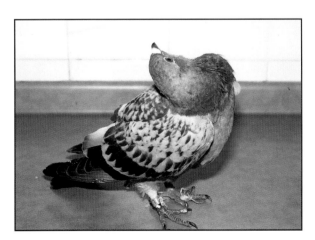

Figure 29.1: Torticollis in a pigeon with paramyxovirus.

Avian paramyxovirus serotype 1 is the causal agent of classical Newcastle disease in poultry. Classical Newcastle disease can occasionally cause nervous signs in pigeons (Stewart, 1971). A pigeon variant of PMV-1 spread from the Middle East into Europe in the early 1980s, causing an epidemic of losses in pigeons and reaching the United Kingdom (UK) in 1983 (Alexander *et al*, 1984a,b). A similar disease of pigeons in Iraq and Egypt in 1978 was initially thought to be the result of a pigeon herpesvirus, but after further virology Kaleta *et al* (1985) later concluded that this was also PMV-1. In 1984 and 1991 disease spread from pigeons to domestic poultry flocks in Britain and Northern Ireland respectively.

Clinical Signs

A large proportion of the pigeons suddenly develop polydipsia and polyuria. The faeces appear as a pool of clear urine surrounding a core of green material. Some birds develop nervous signs, such as loss of balance, inability to pick up feed, torticollis (see Figure 29.1), unilateral or bilateral paralysis of legs or wings, loss of righting reflexes, circling, somersaulting, flying backwards or tremors of the head and neck. The nervous signs are increased if the birds are alarmed. Breeding birds may produce deformed eggs. Reduced egg numbers and reduced hatchability may also occur. Mortality in adults is usually low, but can be high in young birds as a result of secondary malnutrition or kidney failure. Recovery from the diarrhoea and mild nervous signs can take 3-8 weeks. The outcome in birds with severe nervous signs cannot be predicted, but some birds eventually recover. (See also Chapter 25.)

Post-Mortem Findings

Findings at *post-mortem* examination tend to be non-specific, with overall congestion of viscera. Mottling of spleen, pancreas and kidneys may be noted.

Diagnosis

Confirmation of the diagnosis is by the demonstration of PMV-1 in the tissues (brain, intestine) or faeces, or by demonstrating significant serum antibody levels relative to the vaccination history. Virology and serology may give inconclusive results, and material from several pigeons should ideally be submitted. Histopathology may provide supporting evidence of a viral encephalitis and interstitial nephritis.

Differential Diagnosis

Consideration must be given to the other causes of nervous signs discussed in this chapter, in particular paratyphoid (see Table 29.1), and to the causes of diarrhoea described in Chapter 31.

Treatment

Electrolytes in the drinking water are beneficial, and birds with nervous signs should be placed in small groups and assisted to feed and drink. Several different products containing electrolytes are marketed for use in pigeons, including Bio-Lyt (Versele-Laga) and Electroform (Aviform). Some also contain a probiotic, eg. Entrodex (Vydex) and Vitalyte Plus (Vetrepharm). All these products should be used as directed by the manufacturers. Severely affected birds should be culled if they do not show any signs of improvement within two weeks.

Hygiene and the efficient use of approved disinfectants is essential to limit the spread of PMV-1 and to control secondary parasitic conditions. Monitoring of loft faeces for internal parasites and *S. typhimurium* is advisable, with treatment of any concurrent disease. Additional measures may be required by the DVO.

Epidemiology

Despite the availability of inactivated vaccines against pigeon PMV-1, between 1983 and 1993 at least 100 outbreaks occurred in most years, especially in August to November, most often in young, unvaccinated birds (Pennycott, 1994a). Infection is usually acquired during racing or showing or by direct human or bird contact with infected lofts, including stray racing pigeons (Alexander *et al*, 1986). Feral pigeons can provide a reservoir of infection (Pennycott, 1994b).

Disease commonly first appears in unvaccinated, non-racing young birds in the loft, the virus probably having been introduced to the loft by the vaccinated racing birds acting as mechanical carriers. The incubation period can be at least six weeks. Birds vaccinated while incubating the virus may succumb to disease. If the virus numbers in a loft eventually become high, transitory disease may also be seen in fully vaccinated birds. There are therefore circumstances in which clinical disease may appear in vaccinated birds.

Control

In addition to the other statutory control measures against PMV-1 in pigeons, the vaccination of pigeons taking part in shows or races which take place wholly or partly in Britain is now a legal requirement under The Diseases of Poultry Order 1994. In April 1995 there were three approved vaccines, all inactivated and administered by subcutaneous injection - Colombovac PMV (Solvay Duphar), Harkavac (Harkers) and Nobi-Vac Paramyxo (Vetrepharm). Compulsory vaccination may have been responsible for the drop in reported cases in 1994 to 36 infected lofts.

The directions of the manufacturers should be followed, but in general terms, young birds should be vaccinated from 3-4 weeks of age and adults 4-6 weeks before the onset of breeding. Annual revaccination is required. A very small proportion of birds may develop an adverse reaction to the vaccine - small lumps, large subcutaneous abscesses or rapid death immediately or soon after vaccination (Kaleta *et al*, 1989). These losses will be minimised if the instructions of the vaccine manufacturers are followed.

SALMONELLOSIS (PARATYPHOID)

Infection of pigeons with *Salmonella typhimurium* (usually phage types 2 and 99) is often called paratyphoid infection. It is a requirement of the Zoonoses Order 1989 that all isolations of *Salmonella* spp. from pigeons are reported to the State Veterinary Service.

Clinical Signs

Any combination of the following signs may be seen: loss of balance, inability to hold the head in a natural position, difficulty feeding, lying in lateral recumbency, etc. suggest involvement of the brain or inner ear. Loss of appetite, loss of weight and diarrhoea (see Figure 29.2) is frequently seen. Vomiting is less common. The joints of the legs or wings may be hot, painful and swollen, causing the bird to show lameness or to droop a wing. The first signs are often seen in young squabs, with sudden deaths and stunting of survivors. At the same time there may be a rise in the number of embryos dying during incubation (dead-in-shells) and infertile eggs.

Localised manifestations include sinusitis, panophthalmitis, abscesses on the skin, etc.

Post-Mortem Findings

Carcases may be fevered, with dark muscles and

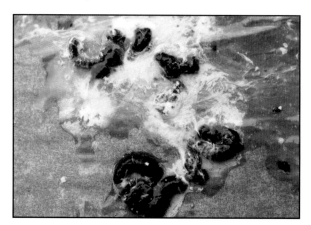

Figure 29.2: Diarrhoea in a pigeon with salmonellosis.

congested blood vessels. There may be splenomegaly and hepatomegaly. Pale granulomata 1-10mm in diameter may be found in the liver, lungs, kidneys and pancreas, and in the wall of the intestine. The mucosa of the intestine may be ulcerated or show focal diphtheritic necrosis. A purulent arthritis affecting one or more joints of the legs or wings is often seen, and in chronic cases there may be substantial periarticular fibrosis. In male birds it is not uncommon to find swelling of one testis, and in adult female birds there may be degeneration of the ovary.

Other lesions include a purulent sinusitis, focal abscesses in the skin and panophthalmitis.

Diagnosis
Confirmation of salmonellosis is usually by isolation of *S. typhimurium* from the tissues or faeces of affected birds, or by culturing the organism from pooled loft faeces. A serum agglutination test can be carried out on blood samples from suspected cases - a positive result indicates exposure to the organism, but not whether the bird is excreting the organism.

Differential Diagnosis (see Table 29.1)
Paratyphoid must be differentiated from the other causes of nervous signs discussed in this chapter, including PMV-1 infection. Other causes of diarrhoea (see Chapter 31), leg/wing problems (see Chapter 27), blindness (see Chapter 25) and neonatal/breeding problems (see Chapter 32) must also be considered.

Treatment
A number of antimicrobials are effective against *S. typhimurium*, usually administered in the drinking water to all the birds in the loft. Preparations include amoxycillin (Vetremox Powder [Vetrepharm] is licensed for use in pigeons) (1g per litre of drinking water for seven days), combined trimethoprim and sulphamethoxazole (20mg trimethoprim/100mg sulphamethoxazole per litre of drinking water for 10 days) and enrofloxacin (200mg per litre of drinking water for 10 days). Furazolidone and furaltadone were also widely used (see later re dangers of overdosing).

Treatment should be combined with disinfection of the loft, feeders and drinkers with an effective but safe disinfectant such as Virkon (Antec), followed by probiotics. Several probiotics are currently marketed for use in pigeons, including Entrodex (Vydex), Proguard (Vetrepharm) and Magic (Stock Nutrition). However, there is considerable debate among the companies as to the merits of the different products, and the range of products on the market is likely to change.

Pooled faeces from the loft should be screened for *S. typhimurium* on a number of occasions following medication to ensure elimination of the organism, with repeat medication if required. Individual birds may receive the antibacterial by crop tube, dropper, tablet or injection if necessary.

Birds with severe involvement of the brain, joints or internal organs should be culled.

Epidemiology
Pigeons can be asymptomatic carriers of *S. typhimurium*, intermittently excreting the organism in the faeces, saliva and crop milk, and in their eggs. Carrier birds are the most likely source of infection, either directly as purchased birds or stray birds, or indirectly by cross contamination during racing, showing or contact with feral pigeons.

Control
General hygiene measures, avoiding overcrowding, the exclusion of stray pigeons, etc. will reduce the dangers of loft contamination. Tudor (1991) suggested that acidification of the loft litter might help to control salmonellosis by preventing the replication of the organism in the environment. These measures should be coupled with routine screening for *S. typhimurium* in faeces from the loft before the onset of breeding.

There is an inactivated vaccine against salmonellosis in pigeons available in some countries. This appears to be beneficial in controlling the reappearance of disease in lofts which have already been infected.

POISONING

The possibility of poisoning should be considered if large numbers of birds simultaneously develop nervous signs, if there is a history of access to potentially poisonous substances (including therapeutics), or if no other explanation can be found for the onset of nervous signs.

Dimetridazole is frequently used to treat trichomoniasis. Incoordination, ataxia, muscle tremors and even death may result from excessive doses (Reece *et al*, 1985). This may also occur if there is increased water consumption, eg. in hot weather or in breeding birds, resulting in an increased intake of dimetridazole. Similar signs may arise following overdosing with furaltadone, or if strong solutions of copper sulphate are used as dips against ectoparasites and fungi.

Pigeons are also at risk from agricultural chemicals because of their diet of cereals, pulses and seeds. Organochlorine pesticides, such as aldrin, dieldrin and DDT, although no longer approved, can result in tremors, muscular spasms and rigidity, convulsions, paralysis and death. Similar signs plus respiratory distress and diarrhoea are seen in poisoning by organophosphorus compounds such as fenitrothion, fonofos and chlorfenvinphos. Metaldehyde poisoning causes nervous signs including ataxia and torticollis.

Racing pigeons may be accidentally exposed to alphachloralose, which is frequently used as a rodenticide and for licensed bird control operations. Hyperaesthesia is followed by incoordination, ataxia and narcosis. Recovery can occur if death from

Table 29.1. A comparison of the clinical signs of PMV-1 and salmonellosis (paratyphoid).

Feature	Comment
Percentage of birds with diarrhoea.	Much higher in PMV-1.
Percentage of birds with nervous signs.	Much higher in PMV-1.
Nature of diarrhoea.	Excess watery urine in PMV-1. Soft, slimy, bulky in paratyphoid.
Nature of nervous signs.	Become more pronounced in PMV-1 when the bird is stressed.
Loss of weight.	More severe in paratyphoid.
Loss of appetite.	More severe in paratyphoid.
Swelling of joints.	A feature of paratyphoid, not of PMV-1.
Mortality in squabs.	Much higher in paratyphoid.

hypothermia is averted. Tudor (1991) commented that numerous pigeon poisoning cases have incriminated herbicides, but that factual evidence is not presented. However, incoordination and death following exposure to monochloroacetate has been reported recently (Anon, 1994).

Pigeons with suspected poisoning should be given warmth, quietness, semi-darkness, a minimum of stimulation and fluids/electrolytes. The crop may be washed out with warm water provided this does not distress the bird, and adsorbents such as activated charcoal and kaolin may be administered by crop tube. Very strong cold tea can be given as a source of tannic acid to help precipitate poisonous metals and alkaloids, preventing their absorption. Diazepam (0.5-1.5mg/kg i/m or p/o) may be given to control convulsions if present. In cases of organophosphorus poisoning, atropine sulphate (0.1mg/kg s/c) should be administered.

HYPOCALCAEMIA SYNDROME

A hypocalcaemia syndrome affecting breeding female pigeons is fairly common; birds develop paresis of the legs and wings. The paresis usually becomes apparent after the first egg has been laid, worsening when the second egg has been laid or is due to be laid. Affected birds cannot fly up to their nestboxes, and they attempt to move by pulling themselves along with their wings (see Figure 29.3).

A large proportion of the breeding birds may be affected, especially if the birds are receiving insufficient calcium or are permanently housed with no access to sunlight or Vitamin D_3.

Treatment is by administration of multivitamins, including Vitamin D_3, via a crop tube or in the drinking water, and ensuring access to calcium in the form of soluble grit or other calcium containing supplements.

There are anecdotal reports of a similar problem affecting both male and female pigeons while feeding their squabs, and in young weaned birds or birds after an exhausting race, in which a good response has been achieved by giving the birds tablets containing 165mg magnesium. However, the accuracy of these reports and of the apparent response to magnesium remains to be confirmed.

Inability to fly and drooping of wings has also been described (De Herdt *et al*, 1994) associated with *Streptococcus bovis* septicaemia, in which treatment with ampicillin (2g/litre of drinking water for seven days) was successful.

VITAMIN B$_1$ (THIAMINE) DEFICIENCY

Thiamine deficiency is sometimes cited in pigeon fancier books as a cause of nervous signs in pigeons, resulting in ataxia, weakness, tremors, opisthotonus and death. In normal circumstances the traditional pigeon diet will contain adequate quantities of thiamine

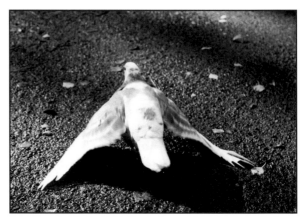

Figure 29.3: Pigeon with hypocalcaemia 'walking' using its wings.

(Tudor, 1991). However, if pigeons become inappetent for other reasons, they may develop a secondary thiamine deficiency. Supportive treatment of pigeons which have a reduced food intake should therefore include multivitamins. (See also Chapter 25.)

REFERENCES

Alexander DJ, Russell PH and Collins MS (1984a) Paramyxovirus type 1 infection of racing pigeons: 1. Characterisation of isolated viruses. *Veterinary Record* **114**, 444.

Alexander DJ, Wilson GWC, Thain JA and Lister SA (1984b) Avian paramyxovirus type 1 infection of racing pigeons: 3. Epizootiological considerations. *Veterinary Record* **115**, 213.

Alexander DJ, Lister SA and Wilson GWC (1986) Avian paramyxovirus type 1 infection of racing pigeons: 5. Continued spread in 1984. *Veterinary Record* **118**, 424.

Anon (1994) Report of the Veterinary Investigation Service. *Veterinary Record* **135**, 422.

DeHerdt P, Ducatelle R, Haesebrouck F, Devriese LA, DeGroote B and Roels S (1994) An unusual outbreak of *Streptococcus bovis* septicaemia in racing pigeons (*Columba livia*). *Veterinary Record* **134**, 42.

Kaleta EF, Alexander DJ and Russell PH (1985) The first isolation of the avian PMV-1 virus responsible for the current panzootic in pigeons. *Avian Pathology* **14**, 553.

Kaleta EF, Bruckner D and Goller H (1989) Acute fatalities following subcutaneous injection of paramyxovirus type 1 vaccines in pigeons. *Avian Pathology* **18**, 203.

Pennycott TW (1994a) Pigeon diseases - results from a Scottish diagnostic laboratory. In: *Proceedings of the Association of Avian Veterinarians Annual Conference 1994*. AAV, Lake Worth.

Pennycott TW (1994b) Avian paramyxovirus type 1 in feral pigeons. *Veterinary Record* **134**, 560.

Reece RL, Barr DA, Forsyth WM and Scott PC (1985) Investigations of toxicity episodes involving chemotherapeutic agents in Victorian poultry and pigeons. *Avian Diseases* **29**, 1239.

Stewart GH (1971) Naturally occuring clinical Newcastle disease in the racing pigeon (*Columba livia*). *Veterinary Record* **89**, 225.

Tudor DH (1991) *Pigeon Health and Disease*. Iowa State University Press, Ames.

CHAPTER THIRTY

Poor Performance and Weight Loss

Frank D W Harper

INTRODUCTION

It is axiomatic that pigeons must be healthy to win races. The veterinary surgeon may be called upon to advise, investigate and resolve problems in flocks with a record of poor performance. Poor results may be caused by subclinical disease, or there may be obvious symptoms of ill health such as weight loss.

PRELIMINARY ASSESSMENT

When birds are presented at the surgery, as much of the background to the problem as is possible should be established by taking a comprehensive history. Where the consultation involves a visit to the loft, much can be learned from direct observation; clinicians who are unfamiliar with racing pigeons may gain considerable insight into the problems encountered by the fancier.

The results and performance of previous years will help to establish the quality of the fancier and the pigeons in question. The problem may be one of unrealistic expectations. In recent years there has been an increasing commercialisation of the sport and many young pigeons of apparently impeccable pedigree are bred or purchased, but subsequent performance falls short of that anticipated.

Most pigeon fanciers are fairly astute and observant. The history is usually reliable, but the practice of 'preventive treatment' with named therapeutics is widely advocated and anecdotal 'cures' (frequently valid) are given currency in the pigeon fancy press. The history should ascertain any current or prior medication used as well as any vaccination programme. The effect of this on clinical interpretation is self-evident, but the degree of response to such treatment can aid the elimination of some differentials. The type of birds involved, particularly the age group, and, in young birds, details of recent imports or purchases can help in the preliminary assessment. History taking has to gather information on factors that cannot be directly observed, such as reduced, selective or increased appetite; polydipsia or other abnormal behaviour; exercise tolerance; numbers lost in training flights or races; stocking rates; and recent changes in loft or management (particularly feeding). Management has many facets and implications: for example, birds allowed full freedom may 'field' and ingest dressed seed. Similarly, access to lichens or roof mosses can cause 'loose droppings' and loss of form.

IDENTIFICATION OF THE PROBLEM

It is likely that the history will indicate the main priorities for investigation, but it must be emphasised that most problems in pigeons are multifactorial and a routine for a comprehensive work up should be developed and adhered to. Wallis (1991) described such a routine (see also Tables 30.1 and 30.2). In addition to an awareness of the probability of a multifactorial aetiology, it is important to remember that a flock is a collection of individuals. A sample needs to be representative. The opportunity may be taken by the owner to present a number of individuals with chronic conditions of no immediate significance to the problem in hand. A representative sample is considered to be 10% of the birds involved, with faeces from 25% of the loft mates. There is, however, a recurrent problem of distinction between affected individual(s) and the flock.

The subtleties of management and racing systems are a specialised interest, but the average practice can render a constructive and rewarding input to the sport in the diagnosis and control of clinical or subclinical disease. Problems most frequently encountered are those involving the respiratory and alimentary systems.

Respiratory System

The respiratory system is considered in detail elsewhere in this manual (see Chapter 28), but a simplistic overview would ascribe the problem to a widespread viral infection (herpesvirus), which persists as a healthy carrier state but with recrudescence under the stress of racing. Primary infection by herpesvirus is mild and self-limiting in most cases, but clinical disease becomes significant when there is association with opportunistic or facultative pathogens, eg. mycoplasmas, bacteria, trichomonads. Other viruses may be involved, as may *Chlamydia psittaci*. Current racing practices make exposure inevitable and subclinical disease is prevalent. This may account for the 'tonic' effect of antibiotics. The concerned clinician should advise against unnecessary and ineffective medication (it is often applied on a single-day basis) where consequent immune suppression could further reduce natural resistance.

Alimentary System

Conditions of the alimentary system, specifically enteritis, are described elsewhere (see Chapter 31). It is probable that similar considerations of stress or immune suppression initiated by viral diseases are important, but most practices would not have the facilities to undertake the necessary investigation. However, the secondary pathogens involved are commonly endoparasites which are readily identified, and response to appropriate treatment can be dramatic.

WEIGHT LOSS ('GOING LIGHT')

Clinical experience does not reflect the popular perception that endoparasitism is synonymous with weight loss or 'going light'. Obvious weight loss is often the result of acute or chronic bacterial infections causing enteritis or granulomatous lesions of the viscera, particularly the liver. Weight loss can be a symptom of other hepatic conditions such as neoplasia or leucosis. Viral hepatitis is a major cause of diarrhoea and weight loss in young birds. In both herpesvirus infection (inclusion body hepatitis) and adenovirus infection, intranuclear inclusions in the hepatocytes can be demonstrated by simple cytology. Differentiation is aided by clinical history; vomiting is a major symptom of adenovirus infection. Candidiasis is common, but is usually a secondary complication.

Endoparasites

Endoparasitism, however, may be more insidious. There may be problems of underperformance and changed faecal aspect (to a green colouration rather that noticeable diarrhoea). Individual birds may handle poorly, losing resilience of the muscle and silkiness of feather. There may be difficulty 'putting weight on' when conditioning for the longer races. Individuals can be acutely ill, show vomiting or weakness and may die, but still hold normal weight. Nevertheless, endoparasites are an important differential. Faecal examination by standard flotation and McMaster technique using saturated salt solution should be routine for enumeration of nematode eggs and coccidial oocysts. Zinc sulphate flotation is not performed as a routine. It usually gives false negatives with cestodes (even in birds known to be infected). These can be identified on direct smears, but the severity of infestation is an important consideration. Direct observation is necessary to identify cestode segments (eggs are rarely seen in the droppings); direct smears can give

an estimation of bacterial and/or yeast levels (see Chapter 6); very fresh samples or cloacal swabs are essential for the detection of fragile protozoans. Some drugs and dosages used for treatment of endoparasites in pigeons are listed in Table 30.3.

Nematodes
Ascaridia spp. and *Capillaria* spp. are the most commonly diagnosed nematodes and an improvement in condition and performance can be expected after treatment of infected birds. In both ascaridiasis and capillariasis, faecal egg counts can be unreliable for diagnosis of infection. In young pigeons or recently infected adults, heavy infections with immature worms may be missed. Furthermore, individuals can be severely infected when the loft average is low. This may indicate different feeding behaviour or, more likely, concurrent disease, eg. hepatitis or salpingitis, in the affected bird.

Ascarids. *Ascaridia columbae* is the main ascarid found in pigeons. The worms (2.5cm long) are easily seen in the faeces, or in the bowel on *post-mortem* examination. There is a direct life cycle. The thick-shelled, ovoid eggs (approximately 90 x 50μm) become infective 16-20 days after they are passed and the prepatent period is 42-45 days. Egg counts of up to 1,000 eggs/g of faeces are assessed as moderate infection, up to 5,000 eggs/g severe infection, and above this very severe (Wallis, 1991). Moderate infection can cause loss of condition and poor performance. In heavy infestation there may be intestinal blockage (vomiting), intestinal perforation (acute illness and early death) or invasion of the bile ducts with liver enlargement (chronic, non-responsive illness).

Capillaria **spp**. Capillariasis is usually due to *Capillaria obsignata*. The life cycle is direct; the ovoid (approximately 50 x 25μm) eggs are thick-shelled with bipolar plugs (see Figure 30.1). The eggs mature in 3-14 days and the prepatent period is 3-4 weeks. More rarely, infection may be due to *C. caudinflata* which has an indirect life cycle with the earthworm as the intermediate host. *Capillaria* spp. may be seen occasionally in faeces samples. The tiny (1cm) hair-like worms are not easily seen on *post-mortem* examination. It is necessary to scrape the bowel and intestinal contents into a fine sieve. The contents should be washed and the residue tipped into water for examination. *Capillaria* spp. are more pathogenic than ascarids. The worms burrow into the bowel wall and produce more dramatic symptoms which may include vomiting. As few as 50 worms can cause the death of an adult pigeon.

Ornithostrongylus quadriradiatus. This parasite is found sometimes and is considered the most pathogenic of the nematodes detected routinely (blood

Table 30.1. Suggested routine for performance screening (or health check).

Examination	Possible observations	Interpretation
Appearance and feathering	Poor quality feather.	Management or nutrition; can be chronic helminthiasis.
	Faecal staining.	Diarrhoea in loft mates.
	Ectoparasites.	Increase in sick birds. Have direct (anaemia in red mites) or indirect effects (disturbed rest).
Body condition	Loss of weight.	Endoparasites, infection, internal granulomata.
	Overweight, fat.	Feeding: subclinical disease reduces exercise and food requirement; weight may increase.
Eyes and nostrils	Stains or exudate.	Respiratory complex.
	Warty lesions.	Pigeon pox.
	Loss of 'chalky' appearance of wattles.	Endoparasites. May be when feeding young or on medicated water.
Oropharynx	Lesions, discolouration, mucopurulent or dried exudate.	Respiratory complex, trichomoniasis, candidiasis, pox.
Respiration	Dyspnoea.	Abdominal conditions, trauma, tracheal fistula, *Syngamus trachea* (gapeworm), aspergillosis.
	Audible rales (need to establish source). A vibratory sound may indicate tracheal trauma; a deep rattle, syringeal oedema. In cases of syringeal aspergilloma the sound is intermediate.	Respiratory disease, trauma. If oedema of syrinx, suspect chlamydiosis.
Abnormal behaviour	Vomiting.	Adenovirus, nematodes, foreign body, moss picking.
	Uvulation/panting.	Overweight, unfit, climatic.
	Sneezing, scratching, yawning.	*Mycoplasma* spp., trichomoniasis.
	Nervous signs.	Paramyxovirus, *Salmonella* spp., toxins and others.
Faecal aspect	Changed (colour and/or consistency).	Endoparasites or feeding.
	True diarrhoea.	Protozoal, viral or bacterial infection.
	Polyuria.	Paramyxovirus, acute salmonellosis, plant toxins, hormonal or metabolic in 'wet feeders', diabetes, nephritis.

Table 30.2. Further investigation for performance screening.

Sample (or consider sampling)	Investigation
Feathers and skin	Microscopic examination of fresh or cleared samples.
Eye and conjunctiva	Impression smears: stain with modified Ziehl-Neelsen (for *C. psittaci*).
Oropharynx	Mucus samples by loop or swab; examine fresh or stained material for *Trichomonas* spp., *Candida* spp., reactive cells and 'normal' bacterial picture. Blood agar culture and sensitivity testing useful, but not all pathogens grow.
Faecal examination	McMaster enumeration is routine for coccidial oocysts and nematode eggs; direct examination of fresh faeces for cestode segments. Very fresh faeces for intestinal *Trichomonas* spp., *Hexamita* spp. and bacterial and fungal overgrowth.
Haematology/serology	Heterophilia, leucopaenia and erythrocyte status can be rapidly assessed, as can PCV and slide agglutination for *Salmonella* spp.
Post-mortem examination (culls or sacrificed birds may not be typical)	Gross pathology and material for further investigation. Impression smears of viscera or air sacs, and cytology, especially of liver, useful.
Specialist laboratory services	As necessary.
Radiography, laparotomy and laparoscopy	More applicable to the individual bird.

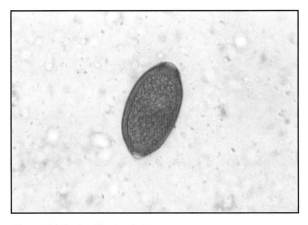

Figure 30.1: *Capillaria obsignata egg.*

sucking, can cause diarrhoea and emaciation). The eggs are thin-shelled (do not confuse with mite eggs) and are embryonated in all but the freshest samples; hatched larvae may sometimes be observed in the sample.

Syngamus trachea **(gapeworm)**. Pigeons may occasionally be infected with gapeworm.

Cestodes
Cestodes are less commonly diagnosed and are not often a flock problem. The life cycle is indirect via molluscs or other intermediaries and usually individu-

als are affected. Affected birds are likely to be returnees after a period spent living wild. When cestodes are a loft problem, it is generally in a moorland locality and in birds allowed to 'field'. Large (*Hymenolepsis*) and microscopic (*Raillietina*) species occur. There may be some lowered exercise tolerance and faecal change (to a pulpy grey/green dropping).

Trematodes
Echinostoma revolutum infection has been reported (Foster, 1991). The parasites cause a rapidly fatal haemorrhagic enteritis of the lower bowel. Diagnosis is on *post-mortem* examination. Foster (1991) suggested that snails might be the intermediate host.

Coccidiosis
Coccidiosis is widely held to be an important cause of enteritis and weight loss in young pigeons: an alternative opinion is that such symptoms are more attributable to other causes. Undoubtedly, a high oocyst count is a common finding in flocks showing poor condition and performance. Wallis (1991) assessed 3,000-20,000 oocysts/g of faeces as moderate, 20,000-50,000 oocysts/g as severe. However, there is little correlation between oocyst count and clinical symptoms. *Eimeria labbeana* and *E. columbarum* are the species commonly encountered and there may be some variation in pathogenicity.

Hexamitiasis

Hexamitiasis is widespread in the UK (Harper, 1991). *Hexamita* spp. may be the cause of enteritis and loss of weight in young birds and may be erroneously diagnosed as coccidiosis. Incidence is highest in midsummer in birds aged 5-9 weeks, usually in second or third round youngsters, ie. birds hatched from later clutches, when mixed with those hatched earlier. The major differential is the adenovirus/*E. coli* complex, where there is no such age relationship.

Diagnosis is dependent upon direct examination (x400 magnification) of very fresh, body warm faeces, cloacal swabs or intestinal scrapings. The rapidly directional protozoan parasites can be recognised in large numbers in affected birds. The parasite is bilaterally symmetrical and lanceolate in shape, measuring about 9 x 3µm - for comparison, approximately the size of an erythrocyte nucleus; erythrocytes are likely to appear in the same field in a sample from an affected bird. There are eight flagella, six anterior and indistinct, two trailing and obvious. No encysted stage has been reported in pigeons nor is there any effective transport medium. Smears can be fixed and stained with acetone/Giemsa but identification from fixed material is not reliable.

Trichomoniasis

The typical lesions of trichomoniasis are caseous masses in the oropharynx (see Figure 30.2); birds may have difficulty swallowing and there can be rapid weight loss. Trichomonads can occur in the bowel in the absence of upper alimentary tract infection, and it is likely that different strains or species are involved. Intestinal trichomonads can produce symptoms similar to, but less severe than, those of hexamitiasis. The slower, larger and less directional *Trichomonas* spp. can be distinguished from *Hexamita* spp., but mixed infection is frequently encountered. The characteristic caseous lesions of the oropharynx seldom occur in the bowel, but they may be found in the liver and, in nestlings or recently fledged birds, in the navel or cloaca (vent canker).

Diagnosis of trichomoniasis may be suggested by the owner where typical caseous lesions have been noticed. Subclinical infection can be of significance in performance screening. Microscopic examination of pharyngeal mucus (swab or loop) or crop smears should be performed. *T. gallinae* is larger (18 x 8µm, but variable) than *Hexamita* spp. and the shape is asymmetric and irregularly ovoid or triangular. There are four free anterior flagella and a single enclosed flagellum at the posterior pole. The beat of the flagella produces a slow, erratic circular motion. Where there is heavy infestation, the mass of parasites can overlap in a mosaic pattern and the flagellar beat and motion is no longer apparent. Trichomonads identified in bowel samples are usually smaller and exhibit a more directional movement.

Trichomonads can be fixed and stained (Romonawski) but the loss of the characteristic flagellar motion makes identification more difficult. Transport/culture medium can be prepared but is not available commercially. Interpretation of the findings is subjective and is based on the number of organisms present and the clinical history. Regular treatment, both curative and preventive, is widely advocated within the fancy and by many practitioners. However, there is evidence that there is variation in virulence and that benign strains can give some protection from the more virulent strains.

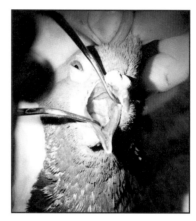

Figure 30.2: *Trichomoniasis lesions in the oropharynx of a pigeon. (Photo courtesy N A Forbes)*

Toxoplasmosis

Toxoplasma spp. and other protozoa are probably more widespread than is realised and may account for the efficiency of sulphonamides in some cases of 'coccidiosis'. Blood parasites seem of little significance in pigeons in the UK.

Traumatic Ventriculitis

Traumatic ventriculitis is common in the early breeding season when nails and wires (from loft alterations) are collected as nesting material and inadvertently swallowed. In a stock loft of captive birds, several birds may be involved and a contagious 'going light' condition suspected. Hens are more commonly affected. Diagnosis is by elimination of other causes and radiography. Retrieval by gluviotomy is seldom possible; the object is usually impacted and penetrating the powerful muscles of the ventriculus. Abdominal surgery (left flank approach) allows direct access to the site. The incision should be into the proventriculus, since reliable closure of the muscular gizzard wall is difficult. However, in many cases there is an established defect or fistula in the gizzard which may be utilised, but must be repaired. Prognosis is reasonable in early cases and where there has been no great damage to other viscera.

Table 30.3. Drugs for treating endoparasites in pigeons.

Drug	Dosage
Anthelmintics	
Cambendazole (Ascapilla*, Chevita)	30mg capsule (75mg/kg) on two consecutive days.
Febantel (Avicas*, Orthopharma)	15mg tablet (37.5mg/kg).
Fenbendazole (Panacur* Hoechst)	8mg capsule (20mg/kg).
Tetramisole (Spartakon*, Harkers)	20mg tablet (50mg/kg).
Piperazine	1g per litre drinking water (ascarids only) (12.5mg/kg).
Ivermectin	200-400mcg orally (variable efficacy).
Praziquantel	50mg tablet (20mg/kg) for cestodes.
Antitrichomonals	
Dimetronidazole (Harkanka*, Harkers)	500mg per litre drinking water of 40% powder for seven days (25mg/kg/day).
Carnidazole (Spartrix*, Harkers)	10mg tablet (25mg/kg) once.
Metronidazole	10g per litre drinking water of 25% powder for five days; 200mg tablets - 100-150mg in total divided over five days** (60mg/kg/day).
Ronidazole 10% Powder	1g per litre drinking water for six days** (12.5mg/kg/day).
Anticoccidials	
Clazuril (Appertex*, Harkers)	2.5mg tablet (6.25mg/kg) once.
Tolzaturil	3ml per litre drinking water of a 2.5% solution for five days (10mg/kg/day).
Furaltadone 20% Powder	2g per litre drinking water for five days (also hexamitiasis) (50mg/kg/day).
Amprol (Coccoid*, Harkers)	28ml of 3.4% solution per 4.5 litres drinking water for seven days (25mg/kg/day) - half strength for extended regime.
Sulphadimidine sodium 33%	10-20ml per 4.5 litres drinking water for five days (also effective for toxoplasmosis).

* Licensed for pigeons.
** Moderate control of hexamitiasis.

REFERENCES

Foster PD (1991) Echinostomatid flukes in pigeons. *Veterinary Record* **129**, 455.
Harper FDW (1991) *Hexamita* species present in some avian species in South Wales. *Veterinary Record* **128**, 130.
Wallis AS (1991) Common conditions of domestic pigeons. *In Practice* **13**, 95. 7

CHAPTER THIRTY ONE

Diarrhoea

Tom W Pennycott

INTRODUCTION

The presence of abnormally soft or fluid faeces in the pigeon loft is one of the commonest problems encountered by pigeon fanciers and their veterinary advisers. This is not surprising, because the appearance of the faeces is readily apparent and is carefully monitored as an indication of the general health of the pigeons.

Normal faeces are often described as green/brown 'marbles' (of intestinal origin) with a 'cap' of white urates from the kidneys. In pigeons in a loft, small downy feathers are often found sticking to the faeces. This is regarded as a sign of good health.

Abnormal faeces can arise if there are problems of the intestinal tract or urinary system, polydipsia or combinations of these factors. Excessively soft or fluid faeces, regardless of the cause, will be considered as 'diarrhoea' in this chapter. Diarrhoea (described by fanciers as wet droppings, watery droppings, the squirts) has become very common in recent years, and some fanciers believe that 'wet/watery droppings' is a single disease rather than a sign of disease.

Clearly there are many potential causes of outbreaks of diarrhoea in racing pigeons. In addition, individual pigeons may have loose faeces for a variety of reasons such as nervousness, neoplasia, foreign bodies in the alimentary tract, diabetes mellitus, etc.

In this chapter, emphasis will be placed on outbreaks of diarrhoea affecting several pigeons in the loft. The commonest causes and combinations will be discussed and, where appropriate, specific treatments will be described.

The overall approach to the management and investigation of an outbreak of diarrhoea in pigeons will be summarised.

PARAMYXOVIRUS I (PMV-1)

One of the commonest causes of diarrhoea in pigeons in recent years is PMV-1 infection. In typical outbreaks there is sudden onset of thirst and profuse diarrhoea. A variety of nervous signs may be present in a proportion of the birds, including tremors, torticollis, drooping of a wing or leg weakness, inability to feed properly, loss of balance, circling and lateral recumbency. All ages of birds may be affected, depending on their immune status.

PMV-1 is discussed fully in Chapters 28 and 29. It is a notifiable disease, and the local Divisional Veterinary Officer of the State Veterinary Service must be informed if the presence of the disease is suspected.

There is no specific treatment for PMV-1. Control is by vaccination.

ADENOVIRUS INCLUSION BODY HEPATITIS

Occasional cases of adenovirus infection have been described in pigeons since 1976, but from the mid-1980s adenovirus as a significant cause of diarrhoea has been reported from continental Europe and from the UK. Uyttebroek and Ducatelle (1991) described the situation in Belgium in 1989 and 1990. A similar picture has been seen in the UK more recently.

There is sudden onset of watery diarrhoea, loss of weight, sometimes failure of the crop to empty, and/or vomiting. Death within 24 hours can occur in severely affected birds. The disease characteristically affects young birds under one year old, and is most common in the months May to August.

Post-mortem examination is often unspectacular, but there may be moderate to marked hepatomegaly (see Figure 31.1) with haemorrhages and pinpoint liver necrosis, and roughened areas on the mucosa of the oesophagus, crop and proventriculus.

There are frequently concurrent infections such as crop candidiasis, chlamydiosis, pigeon pox, hexamitiasis, trichomoniasis, coccidiosis, colisepticaemia, etc.

Diagnosis is based on the histopathological appearance of the liver, in which there is widespread degeneration of hepatocytes and significant numbers of intranuclear inclusions in the hepatocytes. The majority of the inclusions are basophilic, filling most of the nucleus. Eosinophilic inclusions are also seen, surrounded by a halo and marginated nuclear chromatin.

If necessary, virus isolation can be attempted from liver, intestinal contents or faeces.

There is no specific treatment for an adenovirus

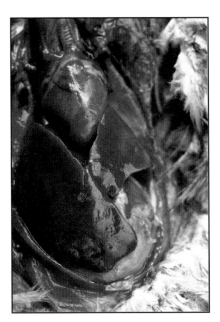

Figure 31.1: *Hepatomegaly in a pigeon with inclusion body hepatitis.*

infection, but concurrent bacterial, chlamydial or parasitic diseases should be identified and treated.

VOMITING SYNDROME 1993

'A new viral infection of quite mammoth proportions affecting mainly young birds all over the country' was reported in *Pigeon Sport* of August 19th, 1993. The condition was characterised by failure of the birds' crops to empty properly, vomiting, excessive drinking and the production of green diarrhoea (Harper and Wallis, 1993). Affected birds were usually under 12 months of age and had often been racing recently. Most birds recovered within 4-6 days. Withholding of food for 24-36 hours, followed by a light diet of a grain such as barley for 2-4 days, was reported to be beneficial. The addition of electrolytes in the drinking water was also helpful.

It seems likely that this 'vomiting syndrome' was the result of an uncomplicated adenovirus infection precipitated by the stress of racing.

HERPESVIRUS INCLUSION BODY HEPATITIS

Pigeon herpesvirus infection can damage the upper respiratory tract, upper digestive tract and the liver. There may be discharges from the eyes and nostrils, and the mouth, pharynx, oesophagus and crop can become coated with yellow, cheesy material. As a result, affected birds have difficulty breathing and may vomit. In addition, affected birds stop eating or eat only small seeds or grains, lose weight, and their droppings become green and fluid (Callinan *et al*, 1979). Death may follow within 48 hours.

Eosinophilic and basophilic intranuclear inclusions are found on histopathological examination of the liver.

This disease is discussed in full in Chapter 28, but should be considered as a possible cause of diarrhoea if mouth lesions are also present in affected birds.

ROTAVIRUS

Rotavirus infections are almost certainly an under-diagnosed cause of diarrhoea in young pigeons. Gough *et al* (1992) demonstrated rotavirus in young pigeons with diarrhoea from three lofts. Other signs included lethargy and loss of appetite, although the birds eventually made a full recovery. The same authors found that 68% of the pigeon sera they tested gave a positive reaction to a microneutralisation test for antibodies to rotavirus.

The virus is characteristic of a Group A avian rotavirus and can be detected by polyacrylamide gel electrophoresis (PAGE), electron microscopy or by latex agglutination tests using commercial kits.

Clearly, rotavirus is widespread in pigeon lofts and must be considered when investigating diarrhoea in pigeons. There is no specific treatment.

CIRCOVIRUS

Recently, a circovirus infection has been described in pigeons between two and three months of age, associated with diarrhoea and poor thrift (Smyth and Carroll, 1995). Histological changes included lymphoid depletion and histiocytosis, and the presence of basophilic intranuclear and intracytoplasmic inclusion bodies in the spleen and the bursa of Fabricius. Macroscopic abnormalities, however, were restricted to the presence of green coloured contents in the digestive tract. The prevalence of circovirus infection remains unclear at the present.

SALMONELLA TYPHIMURIUM (PARATYPHOID)

Infection with *S. typhimurium* (usually phage type 2 or 99) is often called paratyphoid. It is one of the diseases most feared by pigeon fanciers, because many birds may die or need to be culled, because the disease can suddenly flare up again and because the disease can affect the next generation of birds.

Salmonellosis is described fully in Chapter 29. A typically affected loft may have a history of diarrhoea in birds of all ages, with the highest mortality in young birds before weaning. Some birds may show nervous signs, such as torticollis and loss of balance, and there may be swollen joints in the legs and wings. Loss of weight can be rapid. Vomiting may be noted. Poor hatchability with dead-in-shells may be a feature.

Specific treatment is with antibacterial agents - see Chapter 29.

MISCELLANEOUS BACTERIA AND YEASTS

Candida albicans may result in vomiting with or without diarrhoea. A brief description is given in Chapter 25 (see Table 25.3).

The bacteria *Yersinia pseudotuberculosis*, *Streptococcus faecalis*, *Pseudomonas* spp. and *Escherichia coli* may be involved in some outbreaks of diarrhoea, but usually in a secondary role. *Mycobacterium avium* and *Streptococcus bovis* are unusual causes of diarrhoea in pigeons.

HEXAMITA COLUMBAE

Diarrhoea caused by *H. columbae* has become increasingly common in recent years. This flagellated protozoan parasite lives in the duodenum and small intestine of pigeons and is passed in the faeces. Infection is acquired by accidental contamination of food or water with the organisms. Numbers increase in the birds by binary fission.

Hexamitiasis is usually a problem of pigeons in their first year of life, although adult birds may be asymptomatic carriers. Affected birds have loose green faeces (not as watery as PMV-1), are dull and reluctant to exercise, and lose weight. Vomiting or delayed emptying of the crop is seen in some birds. Severely affected birds may die or need to be culled.

Post-mortem examination reveals a dehydrated carcase. The wall of the duodenum and small intestine is thickened and may evert when cut. In many cases a characteristic finding in the intestine is a layer of clear watery mucus surrounding a core of bile-stained semisolid material.

H. columbae can be demonstrated in wet preparations made from very fresh faeces or in wet preparations made from the intestine at *post-mortem* examination. When the wet preparations are examined microscopically (x10 and x25 objectives) the organisms appear as lemon-shaped protozoa rapidly moving in all directions. By contrast, *Trichomonas gallinae* (see later) appear larger and more circular, and move in a more leisurely spiral fashion. The detection of both *H. columbae* and *T. gallinae* becomes very difficult if there is a long time delay between the bird dying or the faecal sample being collected and the examination of the wet preparations microscopically, because the protozoa stop moving and die as their environment cools.

Treatment with metronidazole (single dose of 50mg) followed by 20% furaltadone (8g/4.5 litres drinking water for seven days) has proved successful (Harper, 1991).

TRICHOMONAS GALLINAE

Trichomoniasis, or canker, most commonly affects the mouth, pharynx, oesophagus and crop. The condition is described more fully in Chapter 25.

Depending on the severity of the infection, affected birds may be depressed, have ruffled feathers and may have yellow caseous material on the mucosa of the mouth, pharynx, oesophagus and crop. Similar lesions may be found in the umbilicus and liver of young birds. In addition, affected birds sometimes have diarrhoea, and intestinal wet preparations may reveal motile trichomonads. These must be differentiated from *H. columbae* (see earlier).

Treatment and control measures are described in Chapter 25.

COCCIDIA (see also Chapter 30)

Most pigeons carry small numbers of coccidia (*Eimeria labbeana* and *E. columbarum*) without any ill effects being seen. Moderate to high burdens of coccidia can adversely affect racing performance. Very high numbers in adults may result in some softening of the faeces in addition to unthriftiness and, if young pigeons under five months of age are exposed to large numbers of coccidia, severe diarrhoea may occur, sometimes leading to dehydration and death.

NEMATODES AND CESTODES

Nematodes of the genera *Capillaria* (hairworms) and *Ascaridia* (roundworms) are common in pigeons, especially the former. Moderate burdens result in poor performance, loss of weight and general unthriftiness, and they are discussed in full in Chapter 30. Heavy burdens can cause a mucoid diarrhoea, sometimes with vomiting. The diarrhoea may be blood stained if high numbers of *Capillaria* spp. are involved. If large numbers of second stage *Ascaridia* spp. larvae migrate through the liver simultaneously, the bird may die suddenly and an enlarged, friable, haemorrhagic liver may be found at *post-mortem* examination.

Much less common is the trichostrongyle nematode *Ornithostrongylus quadriradiatus*. A good description of this nematode and the damage it causes can be found in Rose and Keymer (1958). The worms are present in the duodenum and intestine, and are red due to the presence of ingested blood. The worms found by Rose and Keymer measured 5-15mm. Heavy burdens result in a haemorrhagic enteritis.

Many different cestodes (tapeworms) have been recovered from pigeons, the infection being acquired by eating intermediate hosts such as insects and snails. Moderate burdens result in unthriftiness and heavy burdens can cause a mucoid diarrhoea. Tapeworms are seen in racing pigeons less commonly than hairworms or roundworms, but are more common in feral pigeons (Pennycott, 1994)

The treatment and control of nematodes and cestodes is discussed in Chapter 30.

TREMATODES

Occasionally, significant burdens of intestinal flukes of the genera *Echinostoma* and *Echinoparyphium* are found in pigeons, causing a severe, sometimes haemorrhagic, enteritis (Foster, 1991). There is reduced appetite, rapid loss of weight and frequently mortality.

The flukes are 3-22mm long and are easily seen when wet preparations from the intestinal contents are examined microscopically (see Figure 31.2). The intermediate hosts of flukes are snails, tadpoles and small fish. Pigeons acquire the parasites by eating snails, possibly to obtain calcium from the snail shells. The large, thin-walled, ellipsoid fluke eggs are passed in the faeces, but may not be detected using standard saturated salt flotation techniques. Flotation with saturated zinc sulphate improves the recovery rate of fluke eggs.

The possibility of fluke (or tapeworm) burdens should therefore be considered if large numbers of snail shells are found in the crop.

Treatment with praziquantel (12.5mg per pigeon p/o) is usually effective.

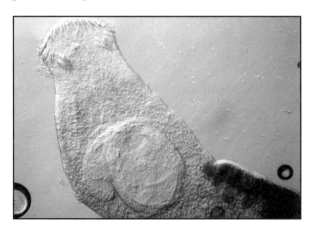

Figure 31.2: Intestinal fluke from the intestinal contents of a pigeon (wet preparation x400)

CHLAMYDIA PSITTACI

Chlamydial infection is widespread in pigeons throughout the world, including the UK (Alexander *et al*, 1989). Commonly known as ornithosis or the ornithosis complex, chlamydiosis is usually associated with respiratory disease or conjunctivitis, often in conjunction with other microorganisms.

However, chlamydiosis can also cause green diarrhoea in pigeons, especially birds under five months of age. Affected birds are depressed and sit hunched up, are anorexic and lose weight. Mortality can be high in young birds. There may be a concurrent ocular or nasal discharge.

At *post-mortem* examination the liver is often swollen, sometimes with necrotic foci and a perihepatitis. Splenomegaly, pericarditis and air sacculitis may be present. In some birds, pallor of the kidney has been

noted, sometimes with urolithiasis or visceral gout.

The presence of chlamydial antigen is best demonstrated using a polymerase chain reaction (PCR) test. Alternatively, an ELISA can be used to detect antigen in liver, spleen or faeces, but false positives may occur, particularly if faeces are tested. Impression smears of liver and spleen stained with modified Ziehl-Neelsen stain can give false negative results and examination of stained faeces is seldom worthwhile.

Chlamydiosis, including treatment and control, is discussed more fully in Chapter 28.

TEN-DAY DIARRHOEA

A diarrhoeic syndrome affecting pigeon squabs around ten days of age has become increasingly common in the UK and continental Europe, and is thought to be nutritional/hormonal in origin.

Under the influence of the hormone prolactin, both parent pigeons become broody and take turns to incubate their eggs. The same hormone causes the epithelium of the parent birds' crops to thicken, and holocrine crop glands begin to produce what is termed crop milk (see Figure 31.3). When hatching occurs, epithelial cells full of lipids are desquamated into the crop, appearing like fatty white/yellow grains of rice. This constitutes the crop milk, and is fed by both parents to the pigeon squabs.

Initially, the crop milk consists of approximately 75% water and high levels of protein and fat. Around ten days after the squabs hatch, the production of crop milk is rapidly reduced and the parents start to feed the young birds an increasing proportion of solid food and water.

On some occasions the parent birds start to drink excessive quantities of water and pump this water into the young birds, causing a diarrhoeic syndrome at around ten days of age. The adult birds themselves often have watery faeces due to the increased water consumption.

Because the young birds are receiving the wrong balance of food and water, and because they are losing electrolytes in the diarrhoea, the young birds stop

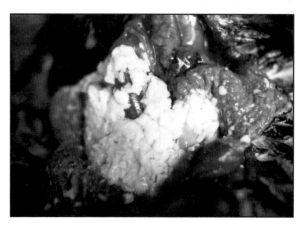

Figure 31.3: Normal crop milk.

growing and are often culled. If adults and young birds are separated at this stage, the water consumption of the adults returns to normal and the diarrhoea in the squabs stops. The underlying reason for the increased water consumption by the adults is unknown, but it may be linked with prolactin levels. If this situation arises, electrolytes (see Chapter 29) should be added to the drinking water of the adult birds. Supplementary feeding of the young birds, for example with Complan, may also be beneficial.

The crop of adult birds producing crop milk is thickened and hyperaemic, and the mucosa is covered by white/yellow material resembling grains of rice. This must not be confused with pathological conditions such as candidiasis, herpesvirus infection, etc.

MANAGEMENT OF AN OUTBREAK OF DIARRHOEA

If there is an outbreak of diarrhoea in the loft, the pigeon fancier and the veterinary adviser must take steps to:
● Prevent the disease spreading to other sections of the loft and to other lofts.
● Provide specific treatment.
● Provide supportive treatment.
● Confirm or refute the possibility that the cause of diarrhoea is the notifiable disease PMV-1. If the presence of PMV-1 is suspected, the DVO of the local Animal Health Office must be informed.
● Reduce the risks of a similar outbreak in future years.

To achieve these objectives it is essential that a diagnosis is made, which invariably requires some laboratory investigation, in addition to clinical examination and history taking (see Chapter 2).
● One or more typically affected birds should be examined, looking for additional signs such as ocular/nasal/oral discharges and lesions inside the mouth.
● Crop swabs should be examined microscopically for *T. gallinae*, and wet preparations from **freshly** voided faeces examined microscopically for *H. columbae*, *T. gallinae*, the eggs of nematodes and trematodes, coccidial oocysts, and tapeworm eggs and segments.
● If no *post-mortem* material is available, a blood sample should be collected from one or more affected birds, primarily for serology for PMV-1 if suspected. Serum can be stored in the deep freeze for additional serology, eg. for salmonellosis and/or chlamydiosis, if required later.
● Affected birds should be placed in isolation and a sample of their faeces collected over a 24 hour period, eg. on greaseproof paper, and a worm egg count, coccidial oocyst count and *S. typhimurium* culture performed. The 24 hour faecal sample can also be tested for PMV-1 if suspected, and retained for additional tests such as *C. psittaci* and rotavirus detection if required later.
● The crop swab tested for *T. gallinae* can be cultured for *Candida albicans*, or impression smears stained with Diff Quik.
● A full *post-mortem* examination of a typically affected bird increases the likelihood of a rapid

Table 31.1. Diarrhoea/vomiting in pigeons - some additional diagnostic pointers.

Feature	Most likely causes
Vomiting in some birds.	Adenovirus inclusion body hepatitis; vomiting syndrome; *H. columbae*; *C. albicans*; *S. typhimurium*; nematodes; poisoning.
Ocular/nasal/oral discharge.	Herpesvirus inclusion body hepatitis; *C. psittaci*; *C. albicans*; *T. gallinae*.
Nervous signs in some birds.	*S. typhimurium*; PMV-1; poisoning.
Mixed ages affected by diarrhoea.	PMV-1 (depending on immune status); *S. typhimurium*; flukes; nematodes and cestodes; herpesvirus; *T. gallinae*; poisoning; ten-day diarrhoea; *C. albicans*.
Predominantly young birds affected by diarrhoea.	*C. psittaci*; *H. columbae*; adenovirus inclusion body hepatitis; vomiting syndrome; rotavirus; coccidia.
Very watery faeces (excess urine).	PMV-1; *C. psittaci*; adenovirus inclusion body hepatitis; herpesvirus inclusion body hepatitis; vomiting syndrome; ten-day diarrhoea.
Blood in faeces.	Flukes; *Capillaria* spp.; *Ornithostrongylus* spp.
Enlarged liver at *post-mortem* examination.	*C. psittaci*; adenovirus inclusion body hepatitis; herpesvirus inclusion body hepatitis; *Ascaridia* spp.; *S. typhimurium*; *T. gallinae*.

diagnosis. Preferably, this should be done on a culled or recently dead bird. Wet preparations from crop, duodenum, mid-intestine and terminal intestine should routinely be examined for *T. gallinae*, *H. columbae*, nematodes, cestodes and trematodes, and viscera cultured for significant bacteria and yeasts including *S. typhimurium*, *C. albicans*, *Y. pseudotuberculosis* and *E. coli*.

Isolation of PMV-1 should be attempted on brain and intestine if this disease is suspected, or else material retained. Intestine, liver and spleen may be tested or retained if chlamydiosis is suspected, and intestinal contents retained for additional virology, eg. for rotavirus, if all other tests are negative.

Liver should be placed in formal saline and histopathology carried out for inclusion body hepatitis. Fixed brain, intestine and kidney may also be valuable if initial investigations into the cause of the diarrhoea are negative or inconclusive.

● Pooled faeces from the loft should be tested for worm eggs, coccidial oocysts and *S. typhimurium*. Surplus faeces could be stored for future investigation for viruses and *C. psittaci*.

In view of the wide range of tests which may be required, and especially if PMV-1 may be involved, consideration should be given to submitting the carcase or live bird to a laboratory of the MAFF Veterinary Investigation Service (England and Wales) or to a laboratory of the Scottish Agriculture College, Veterinary Services (Scotland).

Specific treatment (as outlined for each disease) and future control measures will depend on the diagnosis reached. While these investigations are in progress, supportive measures should be taken. These are discussed in detail in Chapter 24. The provision of a solution of electrolytes is very useful. There are several proprietary electrolytes marketed for pigeons, but in an emergency the human preparation Dioralyte (Rorer Pharmaceuticals Ltd) (1 sachet per 200ml of drinking water) can be given. Multivitamins (especially B vitamins) are helpful and, during the period of convalescence, a course of probiotics will promote the return of the normal gut flora.

While the investigations continue, and possibly after, the birds must not be sent to any shows or races, or undertake training tosses, until they no longer pose a threat to other lofts. Flying around the loft should be discouraged if there are other lofts nearby. Good hygiene and the effective use of disinfectants will help reduce the spread of diarrhoea to other sections of the loft and reduce the likelihood of secondary infections. Identification of the cause of the diarrhoea will also allow the pigeon fancier/veterinary surgeon to devise control measures for the future.

REFERENCES

Alexander DJ, Bevan BJ, Lister SA and Bracewell CD (1989) Chlamydial infection in racing pigeons in Great Britain. A retrospective serological survey. *Veterinary Record* **125**, 239.

Callinan RB, Kefford B, Borland R and Garrett R (1979) An outbreak of disease in pigeons associated with a herpesvirus. *Australian Veterinary Journal* **55**, 339.

Foster PD (1991) Echinostomatid flukes in pigeons. *Veterinary Record* **129**, 455.

Gough RE, Cox WJ and Devoy J (1992) Isolation and identification of rotavirus from racing pigeons. *Veterinary Record* **130**, 273.

Harper FDW (1991) *Hexamita* species present in some avian species in South Wales. *Veterinary Record* **128**, 130.

Harper FDW and Wallis AS (1993) Crop stasis and regurgitation in racing pigeons. *Veterinary Record* **133**, 196.

Pennycott TW (1994) Avian paramyxovirus type 1 in feral pigeons. *Veterinary Record* **134**, 560.

Rose JH and Keymer IF (1958) An outbreak of ornithostrongylosis in domestic pigeons. *Veterinary Record* **70**, 932.

Smyth JA and Carroll BP (1995) Circovirus infection in European racing pigeons. *Veterinary Record* **136**, 173.

Uyttebroek E and Ducatelle R (1991) Epidemiology of adenovirus infection in pigeons. In: *Proceedings of the Association of Avian Veterinarians European Conference, Vienna, 1991*. AAV, Lake Worth.

CHAPTER THIRTY TWO

Breeding Problems and Neonate Diseases

David G Parsons

INTRODUCTION

Problems associated with breeding of pigeons and neonate diseases may not be considered by the fancier to be regular or significant occurrences, but they do occur. It may well be that problems related to breeding increase as the value of the stock birds increases.

NORMAL BREEDING

To understand some of the potential problems, it is important to know the normal breeding cycle. Pigeons lay clutches of two white eggs. Breeding would occur all year round if the environmental conditions were suitable. The fact that the majority do not is a direct result of interference by the fancier separating the sexes. However, so called 'late breds' are a common feature of the sport. These are the young from pairs of birds that have either flown particularly well during the season or are from particularly valuable stock birds. They will generally have been bred to sell.

The breeding season begins with the pairing of the hen and cock birds. This can occur any time after the moult has been completed, ie. December. The timing of pairing will depend on the requirements of the fancier and his method of racing, ie. natural system or the widowhood system (see Chapter 24). The new year's ring numbers are available from January 1st. Only young birds bred that year can be entered for young bird races. Consequently, if the aim is to have the best developed and trained birds for the young bird races (July to September), the closer they are hatched to January 1st the better. This would be the case if adults are flown on the widowhood system (old bird races are from mid-April to the end of July). Pairing would be later (March onwards) if the birds are flown on the natural system.

One section of the loft will contain the nestboxes. The number will depend on the size of the section. Each nestbox will contain a nest bowl, pots for feed and water, and moveable partitions that allow the birds to be confined. The cocks will be introduced and allowed to pick their own nestbox. The fancier will have decided on the pairings and the hen will then be introduced to the cock bird.

The first egg will be laid in the evening about 10 days later. The second egg is laid about one and a half days later in the early afternoon. Incubation commences when the second egg has been laid. Both the cock and the hen take it in turns to incubate the eggs. Candling the egg will reveal infertile eggs. After five days of incubation the blood vessels of the chorioallantoic membrane can be seen. By 10 days the egg will have become opaque as the embryo has grown. At this time the only feature discernible will be the air cell. The first egg will hatch after 18 days and the second egg up to a day later. It may take 15-20 hours for the squab to hatch from the first moment that it is seen to have pipped the eggshell.

The squab is fed predominately on crop milk by the cock and the hen bird for the first seven days of its life. This milk is produced by the cells lining the crop. The changes to the crop begin at about the sixth day of incubation. The crop reaches its greatest thickness by the fifteenth day of incubation, continuing until the squab is seven days of age (resting crop weighs 1.7g; an actively secreting crop weighs 15g). The crop milk consists of 8.6% fat, 12.4% protein, 1.4% minerals and 77.6% water. There is no carbohydrate in crop milk. When the squabs are about four days of age the crop milk will begin to contain some partially digested feed. From about seven days of age the squab will be fed predominately on regurgitated feed.

The squab weighs about 14g on hatching, and it will then rapidly gain weight. By the fourth day it will weigh 63g and at 20 days it will weigh 400g (nearly the adult bodyweight). During this time the juvenile feathers will have developed. The squab is normally weaned at about 24 days of age when the feathering has fully developed.

DISEASES ASSOCIATED WITH BREEDING

The first indications of breeding problems will be failure of the bird to lay or the laying of only one egg; failure to detect embryo development if candling is practised; failure of the eggs to hatch; or early squab mortality. Broadly, the problems can be classified as follows:

● Infertility - failure to lay eggs or failure of embryonic development.
● Contamination - evidence of bacterial or fungal contamination of the egg.
● Embryo mortality - early and late embryonic mortality will be the commonest findings.
● Neonatal mortality - the squabs will fail to thrive or suddenly stop thriving. Dead or moribund squabs should be examined.

The type of problem being experienced can be determined initially by examining eggs and chicks. Unfortunately, many fanciers will present the offending pair of adults without appreciating that they have just disposed of the most useful evidence.

The deficiency diseases described result from experimental work with poultry, but they should be expected to cause similar problems in pigeons.

Infertility

● No eggs or too many eggs. Same sex - sexing pigeons is done on body conformation, hence this could be a problem for the inexperienced fancier. A salpingitis could have resulted from an earlier generalised infection or be the result of stress, eg. inappropriate vaccination of hens between pairing and laying.
● The bird may be too young or too old.
● Too many feathers around the vent. This can interfere with mating. The feathers around the vent should be trimmed.
● Too much disturbance. This may be the result of overcrowding, cracked eggs through constant movement on the nest, fighting for nestboxes and throwing of eggs out of the nest bowls by intruders into the nestbox. This could also result in ectopic eggs.
● Failure to mate. Copulation should have occurred 24-48 hours before the egg is laid in order to ensure fertilisation.
● Too high a temperature, ie. 30°C, will result in lower fertility. However, too cold a temperature, ie. 4°C, coupled with damp, is more likely to be a problem, particularly for matings that occur very early in the year. Increasing day length is also an important stimulus for reproduction. The provision of extra artificial light may be required.
● Both underweight and overweight birds will have reduced fertility. Attention to the diet and regular checks of body condition will avoid this problem. An ample source of fresh water must be available. The fat hen is more likely to develop abdominal hernias, retain the egg or suffer from prolapse of the cloaca or oviduct.
● Deficiencies. Vitamin A - decreased sperm counts, reduced sperm motility, increased numbers of abnormal sperms, irregular laying cycles. Vitamin B_6 (pyridoxine) - poor egg laying. Vitamin D_3 - (thin shells and soft shells) and irregular laying cycles. Vitamin E - testicular degeneration if low levels fed for a prolonged period.
● Nervous disorders. This could result from overzealous use of dimetridazole, pigeon paramyxovirus infection, salmonellosis or cypermethrin dips. The cause must be diagnosed and treated accordingly.
● Infection of the reproductive tract. This could be the result of generalised infection or secondary to a stress in the case of salpingitis.
● Congenital and inherited diseases. Accurate breeding records should indicate if this is likely to be a problem.
● Hormone imbalance, eg. tumours of the ovary or testes.
● Overbreeding. This could lead to inertia of the oviduct and calcium deficiency. This is most likely to be seen in a hen that is on her second or third round of eggs. She may have laid the first egg but not the second. The presenting signs are sudden onset of nervous symptoms and an inability to walk, fly or feed. The author has found that crop tube feeding with Rapidaid (Vetrepharm) (10g/100g bodyweight in two doses over 24 hours) and calcium tablets (0.25 of a 300mg tablet once daily) gives a rapid improvement in this condition. The second egg is then laid. The eggs are discarded. It is several weeks before the hen fully regains normal flight.
● Therapeutics. Sulphonamides are known to predispose to thin shells and poor hatchability. Mebendazole is contraindicated in breeding birds. Ointments that adhere to the vent feathers may be transferred onto the shell, thus blocking the pores and reducing hatchability.
● Eggshell damage. Calcium deficiency in the diet can predispose to thin shells and membrane eggs. The former will permit the hairline cracks and toe holes to be made more easily.

Contamination

Poor nestbox hygiene, loft hygiene and inappropriate nesting materials will predispose to contamination of the eggs. Fresh straw and tobacco stalks are often provided as nesting materials. Hay should not be given because it will rapidly go mouldy and the long strands can wrap themselves around the legs of the squabs. These problems are always worse if there are concurrent shell quality problems. Microbiological examination will identify the causal agents, eg. bacterial (*Escherichia coli*, *Pseudomonas* spp., *Salmonella* spp.) or fungal (*Aspergillus* spp.).

Embryonic Mortality

Early

● Parents not incubating eggs (see Excessive Disturbance).
● Chilling - very cold weather and parents not sitting for long periods.

- Vitamin A deficiency - loss of epithelial membrane structure, hence failure to develop blood vessels and reduced hatchability.
- Biotin deficiency - two peaks of mortality at the beginning and end of incubation. (For lesions see Late Mortality.)
- Vitamin E deficiency - oedema, death.

Mid-term
- Parents not incubating eggs (see Disturbances).
- Thin shells and egg drying out.
- Vitamin B_{12} deficiency - malposition, oedema, curly toes, poor muscling.
- Vitamin B_2 (riboflavin) deficiency - stunted chicks with oedema.

Late
- Parents disturbed during incubation.
- Insufficient humidity because of lack of water for parents.
- *Salmonella typhimurium* infection either in the oviduct or through the eggshell resulting in death.
- Deficiencies (see Table 32.1)
- Inbreeding can result in more malpositioned embryos being found.
- Malposition (see Table 32.2).

NEONATE DISEASES (to 24 days of age)

Bullying

Signs
This is most commonly seen with some parents at weaning. Severe aggressive peck damage can occur to the head resulting in the removal of large areas of skin revealing the skull beneath.

Treatment
Topical treatment with Dermisol Cream (Pfizer) and supportive antibiotic therapy will aid recovery. It is important that the bird is removed to another section of the loft.

Fenbendazole Toxicity
Fenbendazole toxicity results from inappropriate worming with fenbendazole, eg. Panacur Pigeon Capsules (Hoechst). Fanciers worm unnecessarily before the squabs are eight weeks of age. A single capsule given to a 10 day old squab will result in a 'feather duster' type of feathering 7-10 days later due to weakness of the pin feathers. The feathers break at various positions along the shaft depending on their stage of growth when the capsule was administered.

Table 32.1. Effect of various deficiencies on late embryonic mortality

Deficiency	Comments
Vitamin B_6	Poor hatchability.
Vitamin D_3	Stunted chicks, soft bones, chondrodystrophy, poor hatchability.
Vitamin E	Poor hatchability.
Pantothenic acid	Subcutaneous haemorrhages and oedema. The age of mortality depends on the severity of the disease.
Biotin and folic acid (folacin)	Micromelia, syndactylism, bradygnathism, death occurring after pipping of the air cell.
Vitamin K	Haemorrhage and death of the embryo.
Phosphorus	Soft beaks and legs, poor hatchability.
Calcium	Poor hatchability, short thick legs, short wings, short lower mandible, pliable beak and legs, oedema of the neck, bulging forehead, protruding abdomen.
Zinc	Skeletal abnormalities. Wings and legs absent.
Manganese	Short wings and legs, abnormal head, parrot beak, retarded growth, oedema.
Selenium	Poor hatchability, oedema.

Table 32.2. Result of malpositioned embryo.

(Malposition) position of embryo	Result
(1) Head between thighs.	Can result in mortality.
(2) Head in small end of egg.	Death.
(3) Head under left wing.	Death.
(4) Chick rotated so head facing side of egg and not the airspace.	Death.
(5) Feet over head.	Death.
(6) Head over right wing.	Usually hatch.
(7) Small embryo lying across egg.	Death.

Treatment

Euthanasia. Normal feathers would be expected to grow after the next moult. The author has not had the opportunity to wait for this to occur. This problem is completely avoidable and is a direct consequence of failure to read the directions for administration of the drug.

Pigeon Herpesvirus Infection

This should not normally be a cause of mortality because of protection afforded by maternal antibodies. Further details can be found in Chapter 28.

Pigeon Pox

Squabs are infected with pigeon pox virus transmitted from the parents. This could occur as a result of natural infection or a fancier vaccinating adults within six weeks of hatching. Diphtheritic or cutaneous forms may be seen in squabs of about seven days of age. Differential diagnosis should include trichomoniasis and vitamin A deficiency.

Treatment and Control

See Chapters 26 and 28.

Red Mite Infestation

Red mite infestation (*Dermanyssus gallinae*) results in poor growth, lethargy, anaemia and death. Diagnosis may be suspected on *post-mortem* examination but confirmation may require examination of the loft by torchlight at night in order to see the migrating mites.

Treatment

All nestbox materials must be cleaned with an acaracide, eg. Microcarb (Microbiologicals). The squabs can be treated with pyrethrins.

Rickets

Rickets may be caused by deficiency of vitamin D_3, calcium or phosphorus. The signs are lameness, poor growth and death. On *post-mortem* examination the long bones and beak will be very pliable.

Treatment

This condition is a reflection of inadequate parent nutrition. Extra sources of calcium, phosphorus and vitamin D_3 should be provided in the form of vitaminised grit (available from pigeon suppliers).

Salmonellosis

Salmonella typhimurium infection occurs as a result of vertical transmission through the egg or from faecal contamination of the egg. Squabs are particularly susceptible to *S. typhimurium* infection. Infected squabs may hatch weak or die within two days of hatching. Older squabs may show signs of lameness, particularly swollen hocks. Diagnosis can be confirmed on *post-mortem* examination in conjunction with bacteriology.

Treatment

Antibiotic therapy of all affected and in-contact birds should be advised. The choice of antibiotic will depend on the result of sensitivity testing of the isolate. Owners must be made aware that salmonellosis is a zoonosis and that good hygiene precautions are required.

Starvation

Both parents are required to raise two squabs successfully. The loss of one parent will result in poor growth of both birds or starvation of one of the birds.

Treatment

One of the squabs must be fostered out.

Trichomoniasis

Trichomoniasis in squabs is caused by *Trichomonas gallinae*. The typical chronic form (yellow, cheesy deposits in the mouth) may be seen. However, more often, intestinal or liver infections affect the squab, resulting in stunting, enteritis and death. Infection of the navel can occur. Diagnosis is most commonly made on *post-mortem* examination.

Treatment

Early recognition will enable treatment with metronidazole to be instituted. Treatment of the parents whilst they are sitting on the eggs is more appropriate. This will prevent the direct transmission of a heavy infection to the squabs.

Yolk Sac Infection and Omphalitis

This is due to bacterial infection (commonly with *E. coli*) of the egg or one-day-old squab. The signs are poor growth, inanition, lethargy, a poorly healed and inflamed navel, and death within a few days of hatching.

Treatment

Antibiotic treatment of the sibling and possibly the parents. Most importantly, examination of the nestbox hygiene and rectification of any shortcomings.

FURTHER READING

Coles BH (1985) *Avian Medicine and Surgery*. Blackwell Scientific Publications, Oxford.

Arnall L and Keymer IF (1975) *Bird Diseases*. Baillière Tindall, London.

CHAPTER THIRTY THREE

Husbandry and Nutrition

Neil A Forbes and Tony Richardson

TERMINOLOGY AND DESCRIPTION

Birds of the Order Anseriformes include ducks, geese, swans and screamers. When considering waterfowl, flamingos are generally included as they are widely kept in captivity, often in combination with other members of the group. Table 33.1 lists some of the terminology commonly used for the different groups of waterfowl.

Anseriformes differ from most other birds in that the male has an erectile phallus, which may be seen if the cloaca is everted. To determine the sex, birds should be held head downwards between the knees, with the abdomen facing towards the handler. Firm, gentle pressure should be applied with the thumbs in a dorsolateral direction on either side of the cloaca. The female has two small labia-like structures, whilst the male has a definite phallus. The ease of carrying out this procedure varies with respect to the age, breed and sex of the bird, and the season of the year. Care, skill and experience are required, all of which may be gained by practice. Species of waterfowl from tropical areas are sensitive to extreme cold weather and are prone to frost bite and gangrene. These species should be housed during the winter. Others are tolerant of extreme conditions, although it is important that they have access to open (unfrozen) water.

All members of the group have nidifugous young, ie. they are covered in down, and can eat, swim and dive almost immediately following hatching. Young birds may readily be adversely imprinted. This should not be encouraged as it will cause problems when the birds reach sexual maturity (both aggression towards humans and failure to breed with their own species).

A classification of the Family Anatidae together with some silhouette shapes and a brief description is given in Table 33.2.

Flamingos (*Phoenicopteridae*) are considered to be the link between ducks, geese, swans and storks. There are six different species of flamingos, all of which live in groups, sometimes of thousands of birds. They are mainly found in tropical and subtropical climates. Both parents nest build and incubate the single egg. At ten days of age the youngsters join a crèche comprising several young minded by a few adults. The specialised bill, which is held upside down in the water, is used for sieving small particles of food out of the water. Additional carotene is required in their diet in captivity to maintain their bright pink/orange colouration.

The anatomy of Screamers (*Anhimidae*) suggests a close relationship with wildfowl. They will perch in trees, but also wade and swim despite their feet having no webs. Their screaming calls are heard only in tropical and subtropical South America.

The recognition of the different tribes is important, as this in turn dictates the feeding, nesting and mixing requirements of the group in question. Table 33.3 lists some biological data for the commoner species.

Table 33.1. Commonly used terminology for waterfowl.

	Male	**Female**	**< 3 weeks**	**Young**	**First year**
Ducks	Drake	Duck	Downy	Duckling	Juveniles or adolescents
Geese	Gander	Goose	Downy	Gosling	Juveniles or adolescents
Swans	Cob	Pen	Downy	Cygnet	Juveniles or adolescents
Flamingos	Male	Female	Downy	Chick	Juveniles or adolescents

Table 33.2. A simplified classification of the Family Anatidae.
(Adapted with kind permission from the Wildfowl and Wetlands Trust Souvenir Booklet, 1990.)

Sub-Family	Tribe	Genera and species
Anseranatinae	Anseranatini	One species - Magpie Goose. As its Latin name (*Anseranas semipalmata*) suggests, this strange Australian bird has half-webbed feet and is more adapted to living on land than on water. Magpie Geese have a specially lengthened hind claw, which is an adaptation for semi-terrestial life. They nest and rest in trees and, unlike other waterfowl, feed their young with food held in their beak. They are polygamous, often breeding in trios consisting one male and two females. They have a specially elongated trachea, which forms coils, subcutaneously over the pectoral muscles. This adaptation is thought to enable low resonant vocalisation (Johnsgard, 1978).
Anserinae Undergo a complete annual moult after the breeding season. The flight feathers are shed almost simultaneously, so that they are flightless for 3-6 weeks. The front toes are fully webbed in almost all species. In all species the plumage is monomorphic with no iridescent colouration, even of the wing.	Dendrocygnini (Whistling Ducks)	2 genera - 9 species. Named for their whistling call; also known as Tree Ducks, as they often live and nest in or near trees. Sexually monomorphic. Longer legs and more upright stance distinguish these from other groups of ducks.
	Anserini (Swans and true geese)	4 genera - 22 species. Swans and geese are closely related. They are long lived; the sexes are monomorphic. Save for untimely fatalities, they pair for life. The family remains together for the first year. Geese are well adapted to living on land; their legs are longer than swans or ducks and are centrally placed under the body, which facilitates taking off and walking on land.
	Cereopsini (Cape Barren Goose)	1 species.
	Stictonettini (Freckled Duck)	1 species.

Table 33.2. Continued.

Sub-Family	Tribe	Genera and species
Anatinae Most members of this group moult twice a year; hence the breeding (nuptial) and non-breeding (eclipse or winter) plumage are different. Often the male breeding plumage is different from the female, ie. sexually dimorphic. The plumage of the downy young is patterned (often spotted and striped, including the head and neck). Males generally do not help in incubation but may assist in rearing young.	Tadornini (Shelducks and allies) 	5 genera - 14 species. These birds, somewhere between true geese and ducks, are notable for their attractive and distinctive plumage patterns. They have long necks and legs and live mainly on land. Although they look like true geese and eat the same sorts of food, in may respects they are more like ducks. Some are sexually dimorphic, they moult twice a year and have patterned downy young.
	Surface feeding ducks Anatini (dabbling ducks) 	4 genera - 40 species. This group includes all the dabbling ducks including Mallard, that dabble in shallow water for their food. Wigeon are distinct and different in that they graze on short vegetation on land. Mallard, Pintail and Teal often up-end for their food, whilst the Shoveller's wide beak has a ridged edge which is used as a sieve.
	Cairinini (perching ducks and allies) 	9 genera - 13 species. The perching ducks, such as Mandarins and Carolinas (Wood Ducks), are also mainly surface feeders. Most of the perching ducks nest in holes in trees.
	Diving ducks Tachyerini (Steamer Ducks) 	1 genus - 3 species. Steamer Ducks are large ungainly birds on land. Two species are flightless. They are high-speed, long-distance paddlers. Generally found in coastal areas (native to southern South America, including the Falkland Islands).
	Merganettini (Torrent Duck) 	3 species.
	Aythyini (Pochards) 	2 genera - 15 species. Found worldwide. All freshwater ducks, with the exception of the Scaups. Their bodies are short and rounded. Individual species only vary from each other in minor detail.

Table 33.2. Continued.

Sub-Family	Tribe	Genera and species
	Mergini (Mergansers, Scoters and Goldeneyes)	7 genera - 18 species. Found in both fresh water and sea water. They are typically hole nesters. Their favourite foods are shellfish and crustaceans. Mergansers have pointed beaks with tooth-like projections to hold fish securely.
	Somateriini (Eiders)	2 genera - 6 species. These ducks are found in open sea and coastal waters. Males have conspicuous black and white plumage during the breeding season. Females pluck the famous eider down feathers from their breasts to line the nest.
	Oxyurini (Stifftails)	3 genera - 8 species. All species have stiff tail feathers which are used as a rudder and which are most conspicuous during courtship display. Stifftails have extremely large feet and find walking on land very difficult. They hardly ever leave water, even nesting on floating reed platforms.

HUSBANDRY

Handling

Anseriformes are relatively easily restrained. Their primary defences are their beaks, wings and feet, none of which present any grave risk to staff as long as proper training has been received. Handling varies with respect to species. Swans and larger geese should be approached confidently. The neck should be grasped just below the head with the left hand, whilst the right forearm is swiftly placed under and around the body. The bird can be drawn in against the handler's body. With long-legged species, eg. flamingos, great care must be taken to prevent damage to the legs during or after catching. As the bird is picked up with one hand, the legs are grasped with the other, just distal to the intertarsal joints. One finger is kept between the legs at all times in order to prevent pressure damage between the legs.

NB. Care should be taken when handling birds with pointed beaks, eg. herons (Ardeidae). Such birds may use their beaks as weapons. After initial restraint, a ball of bandage should be impaled onto the tip of the beak to prevent it causing any damage.

Hospitalisation

A dry, warm enclosure with non-slip flooring is suitable for brief periods of hospitalisation. Confinement, isolation and proximity to humans are frequently stressful to waterfowl; a quiet, dimly lit enclosure is preferable. During periods of hospitalisation in excess of 48 hours, access to water to swim in and a properly padded floor, eg. butyl rubber matting, should be available. Where birds have become oiled, the waterproofing of the feathers will have become damaged, thus losing the insulation properties and leading to risk of marked hypothermia. In these situations the ambient temperature should initially be maintained at 35-40°C (see Chapter 35).

Encouraging birds to feed voluntarily during hospitalisation is a challenge. Attempts should be made to feed as natural a diet in a manner as close to nature as possible. Although there is considerable variation in the natural diets of different groups of waterfowl, there is also a great diversity within the natural diet of each species (see later). Most hospitalised waterfowl (except specialised eaters) will eat (a choice of) wheat (dry on the ground, and also some submerged in a water bowl) and fresh river weed. If birds are not willing to eat, they should be crop fed with a convalescent type diet, eg. Reanamyl (Rhône Mérieux) or Complan

Table 33.3. Average biological data for some of the commoner species of waterfowl.

Species	Male weight (kg)	Female weight (kg)	Sexual maturity (years)	Clutch size	Incubation period (days)	Longevity (years)	RR *	HR **	CT ***
Mute Swan	12.2	8.9	5	4-8	35-40	25-30	13-40	80-150	40.5
Pink-footed Goose	2.6	2.35	2	3-5	26-27	15-20	13-40	80-150	40.5
Bar-headed Goose	2-3	2-3	2	4-6	27	15-20	13-40	80-150	40.5
Hawaiian Goose	2.2	1.9	2	3-5	29	15-20	13-40	80-150	40.5
Red-breasted Goose	1.3-1.6	1.15	2	3-7	23-25	15-20	13-40	80-150	40.5
European Wigeon	0.7	0.64	1	7-11	23-25	10-15	30-95	180-230	41.0
Mallard	1.26	1.1	1	8-12	23-29	10-15	30-95	180-230	41.0
Common Eider	2.25	2.12	1	3-6	25-30	10-15	30-95	180-230	41.0
Tufted Duck	1.1	1.05	1	6-14	23-25	10-15	30-95	180-230	41.0
Mandarin Duck	0.44-0.55	0.44-0.55	1	9-12	28-30	10-15	30-95	180-230	41.0
Muscovy Duck	2-4	1.1-1.5	1	8-15	35	10.15	30-95	180-230	41.0
European Goldeneye	0.99-1.16	0.7-0.8	1	9-11	27-32	10-15	30-95	180-230	41.0

(From Todd, 1979; Hayes, 1984; Coles, 1985).

RR * = Respiratory rate, breaths per minute.
HR** = Heart rate, beats per minute.
CT*** = Cloacal temperature, degrees Centigrade.

(Crookes Health Care). The provision of a captive decoy or other duck to act as a companion for hospitalised patients will often help stimulate feeding. Great care must be taken, however, to minimise the risk of such a duck acting as a vector for infection. It should only be allowed to mix with healthy (rather than infected) birds, and should be regularly screened for subclinical infection. Waterfowl are generally strong swimmers, but poor walkers. For this reason, if birds are recovering from leg injuries it is particularly important to allow access to water, rather than to force them to weight bear on an injured limb.

Housing

It is necessary to differentiate between domestic wildfowl and ornamental wildfowl.

Domestic wildfowl have been selected over the years for size, growth rate, carcase quality or egg production. They are accustomed to a degree of captivity, are less easily stressed, and may be housed at night to help reduce the risk of predation.

Ornamental wildfowl are commonly kept pinioned in large open pens and have access to a pond or stream. They should not be kept unless the correct facilities are available, as they will be subject to stresses not experienced by domesticated breeds.

Currently, more collections of both domestic and ornamental wildfowl are using highly durable, knotless, nylon mesh netting to enclose pens, eg. Gundry Netting, The Court, Bridport, Dorset DT6 3QU. This has the advantage that it dispenses with the requirement for pinioning of stock and, at the same time, prevents access to the site by feral birds, which may present a major health risk to the captive birds. Pinioning of birds up to 10 days of age may be carried out by lay persons; thereafter, it may only be carried out by a veterinary surgeon who has a complete knowledge of the bird and the collection and believes it to be in the bird's best interest.

Enclosures should not be totally overrun with vegetation. Ingestion of long coarse grass can lead to crop impactions. Although planted aviaries provide shade and nesting materials, dark shaded areas will allow a greater environmental build up of *Mycobacterium avium* if the organism is present. The proportion of land to water will vary with the species. Grazing species, such as geese and swans, require a greater proportion of grazing land. Grazing areas should be cultivated once or twice each year and be thoroughly exposed to sunlight. Gizzard worm ova (*Amidostomum* spp.) and gapeworm ova (*Syngamus* spp. or *Cyathostoma* spp.) overwinter on grass, and present a particular risk to juvenile grazing birds. It is important, therefore, to have fresh grazing each year for juvenile birds (see Quarantine and Disease Control). Geese, in particular, are prone to nibble at any rough surfaces around the water margin; this generally leads to erosion of the bank. Furthermore, the water-land margin is a common area from which dabbling ducks may ingest *M. avium*. For both these reasons many waterfowl keepers use concrete or stone blocks around the water margin. Care should be taken with regard to the texture of the substrate on which the birds will be walking. Rough concrete surfaces may lead to considerable foot trauma and infection; some species, eg. Black Swans, appear particularly prone to this problem.

Ponds should have at least one island; this allows privacy for nesting areas and affords considerable predation control.

Water Quality

Many potential sites for wildfowl collections will already have water in one form or another. The most important factor is that a constant supply of fresh water (it need not be large volumes) is available. Water from a nearby stream, that can be diverted through some pools and returned, can be ideal. Anti-erosion measures should be taken to maintain the integrity of the ponds and not allow the system to become clogged with mud and solids. However, routine de-mudding of ponds will prove necessary, even if only every few years.

Reed bed technology (using *Phragmites australis*) can act as a partial purifier of water. This means that small treatment beds can be installed at the entry and, particularly, the exit points of the water flow of a collection. This is an important factor in obtaining the necessary water abstraction licences from the National Rivers Authority.

SELECTION OF STOCK

There are many considerations that must be taken into account when selecting stock for a waterfowl collection. Irrespective of whether the collection is large or small, there are some basic questions to be answered:
● For what purposes are the birds being kept?
● Which species are the personal favourites of the collector?
● Which species can the collector afford to acquire and keep?
● How much space is available and what is the water quality?
● How much grazing is available if considering a grazing species such as geese?
● Where and when will the birds be acquired?
● Species compatibility?
● Predator risk?
These questions should be considered in the approximate order in which they are stated.

If it is intended to breed birds successfully, good blood lines are important. Stud records should be kept and birds acquired from known backgrounds.

If only a few birds are being kept, it is important to choose a species which is fairly independent, eg. domesticated Mallard.

If wild species are to be kept, other factors must be considered. Having ensured predator control (see later), space availability must be considered. The requirements of the species must be considered; if these are not met the birds will not thrive and may not even survive.

Sea ducks and diving ducks require a deep water area. Dabbling ducks require an expanse of shallow waters edge. Grazers, eg. geese, require adequate grass, not only in the grass growing season but all through the year.

Acquiring birds, either for the first time or as additions and replacements, requires much thought and a little luck. The best time to bring in young birds is as soon as they are fully fledged and at peak bodyweight, usually August or September. This will allow the birds to become accustomed to their new surroundings before the onset of winter. Alternatively, one can wait until early spring when the rigours of winter may have resulted in a need for some replacements. Birds which have not yet fully fledged or are in the process of moulting should not be taken unless particular care in both transport and acclimatisation can be guaranteed.

Although it may seem ideal to keep a varied collection of single pairs, it may be difficult to replace a bird following the death of one of a pair with the correct sub-species. This can lead to mis-pairing and hybridisation. Action that can be taken to avoid hybridisation includes:
● When releasing new birds on to a pond, only allow birds from one species to go off together. Five minutes later release another species, but from another part of the pond, and so on.
● Try to replace a lost bird from a single pair as quickly as possible.
● With most ducks and true geese, keep more than just a single pair, eg. three pairs or three males and four females; immediate replacement of a single lost bird is therefore less critical.
● Avoid too many different species of geese or ducks in one pen, especially sub-species, as interbreeding is likely.
● As far as is possible, rear young birds with their own species.
● Acquiring young replacement birds is preferable.

A replacement adult bird may not have spent its life with birds of the species to which it is to be introduced.
● When releasing a replacement single bird, make sure that it is done in such a way that it cannot fail to meet with the existing bird or birds. They may part, but invariably not for long.
● Try to replace a lost bird with a bird of similar age. This is not so important with geese and less so with most ducks, but care should be taken with swans. Widowed, adult, female swans can be given a young male relatively safely as a mate at any time. The reverse is not true. An aggressive, breeding, male swan will often demand a lifestyle from a first year female that she is not physically equipped to deal with. Her bodyweight can fall and death will often occur. In this situation, and with no adult females available, try to avoid such an introduction until late in the younger bird's second summer. If this results in a male being on its own for too long, introduce the younger bird earlier, but establish the pair in a new area or pond.

Similar actions can be useful with some species of geese. If a young bird is to be added to an established group, eg. five Red-breasted Geese or three Common Eiders, consider adding a young pair instead. Neither of these examples are likely to breed in their first year, but they will keep each other company through both the initial settling down period (during the group investigation) and the subsequent breeding season. They may stay as a pair within the flock, so where possible try to ensure that they are unrelated.
● Checking for different blood lines when acquiring birds is not easy and much has to be taken on trust. Breeders, however, will have a vested interest in keeping the different broods identifiable.

● Check that the birds you are acquiring will fit into your collection. For example, do you have the correct feed necessary for a pair of Hooded Mergansers? Will they be aggressive to other birds, or the opposite?

Species Compatibility

This is a very important aspect of stock selection, in particular when commencing a waterfowl collection. Having considered personal choice and all the previously mentioned criteria, some variation in species selected may be necessary in the interest of achieving harmonious and productive results. Table 33.4 shows species which may not be mixed.

Further Considerations

Some ducks and geese do particularly well in small groups, eg. European Teal, Common Eider, European Goldeneye. Displaying and other behaviour patterns can be observed which may never occur with single pairs.

Stock should be selected to fit the collection area available and for ease of management. Large, less manageable ponds should be stocked with indigenous species, so that if young birds fledge and cannot be caught, there will not be any contravention of the Wildlife and Countryside Act 1981 (as amended 1988 and 1991). More delicate birds should be kept in sheltered areas and not kept at all if the collection is particularly exposed to severe wintry conditions.

Diving ducks should be kept in sufficient numbers on each large pond to try and keep an area ice-free in winter. Other birds will use these areas during the day and only the severest of weather will cause a total freeze.

Table 33.4. Waterfowl species which should not be mixed.

Keep isolated as a single pair	Exceptions	Specific non-mix combinations
Swans, especially Coscoroba Swans Egyptian Geese Shelducks Sheldgeese, especially Andean Geese Crested Ducks	Two pairs of Black Swans may be kept together if the area is large enough, as long as they are released together. Never release a young pair into the territory of an established pair.	Even on large lakes, never mix two pairs of Trumpeter Swans or a pair of Bewick's Swans with a pair of Whistling Swans.
Steamer Ducks Cereopsis Geese Bronze-winged Ducks Pink-eared Ducks Hartlaub's Ducks Comb Ducks Spur-winged Geese White-winged Wood Ducks Musk Ducks New Zealand Teals (Brown Teals or Brown Ducks)	More than one pair of Comb Ducks and White-winged Wood Ducks can be released together if the area is large, but do not release new birds into an existing group.	Hawaiian Geese ('Néné') and Cackling Canada Geese. Avoid keeping any sub-species together.

Noise can be a factor. Some birds have very loud calls and this may be a nuisance both to the keeper and to neighbours.

If stocking for a collection open to the public, consideration must be given to the education and conservation aspects of the birds kept. A mixed group of available ducks exhibited out of context does little for the birds, the keeper or the visitor.

Overcrowding and mixing too many different species are the commonest causes of disaster. Poor planning and husbandry are likely to lead to increased disease incidence and poor productivity.

NUTRITION

Wildfowl kept in captivity need to be fed. Some species which graze, dabble or catch fish will require less feeding, especially in the summer. In most wildfowl collections the number of birds kept is invariably too many to allow 12 month sustainable natural food production, and so feeding is necessary throughout the year. Wheat is an excellent bulk food for wildfowl. Food must be well stored (maximum 16% moisture) close to the point of feeding. Several companies now make proprietary diets for ornamental waterfowl. The range will often include:
● 'Maintenance Pellets' with an approximate protein level of 14% for general non-breeding use.
● 'Breeder's Pellets' with a protein level of 16% for the period prior to and running throughout the laying period.
● 'Duckling or Chicken Starter Crumbs' with a protein level of 20% for young birds in the first 2-3 weeks of life.
● 'Grower or Rearer Pellets' with a protein level of 16% for adolescents and juveniles up to 4-6 months of age. Different diets are advisable for different ages and tribes of birds.

Anseriformes generally have an ability to grow at faster rates than poultry or gamebirds, and this can be a particular problem with the grazers, eg. geese, swans, shelduck and wigeon. These species would normally only eat grass with a protein content of 16-17%. Using feeds with protein levels in excess of this can cause growth defects or kidney damage.

Fish-eating ducks and flamingos need a more specialised, slightly higher protein diet which is also manufactured specifically, eg. Flamingo Food, available from Special Diets Services (SDS), PO Box 705, Witham, Essex CM8 3AD; or Sea Duck Food, available from SDS or Clarke and Butcher, Lion Mills, Soham, Ely CB7 5HJ. These are generally more expensive than the simpler diets.

Additional food stuffs, including various millets and seed, can assist in the rearing process of young Stifftails; small insects (crickets/mealworms) for sea ducks.

Grass is the main requirement of geese and goslings. Supplemental feeding will be required and is beneficial (although not to excess, as excessive growth rates may be detrimental), but access to grazing areas is important and this must be reflected in stocking levels.

QUARANTINE AND DISEASE CONTROL

Whether considering a new site or introducing additional birds to an existing collection, the same rules apply. If wild or feral birds are present, prevention of disease introduction and prevention of spread between pens is of limited value.

When starting a collection every precaution must be taken to prevent the introduction of disease, in particular infectious, chronic, debilitating disease, eg. tuberculosis. The collection may become contaminated prior to clinical signs being apparent. It is possible to set up a significant collection (more than 1,000 birds) of waterfowl by bringing in eggs and small ducklings that have not been exposed to disease. However, this is not an easy option. Wherever possible, juvenile birds less than one-year-old, which have been reared on fresh uncontaminated pasture, should be acquired. Incoming birds should be subjected to a careful clinical examination and prophylactic roundworm therapy, eg, mebendazole (5-15mg/kg daily for two days); mebendazole in feed (120ppm for 14 days); flubendazole in feed (240 ppm for seven days); or ivermectin (200mcg/kg once).

If possible, all birds should be screened for general health status with a blood test. The one single test which will give the greatest information regarding a bird's state of health is the fibrinogen level (normal< 4g/1). Birds with a fibrinogen level above 4g/l who are thin or appear ill in any way should not be introduced into a collection. Ideally, a full blood screen and a *M. avium* ELISA test (see Chapter 39) should be performed.

All incoming birds should be maintained in quarantine accommodation or small groups for at least six weeks. This is not always easy when dealing with small numbers of young birds (because of the fear of imprinting), but it is important. Maintaining a waterfowl collection is similar to maintaining a loft of fit racing pigeons - the health of the collection is paramount, rather than that of the individual. For this reason it is important that thorough *post-mortem* examinations are carried out on all stock which die or are euthanased. Parasitism must be minimised by regular rigorous controls. All breeding adults should be wormed in early spring prior to the breeding season, and all birds should be wormed each autumn. As mentioned earlier, juvenile birds should have access to clean pasture not previously grazed by adult birds.

PREDATION RISK AND CONTROL

Keeping wildfowl in captivity, either as part of a conservation release programme or as a private collection or zoo, is not straightforward. Losing stock to predators is a constant threat and a cause of great anxiety.

A balance between the cost of predation control and the likelihood of predation must be achieved. All control measures should be safe and legal. A collection should be designed to minimise predation risk. Tame birds and those in a sheltered environment are less wary of predation than their wild counterparts.

Foxes

Keeping foxes out is the only reliable method of control. Islands a distance from the bank will provide a safe haven from foxes. Fox-proof fencing needs to be substantial. An ideal fence can be made using the following:
2 rolls of 90cm x 7.5cm 16 gauge galvanised wire netting;
1 roll of 120cm x 2.5cm 16 gauge galvanised wire netting;
3 strands of pulsed electric fencing.

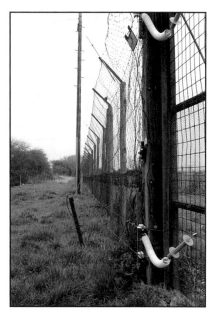

Figure 33.1: Fox-proof fencing.

Construction should be as follows:
Posts are 270cm long with 60cm knocked into the ground. 45cm of angle iron at 45° is projected outwards from the top of the post. One roll of 7.5cm mesh wire is fixed from the extent of the projection via the post head to join with the second roll of 7.5cm mesh, to finish some 75cm above the ground. The roll of 2.5cm mesh wire is joined and continued to the ground. The remaining 45cm is projected underground at 45°, facing outwards. The electric strands should be offset some 22cm from the main fence and placed approximately 20cm, 60cm and 210cm from the ground (see Figure 33.1).

Various methods can be used to fox-proof buildings and gates. Existing, successful systems should be looked at before undertaking fox proofing of a collection.

Mink

Mink are semi-aquatic. They will follow water courses and are therefore difficult to exclude. Trapping, using several Mark 6 Fenn traps (see Figure 33.2) set in tunnels or, preferably, case traps, will remove incoming family groups of mink as they arrive. These traps are best set around the perimeter of the area that houses the collection. Mink should be euthanased humanely, ie. not drowned.

Stoats and Weasels

These animals can and do kill captive waterfowl, though they tend not to kill quite so needlessly as fox and mink. Stoats also take eggs, rolling them one by one from ground nests. Tunnel traps used for mink may be effective, but stoats and weasels are not so water orientated. Ideally, the tunnel traps should be placed near the rearing areas or at the back of overgrown pens.

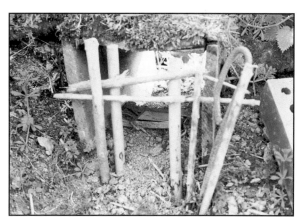

Figure 33.2: Mark 6 Fenn trap.

Cats

Cats tend to be regular visitors, perhaps taking only one bird per visit. Special care should be taken where buildings form part of the perimeter fence, as domestic cats readily climb over walls and roofs. Electric fox-proof fencing is also a deterrent against cats.

Rats

Although mainly posing a hygiene and food stealing threat, rats may kill ducks. Many techniques are used to control rats. Putting poison pellets down holes and trapping are reasonably effective, but only in the short term. Purpose-built bait boxes, which are designed to be safe to other animals and humans, can be used. These boxes should be situated subtly around the site and maintained with a supply of treated food. Mark 4 Fenn traps can also be used.

Aerial Predators

Crows, magpies and owls are the most likely aerial predators in the UK. The only action that one can take against owls is to rear young waterfowl under netting. It is illegal to take more positive action. The same netting will also deter magpies and crows, although they more commonly steal eggs. Numbers of nesting crows and magpies should be controlled in the collection area. Cage trapping is not often successful, as rooks and jackdaws are the species most commonly caught. Herring Gulls and Lesser Black-backed Gulls will often take ducklings. In such a case, shooting an individual may be the solution. They may, however, have been initially encouraged along with other aerial predators by excess food or carrion. A special covered feeding area may be useful.

FURTHER READING

Coles BH (1985) *Avian Medicine and Surgery.* Blackwell Scientific Publications, Oxford.

Hayes MB (1984) *Rehabilitation Guidebook for Birds and Mammals.* Brukner Nature Centre, Ohio.

Johnsgard PA (1978) *Ducks, Geese, and Swans of the World.* University of Nebraska Press, Lincoln and London.

Kear, J (1990) *Man and Wildfowl.* T & AD Poyser, London.

Todd FS (1979) *Waterfowl: Ducks, Geese, and Swans of the World.* Seaworld Press, San Diego.

CHAPTER THIRTY FOUR

Head and Neck Problems

Jason C Waine

INTRODUCTION

Problems affecting the head and neck of waterfowl, both in wild and captive populations, are dominated by injuries caused by collision, fighting and foreign bodies, but also include infections, parasitic infestations, toxaemias and abnormalities of growth. When presented with such problems, the usual features of avian anatomy of this region should be taken into consideration.

ANATOMY

Skull

There are a number of important features which set the avian skull apart from the mammalian skull. There is only a very thin bony septum separating the two orbits. This septum is very close to the brain, making enucleation of the eye a much more dangerous operation than in mammals (see Chapter 15). The articulation between the lower mandible (*rostrum mandibulare*) and the cranium is complex, involving several separate bones and joints. This complexity enables birds to move both the lower mandible and the upper mandible (*rostrum maxillare*) with respect to the cranium (see Figure 34.1). Some of these joints are prone to arthritis.

The quadrate bones rotate rostrally, pushing the jugal arches and the pterygoid bones. The pterygoid bones push the palatine bones rostrally. The palatine bones and jugal arches articulate against the lower edge of the maxillary bone causing it to tilt upwards.

Sinus formation is much more extensive and open, resulting in great weight reduction of the skull compared with mammals, but pneumatisation of the skull is much less than in many other avian Orders.

There is only a single occipital condyle, making the atlanto-occipital joint more mobile than in mammals.

Eyes

The eyes are surrounded by a ring of bony plates - the *annulus ossicularis sclerae*. In Anseriformes this is poorly developed but still provides some support for the eye. The nictitating membrane can extend fully across the cornea. The pupillary size is partially under concious control.

Beak

The beak consists of an upper jaw (*rostrum maxillare*) and a lower jaw (*rostrum mandibulare*). The bony components of the beak are covered by leathery keratin sheaths (rhamphothecae). The rhamphothecae have horny plates at the tips called nails (*unguis maxillaris* and *unguis mandibularis*), which are supported by thickened regions of bone and contain many mechanoreceptor nerve endings. The edges of the rhamphothecae (tomia) have horny lamellae used in apprehension of food, eg. in Shoveler Ducks (used for straining food out of the water) or in Sawbills (used for gripping slippery fish).

Tongue

The tongue is fleshy and muscular and usually adapted for cropping or straining food. It contains bony elements (the rostral basibranchial and entoglossal bones) which are part of the hyoid apparatus (see Figure 34.2). The terminal bones of the hyoid apparatus (the epibranchial bones) curve around the back of the skull and may be exposed in injuries to the skin in this area.

Cervical Vertebrae

The cervical vertebrae vary in number between different species and even within a species, and can reach as many as 25 (in swans).

Oesophagus

The crop is only a simple, spindle-shaped dilation of the oesophagus and is not readily distinguished from the rest of the oesophagus.

Trachea

The trachea has complete cartilaginous rings which overlap giving it greater rigidity than in mammals. The *mons laryngealis*, with the rostral opening of the glottis, is found at the base of the tongue and is clearly visible on examination.

Salivary Glands

Mucus-secreting salivary glands form an almost

Figure 34.1: *Diagramatic representation of the articulation of the maxillary bone with the cranium.*

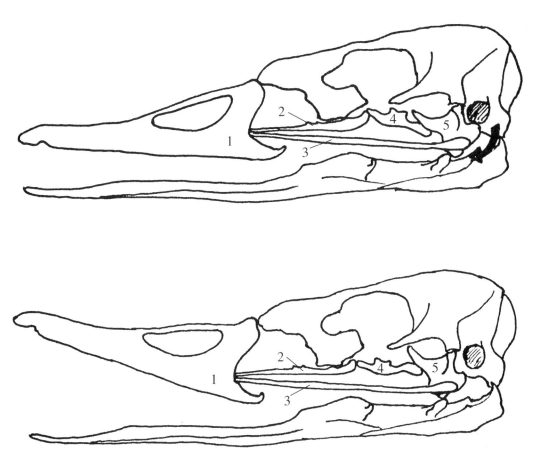

Captions
1. Maxillary bone   2. Palatine bone   3. Jugal arch   4. Pterygoid bone   5. Quadrate bone

The quadrate bones rotate rostrally pushing the jugal arches and the pterygoid bones.
The pterygoid bones in turn push the palatine bones rostrally.
The palatine bones and jugal arches articulate with the lower edge of the maxillary bone causing it to tilt upwards.

continuous layer on the dorsal and ventral surfaces of the oral cavity and in the tongue. The saliva is released through a large number of ducts whose openings are found all over the surface of the oropharynx.

PATHOLOGICAL CONDITIONS

Injuries

Foreign Bodies
Anseriformes, particularly swans, are prone to damage from fishing hooks and line. The plastic wrappers from 'fours' of drink cans can also cause trouble. Hooks are commonly found embedded in the rhamphothecae, the tongue, the skin of the neck, or the oesophagus. Some hooks are very small and may only be revealed by careful examination. Endoscopy may help locate hooks in the oesophagus, although an intractable length of fishing line protruding from the mouth and extending down the throat may indicate the presence of such a hook. Line may be caught on the tongue or beak where it may be very difficult to see but, if left, would cause unpleasant or serious injury. Line may also be anchored by an accumulation of food or by an impacted hook. If the hook cannot readily be dislodged using a fisherman's disgorger, then, after location by palpation or radiography, it can either be removed surgically under local anaesthetic or left in place after cutting the attached nylon as short as possible. A hook caught in the oesophagus usually becomes walled off by fibrosis, rusts away and causes no further trouble. Alternatively, threading the line through a stiff tube, eg. a bovine uterine catheter, may allow the hook to be manipulated and disgorged.

Nylon line commonly becomes entangled around the beak, and routine examination of waterfowl should include this possibility. Line can be completely hidden when it is wrapped tightly around the base of the

Figure 34.2: Dorsal surface of the tongue showing the position of the hyoid bones (Hawaiian Goose).

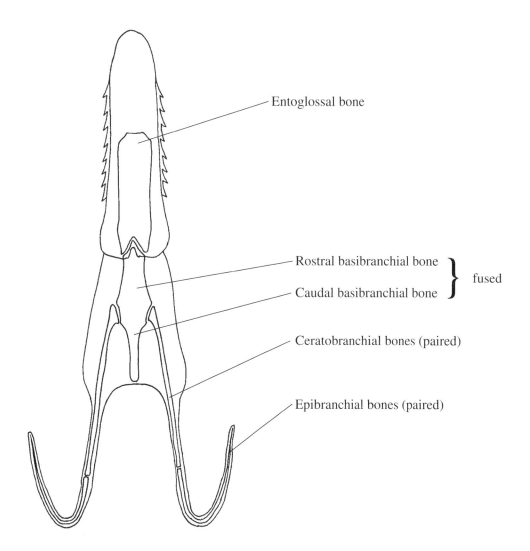

lower mandible. To ensure that this has not occurred, a finger should be run, whilst applying pressure, down the interramal region (the soft tissue joining the rami of the lower mandible) to the throat. Any nylon line present will catch on the finger.

Occasionally, twigs or slivers of wood will be eaten and may impact in the oesophagus, possibly causing serious damage and requiring surgical correction.

Flesh Wounds

Flesh wounds to the head and neck commonly occur and respond well to normal surgical repair. Wounds on the crown may reveal bony spikes which are the ends of the epibranchial bones of the hyoid apparatus: these should be carefully emplaced. In extreme cases, the exposed tips can be removed enabling easier surgical repair. This has no apparent ill effect.

Eye Injuries

Eye injuries are common and may result in blepharospasm (particularly of the nictitating membrane),

conjunctivitis, keratitis (see Figure 34.3), uveitis, hyphema, retrobulbar haemorrhage or total rupture of the eye. The nictitating membrane, which in birds is under conscious control, closes very rapidly making application of drops or ointment to the corneal surface difficult. However, all the common eye applications are suitable. Enucleation of the eyes carries a high risk because of the peculiar anatomy of the avian skull. Ruptured eyes will usually heal with only the precautionary use of antibiotics. The loss of sight in one eye appears to cause waterfowl little trouble: if the eye is left *in situ*, it is less likely to cause problems. A single intrabulbar injection of a therapeutic dose of gentamicin (5mg/kg) will stop fluid production and reduce the risk of infection after rupture of the eye (see Chapter 15).

Fractures

Fractures of the jugal arch, maxilla and mandibles are not uncommon. The end of the *os maxillare*, together with its horny sheath, may be broken off leaving an

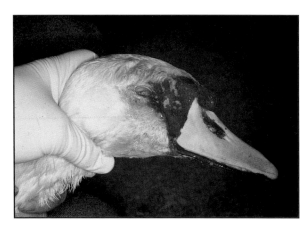

Figure 34.3: Mute Swan with keratitis and epiphora.

'undershot' appearance. Providing the bird can still groom, such damage causes little trouble. The implantation of a prosthesis - a technique for correcting beak damage in a number of avian species - would prove difficult in Anseriformes as the maxilla is paper-thin and offers no firm anchoring point. Jugal arch fractures will usually heal spontaneously to form a false joint that appears to allow normal function.

Damage to the Cervical Air Sac

This allows leakage of air into the subcutaneous loose connective tissue and results in a swelling that can be small and localised, or spectacular and generalised involving not just the neck but the thorax, abdomen and even thighs. This is clinically typical of subcutaneous emphysema. Usually, no action is necessary as the problem is self-limiting. However, cauterising one or two holes about 5mm diameter into the skin over the swelling will allow air to escape. The cauterised hole will heal naturally in 7-10 days by which time the leaking hole in the air sac should also have healed.

Parasitic Diseases

Nasal or Duck Leeches (*Theromyzon tessulatum*)

This is a common parasite infesting the nasal passages, sinuses and mouth of Anseriformes. It can also be found in the periorbital region. Ivermectin (0.02ml/kg or 200mcg/kg bodyweight s/c or i/m) produces a dramatic response.

Feather Lice

A number of species of lice can be found on the feathers of Anseriformes, eg. *Trinoton* spp. or *Anaticola* spp. A heavy louse burden often indicates underlying systemic disease. Some lice are known to inhabit the lacrimal ducts and cause epiphora. Lice also respond to ivermectin (see Chapter 35).

Laryngeal Streptocariasis

Streptocara spp. are nematodes that normally burrow in the mucosa of the oesophagus, proventriculus and ventriculus. There have been reports of these nematodes causing a necrotic, diphtheritic, plaque-like mass overlying and adherent to the pharynx and larynx, thus causing asphyxiation (Mason, 1988).

Trichomoniasis

This is a protozoal disease affecting the upper alimentary tract. Affected birds will loose weight, become listless and inappetent, and may show signs of dyspnoea. A deposit of yellowish-white, cheesy material may be found anywhere from the oropharynx to the proventriculus. The condition can be diagnosed by taking an oesophageal smear from a live or recently dead bird and examining it in isotonic saline under a microscope. Freshly examined trichomonads are highly motile and easily detected. Treatment is with dimetridazole (8g of dimetridazole per 30 litres of drinking water). All affected and in-contact birds should be treated for 12 days.

Infectious Diseases

Candidiasis

This is a yeast infection that may result from poor diet, poor hygiene or the inappropriate use of antibiotics. Spontaneous infection also occurs. Inappetence and loss of condition are the presenting signs and, at autopsy, the mucosa of the oesophagus will be thickened and may be overlayed with soft, white, cheesy deposits. A smear from the mucosa, stained with Lactophenol Blue or Diff Quik, will reveal typical, large, circular organisms. *Candida* spp. infections are particularly common in 'sea ducks', eg. Eiders, Scoters and Long-tailed Ducks, when they have not had access to natural or artificial salt water. It is thought that in these cases the nasal secretions inhibit yeast growth. When the birds are denied access to salt water, the salt glands atrophy and infection is more common. The lesions may occur in the mouth, but are also seen in the conjunctiva and nictitating membrane. Treatment with nystatin (100,000 units [1ml] per 300g bodyweight orally bid for 7-14 days) is usually effective. Nystatin is not absorbed from the alimentary tract, so if it is administered using a crop tube it may be placed distal to some lesions and will therefore not produce a response. Ocular lesions can be treated effectively with topical nystatin preparations, eg. Panalog (Ciba), applied twice daily. Any predisposing problem should also be treated.

Sinusitis

Sinusitis is a common problem in waterfowl, usually affecting the infraorbital sinus and presenting as unilateral or bilateral swelling beneath the eyes. Causative agents include *Mycobacterium* spp., *Pasteurella* spp., *Mycoplasma* spp., *Pseudomonas* spp. (see Figure 34.4), *E.coli* and and influenza A virus. The mucoid contents of the swollen sinuses are usually clear; collection using sterile technique will enable bacterial culture and sensitivity testing to be performed.

However, the majority of cases respond to sinus flushing with enrofloxacin (eg. 2.5% Baytril, Bayer). The bulging sinus should be lanced at the point of maximum swelling and the contents gently 'milked out'. The sinus is then flushed by applying the nozzle of the antibiotic filled syringe to the nasal opening on the same side as the swelling. The opposite nasal opening should be occluded whilst emptying the syringe. As the sinuses are very large, it is important to use adequate amounts of solution, ie. 5ml for a small duck (Teal) up to 30ml for a large swan, and to repeat the procedure daily until the external outline of the sinus(es) has returned to normal and no more mucus is being produced.

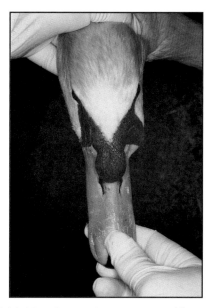

Figure 34.4: *Mute Swan with sinusitis caused by Pseudomonas spp.*

Avian Tuberculosis
Caseous lesions may be present in the oesophagus, pharynx or trachea (see Chapter 39).

Duck Viral Enteritis (Duck Plague)
This is caused by a herpesvirus and can result in severe losses in waterfowl collections. Signs are usually sudden death, but some ailing birds may be found with blood issuing from the vent and, in males, prolapse of the penis. Autopsy reveals classical diphtheresis of the oesophageal mucosa and there may also be sores on the beak and under the tongue (see Chapter 39).

Pox Virus
Typical, brown, pox lesions may be found on the beak, at the commisures, in the gape and in the pharynx or the sinuses (see Chapter 35).

Viral Tracheitis
Adenovirus and paramyxovirus can both cause signs of upper respiratory disease with a tracheitis (see Chapter 37).

Pasteurella anatipestifer
This usually causes a peracute infection with sudden death in ducklings. Clinical cases may show upper respiratory signs including ocular discharge.

Chlamydiosis
As part of a general disease picture, infection with *Chlamydia psittaci* can cause ocular and nasal discharges and dyspnoea. This is not uncommon in Anseriformes. Diagnosis is by ELISA or PCR tests performed on droppings or autopsy material (liver, spleen or air sac wall) (see Chapters 18 and 37).

Avian Cholera
This is caused by *Pasteurella multocida*. Clinical signs include mucoid oral discharges, dyspnoea, diarrhoea or sudden death. It is much less common in this country than in North America, where epizootics affecting wild populations occur annually, often with mortalities numbering hundreds of thousands in one outbreak.

Toxaemias

Lead Poisoning
This is still a common problem in wild Mute Swans and in captive wildfowl collections, despite a ban on split lead shot for fishing. Lead is environmentally persistent and shotgun cartridges are still a widespread source of metallic lead. The clinical picture includes weakness of the neck muscles causing a typical posture with the head resting on the bird's dorsum (see Chapter 38).

Botulism
This causes a clinical appearance very similar to lead poisoning (see Chapter 38).

Incidental Poisons
A number of substances, eg. dimetridazole and organophosphorus pesticides, have been cited in the literature for causing disease with similar signs to lead poisoning (see Chapter 38).

Impactions

Sublingual
This is seen as an obvious sublingual swelling between the tongue and the interramal region. Examination will reveal a ball of impacted food or earth which can be manually removed with ease. If such an impaction is left untreated for a significant period of time, it can lead to permanent dilation of the area which then keeps refilling. Surgical correction may be required.

Oesophageal Impaction Caused by Lead Poisoning
Impaction of the oesophagus as a result of toxaemia causing peristalsis failure is a very common complication

of lead poisoning. The impaction starts in the ventriculus or proventriculus and builds up cranially along the oesophagus until the entire length can be affected. Clearing this impaction can be very difficult and should be undertaken with the bird anaesthetised. External manipulation can be used in mild cases, whilst an ingluviotomy may be helpful when the impaction is more severe.

Oesophageal Impaction Caused by Foreign Bodies

Impacted hooks and/or line in the oesophagus can act as a focus for the accumulation of vegetable matter. This usually presents as a discrete swelling in the mid-oesophageal region. Surgical removal can be performed easily using local anaesthetic only. Care should be taken to suture the oesophagus securely in two layers.

Deformities and Congenital Abnormalities

Torticollis

Radiography may reveal developmental abnormalities of the cervical vertebrae. Apart from the abnormal posture, birds seem little affected by this condition.

Cerebral Lipidosis

This is an hereditary disease in Hawaiian Geese. The clinical picture is one of progressive ataxia, especially of the hindlimbs. *Post-mortem* examination reveals no gross lesions and diagnosis is by histopathological examination of the cerebrum (Wight, 1976).

Beak Deformities

Parvovirus infection has been cited as causing stunted beaks with protruding tongues in ducklings surviving an outbreak (Lu *et al*, 1993).

Tumours

A variety of tumours have been reported affecting the head and neck of waterfowl. These include subconjunctival hibernomas (Murphy *et al*, 1986), dermoids (Busch, 1985) and teratomas (Homer and Riggs, 1991).

REFERENCES AND FURTHER READING

Beer JV (1988) *Diseases of Game Birds and Wildfowl.* The Game Conservancy, Fordingbridge.

Brown MJ, Linton E and Rees EC (1992) Diseases of swans in captivity. *Wildfowl* **43**, 58.

Busch TJ (1985) Bilateral dermoids in a goose. Correspondence. *New Zealand Veterinary Journal* **33**, 189.

Coles BH (1985) *Avian Medicine and Surgery.* Blackwell Scientific Publications, Oxford.

Homer BL and Riggs MW (1991) Cranial teratomas in two domestic ducks (*Anas platyrhynchos domesticus*). *Avian Diseases* **35**, 994.

Keymer IF and Gough RE (1986) Duck virus enteritis (anatid herpesvirus infection) in Mute Swans (*Cygnus olor*). *Avian Pathology* **15**, 161.

King AS and McLelland J (1979) *Form and Function in Birds. Vols. 1 to 4.* Academic Press, London.

King AS and McLelland J (1984) *Birds: Their Structure and Function.* 2nd Edn. Baillière Tindall, London.

Lu YS, Lin DF, Lee YL, Liao YK and Tsai HJ (1993) Infectious bill atrophy syndrome caused by a parvovirus in a co-outbreak with duck viral hepatitis in ducklings in Taiwan. *Avian Diseases* **37**, 591.

Mason RW (1988) Laryngeal streptocariasis causing death from asphyxiation in ducks. *Australian Veterinary Journal* **65**, 335.

McLelland J (1990) *A Colour Atlas of Avian Anatomy.* Wolfe, London.

Murphy CJ, Bellhorn RW and Buyukmihci NC (1986) Subconjunctival hibernoma in a goose. *Journal of the American Veterinary Medical Association* **189**, 1109.

Ochiai K, Jin K, Itakura C, Goryo M, Yamashita K, Mizuno N, Fujinaga T and Tsuzuki T (1992). Pathological study of lead poisoning in Whooper Swans (*Cygnus cygnus*) in Japan. *Avian Diseases* **36**, 313.

Smith GR (1993) Botulism. In: *Diseases and Parasites of Birds. Proceedings of the Autumn Scientific Meeting of the British Ornithologists' Union.* BOU, Tring.

Wight PAL (1976) The histopathology of a cerebral lipidosis in the Hawaiian Goose (*Branta sandvicensis*). *Neuropathology and Applied Neurobiology* **2**, 335.

CHAPTER THIRTY FIVE

Feathers and Skin

Ian Robinson

INTRODUCTION

The feathers of waterfowl can be divided into contour feathers and down feathers. Their basic structure is shown in Figure 35.1.

Contour Feathers

Body Feathers
These are large feathers with a semi-rigid structure. They have a long calamus, a small plumaceous part and large vanes with interlocking barbules. The feathers are arranged in tracts (*pterylae*) separated by relatively bare spaces (*apteria*). The arrangement of these tracts is characteristic for each species.

The function of body feathers is to form a continuous waterproof layer over the body. Although following the approximate shape of the body beneath, they are sufficiently large and rigid to define the outer contour of the bird. Therefore, they create a space for the underlying down feathers, which they protect. In waterbirds particularly (the term waterbird includes all species which live on or near water, and not just Anseriformes), the outer contour can vary significantly from the body shape beneath; the amount and distribution of the downy layer between is responsible for the insulation and buoyancy required for an aquatic lifestyle.

Flight and Tail Feathers
These are very long feathers found on the wings and tail. They have a very long rachis with large, stiff vanes and long barbs with strong barbules. They have little or no plumaceous part. Their function is to produce the outer contour of the wings and tail and, by their size and shape, define the aerodynamic qualities of the bird.

Down Feathers

Down
These have a fluffy vane, a rachis shorter than the longest barb and no barbules. Their function is to provide insulation and buoyancy. The down feathers cover the body below the body contour feathers.

Semiplume
These have a fluffy vane and a rachis longer than the longest barb. They occur along the margins of the feather tracts (*pterylae*).Their function is to provide insulation.

Natal Down
These have a fluffy vane and cover the whole of the newly hatched chick of most waterbirds in a dense layer. They lack barbules on the tips of the central barbs. They provide insulation and waterproofing of the chick until the first moult.

Filoplume
These are found very close to the follicle of each contour feather. They have a long fine shaft with a tuft of barbs at the end. Their follicles have many nerve endings. They are proprioceptive and enable the bird to sense the most effective position for the associated contour feathers.

Hypopennae or Afterfeathers
These are small feathers which project from the distal umbilicus of contour feathers. They provide insulation.

Powder Down
These feathers shed a fine waxy powder of minute keratin granules into the plumage. Their function is to help maintain feather condition. Amongst waterbirds, they are only found in Herons.

Bristles
These feathers have a stiff rachis and few or no barbs. Their follicles are surrounded by encapsulated corpuscles. They are found particularly around the mouth and eyes. Their function is sensory and proprioceptive.

WATERPROOFING

Waterproofing is a characteristic of the structure of contour feathers. The feather vane, with its rows of interlocking barbs and barbules, forms a lattice structure with an airspace between. The size of this airspace is such that an impenetrable air-water interface

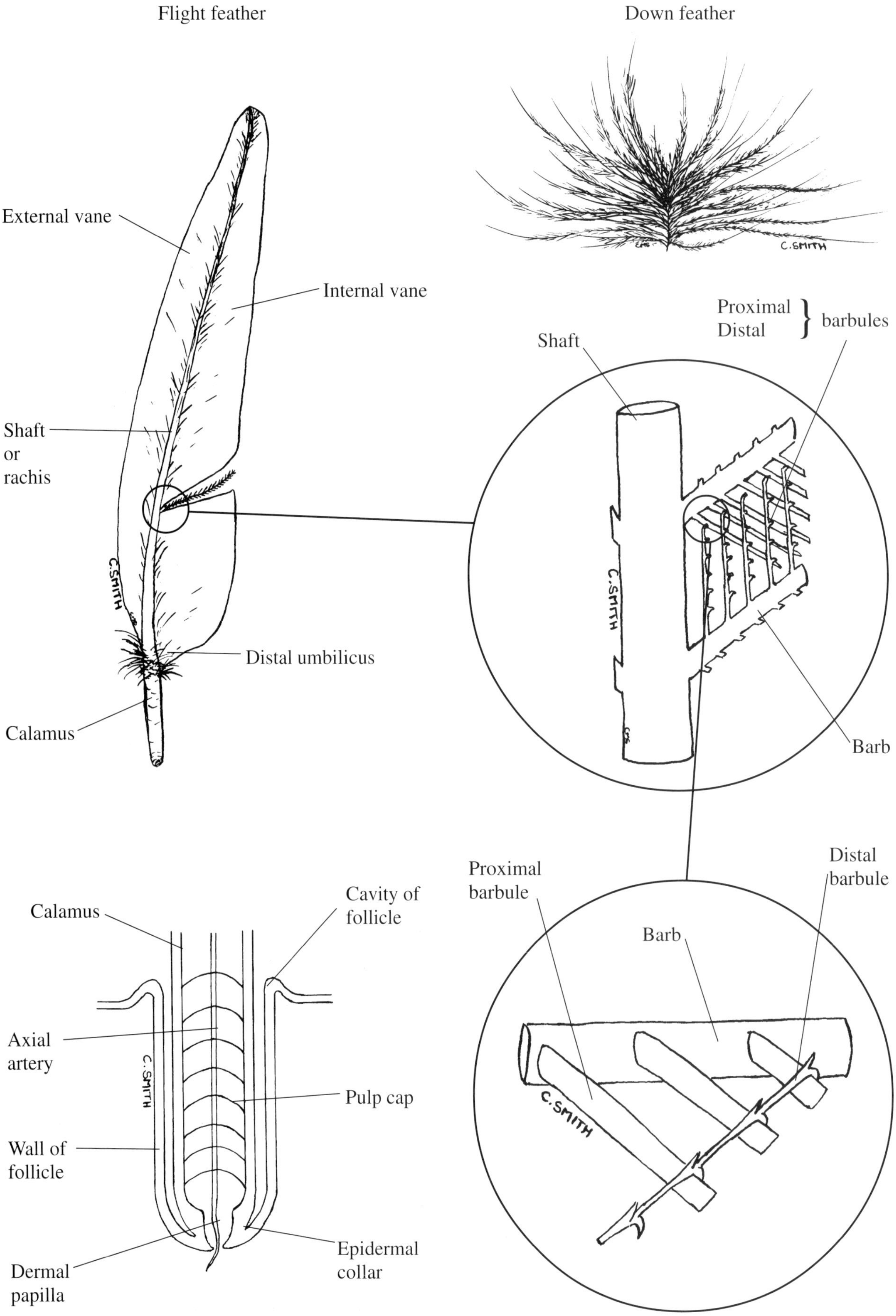

Flight feather

Down feather

External vane

Internal vane

Shaft
or
rachis

Distal umbilicus

Calamus

Shaft

Proximal
Distal } barbules

Barb

Calamus

Cavity of
follicle

Axial
artery

Pulp cap

Wall of
follicle

Epidermal
collar

Dermal
papilla

Proximal
barbule

Distal
barbule

Barb

Figure 35.1: Diagram of contour feather and down feather. (Drawings by Colin Smith.)

is created by surface tension and the feather repels water.

The degree of waterproofing depends on the microscopic anatomy of the feather. Adult Mallard contour feathers have near ideal proportions. Other species may have a less efficient structure: for example, cormorants 'wet out' after prolonged immersion and must leave the water to dry off.

Birds are waterproof because of the intrinsic anatomy of their feathers. Oils play no part in waterproofing.

Moulting

Moulting is the process by which feathers are lost and replaced. The pattern of moulting follows an orderly progression and varies between species. Most adult birds moult once per year after the breeding season, although many species of duck change plumage twice per year (see Chapter 33). Feathers are lost sequentially in order to maintain an adequate body cover at all times. Swans, geese and some ducks loose all flight feathers simultaneously. A period of some weeks of flightlessness follows until the flight feathers regrow. Feathers which become damaged will not be replaced until the next moult. It is therefore essential that feathers are maintained in good condition between moults.

Preening, the Uropygial Gland and Oils

Preening has three functions:

● In order to maintain a waterproof layer, feathers which become disarranged must be reorganised. Barbs and barbules are reunited by pulling the feather between the mandibles, 'zipping' the disordered feather vane together again.

● When feathers are exposed to the environment the keratin they contain gradually dries and becomes brittle. The delicate barbs and barbules can break off and the waterproof structure is lost. Most waterbirds have a well developed uropygial (or preen) gland.

● To spread oil from the uropygial gland to the feathers.

The regular application of oil from the uropygial gland keeps feathers strong and flexible, and prolongs their life. Some oil is also released onto the skin from developing epithelial cells. Naturally produced oils from the uropygial gland are not responsible for waterproofing. However, they do prolong the functional waterproof life of the feathers.

If the uropygial gland is destroyed by trauma or disease, the feathers gradually become dull, dry and brittle. If feather damage is severe, feathers will cease to provide a patent water repellent structure. When the bird moults the new feathers will be waterproof until they too dry out and become damaged.

Ducklings

Artificially reared ducklings in their natal down are very prone to loss of waterproofing due to the poor structure of these feathers. Naturally reared ducklings spend a long time being brooded by their mother (or a parent) and this keeps them clean and dry. This process is difficult to maintain artificially. Unless specialised rearing facilities are available, ducklings are best reared away from water until after their first moult. Water can be provided in drinkers which prevent the ducklings becoming wet, or a bowl of water can be filled with pebbles so that the ducklings can drink but not immerse themselves.

Wet Feather

Waterproofing is dependent on the maintenance of a patent feather structure. Anything which disrupts this can lead to a loss of waterproofing and the soggy appearance known as wet feather. The commonest causes of wet feather are 'shaft lice' (*Holomenopon* spp.) (see later), the prevention of preening (often caused by misguidedly keeping waterfowl away from water, even for a few days), chemical contamination (see later) or biological contamination. Figure 35.2 shows a typical case of wet feather where the bird has been kept in the proximity of Osier Willow trees. These trees are commonly affected by 'sooty mould' (*Cladasporum herbarum*). Mould spores can fall from the trees onto the birds' feathers where they will continue to grow and cause disruption to the waterproofing, thus leading to wet feather. The only solution to the problem is to remove the birds or remove the trees. Once wet feather has occurred, the feather structure will only return to normal following the next moult. Some of the causes of wet feather are listed in Table 35.1.

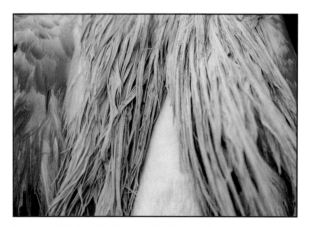

Figure 35.2: *Wet feather in a flamingo. (Photo courtesy Wildfowl and Wetlands Trust)*

TREATMENT OF OILED BIRDS

Before attempting to remove contamination from the feathers of an oiled bird it should be examined clinically and any parenteral symptoms treated. The washing process is stressful. To maintain waterproofing once washed, vigorous preening is required. Only birds that are bright, active and alert should be washed. Good

Table 35.1. Causes of wet feather in waterfowl.

Cause	Clinical signs	Treatment
Lack of preening - sickness - debilitation - behavioural	Feather vanes become disrupted and are not rearranged by preening.	Diagnosis and treatment of underlying problem. Preening can sometimes be stimulated by gently spraying with water.
Soiling of feathers - faecal material - mud - dirty or dusty bedding - plant oils or spores	Feather structure is clogged with dirt.	Correction of environment. Allow access to clean shallow water for bathing and preening (often called 'weathering'). Birds which become waterlogged may drown in water a few centimetres deep.
Chemical contaminants - oil - surfactants	Oil clogs the feather structure and causes them to clump together. Surfactants reduce surface tension and break down the air-water interface in the feather structure.	Light contamination may be treated as for soiling. Heavy contamination requires washing. Sea ducks, sawbills and sea birds rarely respond to weathering and are best washed.
Physical damage to feathers	Interlocking barbs and barbules broken. Lattice structure lost.	If severe and widespread, waterproofing will not return until after the next moult, when new feathers emerge.
Infestation with shaft lice (*Holomenopon* spp.)	Intense irritation causes excessive preening and feather damage.	Diagnose by examining a freshly plucked feather with a hand lens. Treat with acaricides (see later).

veterinary and nursing care before washing and correct timing of the decision to wash are essential for success.

Some sequelae to oil contamination and their treatment are shown in Table 35.2.

Washing Process

Many products and techniques have been tried on oiled birds, from smearing with lard to clothing in woolly vests. Practical experience and *in vitro* testing have shown that the best method is washing in a surfactant solution. The surfactant of choice is Fairy Liquid (Proctor and Gamble). A 2% solution is adequate, but in practice small amounts of neat detergent are applied to difficult residues. Other critical factors are a water temperature of 42°C (range 40-45°C) and a high pressure from the shower used for rinsing (90psi at the shower head is ideal). The water system should be capable of producing water at this temperature and pressure throughout a prolonged washing period. A swan may take over an hour to wash and rinse; a small sea bird or duck 45 minutes. Blown hot air, eg. a fan heater, is ideal for drying washed birds.

A suitable pool with a constant water flow which drains by overflow from the surface (surface skimming) is required for after-care. This will optimise surface tension and ensure that any oil or detergent contamination is quickly removed. Unless these minimum facilities are available, washing should not be attempted.

Two people are required to carry out the washing process: one to hold and one to wash. The bird is immersed in a solution of detergent at 42°C. The holder keeps as much of the bird's body as is possible immersed in the detergent solution whilst presenting the required area of feathers to the washer. The washer rubs the feathers from base to tip between his/her finger and thumb until they are all clean (see Figure 35.3). It is essential that no oil residue is left. The feel of the feather between the fingers in important in assessing cleanliness.

It is important to follow a standard routine so that no feathers are missed. It is usual to start with the head, using a toothbrush or cotton bud if necessary to remove oil from around the nares and inside the beak. The neck and dorsal surface of the body and tail are then cleaned. The bird is rolled onto one side then the other to wash each wing and flank. Finally, the bird is held on its back while the breast feathers and ventral aspect of the tail feathers are washed. Heavily contaminated birds may be washed in this manner two or even three times, discarding heavily soiled detergent solution each time until no more oil comes off the feathers.

The operators must ensure that their hands and clothing, and the working surfaces, are free of detergent contamination before commencing to rinse. Using a shower jet at 42°C and high pressure, the washer rinses against the lie of the feathers until all detergent is

Table 35.2. Sequelae of oil contamination, and suggested treatments.

Sequela	Cause	Clinical signs	Treatment
Hypothermia	Loss of insulating properties of the feathers. Penetration of water to the skin.	Dull, inactive appearance. Shivering. Low body temperature.	Gentle warming, preferably in a stream of warm air, eg. fan heater, followed by maintenance at ambient temperature of 19-21°C.
Diarrhoea	Gastrointestinal irritation by ingested oil.	Visible evidence.	Adsorbants given orally, preferably activated charcoal.
Dehydration	Effect of diarrhoea.	Oval, sunken eyes. Tight inelastic skin. PCV > 60%.	Fluid therapy (see Chapter 3).
Bacterial enteritis	Secondary to gastrointestinal irritation.	Often at *post-mortem examination*.	Prophylactic antibiotics may be given (see Chapter 5). Enrofloxacin (10mg/kg i/m or p/o sid) is effective in most species (best used i/m as birds are often diarrhoeic) .
Haemolytic Heinz body anaemia	Toxic effect of some crude oils. Toxic effects on liver and kidney are not common findings in oil ingestion.	Low PCV (< 30%).	Symptomatic. Haematinics, eg. iron dextran (10mg/kg i/m). Do not release affected birds until PCV returns to within normal range (37-53% for most species) or at least 30%.
Emaciation	Pre-existing subclinical conditions, eg. parasitism. Some lightly oiled sea birds are primarily victims of starvation and emaciation. Oil contamination is a secondary problem.	Clinical examination. Faecal examination.	Treat clinical conditions. Good nutrition (see Chapter 33). Inappetent birds can be fed by stomach tube. Hills A/d diet (mixed with a little water) is suitable for tube feeding most species and can be fed at up to 5% of bodyweight per day split over 3-4 feeds.
Aspergillosis	A sequela of an immune suppression or a contaminated environment and an inadequate ventilation when many birds are housed together.	See Chapter 18.	See Chapter 18.

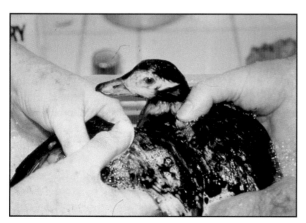

Figure 35.3: *Washing a Long-tailed Duck - feathers rubbed between finger and thumb from base to tip. (Photo courtesy RSPCA Photograph Library)*

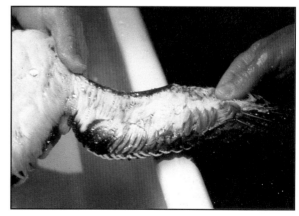

Figure 35.4: *The wing of a Guillemot during the rinsing process. Note the water beading on the feathers. (Photo courtesy Doug Walker, RSPCA)*

removed and water is beading on the feathers. The holder must ensure that contaminated water always flows off the bird away from areas already rinsed. The same methodical routine should be used for rinsing as for washing, taking care that no feathers are missed.

On completion, water should be beading freely on all areas of the bird's plumage (see Figure 35.4). Water from the shower head can be run over the plumage. Any area where water is seen to penetrate the feathers is not 'proofed' and needs further attention. Because of the danger of recontamination the whole body should be rinsed again, concentrating on areas of water penetration. Once completed the bird can be placed in the drying area (see Figure 35.5).

The bird should be left in a current of warm air until dry. Most birds will quickly start to preen. As soon as they are completely dry, birds can be put on water. In practice, birds are usually left overnight and introduced to the pool the following day.

Fish-eating birds should be fed from shallow trays away from the water to ensure the water surface is not contaminated with fish oil. Pool sides should be easy to clean and gently sloping for easy exit if birds become wet.

Once on water it is essential that birds preen. Regular preening will organise remaining disordered barbules and ensure that a patent waterproof layer is regained. Failure of waterproofing can be due to either residual contamination or failure to preen, allowing water to penetrate areas of poor feather structure.

It is usual to retain birds on water for a period to ensure waterproofing is secure. Four to five days is sufficient for most waterfowl, but sea birds may take up to ten days before their plumage shows no water penetration and they are fit for release.

Further Information

Help and advice on oiled birds and oil spill incidents can be obtained from the following sources:
- Royal Society for the Prevention of Cruelty to Ani-

mals (RSPCA) - local helpline. Tel. No: 0990.555999.
- RSPCA Headquarters, Causeway, Horsham, West Sussex RH12 1HG. Tel. No: 01403.264181.
- RSPCA Wildlife Hospital, Little Creek, West Hatch, Taunton, Somerset TA3 5RT. Tel. No: 01823.480156.
- RSPCA Norfolk Wildlife Hospital, Station Road, East Winch, King's Lynn, Norfolk PE32 1NR. Tel. No: 01553.840045.
- RSPCA Stapely Grange Wildlife Hospital, London Road, Stapely, Nantwich, Cheshire CW5 7JW. Tel. No: 01270.610347.

For further information regarding the washing process, a video titled 'Second Chance' is available from RSPCA Headquarters.

EXTERNAL PARASITES

Shaft lice (*Holomenopon* spp.) have been associated with outbreaks of wet feather. However, ectoparasites seldom cause problems in waterfowl. Most waterfowl are asymptomatically infested with lice, which are very mobile within the plumage. Debilitated birds can become heavily infested and require treatment, if only on aesthetic grounds.

Choosing an ectoparasiticide and the method of treatment for waterfowl is similar to other birds (see Chapters 14 and 26). However, if the preparation chosen contains oil, this may destroy the waterproofing of the feathers. Therefore, if such preparations are used, it is advisable to reintroduce the bird to water under close observation.

MISCELLANEOUS SKIN CONDITIONS

Avipox - this papilloma producing virus infection may affect the skin of the feet (see Chapter 36) and the head (especially the commissures of the beak) (see Chapter 34).

Frostbite may cause dry gangrene of the extremities, particularly the feet (see Chapter 36).

Photosensitisation has been reported following ingestion of *Hypericum* spp. berries (Forbes, personal communication). The skin of the legs and feet (except a small band on the left leg of each bird which was covered by an identification ring) became erythematous, oedematous and pruritic. The birds were maintained away from sunlight and, with good nursing, they all made a full recovery in three weeks, except for one bird which died of liver failure.

FURTHER READING

Tseng F (1993) Care of oiled sea birds: a veterinary perspective. In: *Proceedings of the 1993 International Oil Spill Conference*. American Petroleum Institute, Washington DC.

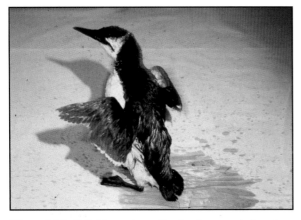

Figure 35.5: A Guillemot immediately after completion of the rinse. Feathers shed water but are in disarray and need to be preened into place (Photo courtesy RSPCA Photograph Library).

CHAPTER THIRTY SIX

Wing and Leg Problems

Patrick N Humphreys

LIMB DEFORMITIES

Anomalies of growth and skeletal deformities are not uncommon in young, fast-growing waterfowl.

Hypovitaminosis D

Hypovitaminosis D can occur when young waterfowl, especially those from low latitudes, are given too high a proportion of protein in their diet. This stimulates the long bones to grow at a rate which requires more vitamin D than can be provided. Therefore, insufficient calcium is absorbed and ossification cannot proceed normally. Shortening of day length or elimination of ultraviolet light may potentiate this problem. Plain wheat and short grass pastures alone are sufficient for normal growth in geese. Feeding a diet containing less than 18% protein to susceptible species will prevent the problem arising.

Developmental Conditions of the Limbs

A particular problem affecting the legs of young flamingos is found in some flocks. It is seen most often in chicks that are hatched later than the main sitting, usually from 'replacement' eggs. These birds grow rapidly; however, the proximal tibiotarsus becomes bowed laterally (see Figure 36.1), the birds become lame, they cease to thrive and they may have to be destroyed on humane grounds. The condition is not present in all flamingo breeding flocks, but is found mostly in Chilean Flamingos, possibly because this species breeds more readily in captivity. The condition was first reported in 1975 and has since been the subject of further research (Humphreys *et al*, 1989). The radiological picture is similar to that seen in classic cases of rickets in man. The precipitating cause of the condition is still obscure: one theory, amongst others, is that these late hatched birds are being fed the crop secretions of more than one pair of adults. The resulting high level of protein in the diet produces excessive rates of growth of the bird's legs and normal mineralisation of the tibial growth plate cartilage does not occur, thus leading to bowing of the proximal tibiotarsus. The syndrome may manifest itself lower down the legs in some long-legged birds, eg. storks and ostriches, but it is likely that the aetiology is the same as for flamingos.

If the wings are affected by this condition, the carpometacarpus rotates laterally, inducing an 'inside-out' appearance, known colloquially as 'slipped wing' or 'angel wing'. Some keepers have had success by strapping up the wing: if this is done while the wing is still growing, the condition is likely to be corrected in 4-7 days. A surgical method of correction involving osteotomy, insertion of an intramedullary pin into the radial metacarpus and realignment of the distal limb has been described (Yeisley, 1993). This procedure achieves a cosmetic appearance at least, but not all cases appear to gain flight capability.

ORTHOPAEDICS

Fractures and dislocations of wings and legs can be repaired using a number of orthopaedic procedures such as pinning, wiring, external coaptation, etc. More information can be found in the relevant chapters in the raptor section of this manual (see Chapters 16 and 17). Blass (1987) gave an excellent review of published work on this subject and he made the valuable point that success in this field is inversely proportional

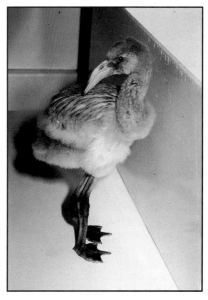

Figure 36.1: *Bowed tibiotarsus in a young flamingo. (Photo courtesy Wildfowl and Wetlands Trust)*

to the time that has elapsed since the original injury. A bird that has been grounded in the wild for some days is likely to be hypoglycaemic and a poor immediate surgical risk.

Treatment of fractures in the limbs of waterfowl may differ from that of raptors as it is not usually so vital to restore flying ability. However, birds such as swans, because of their weight, impose greater strains on their pelvic limbs than ducks.

Fractures in the legs of flamingos and screamers (Anhimidae) are difficult to repair satisfactorily, partly because there is a relatively poor blood supply available and also because patients may be reluctant to stand up after treatment.

Another constraint to surgery is the poor water hygiene and quality commonly available: provision of water is necessary for rehabilitation. Poor water quality can easily give rise to contamination of surgical incisions. The provision of clean water which is changed regularly, as well as sealing of skin wounds, eg. with OpSite Spray (Smith and Nephew), helps prevent infection of wounds from the water.

Best results are achieved using techniques which will allow immediate weight bearing and normal joint function, eg. intramedullary pinning and bone cement, or external fixation (see Chapters 16 and 17).

SHOTGUN TRAUMA

Lameness, wing weakness or bone fractures are commonly due to shotgun trauma. This possibility should not be ignored when assessing a new patient. Many wild birds carry a considerable amount of shot in their bodies: this is inert and does not appear to interfere with normal activity. Radiography should distinguish between inert lead in the body and ingested shot which can cause lead poisoning. A dorsoventral and a lateral view is necessary if doubt exists. Non-enteric lead can, in exceptional circumstances, cause lead poisoning, although this is very rare; however, it does occur occasionally when lead is lodged within the bone marrow (Forbes, personal communication).

PINIONING

This surgical procedure is commonly used as a method of restraint for captive waterfowl. The technique involves amputation of the terminal phalanx of one wing. This will cause the bird to lose balance when it attempts to fly. Pinioning of downies (young waterfowl) is best carried out at 2-3 days of age. No anaesthetic is required. With the bird held upside down in one hand, a sterile pair of scissors is used to cut through the major and minor metacarpal bones just distal to the alula (see Figure 36.2 for anatomical orientation); this will prevent permanently any primary feathers developing on that wing. Only one wing is pinioned. Haemorrhage is slight and may be controlled with silver nitrate if

necessary. Typically, the procedure is carried out by lay persons on birds under ten days of age. There are some adverse welfare implications. Legally, pinioning can only be carried out in adult birds by a veterinary surgeon. However, the procedure does have a role to play in establishing free-flying flocks of geese: a pinioned pair may be the foundation of a flock of their own unpinioned progeny which will subsequently remain in the vicinity. If older birds are to pinioned, either a small volume of local anaesthetic (0.5ml of 1:10 diluted lignocaine) or a general anaesthetic (see Chapter 9) must be used. A tourniquet is placed around the humerus. The feathers are removed from the wing to be pinioned from a level just proximal to the carpal joint to halfway down the metacarpal. The skin is prepared and two sutures of absorbable suture material (sutures a and b) are placed around the proximal metacarpal and the proximal minor metacarpal as shown in Figure 36.2. The skin is incised distal to this point and the soft tissue cleared down to the bone. The two bones are cut proximally as shown, the soft tissue is brought together over the stumps, and the skin is closed with horizontal mattress sutures. There should be no tension on the skin.

Other methods of restraint by interference with the wings, such as propatagiectomy or radial neurectomy, have not proved satisfactory in practice, and have generally been discontinued.

WING WEAKNESS

Inability to fly may be caused by trauma to a wing or by a generalised systemic disease such as botulism, infectious enteritis, duck plague, tuberculosis or lead poisoning (see Chapter 38). Occasionally, septic arthritis of a joint may cause loss of flight, but this is relatively uncommon in waterfowl compared with other groups of birds.

Infected bite wounds to the wings of swans, caused by foxes, are a common problem. These require aggressive therapy as they often result in severe necrotising infected lesions and interference with distal circulation. Bacterial sensitivity testing, broad-spectrum antibiosis, removal of necrotic tissue and twice daily lavage and drainage are essential, together with normal nursing care.

LEG WEAKNESS

Apart from systemic disease, eg. tuberculosis, leg weakness is seen in waterfowl infected with the renal coccidian *Eimeria truncata*. There may also be ataxia with a tendency to tip forward. *E. truncata* infection is most often diagnosed initially on *post-mortem* examination. Treatment must be with a parenterally (rather than an enterically) active drug, eg. clazuril or toltrazuril (see Appendix - Formularies [Waterfowl]). Recovery rates are good except in very severely affected

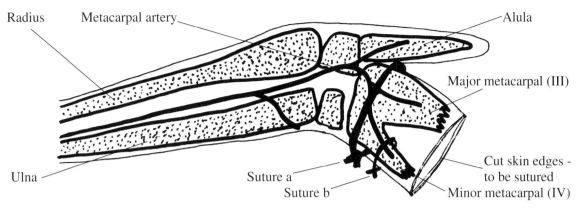

Figure 36.2: Carpal area showing the site for pinioning.

Radius   Metacarpal artery   Alula

Major metacarpal (III)

Cut skin edges - to be sutured

Suture a   Suture b   Minor metacarpal (IV)

Ulna

cases, but return to normal health can take 2-3 weeks. (Ataxia is also seen is cases of lead poisoning.)

Paralysis of the legs, often permanent, may be encountered if long-legged species of birds are transported with their legs folded under their bodies. A necrotising myopathy results. After surgery and during transport these species must have their legs extended or be allowed to stand.

Mycoplasmal Tenosynovitis

Mycoplasmal tenosynovitis is found occasionally (see Figure 36.3). The pathogen involved is *Mycoplasma synoviae*, which is predisposed to by Newcastle disease infection (Blaxland *et al*, 1982). The disease can occur in the acute or chronic form, presenting with anaemia, pallor, breast blisters and respiratory symptoms, or with gross articular and tendon swellings with concurrent lameness. Diagnosis is based on clinical signs and *post-mortem* findings, and on isolation of the pathogen. Treatment of early cases with tylosin, lincomycin or spectinomycin (see Appendix - Formularies [Waterfowl]) may be effective. Tendon or joint swellings may become secondarily infected with other pathogens such as *Staphylococcus* spp. or *Streptococcus* spp.

FOOT PROBLEMS

Frostbite

Certain tropical or near-tropical species of waterfowl, eg. Whistling Ducks and flamingos, are prone to frostbite of the phalanges if exposed to ice or snow when roosting (see Figure 36.4). Geese and ducks frequently sit on their feet in cold weather to keep them warm; this should not be considered to be abnormal behaviour. Frostbite usually causes a dry gangrene of one or more toes which are subsequently lost. In many cases the birds do not appear inconvenienced, but nevertheless birds may die from acute septicaemia or bacterial endocarditis as a result of frostbite. An increase in water temperature and good water hygiene may help prevent frostbite.

Infections

Infections of the feet are common in waterfowl,

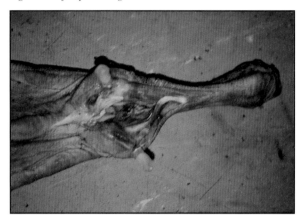

Figure 36.3: Mycoplasmal tenosynovitis. (Photo courtesy N A Forbes)

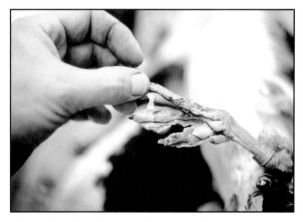

Figure 36.4: Frostbite of the phalanges. (Photo courtesy Wildfowl and Wetlands Trust)

particularly those which are forced to stand on concrete surfaces. The plantar surfaces of the feet of certain species, eg. swans and flamingos, are relatively thin and are easily scratched or bruised. Mixed bacterial infections are found, usually involving the whole plantar surface of the foot (see Figure 36.5).

Bumblefoot occurs most commonly in larger species such as swans (see Figure 36.6), due either to chronic wear, pressure and abrasion (especially when birds have to walk on hard surfaces such as concrete or tarmac, eg. Penguins) or following crash landing on tarmac surfaces as can occur when birds confuse the shimmering surface of a road for a water surface.

Treatment of bumblefoot is similar to that used in raptors (see Chapter 16). The main complication is that the foot cannot be kept dry during the treatment because the web will crack, and if kept off water the bird may stop preening. Conservative treatment should be given initially, comprising increased swimming time, covering rough surfaces with butyl rubber or Astroturf sheets, topical applications of ointments (eg. Preparation H, Whitehall Laboratories), improved diet and supplementation with vitamin A. In severe cases, surgery may be required. Following surgery, the bird should walk only on soft surfaces, eg. grass, for at least four weeks.

Pox virus does occasionally affect the feet of waterfowl as well as their heads (see Chapters 15 and 34), leading to characteristic multiprojectional viral papillomata (see Figure 36.7). The lesions self-heal in 6-8 weeks, although they may become secondarily infected with bacteria in the meantime.

MISCELLANEOUS

Avian tuberculosis, caused by *Mycobacterium avium*, frequently affects bone, producing discrete lesions with or without other systemic tuberculous lesions. Tuberculosis is the commonest cause of lameness in

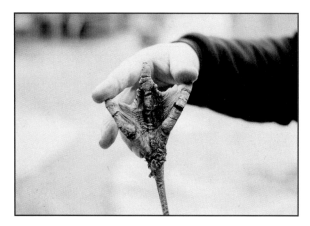

Figure 36.5: Severe cracking and infection in the foot of a flamingo. (Photo courtesy Wildfowl and Wetlands Trust)

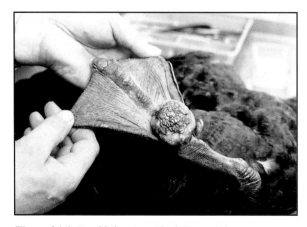

Figure 36.6: Bumblefoot in a Black Swan. (Photo courtesy Wildfowl and Wetlands Trust)

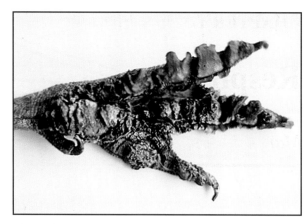

Figure 36.7: Viral papillomata. (Photo courtesy Wildfowl and Wetlands Trust)

many waterfowl collections. Most cases will be in older birds. These birds are likely to be in poor body condition, with little pectoral muscle covering.

Captive geese and ducks frequently live to advanced ages and become liable to a number of degenerative diseases. **Arthritis** may arise secondarily to articular gout or septic arthritis, or be simply due to wear and tear. The species most commonly affected by arthritis of the leg joints are those which are less well adapted to living on, and walking on, land, ie. large ungainly birds such as Steamer Ducks and Muscovy Ducks.

Aflatoxins - these are metabolic products of *Aspergillus flavus*, occurring most commonly in peanut or maize containing feeds. Although the most significant pathology in adult waterfowl is liver cirrhosis, cyanosis of the feet and legs can occur in affected young birds.

REFERENCES AND FURTHER READING

Blass CE (1987) Orthopedics. In: *Companion Bird Medicine*. Ed EW Burr. Iowa State University Press, Ames.

Blaxland JD, Cullen GA, Gordon RF and Jordan FTW (1982) Diseases caused by the bacteria *Mycoplasma* spp. and *Chlamydia* spp. In: *Poultry Diseases*. 2nd Edn. Eds RF Gordon and FTW Jordan. Baillière Tindal, London.

Fowler ME (1986) Ducks, geese, swans and screamers (Anseriformes). In: *Zoo and Wild Animal Medicine*. 2nd Edn. Ed ME Fowler. WB Saunders, Philadelphia.

Humphreys PN, Morgan AJ and Davies BLl (1989) Abnormalities of growth in young Chilean Flamingos (*Phoenicopterus chilensis*). In: *Verhandlungsbericht des 31st Internationalen Symposiums über die Erkrankungen der Zoo und Wildtiere, Dortmund*. Akademie-Verlag, Berlin.

Yeisley CL (1993) Surgical correction of valgus carpal deformities in waterfowl. In: *Proceedings of the Association of Avian Veterinarians Annual Conference 1993*. AAV, Lake Worth.

CHAPTER THIRTY SEVEN

Respiratory Diseases

Martin J Brown and Neil A Forbes

INTRODUCTION

Avian respiratory disease has already been discussed at length (see Chapters 18 and 28). Table 37.1 gives an overview, together with additional details, on diseases specific to waterfowl.

Table 37.1. Overview of respiratory diseases of waterfowl.

Agent	Clinical signs and diagnosis	Treatment and control
Aspergillus fumigatus	Weight loss, respiratory signs in terminal state. Ducks have anatomical variations in the syrinx which should not be misinterpreted as pathological lesions. Swans and geese do not have a syringeal bulla, although many have an elongated or coiled trachea.	Minimise exposure; prophylactic therapy of at-risk species. Penguins particularly susceptible. Diving and sea ducks most susceptible of waterfowl. Infection may occur by feeding mouldy corn or straw. Always commonest in stressed birds, eg. after oiling etc. Eggs can be infected prior to or during incubation. Retrieval of eggs from ground level nests helps to reduce incidence. See Chapter 18 for more details of therapy.
Pasteurella multocida - strains of varying pathogenicity (Humphreys, 1973)	Peracute death, dyspnoea, mucoid oral discharge, diarrhoea. Most species susceptible. Epidemics in captive and wild collections. Diagnosis on signs, history, microbiology. Carrier status birds may break down leading to an outbreak of disease.	Isolate cases, antibiosis, dispose of carcases, vaccination.
Avipoxvirus	Typical (wart like) pox lesions on feet; rarely in pharynx or eyes. Respiratory signs if in pharynx. Mild cases common, rarely serious.	Self-healing. General support and nursing care. Control insect vectors. Fowl or pigeon pox vaccine may be effective; however, not tested and rarely warranted. May be more prevalent in birds with vitamin A deficiency.
Orthomyxovirus	Sinusitis, mucopurulent/caseous (Olsen, 1994). Fowl plague. Captive wildfowl rarely affected. No record of disease in wild.	Improve hygiene, reduce stock levels, nursing care.
Chlamydia psittaci	Conjunctivitis, sinusitis, rhinitis, air sacculitis, diarrhoea, weakness.	Waterfowl are common carriers of this disease, which is a serious pathogen and zoonosis. Treatment by use of chlortetracycline (1,000ppm, ie. 18.2g/kg food, daily for 45 days); or doxycycline (8-25mg/kg p/o bid or 240ppm in food daily for 45 days; or 75mg/kg i/m weekly on six occasions); or enrofloxacin (500ppm in food or 10mg/kg i/m bid for 14 days). Despite medication, no test is available to check that the bird is no longer a carrier. Where collections are open to the public, with children feeding waterfowl by hand etc., this condition should be considered a significant zoonotic risk.

Table 37.1. Continued.

Agent	Clinical signs and diagnosis	Treatment and control
Newcastle disease (paramyxo-virus)	Respiratory, conjunctivitis, gastrointestinal or central nervous signs. Rare in waterfowl.	Vaccination, isolation and nursing of affected birds.
Bacterial/ mycoplasmal sinusitis	Unilateral or bilateral infraorbital swelling (see Chapter 18). Common in some species.	See Chapter 18.
Leeches (*Theromyzon tessulatum*)	Young birds most commonly affected. Causes head shaking, rhinitis, conjunctivitis. Impaired inspiration and sometimes vision. Debilitation, occasionally deaths.	Treat with ivermectin (200mcg/kg s/c or p/o, ie. 0.02ml/kg). Restrict access to water with significant leech infestation.
Air sac mites (*Cytodites nudus*)	Cough, dyspnoea. Seen in trachea and bronchi; rarely cause significant disease.	Treat with ivermectin (200mcg/kg s/c or p/o, repeat three times at 10 day intervals).
Gapeworms (*Cyathostoma bronchialis* and *Syngamus* spp.)	Coughing, depression, sanguinous tracheal mucus. Carrier adults; direct life cycle. Affects goslings.	Treat breeding adults in early spring prior to breeding season: all birds in autumn. Treat with any of the following : ● Mebendazole (5-15mg/kg daily for two days or 120ppm for 14 days). ● Levamisole (25-50mg/kg p/o). ● Ivermectin (200mcg/kg s/c or p/o). ● Flubendazole in food for seven days at 240ppm, ie. 2.4kg/tonne.

REFERENCES

Humphreys PN (1973) Some veterinary aspects of maintaining waterfowl in captivity. *International Zoo Yearbook* **13**, 87.

Olsen JH (1994) Anseriformes. In: *Avian Medicine: Principles and Application*. Eds BW Ritchie, GJ Harrison and LR Harrison. Wingers, Lake Worth.

CHAPTER THIRTY EIGHT

Nervous Diseases

Neil A Forbes

INTRODUCTION

Waterfowl, just as other avian groups, commonly suffer from nervous diseases. The causes of these conditions may be broadly divided into the following categories:
● **Poisons**. Poisons may be exogenous, ie. from outside the body, or endogenous, ie. produced within the body (frequently arising as a consequence of bacterial infections). Exogenous agents may be divided into naturally occurring poisons and man-made poisons.
● **Nutritional/Metabolic**. These are comprised of nutritional deficiencies and metabolic diseases. The latter give rise to abnormally high levels of metabolic by-products.
● **Traumatic**. Waterfowl, particularly larger species such as swans and geese, are less manoeuvrable in flight than smaller species. Therefore, they are more prone to in-flight collisions, especially with power cables. Collisions can give rise directly to nerve damage; however, they frequently result in a 'crash landing' and it is often the landing which causes the majority of nervous signs of traumatic origin. Waterfowl are frequently shot, legally or otherwise. Inevitably, a number of birds will receive non-fatal injuries. Some of these cases will present with nervous signs due to nerve damage (very rarely due to non-enteric lead particles giving rise to lead intoxication).
● **Infectious**. There are a number of common infectious conditions of waterfowl which give rise to acute or chronic nervous signs.
● **Congenital**. These are extremely rare.

Chapter 20 contains a thorough introduction to nervous diseases of birds. Table 38.1 gives a breakdown of causes of nervous conditions in waterfowl. Lead poisoning is dealt with at the end of this chapter.

Table 38.1. Nervous diseases of waterfowl, except for lead poisoning (see later).

Cause	Clinical signs	Diagnosis	Control, comments and prognosis
Endogenous poisons Bacterial, toxaemia.	Lethargy, weakness, acute central nervous signs (CNS).	Toxin tests, microbiology, histopathology.	Rare; spasmodic occurrence; rapidly fatal unless treated early and extensively.
Exogenous poisons Zinc poisoning, ingestion of galvanised wire, coins, etc.	Posterior paralysis, weight loss, anorexia.	Blood levels. Radiography.	As for lead poisoning (see later). Prognosis good if treated before condition is chronic.
Acetylcholinesterase inhibitors, eg. carbamates, malathion, dichlorvos.	Acute onset, many different possible CNS signs. Ataxia, convulsions, blindness, torticollis. May occur with drift from crop spraying or leaking into water course.	Diagnose on clinical signs and history. Blood assay is possible. Acute onset, many different nervous signs. (Acetylcholinesterase inhibition slowly reverses.)	Sedation (diazepam), nursing. Prognosis fair with good nursing. Medicate with atropine (0.1mg/kg i/v or i/m every 3-4 hours) or pralidoxime mesylate (10-40mg/kg) (non-proprietary: contact National Poisons Bureau for availability).

Table 38.1 Continued.

Cause	Clinical signs	Diagnosis	Control, comments and prognosis
Organophosphates, eg, fenthion.	Delayed onset, 1-3 weeks.	Weakness, ataxia, paresis. (Irreversible acetylcholinesterase inhibition).	No specific antidote. Increase fat reserves. Prognosis poor unless signs very mild.
Natural			
Clostridium botulinum, usually toxin type C. Water quality deteriorates in hot weather. Fish or invertebrates die, their carcases acting as a propagator for toxin. Maggots may act as source. Type C toxin does not affect mammals.	Limber neck (bird is not able to lift or support neck properly), acute onset flaccid paralysis of voluntary muscles. Summer or autumn. Sudden death, sometimes in mid-swim; many birds die from drowning. Ducks may be poisoned by ingesting only 2-4 infected maggots.	Clinical signs, history, toxin isolation (Central Veterinary Laboratory, Weybridge) from clotted blood.	If bird can still walk but not fly, good nursing will often be effective. If can swim but not walk, prognosis not so good, but may recover. Standard treatment is oral fluid therapy with activated charcoal and bismuth. If unable to lift neck, require antitoxin. If antitoxin and fluids are used to flush toxin from gut and bloodstream, 75-90% of affected birds may recover (Olsen, 1994). Carcases must be removed from water to prevent further toxin production. Define area of water affected and prevent birds from entering the water; use bird scarers etc. Toxin is stable in the environment. Increasing water flow (autumn floods) will remove toxin from water system.
Algal toxins. Occur in hot water when water flow slow.	Sudden death, blinking of eyes, hypersalivation, repeated swallowing. Prostration.	Clinical signs, presence of pathogenic algae in environment, exclusion of other causes.	Difficult. Increase water flow rate. Use copper sulphate, although this in itself may be toxic. Prognosis poor.
Plant poisons, eg. Oleander.	Ataxia, paralysis. Occurs more frequently in young birds.	CNS toxic plants in environment. If acute poisoning, presence of plant in gastrointestinal tract.	Exclusion of toxic plants from immediate environment of young inexperienced birds. Prognosis is dependent on plant involved and volumes ingested.
Nutritional			
Thiamine deficiency.	Opisthotonus ('star gazing').	Response to therapy.	Beware thiaminase-containing fish fed to fish-eating ducks (Kear, 1973). Treat with thiamine in drinking water (100μg/l). Prognosis good.
Vitamin A deficiency.	Ataxia, paralysis of chicks (Olsen, 1993).	Response to therapy, blood analysis, histopathology.	Good diet. Prognosis good.
Encephalomalacia. Vitamin E/selenium deficiency.	Opisthotonus, muscular dystrophy. Often die < three weeks of age.	Clinical signs, history, response to therapy. Histopathology.	Good diet, no excessive storage period. Prognosis good if treated prior to permanent damage.

Table 38.1 Continued.

Cause	Clinical signs	Diagnosis	Control, comments and prognosis
Metabolic Fatty liver degeneration. Many different causes (infection, toxin, obesity, etc.).	Hepatic encephalopathy. Ataxia, lethargy, fits, tremors.	Biochemistry, liver biopsy. CNS signs; worse shortly after eating (more pronounced in birds fed majority of daily food at one time rather than grazers). *Post-mortem* examination.	Many pet ducks become excessively fat. Prevent obesity and exposure to hepatic pathogens or toxins.
Renal failure.	Ataxia, fits.	Biochemistry. *Post-mortem* examination.	Not common. Prognosis hopeless.
Trauma Vitamin E/selenium deficiency or cellular anoxia and damage.	Capture myopathy. Leg or wing stiffness, weakness, unwilling to walk or fly.	Signs, history, biochemistry, histopathology.	Minimise stress in catching; reduce time restrained. If severe, prognosis grave; if mild, good.
Shooting/trauma. Wire strikes or impact injuries.	Any brain, spinal or peripheral nerve deficits.	Clinical signs, radiology, neurological examination.	Reduction of overhead wires; applying markers on wires. Steroid, manitol, sedation. Require good nursing. Recovery may take up to six weeks.
Infectious Duck viral enteritis (herpesvirus).	Photophobia, ataxia, lethargy, incoordination, tremors, haemorrhage, diarrhoea, nasal discharge. Sudden death.	Occurs April-June. *Post-mortem* examination. Haemorrhage from damaged blood vessels. Bloody enteritis. Necrotic/haemorrhagic ring at oesophageal/ proventricular sphincter. Virus isolation.	Vaccination immediately prior to risk period. May - June (occasionally seen August- October). Prognosis hopeless; usually find birds dead. Vaccinate all risk species prior to risk season. (See Chapter 39).
Duck viral hepatitis (picornavirus).	< 6 weeks of age. Spasmodic contractions of legs, opisthotonus, rapid death.	Diffuse haemorrhage. Virus isolation.	Isolation of affected birds. Vaccination of breeding females. Prognosis for affected birds hopeless.
Avian encephalo-myelitis (picornavirus).	Tremors < 1-2 weeks of age.	Virus isolation.	No treatment. Prognosis hopeless except in very mild cases. Vaccinate.
Goose viral hepatitis (parvovirus).	Ataxia, diarrhoea, coryza. Goslings < 30 days of age (Sandhu, 1986).	Serofibrinous pericarditis, hepatitis, ascites. Virus isolation.	Vaccination of breeding birds.

Table 38.1 Continued.

Cause	Clinical signs	Diagnosis	Control, comments and prognosis
Newcastle disease (paramyxovirus).	CNS, respiratory tract and gastrointestinal tract signs, conjunctivitis.	Not common. History, clinical signs, virus isolation, serology.	Vaccinate.
Salmonella spp.	Incoordination, collapse. Meningitis, septicaemia, enteritis. Nervous signs not common.	Caseous caecal plugs, focal liver necrosis, enteritis. Culture.	Good hygiene, vaccination.
Mycobacterium avium.	Ataxia, weight loss (see Chapters 19 and 39). Hindlimb lameness commonly. CNS signs (rare).	Culture.	Hygiene, screening and eradication, vaccination. Granulomata can form in any site in the body.
Pasteurella anatipestifer.	Paralysis, convulsions, dyspnoea.	Culture.	Vaccination, sensitivity testing and antibiosis. Severity of outbreak and antibiotic sensitivity varies between outbreaks.
Others Developmental abnormalities of cervical vertebrae.	Torticollis, or any signs of incoordination.	Clinical appearance and radiography.	Birds with mild clinical signs often cope well, despite major bony abnormalities. If severe, may require euthanasia.
Hereditary disease of Hawaiian Geese. Arises due to cerebral lipidosis.	Progressive hindlimb ataxia.	Clinical examination, breed line history, no gross lesions *post mortem*. Confirmed on histopathology.	Individual bird identification and careful breed line records should be kept for Hawaiian Geese.

LEAD POISONING

Lead poisoning remains one of the most significant causes of nervous disease in waterfowl. Goode (1981) estimated that as many as 4,000 swans are affected annually in the UK. Lead is ingested whilst feeding (waterfowl normally ingest particulate gravel to aid ventriculus action). Lead pellets may be buried in mud, where fishing or shooting has occurred previously. Waterfowl may ingest small numbers of lead shot intermittently or, in circumstances of reduced water levels, lead previously unavailable may suddenly be ingested in large amounts by large groups of birds, leading to acute outbreaks of severe lead intoxication.

International pressure is growing to ban the use of lead shotgun shot. However, even if this occurs, environmental contamination will lead to continued incidence for many years. Since 1987 the sale and use of lead ledger and split shot under 28gm in weight by fisherman has been banned in the UK. Since this time the incidence of poisonings has reduced markedly (Owen, 1992). Swans with CNS signs should be considered as possible lead poisoning cases.

Diagnosis

The characteristic clinical signs are weight loss, weakness, limb weakness, limber neck (see Figure 38.1) and bright green faeces. Whole body radiography may be of value in recent cases.

However, the grinding action of the ventriculus renders particulate lead into an undiagnostic state in a matter of 1-2 weeks. Chronic cases frequently show dilatation and impaction of the proventriculus, therefore diagnosis may be presumed in the absence of lead particles. Blood lead levels may be assayed on

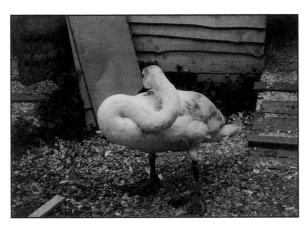

Figure 38.1: Juvenile Mute Swan with typical signs of lead poisoning.

whole EDTA blood (normal <0.4ppm; diagnostic 0.5-2.0ppm; severe >2.0ppm). Haematology may show moderate anaemia (20-38% haematocrit) (Degernes *et al*, 1989). A more recent and more sensitive diagnostic indicator is delta amino levulemic acid dehydrase (ALAD) activity (Degernes, 1995).

Treatment

If particulate lead is present in the ventriculus, it should be removed by gastric lavage (Degernes, 1989). Birds are fasted for 8-12 hours, anaesthetised and suspended by their back legs, inclined (head down) at an angle of 45°. A stomach tube (0.5cm diameter) is passed and held in place in the ventriculus. The ventriculus is irrigated with warm water using a stomach pump. Gravity and water pressure will remove most of the lead. Radiology will indicate if it is all removed. If lead is still present, birds should be allowed to recover and the process repeated the next day. Fragments of lead are usually trapped in crevices in the koilin. Once consciousness is regained and the muscular activity of the ventriculus has returned, the particles will precipitate and be able to be removed the next day when the process is repeated (Forbes, 1993).

All affected birds should receive chelation therapy.

Sodium Calciumedetate (10-40mg/kg i/v or i/m bid for 5-10 days) is effective. However, it has the disadvantage of being potentially nephrotoxic. Meso-2,3-dimercaptosuccinic acid (DMSA, Aldrich Chem Co, USA) is a water soluble heavy metal chelating agent. Dosing at 25-35mg/kg p/o bid five days a week for 3-5 weeks has been shown to be effective. At the time of publication (April 1996) this drug is not available in the UK.

Birds should be monitored closely during therapy by recording weight, behaviour, nervous signs and haematology. If therapy is stopped too early, even if blood lead levels have returned to normal, lead toxicosis can occur again as lead re-enters the circulation from bone and soft tissues.

REFERENCES

Degernes LA (1995) Toxicitites in Waterfowl. *Seminars in Avian and Exotic Pet Medicine* **4(1)**, 15.

Degernes LA, Frank RK, Freeman ML and Redig PT (1989) Lead poisoning in Trumpeter Swans. In: *Proceedings of the Association of Avian Veterinarians Annual Conference 1989*. AAV, Lake Worth.

Forbes NA (1993) Treatment of lead poisoning in swans. *In Practice* **15(2)**, 90.

Goode DA (1981) Lead poisoning in swans. In: *Report of the Nature Conservancy Council Working Group*. NCC, London.

Kear J (1973) Fish for captive waterfowl. *International Zoo Yearbook* **13**, 94.

Olsen JH (1994) Anseriformes. In: *Avian Medicine: Principles and Application*. Eds BW Ritchie, GJ Harrison and LR Harrison. Wingers, Lake Worth.

Owen M (1992) Progress on lead-free shot in the UK: 1991. *Wildfowl* **43**, 223.

Sandhu T (1986) Ducks, geese, swans and screamers: infectious diseases. In: *Zoo and Wild Animal Medicine*. 2nd Edn. Ed ME Fowler. WB Saunders, Philadelphia.

CHAPTER THIRTY NINE

Weight Loss and Enteritis

Martin J Brown and Ruth L Cromie

INTRODUCTION

Waterfowl are generally gregarious by nature and often maintained at high densities in the same area for prolonged periods of time. In these conditions, infectious diseases can frequently cause morbidity and mortality. Captive collections of waterfowl are often frequented by wild and feral birds which may act as vectors of disease.

AVIAN TUBERCULOSIS

Avian tuberculosis is a relatively common disease of captive waterfowl, particularly where the same pens and ponds have been used by birds for many years, allowing a build-up of the causative organism *Mycobacterium avium*. The disease is enzootic in many wild bird populations, particularly gregarious ground dwelling or water feeding species, and these may act initially as sources of infection for captive birds. Infection usually follows oral ingestion of the bacteria from a contaminated environment. As the bacteria live in damp and wet conditions, waterfowl are at particular risk of infection. Even within the Order Anseriformes there are different levels of susceptibility. The disease can cause high rates of mortality in dabbling and diving ducks and swans, ie. those birds which feed predominantly in and around water. Conversely, grazing geese which feed predominantly on dry land suffer lower mortality (Cromie *et al*, 1991). In addition to the genetic make-up of the bird and its feeding behaviour, environmental stresses can affect adversely both the incidence and the pathology of the disease. Although the disease does not have a strongly seasonal distribution and deaths can occur throughout the year, mortality may be precipitated by a stressful event in the bird's life, eg. females may die following breeding when their body condition is low.

The causative organism is slow growing and causes an insidious and chronic wasting disease with a typically slow rate of pathogenesis. Therefore, the disease usually affects older birds; infection in younger birds may indicate a compromised immune system. The slow progress of the disease allows the condition to remain subclinical for many months. Eventually, physical

condition is affected and signs may include some, or all, of the following: weight loss (the sternal keel may become very prominent following atrophy of the pectoral muscles), weakness, lameness, plumage deterioration and diarrhoea. Distension of the abdomen, caused by a build-up of ascitic fluid, may be one of the more specific signs of advanced disease.

At *post-mortem* examination the disease is characterised by caseous necrotic granulomatous lesions which may be minute, miliary or up to several centimetres in size. Typically, these lesions are found in the liver (see Figure 39.1), spleen and intestines, although they can develop in any tissue, probably following intermittent bacillaemia. In advanced cases, coalescing tuberculous masses can all but replace parenchymatous tissue. To confirm the diagnosis, a Ziehl-Neelsen stained smear from a lesion should be prepared. Tuberculous infection is indicated by the presence of numerous acid-fast bacilli.

Although birds as a whole are particularly susceptible to *M. avium* serotypes 1, 2 and 3, serotype 1 is the most common isolate from captive waterfowl.

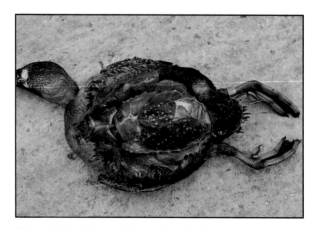

Figure 39.1: African White-backed Duck showing lesions of avian tuberculosis in the liver.

Diagnosis
Ante-mortem diagnosis of avian tuberculosis is notoriously difficult. A thorough physical examination should be carried out. A positive acid-fast stain of faeces may be indicative, although not diagnostic, of infection. The absence of acid-fast rods in stained faeces

does not indicate a non-tuberculous bird, as the bird may not have intestinal lesions or may not be shedding bacilli into the gut at that time. A serological test (ELISA) for the disease in waterfowl has been developed which can detect the disease at an early stage, probably before the bird becomes infectious (Cromie *et al*, 1993; Forbes *et al*, 1993). Unfortunately, at the time of writing this test is not commercially available. On haematological investigation, anaemia, leucocytosis (>18×10^9/l), monocytosis, heterophilia and hyperfibrogenaemia can be indicative of the disease (Hawkey *et al*, 1990). Diagnosis may often be confirmed by viewing lesions on the surface of the liver by laparoscopy under general anaesthesia. This may be useful for particularly valuable birds (Bush *et al*, 1976). (See Chapter 19).

Treatment

M. avium is highly resistant to antituberculous drugs, therefore there is essentially no effective chemotherapy for the disease; however, there have been reports of successful treatment of psittacines using protracted multiple drug combination protocols (Van der Hayden, 1994) (see Chapter 19). A novel immunotherapeutic agent has been used with variable results in medical trials. This therapy has been tried in tuberculous birds at The Wildfowl and Wetlands Trust and also in marsupials with *M. avium* infection at The National Zoological Park, Washington DC, USA.

Control

The protracted pathogenesis of the disease means that birds may shed large numbers of virulent bacilli for considerable periods of time. This, coupled with the bacteria's ability to survive for up to four years outside the host, creates a reservoir of infection, making control of the disease very difficult. Prevention of the disease is imperative.

Management

The best ways to prevent establishment of the disease are by:
● Maintaining well-nourished birds, free from as many stresses as possible.
● Ensuring high standards of hygiene, including incineration of any build-up of organic matter and droppings (attention should be paid to possible sources for spread of infection, eg. footwear of avicultural personnel, wheels of feed barrows, crates, etc.).
● Reducing stocking densities.
● Allowing areas to remain free of birds and then rotating stock.
● Restricting contact between wild and captive birds.
● Strict screening and quarantine of new additions to a collection.

In the event of an outbreak, birds known to be infected and in-contact birds should be euthanased (or possibly isolated if of particular conservation value). As the avian tubercle bacilli can remain viable in soil for considerable periods, an infected area must be decontaminated by removing topsoil, liming and replacing with clean soil. However, even this method may not be adequate. Contamination of eggs from infected females or a contaminated environment is highly unusual.

Vaccination

Currently, there is no commercially available vaccine, although encouraging results have been gained from a vaccine under trial at the Slimbridge Centre of The Wildfowl and Wetlands Trust.

PASTEURELLOSIS

Pasteurellosis, or avian cholera, is a highly infectious bacterial disease caused by *Pasteurella multocida*. Numerous species of wild, domestic and feral birds are susceptible to infection and massive outbreaks of the disease occur regularly among waterfowl in North America. Outbreaks in Europe are less common, but high mortality in wintering waterfowl and in breeding Common Eiders has occurred in Holland (Swennen and Smit, 1991).

Pasteurellosis typically causes sudden high mortality, but occasionally captive waterfowl may develop a chronic wasting disease associated with *P. multocida* infection. Transmission occurs by bird to bird contact, ingestion of bacteria from contaminated environments, and possibly from aerosols generated in the water from bird feeding and preening activity. Survivors of the disease may assume carrier status capable of maintaining the infection between outbreaks. Clinical signs include a mucoid oral discharge, dyspnoea, diarrhoea and sudden death. Affected birds often exhibit loss of balance and may walk or swim in circles.

Diagnosis

Acute mortality combined with gross lesions at *post-mortem* examination, which include petechial haemorrhages on the heart and serous membranes and focal necrosis of the liver, should alert the practitioner to the possibility of pasteurellosis. Heart blood smears stained with methylene blue usually reveal the presence of vast numbers of bacteria exhibiting bipolar staining. *P. multocida* can be readily isolated from the tissues of recently dead birds. It is imperative that laboratory diagnosis is undertaken, as many of the gross lesions are similar to those of duck virus enteritis.

Treatment

Antibiotic therapy using oxytetracycline (200mg/kg i/m), followed by in-feed tetracycline (500mg/tonne feed) is effective. Vaccination is effective in domestic poultry and may be considered in captive waterfowl.

Control

Rigorous collection and incineration of carcases to limit further environmental contamination must be carried out, as *P. multocida* persists in the tissues of dead birds for several weeks. Pond water remains infective for one month and persistence of the organism in decaying carcases and soil may be as long as four months.

YERSINIOSIS

Yersiniosis, or pseudotuberculosis, is a bacterial disease caused by *Yersinia pseudotuberculosis* and characterised by tuberculous-like lesions in many tissues. Numerous species of birds and mammals are susceptible, but waterfowl are affected infrequently. Infection occurs as the result of ingestion of bacteria from a contaminated environment. Clinical signs include weight loss, dyspnoea, diarrhoea, inappetence, reduced mobility and lameness.

Diagnosis

Bacterial cultures from the faeces may assist in diagnosis. *Post-mortem* signs in acute cases include miliary greyish-white foci in the liver and lungs, spleen enlargement and enteritis. In chronic cases, granulomatous lesions may be present in various organs and also in the musculature. Differential diagnosis to exclude tuberculosis and pasteurellosis should be carried out.

Treatment

Antibiotic therapy is seldom successful in chronic cases, but prophylactic treatment of clinically healthy birds in an affected group may be undertaken following sensitivity testing. No reliable vaccine is currently available.

Control

Rodents and wild birds act as reservoirs of infection and should be excluded from food storage areas and bird pens whenever possible.

ENTERITIS

Enteritis is one of the commonest conditions encountered in captive waterfowl and may be viral, bacterial or parasitic in origin. Although it may be the primary condition encountered, enteritis is often a secondary factor associated with other disease conditions, or brought about by stress due to a change in the bird's normal routine or environment. Such stress factors may enhance the virulence of commensal microorganisms which are normally present in the intestinal tract.

Parasitic Enteritis

Several parasitic infections are capable of initiating enteritis in waterfowl and they should be treated with appropriate anthelmintics (see Endoparasites).

Bacterial Enteritis

Enterobacteriaceae are a frequent cause of enteritis in waterfowl. They are Gram-negative bacteria which may be motile or non-motile and, in favourable conditions, are capable of propagation outside the host.

Escherichia coli, an ubiquitous organism, is undoubtedly the most important member of this genus. Numerous serotypes, both pathogenic and non-pathogenic, exist, although only a proportion are of importance as a cause of disease in waterfowl. *Salmonella* spp. have often been isolated from wild birds and outbreaks of salmonellosis in domestic and captive waterfowl are not unusual. Although all strains are a potential threat, *S. typhimurium* has most often been isolated as a causative agent in disease outbreaks. Birds which become infected may act as carriers capable of maintaining the disease for several months without showing signs of clinical infection. *Campylobacter* spp., particularly *C. jejuni*, has been implicated as the cause of disease in many species of birds, including ducks and geese, although the organism is frequently found in the alimentary tract of healthy birds. *Pseudomonas* spp. infections involving both *P. aeruginosa* and *P. hydrophilia* are a common cause of enteritis in waterfowl. Both organisms thrive in wet environments and propagate in water.

Transmission of virtually all these organisms is by the oral route, as all are shed in the faeces. In the case of *E. coli* and *Salmonella* spp., infective dust from dry faeces may cause infection via the respiratory system. Contamination of feedstuffs by rodents or wild birds, or even by humans, is an important consideration. *Salmonella* spp. infections are frequently passed through the egg (see Chapter 40).

Clinical signs of enteritis include diarrhoea, soiling of feathers around the vent, ruffling of plumage, inappetence and rapid weight loss. Young birds often show stunted growth.

Clinicians and staff working with wildfowl collections must be aware of the zoonotic potential of handling waterfowl with diarrhoea (particularly in relation to *Salmonella* spp. and *Campylobacter* spp. infection). Relevant precautions must be taken.

Diagnosis

Diagnosis and subsequent treatment can be based only on successful bacterial culture and antibiotic sensitivity testing. Sterile swabs may be used for the gut contents of freshly dead birds or for the freshly voided faeces of live ones. If there is likely to be a delay between swabbing and culture, the swab should be placed in nutrient broth or a transport medium to prevent desiccation.

Treatment

Antibiotic treatment should be formulated in line with bacteriology and sensitivity test findings. Soluble antibiotics, such as oxytetracycline in drinking water, work well in young ducklings. Access to other sources of water during the treatment should be restricted.

Control

Many outbreaks of bacterial enteritis, particularly in young birds, result from a lack of hygiene in the incubator and in the rearing and food storage areas. Contamination of feed by rodents and wild birds is a common problem and all possible methods of control and prevention should be instigated. Feeding utensils, rearing coops and duckery mats should be cleaned and disinfected daily; incubators must be thoroughly cleaned and fumigated between hatches. Soiled or damp feed should be removed from any area used to house birds, and preferably incinerated. The importance of personal hygiene among avicultural staff cannot be overemphasised. Hot running water and antibacterial soap should be used by all staff handling eggs or birds on each occasion to prevent possible spread of infection. Chlorhexidine applied between handling each batch of birds reduces greatly the risk of cross infection. Footwear and overalls should be disinfected or changed before entering incubation and rearing areas.

Viral Enteritis

Duck Viral Enteritis

Duck viral enteritis (DVE), often referred to as duck plague, is an acute, contagious herpesvirus infection of Anseriformes. The disease has a worldwide distribution and occurs in domestic, ornamental and commercial birds. The only known outbreak in wild waterfowl occurred in 1973 when an estimated 40,000 ducks, mostly Mallards, died at the Lake Andes National Wildlife Refuge in South Dakota, USA. Although all strains of the herpesvirus are antigenically alike, there appears to be a great variation in virulence and consequent mortality. As with other herpesvirus infections, birds which survive primary infection may become carriers, capable of shedding virus for up to four years.

Outbreaks of DVE can occur at any time, but there is a strong seasonal distribution, the disease being most prevalent in late spring and early summer. This marked seasonality of outbreaks is thought to be linked to the stress associated with breeding and the invasion of waterfowl collections by feral birds which may act as carriers during the mating season. Transmission occurs through contact with infected birds or a contaminated environment. In nearly all reported outbreaks, birds had access to water bodies which were frequented by free-flying wild or feral waterfowl.

All waterfowl are susceptible to DVE, but those species most commonly affected are Mallards and Muscovy Ducks; sheldgeese and shelducks (Tadornini) are also highly susceptible. In a limited number of outbreaks, Canada Geese and Mute Swans have experienced high mortality.

Clinical signs of DVE vary but include listlessness, hypersensitivity to light, a bloody nasal discharge, diarrhoea - which may be blood stained - and, in the case of male birds, prolapse of the penis. There is often no prolonged illness associated with the disease and apparently healthy birds may die suddenly with terminal convulsions, the head and neck arched over the back and the tail fanned or raised.

Diagnosis. At *post-mortem* examination there is a great variation in gross lesions, but vascular damage and haemorrhage are usually seen. Petechial haemorrhages are commonly observed on fatty areas of the heart and on the surfaces of the heart muscle (see Figure 39.2). Focal necrosis of the liver and pinhead sized haemorrhages in both liver and pancreas are often present. The lesions with the greatest value when diagnosing DVE are haemorrhagic or necrotic annular bands in the intestine of ducks; these occur where lymphoid tissue is present. In geese and swans these lesions are manifested by haemorrhage in lymphoid discs which are scattered along the intestinal tract (see Figure 39.3).

In addition, diphtheritic-like lesions may be observed on the mucosal surface of the oesophagus; these normally follow the longitudinal folds of the

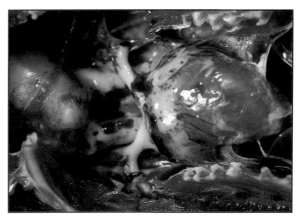

Figure 39.2: Petechial haemorrhages in the heart of a Mallard infected with duck viral enteritis.

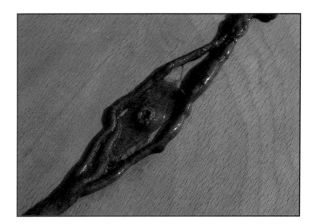

Figure 39.3: Necrosis of lymphoid disc in the intestine of a Barnacle Goose due to duck viral enteritis infection.

oesophageal tissue. Similar lesions may be present in the lower regions of the intestinal tract. Positive diagnosis of DVE can be made only by virus isolation following inoculation of embryonated duck eggs with homogenised tissues. Fresh, chilled liver, kidney and spleen are the preferred tissues, which should be submitted to a specialised laboratory.

Control. Due to the close association of DVE outbreaks with free-flying feral waterfowl, it is important to discourage these birds from established waterfowl collections by limiting available food and nesting sites. In cases where rare or endangered species are kept, it is advisable to prevent access to pens by free-flying birds. This may be achieved by building smaller aviary type housing or by netting over existing enclosures with strong nylon netting. In cases where an outbreak has become established, the prompt removal of carcases and contaminated litter is paramount; both should be incinerated without delay. Footbaths, using MAFF approved disinfectants, and decontamination of footwear, clothing and feeding utensils may limit the spread of the disease between pens. In cases where only a small number of birds survive an outbreak of DVE, euthanasia should be considered, as the remaining birds are likely to be carriers capable of maintaining the disease.

Vaccination. DVE outbreaks have been controlled in commercial, domestic and ornamental waterfowl in Europe and North America by the use of an attenuated live vaccine. At the time of writing (January 1996), there are no commercially available vaccines in the UK. However, the Central Veterinary Laboratories at Weybridge, Surrey, have produced a new vaccine, Anserivac, which is undergoing field trials and showing excellent results. It is hoped that this vaccine will be available in the near future.

ENDOPARASITES

A vast number of metazoan and protozoan parasites have been described from captive and wild waterfowl (McDonald, 1969), but only a limited number have been shown to be pathogenic. Typically, young birds and those debilitated by disease or adverse environmental conditions are most often affected. However, in situations where large numbers of infective hosts or eggs are present, parasitic disease may develop in apparently healthy adult stock. Clinical signs vary, but many endoparasites cause weight loss and inhibition of growth.

Diagnosis and successful treatment can be based only on correct identification of parasite eggs by faecal examination and the identification of mature parasites found during *post-mortem* examination. Useful information on parasitological laboratory techniques can be found in MAFF (1971). An excellent guide to the diagnosis of helminths by faecal examination can be found in Thienpont *et al* (1986).

Table 39.1 describes the most frequently encountered parasitic conditions in waterfowl.

PERITONITIS

Peritonitis, due to an infectious agent or irritant, is an occasional cause of morbidity and mortality in waterfowl. Infection of the peritoneum can become established following an air sac infection, in conjunction with neoplastic or cystic conditions, or due to a penetrating abdominal injury. Severe parasitic infestations can also result in the introduction of flora from the gastrointestinal tract to the peritoneum, eg. following *Acuaria* spp. infestation of the proventriculus, or *Polymorphus* spp. infestation resulting in severe gut wall damage. Waterfowl occasionally develop peritonitis due to perforation of the gastrointestinal tract following ingestion of a sharp foreign body. The presence of foreign bodies, eg. nails, pieces of wire, staples, etc., can be revealed on radiography.

Egg peritonitis is a relatively common cause of death of females both during and after the breeding season. The disease results following retention of an unlaid egg in the oviduct or rupture of a yolk during egg formation.

Clinically, birds appear depressed and display weight loss and inappetence. Leucocyte counts in both blood and peritoneal fluid are raised. Treatment of the disease in waterfowl is considered essentially ineffective, although broad-spectrum antibiotic therapy coupled with peritoneal lavage with antimicrobial agents may be of some value. In the case of a ruptured viscus or presence of foreign bodies, surgical procedures are indicated, although the prognosis is usually poor.

Control
Management of peritonitis requires controlling the causal factors of the primary problem or disease, eg. ensuring no sharp metal objects which can be swallowed are left in pens used by the birds, or taking preventive action to stop the build-up of intestinal parasites by regular use of anthelminthic chemotherapy or environmental management.

OTHER CONDITIONS

Several conditions which may cause weight loss and enteritis in waterfowl have been covered in other chapters. These include lead poisoning (see Chapter 38), aspergillosis (see Chapter 37), candidiasis and sinusitis (see Chapter 34).

Table 39.1. Summary of endoparasites found in waterfowl.

Species and host susceptibility	Clinical signs	Treatment
Nematodes *Amidostomum* spp. and *Epomidostomum* spp. (gizzard worm). Very common debilitating nematodes, especially in geese. Direct infection or by ingestion of transport host (earthworms etc.). Frequently pathogenic in young birds; inhibit growth.	Haemorrhage in gizzard and severe erosion of gizzard lining. Enteritis and diarrhoea, rapid weight loss. Eggs medium size; thin, smooth shell; large numbers of blastomeres.	Ivermectin (200mcg/kg p/o or s/c once); or in-feed mebendazole (1.2g/tonne for 14 days) or flubendazole (2.4kg/tonne for 7 days) prior to breeding season and after summer moult. Rest heavily grazed areas by rotation.
Cyathostoma spp. (see Figure 39.4) and *Syngamus trachea* (gapeworm). Common in young birds, especially geese. Direct infection or by ingestion of transport host (earthworms etc.).	Head shaking and coughing, respiration impaired by mucus in trachea. Bright red nematodes attached to wall of trachea visible by endoscopy. Eggs ovoid, smooth shell. *S. trachea* has operculum at both poles; not visible in those of *Cyathostoma* spp.	Ivermectin (200mcg/kg p/o or s/c once); fenbendazole (20mg/kg p/o once); or mebendazole or flubendazole in feed (see above). Dead parasites and debris remain in respiratory tract. (See Chapters 18 and 37).
Acuaria (*Echinuria*) spp. Debilitating nematode of ducks and swans, rarely seen in geese. Causes high mortality in young birds, especially swans. Infection by ingestion of intermediate host, *Daphnia pulex* (water flea). Typical seasonal (summer) occurrence due to large numbers of *D. pulux* in warm water conditions.	Tumours or nodules containing parasites in proventriculus and at gizzard/proventriculus junction. These may impair passage of food, thus causing starvation. Rapid weight loss, inhibited growth in young birds, enteritis and diarrhoea. Eggs small, ellipsoid, contain single infective larva.	Ivermectin (200mcg/kg p/o or s/c once) or fenbendazole (20mg/kg p/o once). Tumour-like lesions remain after death of parasite. Increase water flow through ponds to discourage build up of *D. pulex*.
Acanthocephalans *Fillicollis anatis* and *Polymorphus* spp. All waterfowl species affected but mortality in Eiders and young swans reported commonly. Infection by ingestion of intermediate host (crustacean), usually *Gammarus* spp. (freshwater shrimp).	Cylindrical non-segmented parasites found in lower small intestine, often bright yellow or orange in colour. May cause gut rupture and peritonitis. Emaciation, enteritis and rapid weight loss.	Ivermectin (200mcg/kg p/o or s/c once); levamisole (25-50mg/kg p/o or s/c once); benzimidazole (eg. fenbendazole) (20mg/kg p/o once). Segregate birds from water areas containing large numbers of intermediate hosts.
Trematodes Numerous species of digenetic flukes with life cycles involving mollusc intermediate hosts. Very few species are pathogenic. Wide range of waterfowl species act as hosts.	Enteritis in lower small intestine. Most species of fluke are found in the intestine, although some species may be found in the respiratory tract.	Praziquantel (10mg/kg i/m, s/c or p/o daily for 14 days). Chlorsulon (20mg/kg p/o three times a week at two week intervals).

Table 39.1. Continued.

Species and host susceptibility	Clinical signs	Treatment
Cestodes Numerous species. *Hymenolepididiae* spp. often found; usually pathogenic only when secondary to other debilitating conditions. Large numbers sometimes found in young birds, especially swans. Freshwater invertebrates act as intermediate hosts.	Found throughout the intestinal tract, including the caeca. They can sometimes be found by cloacal examination of a live bird. May cause enteritis and diarrhoea if present in large numbers.	Praziquantel (10-20mg/kg i/m or s/c, repeat after 10 days). Chlorsulon (20mg/kg p/o three times a week at two week intervals).
Hirudinae *Theromyzon tessulatumn* (duck leech). Attaches itself inside the nasal cavity or conjunctival spaces in a wide range of species.	Head shaking, constant sneezing, conjunctivitis. Leeches often visible in nostrils and attached to conjunctiva. (See Chapter 34). Combination of blood loss and interference with respiration and vision can be debilitating, especially in young birds; mortality can occur.	Physical removal of leeches. Ivermectin (200mcg/kg p/o or s/c once). Restrict access to water areas heavily populated by leeches.
Protozoa Coccidiosis. *Eimeria* spp. rare in intestinal tract, but *E. truncata* often causes renal coccidiosis which may be highly pathogenic in young geese (see Figure 39.5).	Kidneys grossly swollen and mottled with white foci. Affected birds show inappetence, rapid weight loss, lethargy and diarrhoea.	Sulphonamide (25mg/kg p/o bid or 10mg/kg i/m bid). Clazuril (5-10mg/kg p/o every 3rd day on three occasions).
Sarcocystis spp. rare in UK, but found commonly in North American waterfowl.	Muscular weakness, lethargy, death.	Pyrimethamine (0.5mg/kg p/o bid for 30 days).

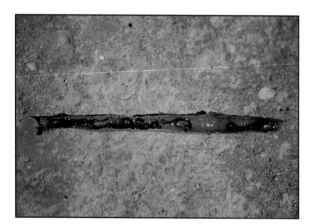

Figure 39.4: *Trachea of a goose showing gapeworm (Cyathostoma bronchialis) infestation.*

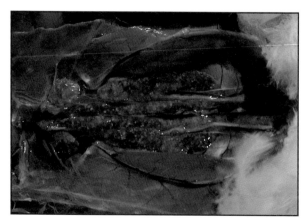

Figure 39.5: *Kidneys of a Lesser Snow Goose showing renal coccidiosis (E. truncata) infection.*

REFERENCES

Bush M, Montali RJ, Smith EE and Peratino WS (1976) Clinical experience with tuberculosis in exotic birds. In: *Mycobacterial Infections of Zoo Animals*. Ed RJ Montali. Smithsonian Institution Press, Washington DC.

Cromie RL, Brown MJ, Price DJ and Stanford JL (1991) Susceptibility of captive waterfowl to avian tuberculosis: the importance of genetic and environmental factors. *Tubercle* **72**, 105.

Cromie RL, Brown MJ, Forbes NA, Morgan J and Stanford JL (1993) A comparison and evaluation of techniques for diagnosis of avian tuberculosis in wildfowl. *Avian Pathology* **22**, 617.

Forbes NA, Cromie RL, Brown MJ, Montali RJ, Bush M and Stanford JL (1993) Diagnosis of avian tuberculosis in wildfowl. In: *Proceedings of the Association of Avian Veterinarians Annual Conference 1993*. AAV, Lake Worth.

Hawkey CM, Kock RA, Henderson GM and Cindery RN (1990) Haematological changes in domestic fowl (*Gallus gallus*) and cranes (Gruiformes) with *Mycobacterium avium* infection. *Avian Pathology* **19**, 223.

McDonald ME (1969) *Catalogue of Helminths of Waterfowl*. United States Department of the Interior, Bureau of Sport Fisheries and Wildlife. Special Scientific Report. Wildlife No. 126. Washington DC.

Ministry of Agriculture Fisheries and Food (1971) Technical Bulletin No. 18. *Manual of Veterinary Parasitological Laboratory Techniques*. Her Majesty's Stationery Office, London.

Swennen C and Smit TH (1991) Pasteurellosis among breeding Eiders (*Somateria mollissima*) in the Netherlands. *Wildfowl* **42**, 94.

Thienpont D, Rochette F and Vanparijs OFJ (1986) Eds. *Diagnosing Helminthiasis by Coprological Examination*. Janssen Research Foundation, Beerse.

Van der Heyden N (1994) Update on avian mycobacteriosis. In: *Proceedings of the Association of Avian Veterinarians Annual Conference 1994*. AAV, Lake Worth.

CHAPTER FORTY

Neonatal Diseases

Neil A Forbes

HATCHERY AND INCUBATION HYGIENE AND TECHNIQUES

The health status of young waterfowl is initiated when the egg is formed and laid. Genetic, infectious, nutritional and husbandry factors all interact from this point. Some breeders will allow birds to incubate naturally; for others, artificial incubation facilitates greater control and a potentially greater production. If eggs are to be artificially incubated, a decision must be taken whether to artificially incubate throughout, in which case eggs should be collected as soon as possible after laying, whilst they are still minimally contaminated, or to allow the female to 'set' the clutch, ie. to incubate it herself for the first 5-7 days. The latter method allows better fertility rates, but also leads to higher rates of egg contamination, which may be a major factor when many eggs are being incubated together, as one infected egg may contaminate the whole incubator. Eggs should be collected in a clean padded receptacle. Storage should be between 15°C and 21°C (LaBonde, 1992) in racks or boxes with the air sac (round end) uppermost. Many breeders will fumigate (in potassium permanganate and formaldehyde), wash or dip eggs (in commercial egg sanitising solutions). Sterilising of eggshells using ultraviolet light (Monachon, 1973) prior to incubation is routinely used by some waterfowl breeders. Waterfowl eggshells are usually more heavily contaminated than other avian species, due to the damp nest sites often chosen by waterfowl. Grossly contaminated or cracked eggs should be discarded. Eggs should not be stored for more than 14 days.

The incubator should be housed in the hatchery, which should itself be a self-contained micro-environment. The hatchery should be easily cleaned and well-ventilated, and be maintained at a constant temperature and humidity. Dust should be kept to a minimum. Hatchery hygiene should be monitored using microbiological settle plates. Blood agar and Sabouraud's medium plates are left open in the hatchery for 10 minutes, then incubated for 24-48 hours to give a bacterial and fungal colony count. This gives an assessment of hatchery hygiene.

Accurate hatchery records detailing numbers of eggs per pair, dates laid, dates incubated, fertility rates, weights during incubation, hatchability and neonatal survivability are essential. Both naturally and artificially incubated eggs should have a hatchability of 85-90%, although this is often not possible due to unavoidable contamination of eggs prior to incubation.

Causes of infertility are as follows:

Parental Factors
● Age.
● Diet (protein, fat, carbohydrate, energy content, calcium and vitamins must all be adequate).
● Antibiotics (many, if used prior to egg laying, will lead to reduced chick hatch weights).
● Concurrent disease.
● Immature/behavioural/social stress/psychological problems.
● Poor parental incubation.
● Clumsy incubation causing repeated egg damage.

Environmental Factors
● Unsuitable nesting sites.
● Dirty, contaminated or unsuitable nest material.
● Inter- or intraspecies aggression which may prevent breeding.
● Insufficient access to food and water.
● Ectoparasites or other disease vectors in the nest.
● Unsuitable macroclimate for that species.
● Unsuitable microclimate (temperature, humidity) of the nest site.
● Toxic substances in the environment (antibiotics, pesticides, herbicides, exhaust gases, etc.).
● Medical, fungal or toxin contamination of the food.

Incubation
● High bacterial contamination of eggs - death or weak offspring.
● Excessive jarring or shaking of eggs - early death or deformations.
● Eggs not laterally positioned, with air cell (round end) up - malformations or malpositions.
● Normal incubation temperature 37.3-37.5°C. Humidity 85%.
● Incubation temperature low - late dead-in-shells, late weak hatchlings.
● Incubation temperature too high - death, weak,

small, dehydrated, unretained yolk sac.
● Humidity too low - lower egg weight; weak, dehydrated, calcium deficient young.
● Humidity too high - large, unretained yolk sac; wet young, may asphyxiate.

Candling Eggs

Eggs should be candled first at 6-7 days. The importance of candling is that it identifies and allows the removal of cracked, infected or non-viable eggs. Moreover, it allows early detection of failed development. Assessment of the stage of egg failure greatly facilitates determination of the cause of the failure. All 'dead-in-shells', ie. fertile eggs which fail to hatch following incubation, should be fully investigated irrespective of the stage of death. Egg deaths may be divided predominantly into early (0-5 days from start) and late (perihatching) deaths. Early deaths are most likely to be caused by faulty incubation temperature, jarring and inbreeding, whilst late deaths are likely to be caused by faulty humidity, temperature or turning. Infection of eggs before or after egg laying can lead to early or late death, or weak young.

Egg Weights

Eggs should lose 12-13% of their initial weight by pipping. At least a sample of individually identified eggs should be weighed at intervals during incubation. A graph is plotted for each egg. The initial weight and target hatch weight are marked, with the incubation period being the interval between the two points. At each weighing, the new weight is entered on the graph and compared with the projected ideal weight loss for that stage of incubation. If the weight is too high, the humidity is too high and should be reduced, and *vice versa*. There may be problems when incubating eggs of different size or shells of differing porosity in the same incubator, as each will require different humidity control.

NEONATAL CARE

Most species are precocial and eat readily for themselves after hatching. Food and grit should be given within 24 hours of hatching. A starter or chick crumb with a protein level of 20% should be given for the initial 2-3 weeks. Thereafter, a grower ration with a protein level of 16% is suitable for most species up to 4-6 months of age. Young waterfowl are very active. Water for bathing should be provided within 24 hours of hatching. This should be in shallow pebble-filled bowls to prevent the young birds from drowning. A typical duckling brooder is shown in Figure 40.1.

Hay, straw, shavings, newspaper, etc. should not be used for bedding; it may tangle around feet, be eaten and cause impaction, or act as a source of *Aspergillus* spp. infection. Plastic matting or artificial grass, eg. Astroturf, is suitable.

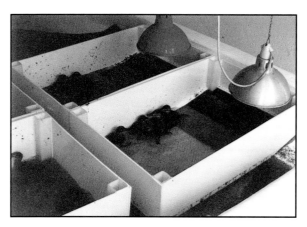

Figure 40.1: *Typical duckling brooder.*

Some young may be reluctant to eat and suffer 'starve out'. In ducks this occurs at 7-14 days, later than in other species. Green and yellow colours appear to be powerful triggers to elicit feeding (Kear, 1986). Birds that are reluctant to eat may be encouraged by crèche rearing, feeding greens or sprinkling hard boiled egg on compounded food. Fresh greens are particularly important for young swans and geese.

The brooder temperature should be 32-34°C and be decreased by 3°C weekly until the young are five weeks of age. Ducklings appear to thrive best if provided with a temperature gradient, ie. a heat source which they can opt to be close to or move away from. Young ducklings should never be allowed to become chilled. If warmed to normal body temperature they will recover initially, but will frequently suffer gastrointestinal or septicaemic disease soon afterwards.

Overcrowding and mixing of different age groups should be avoided. If birds are to be pinioned this should be carried out at 2-5 days of age. Young birds are ready to go outside at 3-5 weeks of age, depending on the weather. First year birds should be reared in clean, well drained, covered enclosures, with access to clean shallow water. Although waterfowl are precocial (and hence relatively self-sufficient), young waterfowl feathers are not water resistant. Excessive swimming or rain will rapidly cause waterlogging, chilling and death.

DISEASES OF NEONATE AND GROWING WATERFOWL

Musculoskeletal diseases are relatively common in developing birds. Lack of exercise and diets with excessive protein levels have been implicated in 'angel wing' (see Chapter 36), splay leg and splayed flexor tendon (perosis). Growth rates should not be excessive, particularly in geese and swans whose natural diet (predominantly grass) is lower in protein. Table 40.1 summarises the main infectious diseases of neonate/young waterfowl.

Table 40.1 Infectious and parasitic diseases of neonate/young waterfowl.

Aetiology	Clinical signs	Diagnosis	Comments and therapy
Duck viral hepatitis (picornavirus)	Lethargy, convulsions, opisthotonus, death in ducklings up to six weeks of age.	*Post mortem*: liver, kidney and spleen enlarged; petechial haemorrhages.	Wild birds act as vectors or fomites. High mortality. Vaccination of breeders in risk areas.
Goose viral hepatitis (parvovirus)	Fibrinous plaques under the tongue, coryza, diarrhoea and ataxia. Mortality 100% in birds under 20 days; resistant once 70 days old.	*Post mortem*: serofibrinous pericarditis, ascites, hepatomegaly, with petechiation and necrotic foci.	Vaccination of breeding stock at 3-6 week intervals prior to breeding. The virus is highly temperature labile (LaBlonde, 1992).
Pasteurella anatipestifer	Lethargy, anorexia, ocular discharge, torticollis, green diarrhoea in birds 1-8 weeks of age. Acute disease in young birds. Older birds may suffer a more chronic form.	Clinical signs, microbiology. Fibrinous air sacculitis, hepatitis and meningitis.	Medicate in water or food with lincomycin (10g/15 litres of water for 5-7 days); tetracyclines (37g [nine teaspoonfuls]/15 litres of water for 5-7 days); amoxycillin (5g/15 litres water - medicated water should be provided on alternate days for three days, ie. two days of medication).
Salmonella spp.	Depression, septicaemia, enteritis, acute death.	Clinical or *post-mortem* signs, bacterial isolation. Most bacterial infections cause an acute or peracute fulminating septicaemia and death.	Transmission from carrier birds; exacerbated in crowded conditions. Antibiotic sensitivity testing and medication is necessary. Good hygiene and minimising stress will reduce incidence. The use of probiotics in the first 14 days of life reduces the incidence of bacteraemia and septicaemia.
Escherichia coli	Depression, inappetence, enteritis, weight loss, septicaemia, death.		
Listeria spp.	Chronic wasting and nervous signs.		
Erysipelas spp.	Depression, inappetence, diarrhoea or an acute, highly fatal haemorrhagic enteritis.		
Pseudomonas spp.	Acute inappetence, weight loss, septicaemia and death.		
Mycoplasma spp.	Infectious sinusitis, high morbidity, low mortality.	Nasal discharge, conjunctivitis, stunted growth. Difficult to culture.	Respond well to tylosin (nasal flush 100mg in 10ml saline daily for 10 days, or 20mg/kg i/m tid for seven days, or one half teaspoonful per litre drinking water for seven days).
Aspergillus spp.	Causes brooder pneumonia in young stock. Prevalent in poorly ventilated, humid overcrowded brooder accommodation.	*Post mortem*: fungal lesions (see Chapter 18).	Improve husbandry. Prophylaxis of susceptible species.

Table 40.1 Continued.

Aetiology	Clinical signs	Diagnosis	Comments and therapy
Cyathostoma spp.	Both worms common in cygnets and goslings grazing on pasture grazed by infected birds the previous season.	'Gaping', stretching or rubbing neck; respiratory signs in severe cases.	Both parasites may cause clinical disease from 10 days of age onwards. Treatment with ivermectin or benzimidazoles is effective (see Chapter 33).
Amidostomum spp. and other ascarids		Weakness, anaemia, malfunction of gizzard. Fine hair-like worms found under the koilin.	
Coccidiosis	Not as common as in poultry. May cause acute haemorrhagic enteritis. Standard poultry prophylactic levels may be toxic. Only treat if clinical disease confirmed.	Faecal or *post-mortem* diagnosis.	Treat with pyrimethamine and sulphaquinoxaline (60mg/l of drinking water, three days on, two days off, three days on) or clazuril (5-10mg/kg p/o every 3rd day on three occasions).

REFERENCES

Kear J (1986) Ducks, geese, swans, and screamers: feeding and nutrition. In: *Zoo and Wild Animal Medicine*. 2nd Edn. Ed ME Fowler WB Saunders, Philadelphia.

LaBonde J (1992) The medical and surgical management of domestic waterfowl collections. In: *Proceedings of the Association of Avian Veterinarians Annual Conference 1992*. AAV, Lake Worth.

Monachon G (1973) Sterilising goose eggshells with ultraviolet light. In: *International Zoo Yearbook*. Ed N Duplaix-Hall. Zoological Society of London, London.

APPENDIX - FORMULARIES

The three formularies list the generic drugs mentioned in the raptor, pigeon and waterfowl sections of this manual together with an example(s) of the trade name(s) and manufacturer(s) current at the time of publication*. In the case of drugs which are produced by several companies, eg. some of the antibiotics, the trade name and manufacturer favoured by the author(s) is shown. The dosage(s) and route(s) of administration shown is the standard one for treatment of the particular group of birds, but in some instances different doses are required for specific conditions and these can be found in the relevant chapter(s).

* The trade names and/or manufacturers names shown in italics are for equivalent products which are available in North America. Some of the generics listed have the same trade name in North America as in the UK. The editors are grateful to Dr Michael Doolen DVM of the Avian and Exotic Animal Hospital, Oakhurst, New Jersey for providing this additional information.

RAPTORS

Generic	Trade name(s) and manufacturer(s)	Dosage(s) and route(s)	Main indications
Antibacterial agents			
Amikacin	Amikin (Bristol-Meyers) *(Amiglyde, Aveco)*.	15mg/kg bid i/m for 5-10 days.	Bacterial infections resistant to other antibiotics, eg. bumblefoot.
Amoxycillin	Many alternatives. Short-acting injection. Long-acting injection.	 150mg/kg i/m bid for 5-7 days. 150mg/kg i/m sid for 5-7 days.	Sensitive bacterial infections. Not good for bumblefoot due to lack of penetration.
	Tablets/solution.	150mg/kg p/o bid for 5-7 days.	
Carbenicillin	Pyopen (Link) *(Geopen, Roerig)*.	100-200mg/kg i/m tid for 3-5 days.	Bacterial infections resistant to other antibiotics, eg. *Pseudomonas* spp. and *Proteus* spp.
Cephalexin	Ceporex (Mallinckrodt) *(Keflex, Dista)*.	40-100mg/kg i/m or p/o, tid or qid, for 3-5 days.	Sensitive bacterial infections.
Chloramphenicol	Chloramphenicol Injection (Willows Francis; *[Fort Dodge; Parke-Davis]*).	50mg/kg i/m tid for 3-5 days.	Very rarely indicated. Oral treatment likely to cause emesis. Can result in rapid anaemia and collapse.
Clavulanate-potentiated amoxycillin	Synulox (Pfizer) *(Clavamox, SmithKline Beecham)*.	150mg/kg p/o bid for 5-7 days.	Sensitive bacterial infections. Injection can cause renal failure in dehydrated raptors.
Clindamycin	Antirobe Capsules (Upjohn).	50mg/kg p/o bid for 7-10 days.	Osteomyelitis and tendon sheath infections. Has been used for up to 12 weeks without ill effects.

Generic name	Trade name(s) and manufacturer(s)	Dosage(s) and route(s)	Main indications
Cloxacillin	Amplicox Syrup/Capsules (SmithKline Beecham) *(Cloxapen, SmithKline Beecham; Tegopen, Bristol).*	250mg/kg p/o bid for 7-10 days.	Sensitive bacterial infections, especially bumblefoot.
Co-trimazine (trimethoprim + sulphadiazine)	Cosumix Plus Soluble Powder (Ciba); Duphatrim Poultry Suspension (Solvay Animal Health); Tribrissen Piglet Suspension (Mallinckrodt) *(Bactrin, Roche).*	12-60mg/kg (combined constituents) p/o bid for 5-7 days.	Sensitive bacterial infections, especially nephritis, bacterial hepatitis and septicaemia in neonates. Do not use in dehydrated birds. Do not overdose, but safe at these levels even when renal infection is present.
	Duphatrim 24% Injection (Solvay Duphar).	30mg/kg s/c bid for 5-7 days.	
Doxycycline	Ronaxan Tablets (Rhône Mérieux) *(Henry Schein; Roerig)*	50mg/kg p/o bid for 3-5 days (for 45 days for chlamydiosis).	Sensitive bacterial infections, especially chlamydiosis.
Enrofloxacin	Baytril 2.5% or 5% Injection, Baytril 2.5% Oral Suspension, Baytril 10% Solution, Baytril Tablets (Bayer) *(Baytril 2.7%, Haver/Diamond).*	10-15mg/kg i/m or p/o bid for 5-7 days.

Baytril 10% Solution can be used either in water or p/o undiluted in food. | Sensitive bacterial infections. I/m or p/o route can cause emesis if the bird has eaten in previous six hours. Useful for bacterial hepatitis or septicaemia in neonates. Used widely in growing chickens and poultry of all ages without any incidence of articular cartilage problems: at normal therapeutic levels (10-15mg/kg bid) it is unlikely to produce joint deformity in neonatal raptors (or in pigeons or waterfowl). |
		4mg in 20ml saline for a 1kg bird - daily nasal flushing for 10 days.	Treatment of sinusitis.
Lincomycin	Lincocin Injection/Tablets (Upjohn).	50-75mg/kg i/m or p/o bid for 7-10 days.	Bumblefoot, osteomyelitis. Has been used at this level by the authors for up to 12 weeks without ill effect.
		0.25-0.5ml by intra-articular injection daily for 7-10 days.	Septic arthritis.
Marbofloxacin	Marbocyl (Univet).	15mg/kg p/o bid for 5-7 days.	As for enrofloxacin but less likely to cause emesis.

Generic name	Trade name(s) and manufacturer(s)	Dosage(s) and route(s)	Main indications
Metronidazole	Flagyl Tablets (Rhône-Poulenc Rorer) *(Flagyl, Searle)*.	50mg/kg p/o sid for 5 days.	Anaerobic infections (and trichomoniasis).
Oxytetracycline	Various injections and tablets.	25-50mg/kg i/m or p/o tid for 5-7 days.	I/m injection may cause significant muscle necrosis.
	Long-acting injection.	200mg/kg i/m daily.	
Piperacillin	Pipril (Lederle) *(Pipracil, Lederle)*.	100mg/kg i/v or i/m bid for 5-7 days.	Sensitive bacterial infections, especially bumblefoot.
Tobramycin	Nebcin Injection (Lilly).	5-10mg/kg i/m bid for 5-7 days.	Least nephrotoxic of all current aminoglycosides.
		0.25-0.5ml by intra-articular flush daily for 7-10 days.	Septic arthritis.
Tylosin	Tylan Injection (Elanco) *(Butler)*.	30mg/kg i/m bid for 3 days.	Mycoplasmosis.
Antifungal agents Amphotericin B	Fungizone (Squibb) *(Bristol-Meyers)*.	1.5mg/kg i/v tid for 7 days.	Aspergillosis. Highly nephrotoxic if bird dehydrated. Give 15ml/kg fluid i/v with each dose.
		1mg/kg i/t bid for 12 days then every other day for 5 weeks.	Syringeal aspergilloma.
	Fungilin Suspension (Squibb).	0.25-1ml p/o daily for 4-5 days.	Candidiasis. Especially in young neonates as not absorbed from the alimentary tract.
Enilconazole	Imaverol (Janssen) *(Clinaform, Sterwin)*.	Dilute 1:10; 0.5ml/kg i/t daily for 7-14 days.	Syringeal aspergilloma.
		Dilute 1:10; apply topically bid for 3-4 weeks.	Cutaneous aspergillosis/candidiasis.
Fluconazole	Flucon (Pfizer) *(Diflucan, Roerig)*.	2-5mg/kg p/o sid for 7 days.	Aspergillosis.
Flucytosine	Alcobon (Roche) *(Ancobon, Roche)*.	20-30mg/kg p/o qid for 20-90 days.	Aspergillosis.
Itraconazole	Sporanox Capsules (Janssen).	10mg/kg p/o sid for 7-10 days for prophylaxis or bid for 4-6 weeks for therapy.	Aspergillosis.

Generic	Trade name(s) and manufacturer(s)	Dosage(s) and route(s)	Main indications
Ketoconazole	Nizoral (Janssen).	25mg/kg i/m bid for 7 days.	Aspergillosis. More hepatotoxic than itraconazole. Has been used safely for periods of up to one month.
Nystatin	Nystan Oral Suspension (Lagap) *(Myco 20, Squibb)*.	300,000 units (3ml)/kg p/o bid for 7 days.	Candidiasis.
Antiprotozoal agents Carnidazole	Spartrix (Harkers) *(Wildlife Laboratories)*.	25mg/kg once.	Trichomoniasis.
Clazuril	Appertex (Harkers).	5-10mg/kg p/o every 3rd day on 3 occasions.	Coccidiosis.
Co-trimazine (trimethoprim + sulphadiazine)	Cosumix Plus Soluble Powder (Ciba); Duphatrim Poultry Suspension (Solvay Animal Health *(Bactrin, Roche)*.	60mg/kg (combined constituents) p/o bid 3 days on, 2 days off, 3 days on.	Coccidiosis. Do not use in dehydrated birds.
	Duphatrim 24% Injection (Solvay Duphar).	30mg/kg s/c bid 3 days on, 2 days off, 3 days on.	
Metronidazole	Flagyl Tablets (Rhône-Poulenc Rorer) *(Flagyl, Searle)*.	50mg/kg p/o daily for 5 days.	Trichomoniasis.
Pyrimethamine	Daraprim (Glaxo-Wellcome).	0.25-0.5mg/kg p/o bid for 30 days.	*Sarcocystis* spp, toxoplasmosis.
Toltrazuril	Baycox (Bayer) *(Bayvet)*.	10mg/kg p/o 3 times on alternate days.	Coccidiosis.
Endoparasiticides Chlorsulon	Curatrem (MSD Agvet).	20mg/kg p/o 3 times at 2 week intervals.	Control trematodes and cestodes.
Fenbendazole	Panacur 2.5% or 10% Liquid, 8mg Capsules (Hoechst).	100mg/kg p/o once.	Control nematodes.
		20mg/kg p/o daily for 14 days.	Control *Serratospiculum* spp.
		20mg/kg p/o daily for 5 days.	Control *Capillaria* spp.
Ivermectin	Ivomec 1% Cattle Injection (MSD Agvet).	200mcg/kg i/m, s/c or p/o, once.	Control nematodes.

Generic names	Trade name(s) and manufacturer(s)	Dosage(s) and route(s)	Main indications
Levamisole	Various, eg. Levacide (Norbrook) *(Ripercol-L, American Cyanamid)*.	10-20mg/kg s/c once.	Control nematodes.
		20mg/kg p/o once.	Control nematodes.
		40mg/kg p/o once.	Control *Capillaria* spp.
Mebendazole	Mebenvet (Janssen) *(Telmin, Pitman-Moore)*.	20mg/kg p/o daily for 14 days.	Control *Serratospiculum* spp.
Praziquantel	Droncit (Bayer) *(Bayvet)*.	5-10mg/kg s/c or p/o once.	Control cestodes.
		5-10mg/kg s/c or p/o for 14 days.	Control trematodes.
Pyrantel	Strongid (Pfizer) *(Nemex, Pfizer)*.	20mg/kg p/o once.	Control nematodes.
Ectoparasiticides Cypermethrin	Dy-Sect (Deosan).	Dilute to 2% (avoid contact with bare skin).	Treatment of premises infested with *Dermanyssus* spp.
Fipronyl	Frontline (Rhône Mérieux).	Spray direct onto skin. One treatment usually sufficient. Repeat after one month if required.	All ectoparasites. Beware drying action of alcohol on feather structure - may reduce durability of the feathers.
High cis permethrin	Harker's Louse Powder, (Harker) *(Generic)*.	Topical application.	Ectoparasite control.
Ivermectin	Ivomec 1% Cattle Injection (MSD Agvet)	200mcg/kg s/c or percutaneous. Repeat after 14 days.	Control sucking ectoparasites. eg. *Cnemidocoptes* spp., *Dermanyssus* spp.
Malathion	Duramitex (Harkers) *(Generic)*.	Dilute to 0.93% - paint or spray onto perches.	Treatment of premises infested with *Dermanyssus* spp.
Piperonyl butoxide/ pyrethrin	Ridmite Powder (Johnson).	Topical dusting. Repeat after 3 weeks.	Control lice, hippoboscids.
Sedatives/ tranquillisers/ anaesthetics Diazepam	Valium (Roche).	0.5-1mg/kg i/v or i/m, bid or tid as required.	Control of fits.
Isoflurane	Isoflo (Mallinckrodt).	Inhalation anaesthetic.	Extremely safe. Anaesthetic of choice.

Generic names	Trade name(s) and manufacturer(s)	Dosage(s) and route(s)	Main indications
Ketamine	Ketaset (Willows Francis); Vetalar (Upjohn) *(Ketaset, Fort Dodge/Aveco; Ketalar,Parke-Davies).*	100mg/kg in a 30g piece of meat.	Sedation to catch an escaped bird.
		5-15mg/kg i/m.	Reversible anaesthetic in combination with medetomidine.
Medetomidine	Domitor (Pfizer).	150-350mcg/kg i/m.	Reversible anaesthetic (by equal volume of Antesedan) in combination with ketamine.
Midazolam	Hypnovel (Roche) *(Versed, Roche).*	0.5-1mg/kg i/v or i/m tid.	Control of fits; shorter duration than diazepam.
Topical preparations Granuflex	Granuflex (Convatec-Squibb).	Apply to area of skin deficit. Change every 3-7 days until re-epithelialisation occurs and the epidermis is strongly repaired.	Sterile, padded, adherent hydrocolloidal dressing. Cut to correct size. May be taped or sutured in position. Promotes epithelialisation.
		Change every 7-10 days.	Protection of wounds from trauma or mutilation.
Non-adhesive dressing	Vetrap (3M); Coflex (Millpledge).	Application of dressings.	Cause no damage to feather structure. Hence are useful for application over feathered areas.
Oil of Evening Primrose	Oil of Evening Primrose Hand Cream (Efamol).	Apply topically once daily to effect.	Local effect preferable to that achieved by oral therapy.
Oil of proflavine	Proflavine Cream (Loveridge).	Apply topically to wounds sid or bid to effect.	Very safe. Stimulates granulation. May cause yellow colouration of urates.
Paragon	Zinc Oxide Tape (Smith and Nephew).	Adhesive dressing.	Apply direct to skin, but be careful not to cause vascular obstruction from potential tourniquet effect.
Povidone-iodine	Pevidine Surgical Scrub (BK); Vetasept (Animalcare).	Topical use. Apply and wash off after 3 minutes.	Very safe cleansing agent for open wounds.
Propylene glycol, malic acid, benzoic acid, salicylic acid	Dermisol (Pfizer).	Topical application sid or bid to effect.	Removes skin debris, scabs and crusts. Also antiseptic. Very safe.
Sodium fusidate	Fucidin (Leo).	Topical. Apply sparingly bid to effect.	Antibacterial, particularly *Staphylococcus* spp. Useful for mild/early bumblefoot and other skin lesions. Reported to penetrate intact skin.

Generic name	Trade name(s) and manufacturer(s)	Dosage(s) and route(s)	Main indications
Sodium fusidate /hydrocortisone	Fucidin H (Leo).	Topical. Apply sparingly bid to effect.	Antibacterial, particularly *Staphylococcus* spp., plus anti-inflammatory action. Reported to penetrate intact skin. Excess application will cause polydipsia.
Miscellaneous			
Atropine	Atropine Injection (C-Vet).	0.1mg/kg i/v or i/m every 3-4 hours.	Acetylcholinesterase poisoning, eg. carbamates.
Biotin	Biotin Tablets (Arnolds) *(Generic)*.	50mcg/kg p/o daily for 30-60 days.	Aid in beak or claw regrowth.
Calcium gluconate or borogluconate 10%	Various.	1-5ml/kg i/v slowly or s/c once.	Initial treatment of hypocalcaemia, hypocalcaemic fits and eggbinding.
Clofazimine	Lamprene Tablets (Geigy).	1.5mg/kg p/o sid for 3 months to 1 year.	Tuberculosis in combination with enrofloxacin, cycloserine and ethambutol. **NB.** Beware zoonotic risk of *M. avium* infection.
Cycloserine	Seromycin Pulvules (Lilly).	5mg/kg p/o bid for 3 months to 1 year.	Tuberculosis in combination with enrofloxacin, clofazamine and ethambutol. **NB.** Beware zoonotic risk of *M. avium* infection.
D-penicillamine	Distamine (Dista) *(Cuprimine, Merk; Depen, Wallace; Titratabs, Wallace)*.	55mg/kg p/o bid for 7-14 days.	Heavy metal poisoning.
Dexamethasone	Dexafort (Intervet).	2mg/kg sid for 2 days only.	Treatment of shock, or anti-inflammatory.
Dinoprost	Lutalyse (Upjohn).	0.02-0.1mg/kg topically onto cloacal mucosa, once.	Eggbinding.
Doxapram	Dopram Injection (Willows Francis) *(Fort Dodge)*.	10mg/kg i/v once.	Respiratory stimulant.
Essential fatty acids	Dermplus Liquid (C-Vet).	0.5ml/kg p/o daily for 50 days or indefinitely.	Pruritic dermatitis (atopy).
Ethambutol	Myambutol Tablets (Lederle).	20mg/kg p/o bid for 3 months to 1 year.	Tuberculosis in combination with enrofloxacin, clofazamine and cycloserine. **NB.** Beware zoonotic risk of *M. avium* infection.

Generic name	Trade name(s) and manufacturer(s)	Dosage(s) and route(s)	Main indications
Flunixin	Finadyne (Schering-Plough) (*Banamine, Schering-Plough*).	1-10mg/kg i/m sid for 1-5 days only.	Pain control, arthritis.
Frusemide (Furosemide)	Lasix Injection (Hoechst).	1.5mg/kg i/m qid as required.	Diuretic.
Iron dextran	Vet Iron Injection (Animalcare) (*Butler, Lextron, Vedco*).	10mg/kg i/m. Repeat after 1 week if required.	Haemopoiesis.
Isoxsuprine	Navicox (Univet).	5-10mg/kg p/o sid for 20-40 days.	Wing tip oedema, dry gangrene syndrome.
Ketoprofen	Ketofen (Rhône Mérieux) (*Fort Dodge/Aveco*).	1mg/kg i/m sid for 1-10 days.	Pain relief, arthritis.
Magnesium sulphate crystals	Magnesium Sulphate (various).	0.5-1g/kg p/o sid for 1-3 days.	Increase gut motility to aid passage of lead if present in intestine.
Metoclopramide	Emequell (Pfizer) (*Reglan, Robins*).	2mg/kg i/v or i/m tid as required.	Anti-emetic. Control of gut stasis, eg. sour crop.
Oxytocin	Oxytocin S (Intervet); Oxytocin (Leo) (*Butler, Lextron, Vedco*).	3-5 IU/kg i/m.	Eggbinding.
Pralidoxime chloride	Contact National Poisons Bureau regarding availability (*Protopam, Wyeth-Ayerst*).	100mg/kg i/m. Repeat once after 6 hours.	Organophosphate and acetylcholinesterase poisoning, eg. carbamates.
Propentofylline	Vivitonin (Hoechst).	5mg/kg p/o bid for 20-40 days.	Wing tip oedema, dry gangrene syndrome.
Sodium calciumedetate	Sodium Calciumedetate (Strong) (Animalcare) (*Calcium Disodium Versenate, 3M Pharmaceuticals*).	10-40mg/kg i/v or i/m bid for 5-10 days.	Lead and other heavy metal poisoning. Dilution not required.
Thiamine	Thiamine Compound Tablets (Rhône Poulenc Rorer) (*Generic*).	1-50mg/kg p/o sid for 7 days or indefinitely.	Control of thiamine responsive fits.
Thyroxine	Soloxine Tablets (Vet-2-Vet) (*Butler*).	Birds weighing 750-1000g, eg. female Red-tailed Hawk: 25mcg sid for 7 days, 50mcg sid for 7 days, 75mcg sid for 7 days, 50mcg sid for 7 days, 25mcg sid for 7 days.	Stimulate a moult. Scale dose up or down by up to 50% for larger or smaller birds.

Generic name	Trade name(s) and manufacturer(s)	Dosage(s) and route(s)	Main indications
Vitamin A	Various Injections.	Maximum 20,000 IU/kg i/m weekly as required.	Hypovitaminosis A. Increase skin healing, eg. bumblefoot.
Vitamin B complex	Various Injections.	Sufficient to give 10-30mg/kg of thiamine. Repeat weekly as required.	Stimulate appetite. General health. Control of thiamine responsive fits.
Vitamin E/ selenium	Dystosel (Upjohn) *(Seletoc, Schering-Plough).*	0.05mg selenium + 3.4 IU vitamin E s/c. Repeat once after 72 hours.	Vitamin E/selenium deficiency.

PIGEONS

The pigeon fancier is much less likely to take the necessary time and trouble nursing sick birds than would be the case with keepers of cage and aviary birds or raptors. Isolation of affected birds may prove difficult. Hospital cages are not commonly available and so restriction in a basket will often be necessary. The fancier will require advice with regard to providing an extra source of heat. Hand feeding may be practised. Rapid Aid (Vetrepharm) has been found to be useful and effective. Subsequently, soaking a few peas and beans for about one hour so that they soften will make forced feeding easier and more acceptable. Administration of medicines via injection, tablets or drinking water will depend on the number of birds involved or susceptible. Following treatment with antibiotics, recuperation may be aided by giving additional multivitamins and probiotics.

Generic	Trade name(s) and manufacturer(s)	Dosage(s) and route(s)	Main indications
Antibacterial agents Amoxycillin trihydrate	Amoxinsol 150 Injection (Univet); Amoxinsol LA (Univet).	150mg/kg i/m or s/c daily for 5 days; every other day if using long acting preparation.	Susceptible infections, eg. paratyphoid.
	Betamox 40mg Tablets (Norbrook); Amoxypen 40mg Tablets (Mycofarm).	40mg/kg p/o bid for 5 days.	
	Vetremox Powder for Poultry/ Pigeons (Vetrepharm).*	1-1.5g per litre drinking water for 5-7 days.	
Chlortetracycline	Aureomycin Soluble Powder (Cyanamid).	130mg activity per litre drinking water for 5-8 days (2.4g Powder/l).	Susceptible infections.
		400mg activity per litre drinking water for 5-8 days (7.25g Powder/l).	Mycoplasmal infections.
		400mg activity per litre drinking water for 21 days (7.25g Powder/l).	Chlamydial infections.
	Aureomycin Ophthalmic Ointment (Cyanamid).	Apply to affected eye bid for 7 days.	Chlamydial infections.

Generic	Trade name(s) and manufacturer(s)	Dosage(s) and route(s)	Main indications
Doxycycline	Ronaxan 20mg Tablets (Rhône Mérieux) *(Henry Schein; Roerig)*.	1 tablet daily for 5-7 days (40mg/kg).	Respiratory infections.
Enrofloxacin	Baytril 10% Oral Solution (Bayer) *(Baytril 2.7%, Haver/Diamond)*.	150mg per litre drinking water for up to 10 days; may need 300mg per litre to prevent reappearance of infection.	Paratyphoid.
	Baytril 10% Injection (Bayer).	20mg/kg i/m or s/c initially, followed by oral treatment.	
Erythromycin	Erythrocin Soluble (11.56g erythromycin activity/70g sachet) (Sanofi) *(Lextron)*.	13-26mg erythromycin activity per litre drinking water for 3 days (1.5g Powder/l).	Susceptible infections, mycoplasmal infections.
Furaltadone	Furaltadone 20% Soluble Powder (Vetrepharm).	400mg furaltadone activity per litre drinking water for 10 days, ie. 2g Powder per litre. (**NB**. Overstrength solutions can kill birds in a few minutes; possibility of toxicity if prolonged treatment.)	Susceptible infections.
Lincomycin HCl 33.3%/ spectinomycin 66.7%	Linco-Spectin 100 Soluble Powder (Upjohn).	50mg (16.7mg lincomycin/33.3mg spectinomycin)/kg for 3-7 days, ie. 1g Powder per litre drinking water.	Susceptible infections, mycoplasmal infections.
Oxytetracycline dihydrate	Oxycare 50mg Tablets (Animalcare).	One tablet daily for 5-7 days.	Chlamydial infections.
	Terramycin Injection (Pfizer).	0.1-0.5ml/kg on alternate days for 21 days in conjunction with oral tetracycline.	
Tetracycline HCl 80%	Tetsol 800 (C-Vet) *(Generic)*.	1g/1.5 litres drinking water for 5-7 days (60mg/kg).	Chlamydial infections.
Tiamulin	Tiamutin 12.5% Solution (Leo Laboratories) *(Denaquard)*.	225mg (2ml) per litre drinking water for 6 days.	Susceptible infections, mycoplasmal infections.
Tylosin	Tylan Soluble Powder (100g tylosin activity per bottle) (Elanco) *(Butler)*.	550mg tylosin activity per litre drinking water for 3 days (activity approx 100%).	Susceptible infections, mycoplasmal infections.

Generic	Trade name(s) and manufacturer(s)	Dosage(s) and route(s)	Main indications
Antifungal agents Griseofulvin	Grisovin 125mg Tablets (Mallinckrodt).	10mg/kg for 21 days as a crushed tablet suspension pipetted directly into the crop (plus appropriate warning).	Dermatophytosis.
	Grisol-V Powder (Univet).	10mg activity/kg for 7 days.	
Ketoconazole	Nizoral Suspension (Janssen).	3mg/kg daily for 7-21 days pipetted into the crop.	Candidiasis, fungal infections.
Nystatin	Nystan Oral Suspension (Lagap) (*Myco 20, Squibb*).	20,000 units into the crop by pipette daily for 7 days.	Candidiasis.
Antiviral agent Acyclovir	Zovirax Suspension (200mg/ml) (Glaxo-Wellcome).	Dilute 5ml suspension with 35ml water - give 1ml tid for 7 days by pipette into the crop.	Herpesvirus infection.
Antitrichomonal agents Aminothiazole	Tricoxine (Fabry).	5ml per litre drinking water for 7 days.	Susceptible trichomonads. **NB**. Avoid overdosing.
Carnidazole	Spartrix 10mg Tablets (Harkers) (*Wildlife Laboratories*).*	0.5-1 tablet once, ie. 12.5-25 mg/kg. Use in conjunction with dimetridazole in rest of the loft.	Susceptible trichomonads.
Dimetridazole (may not be available once current stocks run out)	Harkanka 40% Powder (Harkers)*; Emtryl Prescription (40%) Soluble Powder (Rhône Mérieux).	666mg powder per litre drinking water for 7-12 days (beware field resistance to this drug).	Susceptible trichomonads. **NB**. Avoid overdosing. Beware hot weather and if nursing young.
Metronidazole	Metronidazole 200mg Tablets (Centaur) (*Flagyl, Searle*).	10g powder per litre drinking water for 5 days.	Susceptible trichomonads. **NB**. Also gives moderate control of hexamitiasis.
	Metronidazole 25% Powder (Vetrepharm).	100-150mg in total over 5 days.	
Ronidazole	Ronidazole 10% Powder BP.	1g powder per litre drinking water for 6 days, ie. 12.5mg/kg/day.	Susceptible trichomonads. **NB**. Also gives moderate control of hexamitiasis.

Generic	Trade name(s) and manufacturer(s)	Dosages and route(s)	Main indications
Tetracycline plus furaltadone	None.	400mg tetracycline + 400mg furaltadone per litre drinking water for 7 days. Avoid in adults feeding young less than 10 days of age.	Trichomoniasis (also hexamitiasis).
Anticoccidial agents Amprol	Coccoid 3.4% Solution (Harkers)* *(Corid, MSD Agvet).*	28ml per 4.5 litres drinking water for 7 days, ie. 25mg/kg. Use half strength for extended regimen.	Coccidiosis.
Clazuril	Appertex 2.5mg Tablets (Harkers).*	One tablet/bird single dose, ie. 6.25mg/kg.	Coccidiosis.
Furaltadone	Furaltadone 20% Soluble Powder (Vetrepharm).	2g Powder per litre drinking water for 5 days, ie. 50mg/kg.	Coccidiosis. Also hexamitiasis.
Sulphadimidine sodium 33.3%	Vesadin (Rhône Mérieux); Intradine (Norbrook); Bimadine (Bimeda).	10-20ml per litres drinking water for 5 days (or 3 days on, 2 days off, 3 days on, 2 days off, 3 days on).	Coccidiosis. May be effective against toxoplasmosis.
Toltrazuril	Baycox 2.5% Solution (Bayer) *(Baycox, Bayvet).*	5ml per litre drinking water for 5 days, ie. 10mg/kg.	Coccidiosis.
Anthelmintics Cambendazole	Ascapilla 30mg Capsules (Chevita)* *(Equiben, MSD Agvet).*	75mg/kg on two consecutive days.	Ascariasis and capillariasis.
Febantel	Avicas 15mg Tablets (Orthopharma)* *(Rintal Suspension, Miles).*	37.5mg/kg p/o single dose.	
Fenbendazole	Panacur 8mg Capsules (Hoechst).*	One capsule/pigeon over eight weeks of age, single dose.	
Ivermectin	Ivomec 1% Injection (MSD Agvet).	200-400mcg p/o (variable efficacy).	For nematodes.
Levamisole	Levacide 7.5% Injection (Norbrook).	0.1ml i/m once. Can repeat after 7 days.	Crop capillariasis.
		5ml per litre drinking water as sole source of water over 24 hours. Repeat seven days later.	Loft treatment of capillariasis and ascariasis. Follow-up to parentenal treatment.
Piperazine	Expelix Piperazine Citrate Elixir BP (750mg/ml) *(Wazine 34, Salisbury).*	1g per litre drinking water (equiv to 12.5mg/kg).	Ascarids only.

Generic	Trade name(s) and manufacturer(s)	Dosage(s) and route(s)	Main indications
Praziquantel	Droncit 50mg Tablets (Bayer) *(Bayvet)*.	20mg/kg p/o single dose.	For cestodes
Tetramisole	Spartakon 20mg Tablets (Harkers).*	50mg/kg p/o single dose.	
Ectoparasiticides Cypermethrin 5% concentrated	Barricade (Lever).	Spray or dip with 1:100 dilution.	Lice, mites.
Ivermectin	Ivomec 1% Injection for Cattle (MSD Agvet).	Dilute 1:9 in sterile water just before use. Give 200mcg (0.2ml)/kg i/m.	Lice, mites.
	Ivermectin 0.8% w/v in Propylene Glycol (Vetrepharm).	Apply one drop to the skin once a week for three weeks.	
Permethrin	Companion Flea Powder (Battle, Haywood & Bower) *(Generic)*.	Dusting powder.	Fleas, lice.
Vaccines Paratyphoid	Emergency licensed vaccines available (Bespoke - Specialist Laboratories).	Usually 0.25ml i/m.	Persistent loft problem with paratyphoid.
Pigeon pox	Pigeon Pox Vaccine (Living) Nobilis (Intervet; distributed by Vetrepharm).*	Topical application onto 6-8 exposed feather follicles. For routine prophylaxis vaccinate young birds before racing; vaccinate old birds at least six weeks before pairing. **NB**. Vaccinated birds are infectious until the vaccine lesions have healed. Beware cocks fighting. Vaccine gives excellent immunity.	Pigeon pox.
PMV-1	Colombovac PMV (Solvay Duphar Veterinary).*	0.2ml s/c.	PMV-1. **NB**. Choose vaccination site carefully. Avoid vascular trauma.
	Hartavac (Harkers).*	0.2ml s/c.	
	Nobi-Vac Paramyxo (Intervet; distributed by Vetrepharm).*	0.25ml s/c.	
Miscellaneous Brewers yeast	Dried Yeast Tablets BP 300mg (Lloyds Chemists).	1 tablet crushed over feed/10 birds/ day during the moult.	Brittle feathers if suspect possible nutritional aetiology.
Calcium gluconate 10%	Calcium Sandoz Injection (10ml Ampoules) (Sandoz) *(SmithKline Beecham, Font Dodge)*.	0.1-0.2ml (25-50mg)/kg s/c or slow i/v injection.	Post-laying paralysis.

Generic	Trade name(s) and manufacturer(s)	Dosage(s) and route(s)	Main indications
Diclophenac	Voltarol 25mg Tablets (Geigy).	12.5mg p/o as a single dose.	Arthritis.
Dimethylsulphoxide (DMSO)	Fluvet DMSO (Univet) *(DOMOSO, Syntex).*	Topical application.	Reduce swelling of lower limbs (trauma). Carrier for steroids.
Electrolytes	Liquid Lectade (Pfizer).	1:11.5 in water.	Support in infectious diseases and stress.
Essential fatty acids	Vetreplume (Vetrepharm).	5ml per 1kg feed once weekly.	Improve feather quality.
Glucose polymer	Energix (Vetrepharm).	15g per litre drinking water for 4 days.	Racing pigeon tonic.
Ketoprofen	Ketofen 1% Injection (Rhône Mérieux) *(Font Dodge/Aveco).*	0.1ml i/m or s/c, sid or bid on two consecutive days.	Arthritis.
Liquid iron	Ferripar (Vetrepharm).	2ml per 2kg feed daily for 3 days, then once weekly.	Racing pigeon tonic.
Live probiotic	Proguard (Vetrepharm) *(Armedexan, Schering; Ferrextan, Fort Dodge).*	8g per litre drinking water for 5 days.	Aid in recovery from disease.
Minerals/vitamin B_1	Vetreplex (Vetrepharm).	10g per 3.5 litres drinking water once weekly.	Nutritional supplement.
Probiotic	Vitalyte Plus (Vetrepharm).	One 2.5ml scoop per 3.4 litres drinking water.	Nutritional supplement.
Soluble multivitamins	Duphasol (Solvay Duphar Veterinary).	1g per litre drinking water for 5-7 days or one day per week.	Support in infectious disease. Nutritional dermatitis.
Triamcinolone/ neomycin/ thiostrepton/ nystatin	Panalog Ointment (Ciba).	1 drop into the eye bid for 3-5 days.	Conjunctivitis, 'one-eyed cold'.

* Products licensed for pigeons.

Vaccinating Racing Pigeons

Introduction
Pigeons can be vaccinated against three diseases, pigeon paramyxovirus infection (PMV-1), pigeon pox, and paratyphoid (emergency vaccine).

All the pigeons in the loft may need to be vaccinated at one time: this may well involve several hundreds of birds. In a well organised system it is possible to vaccinate one hundred pigeons against both PMV-1 infection and pigeon pox in one hour. Vaccinating guns are used and one needle may be used to vaccinate 25 or more birds. Good vaccinating practices are required. Whilst it may not be the veterinary surgeon who carries out the vaccinating, it is his/her responsibility to ensure that the pigeon owner is aware of the correct procedures.

Key Points
Poor vaccination practices occur which may result in the death of the pigeon or susceptibility to natural infection.

Injection Abscesses
This is a clinical problem that is reported occasionally.

One level 5ml measure is the equivalent of:	Amount of drinking water to which a 5ml measure is added	Duration of treatment
Amoxycillin 100% - 2g	1.3 litres (2 pints)	3 days
Copper Sulphate (Anhyd) - 5g	9 litres (2 gallons)	3 times on alternate days
Emtryl Soluble 40% - 2.25g	3.4 litres (6 pints)	7 days
Erythrocin Soluble Powder - 3.25g	2.27 litres (4 pints)	3 days
Furaltadone 20% Powder - 2g	1 litre (1.75 pints)	5-7 days
Linco-Spectin 100 Powder - 3g	3.7 litres (6.5 pints)	3-5 days
Tetracycline 50% Powder - 3g	5.7 litres (1.2 gallons)	7 days
Tylan Soluble Powder - 2.5g	5.1 litres (9 pints)	3 days

Injection abscesses are the result of faecal contamination of the needle. The needle can be contaminated by two methods:

● The needle is dropped on to pigeon faeces. A limited number of needles will be supplied with a bottle of vaccine and if it is the last needle that is dropped, there is little choice but to continue with that needle.

● Catching and holding the pigeon will inevitably result in the handler's hands becoming contaminated with faeces. A fancier will often spit on a faeces covered identification ring in order to clean it so that the number can be read and checked against the vaccinating record sheet. The same fingers may then be used to pull back the feathers to allow the vaccinator to see the injection site. This simple and normal procedure can quickly contaminate the skin.

Clinical signs associated with injection abscesses. The abscess is detected from about 7-18 days after vaccination depending on the vigilance of the owner. It may occur more frequently as a subclinical problem that is responsible for leaving pigeons 'under par'. The initial signs are lethargy, inappetence, reluctance to fly and a hunched up appearance. The feathers over the injection site may be seen to be standing up as the swelling enlarges. If left untreated, the abscess will enlarge and the bird may die.

Bacteriology. In one investigation, aerobic and anaerobic cultures from injection abscesses yielded *Streptococcus faecalis*. In addition, *Clostridium perfringens*, *Bacteroides oralis* and *Escherichia coli* were isolated.

The first two, which are toxin producers, were recovered from birds that had died. These organisms are all associated with faecal contamination.

A further small study of the skin of eight healthy pigeons from four lofts failed to yield any anaerobes, but four cultures of *Staphylococcus epidermidis* were isolated. The remaining four cultures were sterile. However, examination of the skin of four birds from a loft with a wet dropping problem yielded positive aerobic cultures of *Strep. faecalis*, *Staph. epidermidis* and *Lactobacillus* spp. from all the birds (Dr A-M Farmer, personal communication). All inactivated vaccines contain adjuvants. The injection of bacteria with the vaccine is likely to predispose to abscess formation.

Vaccination Site
There is an extensive subcutaneous venous plexus (*plexus subcutaneous collaris*) which extends caudally and laterally down the neck, terminating at the base of the neck. Mortality has resulted from the inadvertent intravenous injection of inactivated adjuvanted vaccines into this plexus. This usually occurs within one hour of vaccination. Therefore, when administrating inactivated vaccines, it is important to inject as near to the base of the neck as possible, with the needle pointing caudally.

Aseptic Technique
The use of surgical spirit at the injection site has two major benefits. Firstly, it sanitises the injection site. Secondly, it dampens the feathers around the vaccination site resulting in a clear view for administration of the vaccine. Surgical spirit does not stain the feathers and it will rapidly evaporate in warm weather. Birds are sometimes caught more than once when a loft of birds is being vaccinated; these can be recognised by the spirit mark (or by the ring number).

One needle will often be used to vaccinate several pigeons (one to several hundred). The importance of sanitising the needle between birds should be stressed. This can easily be done using a sponge soaked in surgical spirit contained in a small pot. Nobi-Vac Paramyxo Vaccine and Columovac PMV Vaccine are supplied with stericaps for the vials. Nobi-Vac Paramyxo Vaccine is supplied with a spirit pot.

Points to Watch
- Owners should be advised that the birds should

not be exercised on the day of vaccination. Birds that have been given live pigeon pox vaccine should not be mixed with non-vaccinated birds for six weeks.
- Do not vaccinate unhealthy birds.
- Be aware of the possibility of injection abscesses.
- Retained eggs may occur in hens vaccinated during the breeding season.
- Pigeon pox vaccine should not be applied to a bleeding feather follicle, nor to young birds with pin feathers. Vaccination will 'take' around pin feathers without the need for feather plucking (Parsons, personal observation).

WATERFOWL

Generic	Trade name(s) and manufacturer(s)	Dosage(s) and route(s)	Main indications
Antibacterial agents Amoxycillin	Amoxinsol 50 Soluble Powder (Univet).	1g/3 litres drinking water. Medicated drinking water should be provided on alternate days for 3 days, ie. 2 days of medication.	Sensitive bacterial infections.
Chlortetracycline	Aureomycin Soluble Powder (Cyanamid).	1,000ppm (18.2g/kg feed) in feed for 45 days.	Chlamydiosis.
Co-trimazine (trimethroprim + sulphadiazine)	Cosumix Plus Soluble Powder (Ciba); Duphatrim Poultry Suspension (Solvay Animal Health) *(Bactrin, Roche)*.	1ml/5 litres drinking water for 5-7 days.	Sensitive bacterial infections.
Doxycycline	Ronaxan Tablets (Rhône Mérieux) *(Henry Schein, Roerig)*.	50mg/kg p/o bid for 3-5 days (45 days for chlamydiosis) or 240ppm in feed for 45 days.	Sensitive bacterial infections, especially chlamydiosis.
	Steriject (Pfizer).	75mg/kg i/m once weekly for 6 weeks.	Chlamydiosis.
Enrofloxacin	Baytril 2.5% or 5% Injection, 2.5% or 10% Oral Solution, or Tablets (Bayer) *(Baytril 2.7%, Haver/Diamond)*.	10-15mg/kg i/m or p/o bid for 5-7 days.	Sensitive bacterial infections. Useful for bacterial hepatitis or septicaemia in neonates. Used widely in growing chickens and poultry of all ages without any incidence of articular cartilage problems: at normal therapeutic levels (10-15mg/kg bid) it is unlikely to produce joint deformity in neonatal waterfowl (or in raptors or pigeons).
		4mg in 20ml saline for a 1kg bird - daily nasal flushing for 10 days.	Treatment of sinusitis.
		500ppm in feed for 45 days.	Chlamydiosis.

Generic	Trade name(s) and manufacturer(s)	Dosage(s) and route(s)	Main indications
Lincomycin	Lincocin Soluble Powder (Upjohn).	10g/5 litres drinking water for 5-7 days.	Pasteurellosis, mycoplasmal tenosynovitis.
Lincomycin/ spectinomycin	Linco-Spectin 100 Soluble Powder (Upjohn).	3g/4 litres drinking water for 3-7 days.	Mycoplasmal tenosynovitis, sinusitis.
Oxytetracycline	Various long-acting injections.	200mg/kg i/m daily for 5-7 days.	Pasteurellosis and other sensitive bacterial infections.
	Terramycin Soluble Powder (Pfizer).	37g/15 litres drinking water for 5-7 days.	
Tylosin	Tylan 50 or 200 Injection (Elanco) *(Butler)*.	20-30mg/kg i/m tid for 3-7 days; or100mg in 10ml saline, daily nasal flush for 10 days.	Mycoplasmosis.
	Tylan Tablets (Elanco).	20mg/kg p/o tid for 3 days.	
	Tylan Soluble Powder (Elanco).	2.5g/5 litres drinking water for 3 days.	
Antifungal agents Itraconazole	Sporanox Capsules (Janssen).	10mg/kg p/o sid for 7-10 days for prophylaxis, or bid for 4-6 weeks for therapy.	Aspergillosis.
Nystatin	Nystan Oral Suspension (Lagap) *(Myco 20, Squibb)*.	300,000 units (3ml)/kg p/o bid for 7 days.	Candidiasis.
Antiprotozoal agents Clazuril	Appertex (Harkers).	5-10mg/kg p/o every 3rd day on 3 occasions.	Coccidiosis.
Co-trimazine (trimethoprim + sulphadiazine)	Cosumix Plus Soluble Powder (Ciba); Duphatrim Poultry Suspension (Solvay Animal Health) *(Bactrin, Roche)*.	60mg/kg (combined constituents) p/o bid, 3 days on, 2 days off, 3 days on.	Coccidiosis. Do not use in dehydrated birds.
	Duphatrim 24% Injection (Solvay Duphar).	30mg/kg s/c, 3 days on, 2 days off, 3 days on.	
Pyrimethamine	Daraprim (Glaxo-Wellcome).	0.25-0.5mg/kg p/o bid for 30 days.	*Sarcocystis* spp., toxoplasmosis.
Pyrimethamine/ sulphaquinoxaline	Microquinox (C-Vet Livestock Products).	60mg/litre drinking water, 3 days on, 2 days off, 3 days on.	Coccidiosis.

Generic	Trade name(s) and manufacturer(s)	Dosage(s) and route(s)	Main indications
Toltrazuril	Baycox (Bayer) *(Bayvet)*.	1ml of 2.5% solution/2 litres drinking water for 48 hours.	Coccidiosis.
Endoparasiticides Chlorsulon	Curatrem (MSD Agvet).	20mg/kg p/o 3 times at 2 week intervals.	Control cestodes and trematodes.
Fenbendazole	Panacur 2.5% or 10% Liquid, 8mg Capsules (Hoechst).	20mg/kg p/o once.	Control nematodes.
Flubendazole	Flubenvet (Janssen).	240ppm (2.4kg/tonne) in feed for 7 days.	Control nematodes.
Ivermectin	Ivomec 1% Cattle Injection (MSD Agvet).	200mcg/kg s/c or p/o once.	Control nematodes, and nasal or duck leeches.
Levamisole	Various, eg. Levacide (Norbrook) *(Ripercol-L, American Cyanamid)*.	25-50mg/kg s/c once.	Control nematodes.
Mebendazole	Mebenvet (Janssen) *(Telmin, Pitman-Moore)*.	5-15mg/kg p/o daily for 2 days.	Control *Syngamus* sp.
		120ppm (1.2g/tonne) in feed for 14 days.	Control nematodes.
Praziquantel	Droncit (Bayer) *(Bayvet)*.	10-20mg/kg s/c or p/o. Repeat after 10 days.	Control cestodes.
		10mg/kg s/c or p/o daily for 14 days.	Control trematodes.
Miscellaneous Atropine	Atropine Injection (C-Vet).	0.1mg/kg i/v or i/m every 3-4 hours.	Anticholinesterase poisoning, eg. carbamate.
D-penicillamine	Distamine (Dista) *(Cupramine, Merk; Depen, Wallace; Titratabs, Wallace)*.	55mg/kg p/o bid for 7-14 days.	Heavy metal poisoning.
Dexamethasone	Dexafort (Upjohn).	2mg/kg sid for 2 days only.	Treatment of shock, or anti-inflammatory.
Diazepam	Valium (Roche).	0.5-1mg/kg i/v or i/m, bid or tid, as required.	Control of fits.
Dinoprost	Lutalyse (Upjohn).	0.02-0.1mg/kg i/m or topically onto cloacal mucosa, once.	Eggbinding.

Generic	Trade name(s) and manufacturer(s)	Dosage(s) and route(s)	Main indications
Doxapram	Dopram Injection (Willows Francis) *(Robins)*.	10mg/kg i/v once.	Respiratory stimulant.
Iron dextran	Vet Iron Injection (Animalcare) *(Butler, Lextron, Vedco)*.	10mg/kg i/m. Repeat in 1 week.	Haemopoiesis.
Ketoprofen	Ketofen (Rhône Mérieux) *(Fort Dodge/Aveco)*.	1mg/kg i/m sid for 1-10 days.	Pain relief, arthritis.
Magnesium sulphate crystals	Magnesium Sulphate (various).	0.5-1g/kg p/o sid for 1-3 days.	Increase gut motility. Aid passage of lead if present in intestines.
Metoclopramide	Emequell (Pfizer) *(Reglan, Robins)*.	2mg/kg i/v or i/m tid as required.	Anti-emetic. Control of gut stasis, eg. sour crop.
Oxytocin	Oxytocin S (Intervet); Oxytocin (Leo) *(Butler, Lextron, Vedco)*.	3-5 IU/kg i/m.	Eggbinding.
Pralidoxime mesylate	Contact National Poisons Bureau regarding availability *(Protopam, Wyeth-Ayerst)*.	100mg/kg i/m. Repeat once after 6 hours.	Organophosphate and acetylcholinesterase poisoning, eg. carbamate.
Sodium calciumededate	Sodium Calciumedetate (Strong) (Animalcare) *(Calcium Disodium Versonate, 3M Pharmaceuticals)*.	10-40mg/kg i/v or i/m bid for 5-10 days.	Lead poisoning. No need to dilute.

INDEX

Example Index page numbers: **61** = main section, *230* = illustration, 150 = general/raptor, 242 = pigeon, 293 = waterfowl

Example Index page numbers: **61** = main section, *230* = illustration, 150 = general/raptor, 242 = pigeon, 293 = waterfowl

Example Index page numbers: **61**= main section, *230* = illustration, 150 = general/raptor, <u>242</u> = pigeon, <u>293</u>= waterfowl

Example Index page numbers: **61** = main section, *230* = illustration, 150 = general/raptor, <u>242</u> = pigeon, <u>293</u> = waterfowl

Example Index page numbers: **61** = main section, *230* = illustration, 150 = general/raptor, <u>242</u> = pigeon, <u>293</u> = waterfowl